CONNECT CORE CONCEPTS IN HEALTH

Brief

FIFTEENTH EDITION

Paul M. Insel
Stanford University

Walton T. Roth
Stanford University

Claire E. Insel
California Institute of Human Nutrition

CONNECT CORE CONCEPTS IN HEALTH: BRIEF, FIFTEENTH EDITION

Published by McGraw-Hill Education, 2 Penn Plaza, New York, NY 10121. Copyright © 2018 by McGraw-Hill Education. All rights reserved. Printed in the United States of America. Previous editions © 2016, 2014, and 2012. No part of this publication may be reproduced or distributed in any form or by any means, or stored in a database or retrieval system, without the prior written consent of McGraw-Hill Education, including, but not limited to, in any network or other electronic storage or transmission, or broadcast for distance learning.

Some ancillaries, including electronic and print components, may not be available to customers outside the United States.

This book is printed on acid-free paper.

1 2 3 4 5 6 7 8 9 LMN 21 20 19 18 17

ISBN 978-1-259-70274-7
MHID 1-259-70274-X

Chief Product Officer, SVP Products & Markets: *G. Scott Virkler*
Vice President, General Manager, Products & Markets: *Michael Ryan*
Vice President, Content Design & Delivery: *Betsy Whalen*
Managing Director: *Gina Boedeker*
Director, Product Development: *Meghan Campbell*
Lead Product Developer: *Rhona Robbin*
Product Developer: *Kirstan Price*
Marketing Manager: *Philip Weaver*
Editorial Coordinator: *Carmen Delamboye*
Digital Product Analyst: *Susan Pierre-Louis*
Director, Content Design & Delivery: *Terri Schiesl*
Program Manager: *Marianne Musni*
Content Project Managers: *Rick Hecker; Katie Klochan*
Buyer: *Jennifer Pickel*
Design: *David Hash*
Content Licensing Specialists: *Melissa Homer; Melisa Seegmiller*
Cover Image: *VisualCommunications/E+/Getty Images*
Compositor: *Aptara®, Inc.*
Printer: *LSC Communications*

Library of Congress Cataloging-in-Publication Data

Insel, Paul M., author. | Roth, Walton T., author. | Insel, Claire E., author.
Connect core concepts in health: brief / Paul M. Insel, Stanford
    University, Walton T. Roth, Stanford University, Claire E. Insel,
    California Institute of Human Nutrition.
Brief, fifteenth edition. | New York, NY: McGraw-Hill Education, [2017]
LCCN 2016048862| ISBN 9781259702747 (loose-leaf) | ISBN
    125970274X (loose-leaf)
LCSH: Health. | BISAC: HEALTH & FITNESS / General.
LCC RA776 .C83 2017 | DDC 613—dc23 LC record available at
https://lccn.loc.gov/2016048862

mheducation.com/highered

BRIEF CONTENTS

CONTENTS

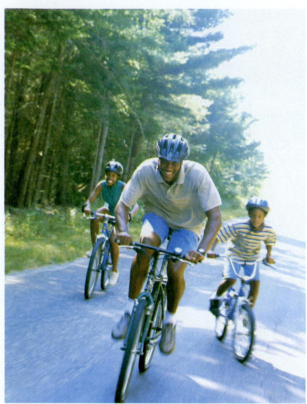
© Tom Stewart/Getty Images

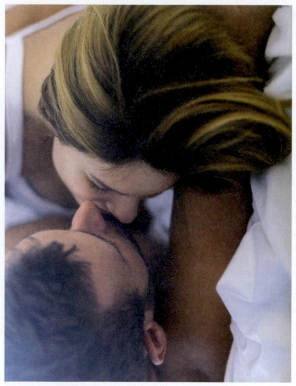

© Katarzyna Bialasiewicz/Getty Images

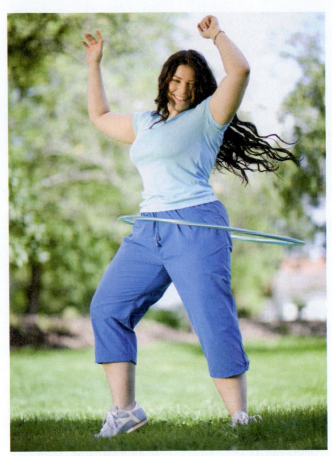
© Cultura Creative (RF)/Alamy RF

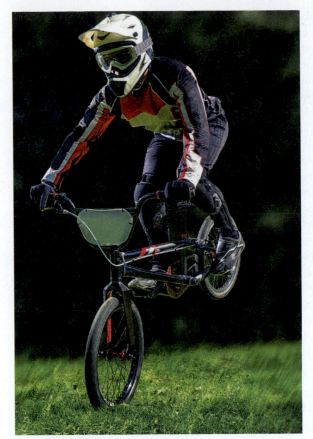
© Alina Shpak/123RF

LEARN WITHOUT LIMITS

CONNECT IS PROVEN EFFECTIVE

McGraw-Hill Connect® is a digital teaching and learning environment that improves performance over a variety of critical outcomes; it is easy to use; and it is proven effective. Connect empowers students by continually adapting to deliver precisely what they need, when they need it, and how they need it, so your class time is more engaging and effective. Connect for *Connect Core Concepts in Health* offers a wealth of interactive online content, including Wellness Worksheets and other self-assessments, video activities on timely health topics, and practice quizzes with immediate feedback.

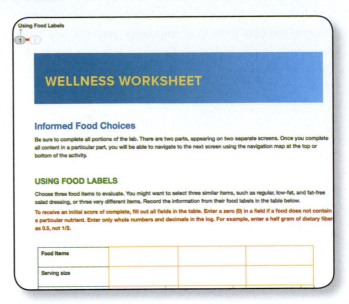

ADDITIONAL ADVANCED CAPABILITIES OF CONNECT

Available within Connect, **SmartBook®** makes study time as productive and efficient as possible by identifying and closing knowledge gaps. SmartBook is powered by the proven **LearnSmart®** engine, which identifies what an individual student knows and doesn't know based on the student's confidence level, responses to questions, and other factors. LearnSmart builds an optimal, personalized learning path for each student, so students spend less time on concepts they already understand and more time on those they don't. As a student engages with SmartBook, the reading experience continuously adapts by highlighting the most impactful content a student needs to learn at that moment in time. This ensures that every minute spent with SmartBook is returned to the student as the most value-added minute possible. The result? More confidence, better grades, and greater success.

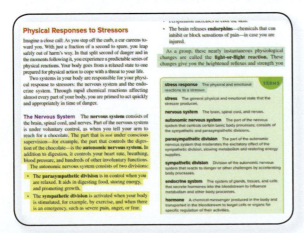

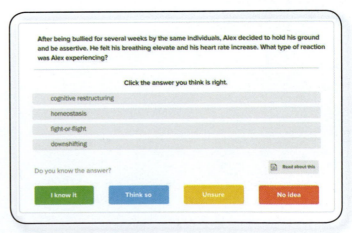

Mc Graw Hill Education connect INSIGHT

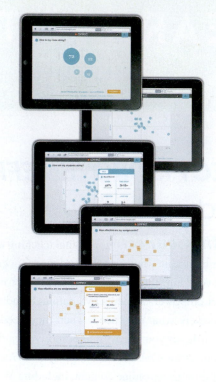

Connect Insight® is Connect's new one-of-a-kind visual analytics dashboard—now available for both instructors and students—that provides at-a-glance information regarding student performance, which is immediately actionable. By presenting assignment, assessment, and topical performance results together with a time metric that is easily visible for aggregate or individual results, Connect Insight gives the user the capability to take a just-in-time approach to teaching and learning, which was never before available. Connect Insight presents data that empowers students and helps instructors improve class performance in a way that is efficient and effective.

PROVEN, SCIENCE-BASED CONTENT

McGraw-Hill's digital teaching and learning tools are built on the solid foundation of *Connect Core Concepts in Health*'s authoritative, science-based content. *Connect Core Concepts in Health* is written by experts who work and teach in the fields of exercise science, medicine, physical education, and health education. *Connect Core Concepts in Health* provides accurate, reliable, current information on key health and wellness topics, while also addressing issues related to mind–body health, research, diversity, and consumer health. The pedagogical program for the 15th edition maintains important features on behavior change, personal reflection, critical thinking, and other key content and skills.

Take Charge boxes challenge students to take meaningful action toward personal improvement.

Critical Consumer sections help students to navigate the numerous and diverse set of health-related products currently available.

Diversity Matters features discuss the ways that our personal backgrounds influence our health strengths, risks, and behaviors.

Wellness on Campus sections focus on health issues, challenges, and opportunities that students are likely to encounter on a regular basis.

Behavior Change Strategy sections offer specific behavior management/modification plans related to the chapter topic.

Ask Yourself: Questions for Critical Thinking and Reflection encourage critical reflection on students' own health-related behaviors.

Quick Stats sections, updated for the 15th edition, focus attention on particularly striking statistics related to the chapter content.

Tips for Today and the Future end each chapter with a quick, bulleted list of concrete actions readers can take now and in the near future.

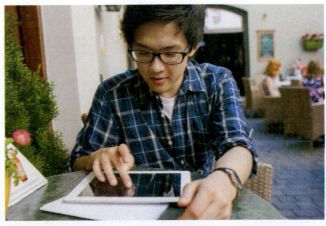
© Jakub Zak/Shutterstock

WHAT'S NEW IN CONNECT CORE CONCEPTS IN HEALTH, 15TH EDITION?

UPDATES INFORMED BY STUDENT DATA

Changes to the 15th edition reflect new research findings, updated statistics, and current hot topics that impact students' wellness behaviors. Revisions were also guided by student performance data collected anonymously from the tens of thousands of students who have used LearnSmart with *Connect Core Concepts in Health*. Because virtually every text paragraph is tied to several questions that students answer while using LearnSmart, the specific concepts that students are having the most difficulty with can be pinpointed through empirical data.

Aggregated student performance data collected anonymously from LearnSmart helps pinpoint concepts students find most challenging, guiding revisions to the text and Connect program.

Sleep and Stress Stress hormone levels in the bloodstream vary throughout the day and are related to sleep patterns. Peak concentrations occur in the early morning, followed by a slow decline during the day and evening. Concentrations return to peak levels during the final stages of sleep and in the early morning hours. Stress hormone levels are low during non-REM sleep and increase during REM sleep. With each successive sleep cycle during the night, REM sleep lasts a little longer. This increase in REM sleep duration with each sleep cycle may underlie the progressive increase in circulating stress hormones during the final stages of sleep.

Even though stress hormones are released during sleep, it is the *lack* of sleep that has the greatest impact on stress. In someone who is suffering from **sleep deprivation** (not getting enough sleep over time), mental and physical processes steadily deteriorate. A sleep-deprived person experiences headaches, feels irritable, is unable to concentrate, and is more prone to forgetfulness. Poor-quality sleep has long been associated with stress and depression.

CHAPTER-BY-CHAPTER LIST OF CHANGES

Chapter 1: Taking Charge of Your Health

- New *Take Charge* feature: Life Expectancy and the Obesity Epidemic; new section on the Affordable Care Act
- New information on qualities and behaviors associated with each dimension of wellness
- Updated information on making life changes, on financial wellness, on key wellness issues for college students, and on health disparities, including updated *Diversity Matters* feature: Moving Toward Health Equality
- Updated statistics on leading causes of death in the U.S., key contributors to death among Americans,

progress toward Healthy People 2020 targets, and deaths attributed to low educational attainment, poverty, and income inequality

Chapter 2: Stress: The Constant Challenge

- New major section on sleep and its role in stress, including a new *Behavior Change Strategy*: Taking Control of Your Sleep and a new *Take Charge* feature: Digital Devices: Help or Harm for a Good Night's Sleep?
- New information on motivation's influence on health, on connectedness and health, and on gender and stress; updated information on steps for managing stress

- Updated *Diversity Matters* feature: Diverse Populations, Discrimination, and Stress; *Wellness on Campus* feature: Coping with News of Traumatic Events; *Take Charge* feature: Mindfulness Meditation

Chapter 3: Psychological Health
- Updated information on defense mechanisms, mood disorders, professional help, and suicide
- Updated *Diversity Matters* feature: Ethnicity, Culture, and Psychological Health and *Wellness on Campus* feature: Deliberate Self-Harm
- New and updated statistics on the prevalence of selected psychological disorders, on suicide methods, and on the prevalence of suicidal thoughts

Chapter 4: Intimate Relationships and Communication
- Updated information on gender roles, sexual orientation, and gender identity in relationships
- New and updated statistics on marital status, median age of marriage, married women in the labor force, Americans' attitudes towards gay relationships, online dating, cohabitation, and single-parent families
- Updated information on digital communication and social networks and on strategies of strong families
- Updated *Wellness On Campus* feature: Hooking Up and *Diversity Matters* feature: Marriage Equality

Chapter 5: Sexuality, Pregnancy, and Childbirth
- New coverage related to the Zika virus
- Updated *Diversity Matters* feature: Genital Alteration, *Critical Consumer* feature: Home Pregnancy Tests, and *Take Charge* feature: Physical Activity during Pregnancy
- Updated information on differentiation of an embryo, intersex, gender roles, sexual orientation, gender identity, commercial sex, treatments for female hypoactive sexual desire disorder, and prenatal care
- Updated statistics on the infertility, fetal alcohol syndrome, depression during pregnancy, hospital vs. at-home births in the U.S., breastfeeding, and premature births, low birth weight, and infant mortality

Chapter 6: Contraception and Abortion
- Updated information on use and effectiveness of con-traceptive methods, legal restrictions and state-specific requirements for abortion, and the public debate about abortion

- Updated *Diversity Matters* feature: Barriers to Contraceptive Use; updated statistics on pregnancy, birth, and abortion rates
- New information about the history of abortion, safety of abortions, and medical vs. aspiration abortion

Chapter 7: Drug Use and Addiction
- New information on Internet gaming disorder
- Updated statistics on drug overdose deaths, nonmedical drug use among Americans, heroin use and deaths, drugs and their potential for substance use disorder and addiction, drug use among college students, workplace drug testing, and on state and federal prison inmates serving time for drug offenses
- Updated information on diagnosing misuse and addiction, risk factors for drug misuse and addiction, commonly misused drugs and their effects, and marijuana legalization, medical uses for marijuana, and long-term effects of using marijuana
- Updated *Diversity Matters* feature: Drug Use and Race/Ethnicity

Chapter 8: Alcohol and Tobacco
- New and updated information about alcohol absorption, e-cigarettes, tobacco additives, tolerance and withdrawal, and economic costs of cigarettes
- Updated *Wellness on Campus* features: Alcoholic Energy Drinks: The Dangers of Being "Drunk and Wide Awake"; Peer Pressure and College Binge Drinking
- Updated statistics on alcohol use disorder and suicide, drunk driving, binge drinking and heavy alcohol use, fetal alcohol syndrome, arrests for drug and alcohol-related offenses, alcohol use's contribution to violent crimes, deaths among nonsmokers due to environmental tobacco smoke, demographics of smokers, and total health care costs of smoking

Chapter 9: Nutrition Basics
- New section on the Dietary Guidelines for Americans 2015–2020; new information on calorie labeling for restaurants and vending machines
- Updated information on added sugars, dietary fat, energy needs, supporting healthy eating patterns, how the U.S. diet compares to recommendations, the DASH eating plan, biotech crops, and food safety

- New *Take Charge* feature: Positive Changes to Meet Dietary Guidelines; updated *Take Charge* feature: Fats and Health; updated *Critical Consumer* feature: Using Food Labels

Chapter 10: Exercise for Health and Fitness
- New information on the health benefits of exercise, the risks of sedentary time, and core training
- New *Take Charge* feature: Move More, Sit Less, and updated *Critical Consumer* feature: What to Wear
- Updated information on target heart rate range, core muscles, and sex differences in muscular strength

Chapter 11: Weight Management
- Updated information on energy intake, dietary patterns, and sleep as lifestyle factors for weight management; safety and effectiveness of common over-the-counter weight loss pills; and prescription weight loss drugs
- New information on gut microbiota, eating disorders, and positive body image
- Updated statistics on the prevalence of obesity and annual spending on weight loss efforts
- Updated *Wellness on Campus* feature: The Freshman 15: Fact or Myth?; *Critical Consumer* feature: Are all Calories and Dietary Patterns Equal for Weight Loss?

Chapter 12: Cardiovascular Health and Cancer
- New information on treatments for high blood pressure, medications for high cholesterol, and e-cigarettes and their relationship to cardiovascular disease
- Updated statistics on the prevalence of overall CVD, high cholesterol, heart attack and stroke deaths, CVD deaths attributed to tobacco use, annual cancer cases and deaths, five year cancer survival rates, and cancer deaths caused by lifestyle factors
- Updated information on early detection of cancer, foods that increase risk of colorectal cancer, recommendations for mammography, skin cancer treatments

Chapter 13: Immunity and Infection
- New coverage of Zika disease and new information on climate change and allergies
- Updated information on HPV, Ebola, West Nile virus, *E. Coli*, hantavirus, hepatitis B, syphilis, and trichomoniasis; on vaccination efficacy and rates; and on HIV diagnosis and treatment
- Updated statistics on the H5N1 virus, tuberculosis, polio, tickborne infections, pertussis, HIV, STIs, HPV vaccination, and antibiotic resistance

- Updated *Diversity Matters* feature: HIV/AIDS around the World, and *Critical Consumer* feature: Getting an HIV Test

Chapter 14: Environmental Health
- New information on pesticides, preventing air and chemical pollution, the 2015 UN Climate Change Conference, and the effects on children whose mothers were exposed to air pollution while pregnant
- Updated information on carbon dioxide levels, climate change, and the hole in the ozone layer
- Updated statistics on world population growth, deaths from air pollution, and trash generated in America

Chapter 15: Conventional and Complementary Medicine
- New information on integrative health, evaluating complementary and alternative therapies, acupuncture, types of research studies, placebo effect, medical specialties, and key concepts in health care insurance coverage
- Updated statistics on the number of Americans using complementary and alternative therapies
- Updated *Critical Consumer* feature: Choosing a Health Insurance Plan

Chapter 16: Personal Safety
- New information on head injuries in contact sports
- New and updated information on preventing acquaintance rape
- Updated *Wellness on Campus* feature: Cell Phones and Distracted Driving and *Diversity Matters* feature: Injuries among Young Men
- New and updated statistics on deaths and costs of injuries, leading causes of deaths from unintentional injuries, deaths from motor vehicle crashes in the U.S., use of seat belts, bicycle helmet laws, pedestrian injuries, gun ownership, sexual assaults, arrests, and violent crimes

Chapter 17: The Challenge of Aging
- Updated statistics and information on the number of older Americans, life expectancy, living arrangements of people 65 and older, Social Security benefits, hospice, and organ transplants
- Updated information on defining and learning about death, physician assisted death and voluntary active euthanasia, and helping children cope with loss
- New *Take Charge* feature: Surviving the Violent Death of a Loved One; updated *Critical Consumer* feature: A Consumer Guide to Funerals

create™

McGraw-Hill Create® is a self-service website that allows you to create customized course materials using McGraw-Hill Education's comprehensive, cross-disciplinary content and digital products. You can even access third-party content such as readings, articles, cases, videos, and more.

- Select and arrange content to fit your course scope and sequence
- Upload your own course materials
- Select the best format for your students—print or eBook
- Select and personalize your cover
- Edit and update your materials as often as you'd like

Experience how McGraw-Hill Education's Create empowers you to teach your students your way: http://www.mcgrawhillcreate.com.

Campus

McGraw-Hill Campus® is a groundbreaking service that puts world-class digital learning resources just a click away for all faculty and students. All faculty—whether or not they use a McGraw-Hill title—can instantly browse, search, and access the entire library of McGraw-Hill instructional resources and services, including eBooks, test banks, PowerPoint slides, animations, and learning objects—from any Learning Management System (LMS), at no additional cost to an institution. Users also have single sign-on access to McGraw-Hill digital platforms, including Connect, Create, and Tegrity, a fully automated lecture caption solution.

INSTRUCTOR RESOURCES

Instructor resources available through Connect for *Connect Core Concepts in Health* include a Course Integrator Guide, Test Bank, Image Bank, and PowerPoint presentations for each chapter. A static PDF version of the interactive Wellness Worksheets offered in Connect is also available.

ACKNOWLEDGMENTS

Connect Core Concepts in Health, 15th edition, has benefited from the thoughtful commentary, expert knowledge, and helpful suggestions of many people. We are deeply grateful for their participation in this project.

Academic Contributors

Steve Flowers, MA, LMFT
Mindfulness Based Stress Reduction Program at Enloe Medical Center
Stress: The Constant Challenge

Heidi Roth, MD
University of North Carolina–Chapel Hill
Sleep Medicine

Michael Joshua Ostacher, MD, MPH, MMSc
Stanford University School of Medicine
Psychological Health

Inge Hansen, PsyD
Stanford University
Intimate Relationships and Communication

Christine Labuski, PhD
Virginia Polytechnic Institute and State University
Sex and Your Body

Kamilee Christenson, MD
Stanford University
Contraception

Anna Altshuler, MD, MPH
California Pacific Medical Center
Abortion

Jeroen Vanderhoeven, MD
Swedish Medical Center
Pregnancy and Childbirth

Chwen-Yuen Angie Chen, MD, FACP, FASAM
Internal and Addiction Medicine, Stanford University
Drug Use and Addiction

Johanna Rochester, PhD
The Endocrine Disruption Exchange
Tobacco Use
Environmental Health

Melissa Bernstein, PhD, RD, LD
Rosalind Franklin University of Medicine and Science
Nutrition Basics

Tom Fahey, EdD
California State University–Chico
Exercise for Health and Fitness

Kim McMahon, MS, RD, LD
Benedictine University and Logan College
Weight Management

Jonathan Schwartz, MD
Stanford University School of Medicine
Cardiovascular Health

Somasundaram Subramaniam, MD, MS
Swedish Cancer Institute
Cancer

Martha Zuniga, PhD
University of California—Santa Cruz
Immunity and Infection

Candice J. McNeil, MD, MPH
Wake Forest University Health Sciences
Sexually Transmitted Infections

Robert Jarski, PhD, PA
School of Health Sciences, Oakland University
Conventional and Complementary Medicine

Marcia Seyler, MPhil
Aging: A Vital Process

Nancy Kemp, MD, MA
Green Valley Hospice
Dying and Death

Academic Advisors and Reviewers for the 15th Edition

Ronald Baldwin, Beaufort County Community College
Kathy Bingham, Antelope Valley College
Mia M. Botkin, Moreno Valley College
Paula Congleton, Santa Barbara City College
Wendy Frappier, Minnesota State University Moorhead
James Metcalf, George Mason University
Kristin Newton, Gardner-Webb University
Jodi Rees, Indiana State University
Scott Rogers, College of Southern Idaho
Richard Scheidt, Fresno City College
Carol Sloan, Henry Ford College
Teresa K. Snow, Georgia Institute of Technology
Susan Stockton, University of Central Missouri
B. Denise Stokich, University of Nevada, Reno
Robert O. Walsh, Utah Valley University
Heidi Wiedenfeld, Texas Tech University

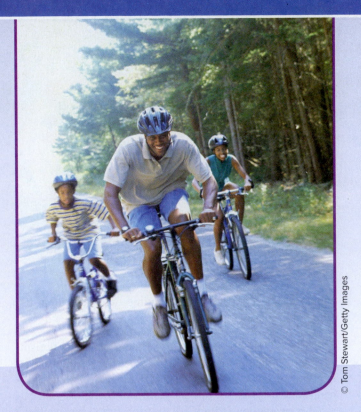

© Tom Stewart/Getty Images

Taking Charge of Your Health

CHAPTER OBJECTIVES

- Define wellness as a health goal
- Explain two major efforts to promote national health
- List factors that influence wellness
- Explain methods for achieving wellness through lifestyle management
- List ways to promote lifelong wellness for yourself and your environment

The next time you ask someone, "How are you?" and you get the automatic response "Fine," be grateful. If that person had told you how he or she actually felt—physically, emotionally, mentally—you might wish you had never asked. Your friend might be one of the too many people who live most of their lives feeling no better than just all right, or so-so, or downright miserable. Some do not even know what optimal wellness is. How many people do you know who feel great most of the time? Do you?

WELLNESS AS A HEALTH GOAL

Generations of people have viewed good health simply as the absence of disease, and that view largely prevails today. The word **health** typically refers to the overall condition of a person's body or mind and to the presence or absence of illness or injury. **Wellness** expands this idea of good health to include living a rich, meaningful, and energetic life. Beyond the simple presence or absence of disease, wellness can refer to optimal health and vitality—to living life to its

fullest. Although we use the words *health* and *wellness* interchangeably, they differ in two important ways. *Health* can be determined or influenced by factors beyond our control, such as our genes, age, and family history. *Wellness* is determined largely by the conscious decisions we make about how we live. These decisions affect the **risk factors** that contribute to disease or injury. We cannot control risk factors such as age and family history, but we can control lifestyle behaviors.

Dimensions of Wellness

Figure 1.1 shows the nine dimensions of wellness. These dimensions are interrelated and may affect each other, as the

TERMS

health   The overall condition of body or mind and the presence or absence of illness or injury.

wellness   Optimal health and vitality, encompassing all the dimensions of well-being.

risk factor   A condition that increases your chances of disease or injury.

FIGURE 1.1 **The wellness continuum.**
The concept of wellness includes vitality in
a number of interrelated dimensions, all of
which contribute to wellness.

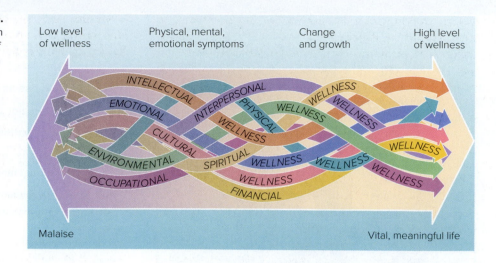

following sections explain. Figure 1.2 lists specific qualities and behaviors associated with each dimension.

Physical Wellness   Your physical wellness includes not just your body's overall condition and the absence of disease but also your fitness level and your ability to care for yourself. The higher your fitness level, the higher your level of physical wellness. Similarly, as you develop the ability to take care of your own physical needs, you ensure greater physical wellness. The decisions you make now, and the

habits you develop over your lifetime, will determine the length and quality of your life.

Emotional Wellness   Trust, self-confidence, optimism, satisfying relationships, and self-esteem are some of the qualities of emotional wellness. Emotional wellness is dynamic and involves the ups and downs of living. No one can achieve an emotional "high" all the time. Emotional wellness fluctuates with your intellectual, physical, spiritual, cultural, and interpersonal health. Maintaining emotional wellness

---

PHYSICAL WELLNESS
- Eating well
- Exercising
- Avoiding harmful habits
- Practicing safer sex
- Recognizing symptoms of disease
- Getting regular checkups
- Avoiding injuries

EMOTIONAL WELLNESS
- Optimism
- Trust
- Self-esteem
- Self-acceptance
- Self-confidence
- Ability to understand and accept one's feelings
- Ability to share feelings with others

INTELLECTUAL WELLNESS
- Openness to new ideas
- Capacity to question
- Ability to think critically
- Motivation to master new skills
- Sense of humor
- Creativity
- Curiosity
- Lifelong learning

INTERPERSONAL WELLNESS
- Communication skills
- Capacity for intimacy
- Ability to establish and maintain satisfying relationships
- Ability to cultivate a support system of friends and family

CULTURAL WELLNESS
- Creating relationships with those who are different from you
- Maintaining and valuing your own cultural identity
- Avoiding stereotyping based on race, ethnicity, gender, religion, or sexual orientation

SPIRITUAL WELLNESS
- Capacity for love
- Compassion
- Forgiveness
- Altruism
- Joy and fulfillment
- Caring for others
- Sense of meaning and purpose
- Sense of belonging to something greater than oneself

ENVIRONMENTAL WELLNESS
- Having abundant, clean natural resources
- Maintaining sustainable development
- Recycling whenever possible
- Reducing pollution and waste

FINANCIAL WELLNESS
- Having a basic understanding of how money works
- Living within one's means
- Avoiding debt, especially for unnecessary items
- Saving for the future and for emergencies

OCCUPATIONAL WELLNESS
- Enjoying what you do
- Feeling valued by your manager
- Building satisfying relationships with coworkers
- Taking advantage of opportunities to learn and be challenged

FIGURE 1.2   **Qualities and behaviors associated with the dimensions of wellness.** Carefully review each dimension and consider your personal wellness strengths and weaknesses.

requires exploring thoughts and feelings. *Self-acceptance* is your personal satisfaction with yourself—it might exclude society's expectations—whereas *self-esteem* relates to the way you think others perceive you; *self-confidence* can be a part of both acceptance and esteem. Achieving emotional wellness means finding solutions to emotional problems, with professional help if necessary.

Intellectual Wellness   Those who enjoy intellectual wellness continually challenge their minds. An active mind is essential to wellness because it detects problems, finds solutions, and directs behavior. Throughout their lifetimes people who enjoy intellectual wellness never stop learning. Often they discover new things about themselves.

Interpersonal Wellness   Satisfying and supportive relationships are important to physical and emotional wellness. Learning good communication skills, developing the capacity for intimacy, and cultivating a supportive network are all important to interpersonal (or social) wellness. Social wellness requires participating in and contributing to your community and to society.

Cultural Wellness   Cultural wellness refers to the way you interact with others who are different from you in terms of ethnicity, religion, gender, sexual orientation, age, and customs (practices). It involves creating relationships with others and suspending judgment on others' behavior until you have lived with them or "walked in their shoes." It also includes accepting, valuing, and even celebrating the different cultural ways people interact in the world. The extent to which you maintain and value cultural identities is one measure of cultural wellness.

Spiritual Wellness   To enjoy spiritual wellness is to possess a set of guiding beliefs, principles, or values that give meaning and purpose to your life, especially in difficult times. The spiritually well person focuses on the positive aspects of life and finds spirituality to be an antidote for negative feelings such as cynicism, anger, and pessimism. Organized religions help many people develop spiritual health. Religion, however, is not the only source or form of spiritual wellness. Many people find meaning and purpose in their lives through their loved ones or on their own—through nature, art, meditation, or good works.

Environmental Wellness   Your environmental wellness is defined by the livability of your surroundings. Personal health depends on the health of the planet—from the safety of the food supply to the degree of violence in society. Your physical environment can support your wellness or diminish it. To improve your environmental wellness, you can learn about and protect yourself against hazards in your surroundings and work to make your world a cleaner and safer place.

Financial Wellness   Financial wellness refers to your ability to live within your means and manage your money in a way that gives you peace of mind. It includes balancing your income and expenses, staying out of debt, saving for the future, and understanding your emotions about money. See the "Financial Wellness" box.

Occupational Wellness   Occupational wellness refers to the level of happiness and fulfillment you gain through your work. Although high salaries and prestigious titles are gratifying, they alone may not bring about occupational wellness. An occupationally well person enjoys his or her work, feels a connection with others in the workplace, and takes advantage of the opportunities to learn and be challenged. Another important aspect of occupational wellness is recognition from managers and colleagues. An ideal job draws on your interests and passions, as well as your vocational skills, and allows you to feel that you are making a contribution in your everyday work.

New Opportunities for Taking Charge

Wellness is a fairly new concept. One hundred and fifty years ago, Americans considered themselves lucky just to survive to adulthood. A boy born in 1850, for example, could expect to live only about 38 years and a girl, 40 years. **Morbidity** and **mortality rates** (rates of illness and death, respectively) from common **infectious diseases** (such as pneumonia, tuberculosis, and diarrhea) were much higher than Americans experience today.

By 1980, **life expectancy** nearly doubled, due largely to the development of vaccines and antibiotics to fight infections, and to public health measures such as water purification and sewage treatment to improve living conditions (Figure 1.3). But even though life expectancy has increased, poor health will limit most Americans' activities during the last 15% of their lives, resulting in some sort of **impaired life** (Figure 1.4). Today a different set of diseases has emerged as our major health threat: Heart disease, cancer, and chronic lower respiratory diseases are now the three leading causes

TERMS

morbidity rate   The relative incidence of disease among a population.

mortality rate   The number of deaths in a population in a given period; usually expressed as a ratio, such as 75 deaths per 1000 members of the population.

infectious disease   A disease that can spread from person to person, caused by microorganisms such as bacteria and viruses.

life expectancy   The period of time a member of a given population is expected to live.

impaired life   The period of a person's life when he or she may not be able to function fully due to disease or disability.

TAKE CHARGE
Financial Wellness

Researchers surveyed nearly 90,000 college students about their financial behaviors and attitudes. According to results released in 2016, a large percentage of students feel less prepared to manage their money than to handle almost any other aspect of college life. They also express distress over their current and future financial decisions. Front and center in their minds is how to manage student loan debt. *Financial wellness* means having a healthy relationship with money. Here are strategies for establishing that relationship:

Follow a Budget

A budget is a way of tracking where your money goes and making sure you're spending it on the things that are most important to you. To start one, list your monthly income and expenditures. If you aren't sure where you spend your money, track your expenses for a few weeks or a month. Then organize them into categories, such as housing, food, transportation, entertainment, services, personal care, clothes, books and school supplies, health care, credit card and loan payments, and miscellaneous. Knowing where your money goes is the first step in gaining control of it.

Now total your income and expenditures and examine your spending patterns. Use this information to set guidelines and goals for yourself. If your expenses exceed your income, identify ways to make some cuts. For example, if you spend money going out at night, consider less expensive options like having a weekly game night with friends or organizing an occasional potluck.

Be Wary of Credit Cards

Students have easy access to credit but little training in finances. The percentage of students who have access to credit cards has increased from 28% in 2012 to 41% in 2015. This increase in credit card use has also correlated with an increase in paying credit card bills late, paying only the minimum amount, and having larger total outstanding credit balances.

Shifting away from using credit cards and toward using debit cards is a good strategy for staying out of debt. Familiarity with financial terminology helps as well. Basic financial literacy with regard to credit cards involves understanding terms like *APR* (annual percentage rate—the interest you're charged on your balance), *credit limit* (the maximum amount you can borrow), *minimum monthly payment* (the smallest payment your creditor will accept each month), *grace period* (the number of days you have to pay your bill before interest or penalties are charged), and *over-the-limit* and *late fees* (the amounts you'll be charged if you go over your credit limit or your payment is late).

Manage Your Debt

A 2015 study indicated that graduating college students often had debts of $35,000—and this amount is expected to rise. When it comes to student loans, having a direct, personal plan for repayment can save time and money, reduce stress,

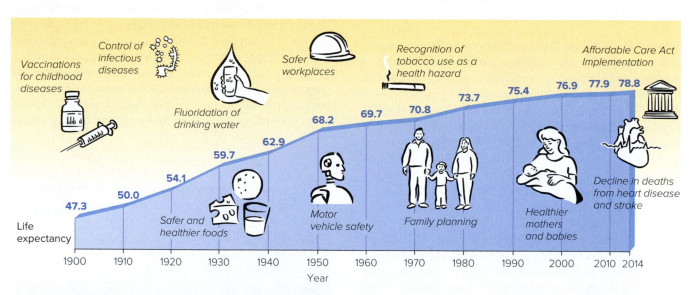

FIGURE 1.3 Public health, life expectancy, and quality of life. Public health achievements during the 20th century are credited with adding more than 25 years to life expectancy for Americans, greatly improving quality of life, and dramatically reducing deaths from infectious diseases. Public health improvements continue into the 21st century, including greater roadway safety and a steep decline in childhood lead poisoning. In 2013, the government mandated that all Americans be covered by health insurance, a protection already long established in most other industrialized countries.

SOURCES: Kochanek, K.D., et al. 2016. Deaths: Final data for 2014. *National Vital Statistics Reports* 65(4); Centers for Disease Control and Prevention. 2011. Ten great public health achievements—United States, 2001–2010. *MMWR* 60(19): 619–623; Centers for Disease Control and Prevention. 1999. Ten great public health achievements—United States, 1900–1999. *MMWR* 48(50): 1141.

and help you prepare for the future. However, only about 10% of students surveyed feel they have all the information needed to pay off their loans. Work with your lender and make sure you know how to access your balance, when to start repayment, how to make payments, what your repayment plan options are, and what to do if you have trouble making payments. Information on managing federal student loans is available from https://studentaid.ed.gov/sa/.

If you have credit card debt, stop using your cards and start paying them off. If you can't pay the whole balance, try to pay more than the minimum payment each month. It can take a very long time to pay off a loan by making only the minimum payments. For example, paying off a credit card balance of $2000 at 10% interest with monthly payments of $20 would take 203 months—nearly 17 years. Check out an online credit card calculator like http://money.cnn.com/calculator/pf/debt-free/. If you carry a balance and incur finance charges, you are paying back much more than your initial loan.

Start Saving

If you start saving early, the same miracle of compound interest that locks you into years of credit card debt can work to your benefit (for an online compound interest calculator, visit http://www.interestcalc.org). Experts recommend "paying yourself first" every month—that is, putting some money into savings before you pay your bills. You may want to save for a large purchase, or you may even be looking ahead to retirement. If you work for a company with a 401(k) retirement plan, contribute as much as you can every pay period.

Become Financially Literate

Most Americans have not received any basic financial training. For this reason, the U.S. government has established the Financial Literacy and Education Commission (MyMoney.gov) to help Americans learn how to save, invest, and manage money better. Developing lifelong financial skills should begin in early adulthood, during the college years, if not earlier, as money-management experience appears to have a more direct effect on financial knowledge than does education. For example, when tested on their basic financial literacy, students who had checking accounts had higher scores than those who did not.

SOURCES: Smith, C., and G. A. Barboza. 2013. The role of trans-generational financial knowledge and self-reported financial literacy on borrowing practices and debt accumulation of college students. Social Science Research Network (http://ssrn.com/abstract=2342168); Plymouth State University. 2013. *Student Monetary Awareness and Responsibility Today!* (http://www.plymouth.edu/office/financial-aid/smart/); U.S. Financial Literacy and Education Commission. 2013. MyMoney.gov (http://www.mymoney.gov); Sparshott, J. 2015. Congratulations, Class of 2015. You're the most indebted ever (for now). *Wall Street Journal,* May 8, 2015 (http://blogs.wsj.com/economics/2015/05/08/congratulations-class-of-2015-youre-the-most-indebted-ever-for-now/); EverFi. 2016. *Money Matters on Campus: Examining Financial Attitudes and Behaviors of Two-Year and Four-Year College Students* (www.moneymattersoncampus.org).

of death for Americans (Table 1.1). An obesity epidemic, beginning in the late 1970s, has also spurred predictions that American life expectancy will decline within the next several decades (see box "Life Expectancy and the Obesity Epidemic" on p. 8). Obesity and poor eating habits can lead to all of the major **chronic diseases.**

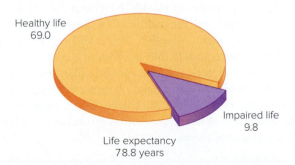

FIGURE 1.4 Quantity of life versus quality of life. Years of healthy life as a proportion of life expectancy in the U.S. population.

SOURCE: Kochanek, K. D., et al. 2016. Deaths: Final data for 2014. *National Vital Statistics Reports* 65(4). National Center for Health Statistics. 2012. *Healthy People 2010 Final Review.* Hyattsville, MD: National Center for Health Statistics.

The good news is that people have some control over whether they develop chronic diseases. People make choices every day that increase or decrease their risks for such diseases. For example, each of us can take personal responsibility for **lifestyle choices** regarding smoking, diet, exercise, and alcohol use. Table 1.2 shows the estimated number of annual deaths tied to selected underlying causes. For example, the estimated 90,000 deaths tied to alcohol includes deaths due directly to alcohol poisoning as well as a proportion of deaths from causes such as liver cancer and injuries. Similarly, sexual behavior is linked to a proportion of all deaths from HIV/AIDS and cervical cancer. As Table 1.2 makes clear, lifestyle factors contribute to many deaths in the United States.

chronic disease A disease that develops and continues over a long period, such as heart disease, cancer, or diabetes.

TERMS

lifestyle choice A conscious behavior that can increase or decrease a person's risk of disease or injury; such behaviors include smoking, exercising, and eating a healthful diet.

Table 1.1 — Leading Causes of Death in the United States, 2013

RANK	CAUSE OF DEATH	NUMBER OF DEATHS	PERCENTAGE OF TOTAL DEATHS	LIFESTYLE FACTORS
1	Heart disease	614,348	23.4	D I S A
2	Cancer	591,699	22.5	D I S A
3	Chronic lower respiratory diseases	147,101	5.6	■ ■ S ■
4	Unintentional injuries (accidents)	136,053	5.2	■ I S A
5	Stroke	133,103	5.1	D I S A
6	Alzheimer's disease	93,541	3.6	■ ■ S ■
7	Diabetes mellitus	76,488	2.9	D I S ■
8	Influenza and pneumonia	55,227	2.1	D I S A
9	Kidney disease	48,146	1.8	■ ■ S ■
10	Intentional self-harm (suicide)	42,773	1.6	■ ■ ■ A
11	Septicemia (systemic blood infection)	38,940	1.5	■ ■ ■ A
12	Chronic liver disease and cirrhosis	38,170	1.5	■ ■ ■ A
13	Hypertension (high blood pressure)	30,221	1.2	D I S A
14	Parkinson's disease	26,150	1.0	■ ■ ■ ■
15	Lung inflammation due to solids and liquids	18,792	0.7	■ ■ ■ A
	All other causes	535,666		■ ■ ■ ■
	All causes	2,626,418	100.0	■ ■ ■ ■

Key

D — Diet plays a part.

I — Inactive lifestyle plays a part.

S — Smoking plays a part.

A — Excessive alcohol use plays a part.

NOTE: Although not among the overall top 15 causes of death, HIV/AIDS (6,721 deaths in 2014) is a major killer. In 2014, HIV/AIDS was the 13th leading cause of death for Americans aged 15–24 years and the 8th leading cause of death for those aged 25–34 years.

SOURCE: Kochanek, K. D., et al. 2016. Deaths: Final data for 2014. *National Vital Statistics Reports* 65(4).

The need to make good choices is especially true for teens and young adults. For Americans aged 15–24, for example, the leading cause of death is unintentional injuries (accidents), with the greatest number of deaths linked to car crashes (Table 1.3). Factors that influence wellness, including the choices we can all make to promote it, are discussed later in this chapter.

Ask Yourself

QUESTIONS FOR CRITICAL THINKING AND REFLECTION

How often do you feel exuberant? Vital? Joyful? What makes you feel that way? Conversely, how often do you feel downhearted, de-energized, or depressed? What makes you feel that way? Have you ever thought about how you might increase experiences of vitality and decrease experiences of discouragement?

PROMOTING NATIONAL HEALTH

Wellness is a personal concern, but the U.S. government has financial and humanitarian interests in it, too. A healthy population is the nation's source of vitality, creativity, and wealth. Poor health drains the nation's resources and raises health care costs for all. The primary **health promotion** strategies at the government and community levels are public health policies and agencies that identify and discourage unhealthy and high-risk behaviors and that encourage and provide incentives for positive health behaviors. At the federal level in the United States, the National Institutes of Health (NIH) and the Centers for Disease Control and Prevention (CDC) are charged with promoting the public's health. These and other agencies translate research results into interventions and communicate research findings to health care providers and the public. There are also health promotion agencies and programs at the state, community, workplace, and college levels. Take advantage of health promotion resources at all levels that are available to you.

health promotion The process of enabling people to increase control over their health and its determinants, and thereby improve their health. TERMS

Table 1.2 — Key Contributors to Deaths among Americans

	ESTIMATED NUMBER OF DEATHS PER YEAR	PERCENTAGE OF TOTAL DEATHS PER YEAR
Tobacco	480,000	18.3
Diet/activity patterns (obesity)*	400,000	15.2
Alcohol consumption	90,000	3.4
Microbial agents**	80,000	3.0
Firearms	30,000	1.1
Illicit drug use***	25,000+	1.0
Motor vehicles	20,000	0.8
Sexual behavior****	15,000	0.6

*The number of deaths due to obesity is an area of ongoing controversy and research. Recent estimates have ranged from 112,000 to 400,000.

**Microbial agents include bacterial and viral infections, such as influenza, pneumonia, and hepatitis. Infections transmitted sexually are counted in the "sexual behavior" category, including a proportion of deaths related to hepatitis, which can be transmitted both sexually and nonsexually.

***Drug overdose deaths have increased rapidly in recent years, making it likely that this estimate will rise.

****Estimated deaths linked to sexual behavior includes deaths from cervical cancer and sexually acquired HIV, hepatitis B, and hepatitis C.

SOURCES: Kochanek, K. D., et al. 2016. Deaths: Final data for 2014. *National Vital Statistics Reports* 65(4), National Research Council, Institute of Medicine. 2015. *Measuring the Risks and Causes of Premature Death: Summary of Workshops.* Washington, DC: National Academies Press; Stahre, M., et al. 2014. Contribution of excessive alcohol consumption to deaths and years of potential life lost in the United States. *Preventing Chronic Disease: Research, Practice, and Policy* 11: 130293; U.S. Department of Health and Human Services. 2014. *The Health Consequences of Smoking—50 Years of Progress: A Report of the Surgeon General.* Atlanta, GA: U.S. Department of Health and Human Services, Centers for Disease Control and Prevention.

The Affordable Care Act

The Affordable Care Act (ACA), also called "Obamacare," was signed into law on March 23, 2010, and upheld by the Supreme Court in 2012 and 2015. The new law requires most people to obtain health insurance or pay a federal penalty. Here is a brief summary of the new law:

Coverage

- Health plans can no longer deny or limit benefits due to a preexisting condition.
- If you are under 26, you may be eligible to be covered under your parent's health plan.
- Insurers can no longer cancel your coverage because of honest mistakes in your application.
- If your plan denies payment, you are guaranteed the right to appeal.

Table 1.3 — Leading Causes of Death among Americans Aged 15–24, 2014

RANK	CAUSE OF DEATH	NUMBER OF DEATHS	PERCENTAGE OF TOTAL DEATHS
1	Unintentional injuries (accidents):	11,836	41.1
	Motor vehicle	6,959	24.2
	All other unintentional injuries	4,877	16.9
2	Suicide	5,079	17.6
3	Homicide	4,144	14.4
4	Cancer	1,569	5.4
5	Heart disease	1,199	4.2
	All causes	28,791	100.0

SOURCE: Kochanek, K. D., et al. 2016. Deaths: Final data for 2014. *National Vital Statistics Reports* 65(4).

Costs

- Lifetime dollar limits are not permitted on most benefits you receive.
- Insurance companies must now publicly justify rate hikes.
- Your premium dollars must be spent primarily on health care—not administrative costs.

Care

- Recommended preventive health services are covered with no copayment.
- From your plan's network, you can choose the primary care doctor you want.
- You can seek emergency care at a hospital outside your health plan's network.

Finding a Plan   Under the ACA, health insurance marketplaces, also called health exchanges, facilitate the purchase of health insurance in every state. The health exchanges provide a selection of government-regulated health care plans that students and others may choose from. Those who are below income requirements are eligible for federal help with the premiums.

Benefits to College Students   The ACA permits students to stay on their parents' health insurance plans until age 26—even if they are married or have coverage through an employer. Students not on their parents' plans who do not want to purchase insurance through their schools can do so through a health insurance marketplace.

If you're under 30, you have the option of buying a "catastrophic" health plan. Such plans tend to have low premiums but require you to pay all medical costs up to a certain amount,

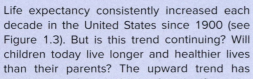

Life expectancy consistently increased each decade in the United States since 1900 (see Figure 1.3). But is this trend continuing? Will children today live longer and healthier lives than their parents? The upward trend has slowed, and some researchers point to the significant increase in obesity among Americans as a potential cause. According to estimates released in 2016, 35% of American men and 40% of American women are obese. The problem isn't confined to the United States: The World Health Organization estimates that 2 billion adults worldwide are overweight or obese.

Along with increases in obesity come increased rates of diabetes, chronic liver disease, heart disease, stroke, and other chronic diseases that are leading causes of death. Of course, medical interventions for these conditions have improved over time, lessening the impact of obesity to date. Still, medical treatments may be reaching their limits in preventing early deaths related to obesity. Moreover, people are becoming obese at earlier ages, exposing them to the adverse effects of excess body fat over a longer period of time. The magnitude of the obesity problem has brought predictions that an overall decline in life expectancy will take place in the United States by the mid-21st century.

What can be done? For an individual, body composition is influenced by a complex interplay of personal factors, including heredity, metabolic rate, hormones, age, and dietary and activity habits. But many outside forces—social, cultural, and economic—shape our behavior, and some experts recommend viewing obesity as a public health problem that requires an urgent and coordinated public health response. A response in health care technology such as gastric bypass surgery, medications, and early screening for obesity-related diseases has helped in the past, but if obesity trends persist, especially among children, average life spans may begin to decrease.

What actions might be taken? Suggestions from health promotion advocates include the following:

- Change food pricing to promote healthful options; for example, tax sugary beverages and offer incentives to farmers and food manufacturers to produce and market affordable healthy choices and smaller portion sizes.

- Limit advertising of unhealthy foods targeting children.

- Require daily physical education classes in schools.

- Fund strategies to promote physical activity by creating more walkable communities, parks, and recreational facilities.

- Train health professionals to provide nutrition and exercise counseling, and mandate health insurance coverage for treatment of obesity as a chronic condition.

- Promote expansion of worksite programs for improving diet and physical activity habits.

- Encourage increased public investment in obesity-related research.

In addition to indirectly supporting these actions, you can directly do the following:

- Analyze your own food choices, and make appropriate changes. Nutrition is discussed in detail in Chapter 9, but you can start by shifting away from consuming foods high in sugar and refined grains.

- Be more physically active. Take the stairs rather than the elevator, ride a bike instead of driving a car, and reduce your overall sedentary time.

- Educate yourself about current recommendations and areas of debate in nutrition.

- Speak out, vote, and become an advocate for healthy changes in your community.

See Chapters 9–11 for more on nutrition, exercise, and weight management.

SOURCES: Flegal, K. M., et al. 2016. Trends in obesity among adults in the United States, 2005–2014. *JAMA* 315(21): 2284–2291. Ludwig, D. S. 2016. Lifespan weighed down by diet. *JAMA* (published online April 4, 2016, DOI: 10.1001/jama.2016.3829); Olshansky, S. J., et al. 2005. A potential decline in life expectancy in the United States in the 21st century. *New England Journal of Medicine* 352(11): 1138–1145; National Center for Health Statistics. 2016. *Health, United States, 2015: With Special Feature on Racial and Ethnic Health Disparities.* Hyattsville, MD: National Center for Health Statistics; International Food Policy Research Institute. 2016. *Global Nutrition Report 2016: From Promise to Impact: Ending Malnutrition by 2030.* Washington, DC: International Food Policy Research Institute; U.S. Department of Agriculture. 2015. *Scientific Report of the 2015 Dietary Guidelines Advisory Committee* (http://www.health.gov/dietaryguidelines /2015-scientific-report).

usually several thousand dollars. The insurance company would pay for essential health benefits over that amount.

Students whose income is below a certain level may qualify for Medicaid. Check with your state. Individuals with nonimmigrant status, which includes worker visas and student visas, qualify for insurance coverage through the exchanges. You can browse plans and apply for coverage at HealthCare.gov.

The Healthy People Initiative

The national Healthy People initiative aims to prevent disease and improve Americans' quality of life. *Healthy People* reports, published each decade since 1980, set national health goals based on 10-year agendas. The initiative's most recent iteration, *Healthy People 2020,* was released to the public in 2010 and envisions "a society in which all people live long, healthy lives" and proposes the eventual achievement of the following broad national health objectives:

- Eliminate preventable disease, disability, injury, and premature death.
- Achieve health equity, eliminate disparities, and improve the health of all groups.
- Create social and physical environments that promote good health for all.
- Promote healthy development and healthy behaviors across every stage of life.

In a shift from the past, *Healthy People 2020* emphasizes the importance of health determinants—factors that affect the health of individuals, demographic groups, or entire populations. Health determinants are social (including factors such as ethnicity, education level, or economic status) and environmental (including natural and human-made environments). Thus one goal is to improve living conditions in ways that reduce the impact of negative health determinants.

Examples of individual health-promotion goals from *Healthy People 2020,* along with estimates of how well Americans are tracking toward achieving those goals, appear in Table 1.4.

Health Issues for Diverse Populations

We all need to exercise, eat well, manage stress, and cultivate positive relationships. We also need to protect ourselves from disease and injuries. But some of our differences—both as individuals and as members of groups—have important implications for wellness. These differences can be biological (determined genetically) or cultural (acquired as patterns of behavior through daily interactions with family, community, and society); many health conditions are a function of biology and culture combined.

As described in the previous section, eliminating health disparities is a major focus of *Healthy People 2020*. But not all health differences between groups are considered **health disparities,** which are those differences linked with social, economic, and/or environmental disadvantage. They affect groups who have systematically experienced greater obstacles to health based on characteristics that are historically linked to exclusion or discrimination. For example, the fact that women have a higher rate of breast cancer than men is a health *difference* but is not considered a disparity. In contrast, the higher death rates from breast cancer for black women compared with non-Hispanic white women is considered a health disparity.

You share patterns of influences with certain others, and information about those groups can help you identify areas that may be of concern to you and your family. *Healthy People 2020* tracks health status and behaviors in relation to a number of demographic dimensions, including sex and gender, race and ethnicity, income and educational attainment, disability status, geographic location (rural and urban), and sexual orientation and gender identity. These are broad categories, and you should consider whether and to what degree issues associated with a particular group are relevant for you.

Sex and Gender   *Sex* refers to the biological and physiological characteristics that define men, women, and intersex people. In contrast, *gender* encompasses how people identify themselves and also the roles, behaviors, activities, and attributes that a given society considers appropriate for them. A person's gender is rooted in biology and physiology, but it is also shaped by how society responds to individuals based on their sex. (See Chapters 4 and 5 for more on sex, gender, and gender roles.) Examples of gender-related characteristics that affect wellness include the higher rates of smoking and drinking found among men and the lower earnings found among women (compared with men doing similar work). Although men are more biologically likely than women to suffer from certain diseases (a sex issue), men are less likely to visit their physicians for regular exams (a gender issue). Men have higher rates of death from injuries, suicide, and homicide, whereas women are at greater risk for Alzheimer's disease and depression. On average, men and women also differ in body composition and certain aspects of physical performance.

health disparity   A health difference linked to social, economic, or environmental disadvantage that adversely affects a group of people.   **TERMS**

Table 1.4	Progress toward *Healthy People 2020* Targets			
	BASELINE (% IN 2008)	MOST RECENT (% IN 2013–2014)	TARGET (% BY 2020)	PROGRESS TOWARD GOAL
Increase proportion of people with health insurance	83.2	86.7	100.0	Significant progress
Help adults with hypertension get blood pressure under control	43.7	48.9	61.2	Significant progress
Reduce proportion of obese adults	33.9	37.7	30.5	Getting worse
Reduce proportion of adults who drank excessively in past 30 days	27.1	26.9	24.4	Insignificant progress
Increase proportion of adults who meet federal guidelines for exercise	18.2	21.3	20.1	Target met
Reduce proportion of adults who use cigarettes	20.6	17.0	12.0	Significant progress

SOURCE: U.S. Department of Health and Human Services. *Healthy People 2020* data search (https://www.healthypeople.gov/2020/data-search/Search-the-Data).

Race and Ethnicity   Among America's racial and ethnic groups, striking disparities exist in health status, access to and quality of health care, and life expectancy. However, measuring the relationships between ethnic or racial backgrounds and health issues is complicated for several reasons. First, separating the effects of race and ethnicity from socioeconomic status is difficult. In some studies, controlling for social conditions reduces health disparities. For example, a study from the Exploring Health Disparities in Integrated Communities project found that in a racially integrated community where blacks and whites had the same earnings, disparities were eliminated or reduced in the areas of hypertension, female obesity, and diabetes.

In other studies, even when patients shared equal status in terms of education and income, insurance coverage, and clinical need, disparities in care persisted. For example, compared with non-Hispanic whites, blacks and Hispanics are less likely to get appropriate medication for heart conditions or to have coronary artery bypass surgery; they are also less likely to receive kidney transplants or dialysis.

Second, the classification of race (a social construct) itself is complex. How are participants in medical studies classified? Sometimes participants choose their own identities; sometimes the physician/researcher assigns identities; sometimes both parties are involved in the classification; and sometimes participants and researchers may disagree.

Despite these limitations, it is still useful to identify and track health risks among population groups. Some diseases are concentrated in certain gene pools, the result of each ethnic group's relatively distinct history. Sickle-cell disease, for example, is most common among people of African ancestry. Tay-Sachs disease tends to afflict people of Eastern European Jewish heritage and French Canadian heritage. Cystic fibrosis is more common among Northern Europeans.

In addition to biological differences, many cultural differences occur along ethnic lines. Ethnic groups vary in their traditional diets; the fabric of their family and interpersonal relationships; their attitudes toward tobacco, alcohol, and other drugs; and their health beliefs and practices. All these factors have implications for wellness.

In tracking health status, the federal government collects data on what they define as five race groups (African American/black, American Indian or Alaska Native, Asian American, Native Hawaiian or Other Pacific Islander, and white) as well as two categories of ethnicity (Hispanic or Latino; not Hispanic or Latino); Hispanics may identify as being of any race group. Other researchers may use these or similar designations. Health concerns have been identified for each of the broad ethnic or racial minority groups.

- *African Americans* have the same leading causes of death as the general population, but they have a higher infant mortality rate and lower rates of suicide and osteoporosis. Health issues of special concern for African Americans include high blood pressure, stroke, diabetes, asthma, and obesity. African American men are at significantly higher risk of prostate cancer than men in other groups.

- *American Indians and Alaska Natives* typically embrace a tribal identity, such as Sioux, Navaho, or Hopi. American Indians and Alaska Natives have lower death rates from heart disease, stroke, and cancer than the general population, but they have higher rates of early death from causes linked to smoking and alcohol use, including injuries and cirrhosis. Diabetes is a special concern for many groups.

- *Asian Americans* include people who trace their ancestry to countries in the Far East, Southeast Asia, or the Indian subcontinent, including Japan, China, Vietnam, Laos, Cambodia, Korea, the Philippines, India, and Pakistan. Asian Americans have lower rates of coronary heart disease and obesity. However, health differences exist among these groups. For example, Southeast Asian American men have higher rates of smoking and lung cancer, and Vietnamese American women have higher rates of cervical cancer.

- *Native Hawaiian and other Pacific Islander Americans* trace their ancestry to the original peoples of Hawaii, Guam, Samoa, and other Pacific Islands. Pacific Islander Americans have a higher overall death rate than the general population and higher rates of diabetes and asthma. Smoking and obesity are special concerns for this group.

- *Latinos* are a diverse group, with roots in Mexico, Puerto Rico, Cuba, and South and Central America. Many Latinos are of mixed Spanish and American Indian descent or of mixed Spanish, Indian, and African American descent. Latinos on average have lower rates of heart disease, cancer, and suicide than the general population; areas of concern include gallbladder disease, obesity, diabetes, and lack of health insurance.

Why do these disparities exist? Poverty and low educational attainment are key factors underlying ethnic health disparities, but they do not fully account for the differences. Access to appropriate health care can be a challenge, even as the Affordable Care Act has reduced the number of uninsured Americans. Non-white racial and ethnic groups, regardless of income, may live in areas that are medically underserved, with fewer sources of high-quality or specialist care. Language and cultural barriers, along with racism and discrimination, can also prevent people from receiving appropriate health services.

Not all the news is bad, however. Progress is being made on reducing health disparities and in developing effective strategies to tackle health issues that disproportionately affect specific population groups. See the box "Moving toward Health Equity."

Income and Education   Income and education are closely related. Groups with the highest poverty rates and least education have the worst health status. They have higher rates of infant mortality, traumatic injury, violent death, and many diseases, including heart disease, diabetes, tuberculosis, HIV infection, and some cancers. They are also more likely to eat poorly, be overweight, smoke, drink, and use drugs. And to complicate and magnify all these factors, they are also exposed to more day-to-day stressors and have

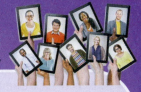

In 2016, the National Center for Health Statistics released a special review of progress on racial and ethnic health disparities over a 15-year period. Although disparities persist, the gaps have shrunk in many key measures of health conditions, health behaviors, and access to and use of health care. Examples include the following:

• The life expectancy gap between whites and blacks dropped from 5.9 years to 3.4 years.

• The percentage of adults without health insurance declined among all groups following the passage of the Affordable Care Act, with the greatest improvement seen among Latinos.

• Infant mortality rates dropped among all groups; the largest declines were for the two groups with the highest rates—African Americans and American Indian or Alaska Natives.

One key goal for collecting data by demographic characteristics is to better identify the population groups at risk and to target those groups with tailored strategies specifically designed to reduce health disparities. A 2016 report from the CDC highlighted a variety of successful interventions (see table).

Public health professionals hope to identify and implement more such programs that promote health equity and help ensure that all Americans live long and healthy lives. You can help by supporting health promotion programs in your community.

SOURCES: National Center for Health Statistics. 2016. *Health, United States, 2015: With Special Feature on Racial and Ethnic Health Disparities.* Hyattsville, MD: National Center for Health Statistics; Centers for Disease Control and Prevention. 2016. *Selected CDC-Sponsored Interventions, United States, 2016* (http://www.cdc.gov/minorityhealth /strategies2016/index.html).

TARGETED POPULATION	INTERVENTION AND RESULTS
Black and Hispanic children	Case management and home visits by community health workers **decreased asthma-related hospitalizations.**
Non-white racial/ethnic groups	Expanded vaccination recommendations **eliminated some disparities in hepatitis A disease.**
People living with disabilities	Curriculum for living well with a disability **improved quality of life.**
Men who have sex with men	Personalized counseling **reduced HIV risk behaviors.**
American Indian and Alaska Native populations	Tribally driven efforts to reclaim traditional food systems **facilitated dialogue about health.**
Low-income populations and Alaska Natives	Client and provider reminders and patient navigators **increased colorectal cancer screening rates.**
Youth in high-risk communities	Programs and policies supporting better neighborhood conditions **reduced violence.**
Hispanic and Latino immigrant men	Lay health advisors **reduced HIV risk behaviors.**

less access to health care services. Researchers estimate that about 250,000 deaths per year can be attributed to low educational attainment, 175,000 to individual and community poverty, and 120,000 to income inequality.

Disability   People with disabilities have activity limitations or need assistance due to a physical or mental impairment. About one in five people in the United States has some level of disability, and the rate is rising, especially among younger segments of the population. People with disabilities are more likely to be inactive and overweight. They report more days of depression than people without disabilities. Many also lack access to health care services.

Geographic Location   About one in four Americans currently lives in a rural area—a place with fewer than 10,000 residents. People living in rural areas are less likely to be physically active, use seat belts, or obtain screening tests for preventive health care. They have less access to timely emergency services and much higher rates of some diseases and injury-related deaths than people living in urban areas. They are also more likely to lack health insurance. Children living in dangerous neighborhoods—rural or urban—are less likely to play outside and are four times more likely to be overweight than children living in safer areas.

Sexual Orientation and Gender Identity   Lesbian, gay, bisexual, and transgender (LGBT) health was added as a new topic area in *Healthy People 2020*. Questions about sexual orientation and gender identity have not been included in many health surveys, making it difficult to estimate the number of LGBT people and to identify their special health needs. However, research suggests that LGBT individuals may face health disparities due to discrimination and denial of their civil and human rights. LGBT youth have high rates of tobacco, alcohol, and other drug use as well as an elevated risk of suicide; they are more likely to be homeless and are less likely to have health insurance and access to appropriate health care providers and services.

FACTORS THAT INFLUENCE WELLNESS

Optimal health and wellness come mostly from a healthy lifestyle—patterns of behavior that promote and support your health and promote wellness now and as you get older. In the pages that follow, you'll find current information and suggestions you can use to build a healthier lifestyle; also, see the "Wellness Matters for College Students" box.

Our behavior, family health history, environment, and access to health care are all important influences on wellness. These factors, which vary for both individuals and groups, can interact in ways that produce either health or disease.

Health Habits

Research continually reveals new connections between our habits and health. For example, heart disease is associated with smoking, stress, a hostile attitude, a poor diet, and being sedentary. Poor health habits take hold before many Americans reach adulthood.

Other habits, however, are beneficial. Regular exercise can help prevent heart disease, high blood pressure, diabetes, osteoporosis, and depression. Exercise can also reduce the risk of colon cancer, stroke, and back injury. A balanced and varied diet helps prevent many chronic diseases. As we learn more about how our actions affect our bodies and minds, we can make informed choices for a healthier life.

Heredity/Family History

Your **genome** consists of the complete set of genetic material in your cells—about 25,000 genes, half from each of your parents. **Genes** control the production of proteins that serve both as the structural material for your body and as the regulators of all your body's chemical reactions and metabolic processes. The human genome varies only slightly from person to person, and many of these differences do not affect health. However, some differences have important implications for health, and knowing your family's health history can help you determine which conditions may be of special concern for you.

Errors in our genes are responsible for about 3500 clearly hereditary conditions, including sickle-cell disease and cystic fibrosis. Altered genes also play a part in heart disease, cancer, stroke, diabetes, and many other common conditions.

However, in these more common and complex disorders, genetic alterations serve only to increase an individual's risk, and the disease itself results from the interaction of many genes with other factors. An example of the power of behavior and environment can be seen in the more than 60% increase in the incidence of diabetes that has occurred among Americans since 1990. This huge increase is not due to any sudden change in our genes; it is the result of increasing rates of obesity caused by poor dietary choices and lack of physical activity.

Environment

Your environment includes substances and conditions in your home, workplace, and community. Are you frequently exposed to environmental tobacco smoke or the radiation in sunlight? Do you live in an area with high rates of crime and violence? Do you have access to nature?

Today environmental influences on wellness also include conditions in other countries and around the globe, particularly weather and climate changes occurring as a result of global warming. In the past few years, climate change has attracted much attention worldwide. Most climate scientists agree that human activity—specifically, the burning of fossil fuels for energy and the release of greenhouse gases into the atmosphere—has caused changes that are raising Earth's temperature and threatening the health of the planet and its living systems. The evidence includes melting ice caps, shifting weather patterns, and the threatened extinction of species. Scientists are trying to determine how high Earth's temperature can climb before damage becomes irreversible.

Access to Health Care

Adequate health care helps improve both quality and quantity of life through preventive care and the treatment of disease. For example, vaccinations prevent many dangerous infections, and screening tests help identify key risk factors and diseases in their early treatable stages. As described earlier, inadequate access to health care is tied to factors such as low income, lack of health insurance, and geographic location. Cost is one of many issues surrounding the development of advanced health-related technologies.

Personal Health Behaviors

In many cases, behavior can tip the balance toward good health, even when heredity or environment is a negative

TERMS

genome The complete set of genetic material in an individual's cells.

gene The basic unit of heredity, containing chemical instructions for producing a specific protein.

Most college students, in their late teens and early twenties, appear to be healthy. But appearances can be deceiving. Each year, thousands of students lose productive academic time to physical and emotional health problems—some of which can continue to plague them for life.

The following table shows the top 10 health issues affecting students' academic performance, according to the fall 2015 American College Health Association–National College Health Assessment II.

HEALTH ISSUE	STUDENTS AFFECTED (%)
Stress	30.3
Anxiety	23.7
Sleep difficulties	20.4
Depression	14.6
Cold/flu/sore throat	13.5
Concern for a friend/family member	10.0
Relationship difficulties	8.6
Attention deficit/hyperactivity disorder	6.0
Death of a friend/family member	5.5
Sinus or ear infection, strep throat, bronchitis	4.7

Each of these issues is related to one or more of the dimensions of wellness, and most can be influenced by choices students make daily. Although some troubles—such as the death of a friend or family member—cannot be controlled, students can moderate their physical and emotional impact by choosing healthy behaviors. For example, there are many ways to manage stress, the top health issue affecting students (see Chapter 2). By reducing unhealthy choices (such as using alcohol to relax) and by increasing healthy choices (such as using time management and relaxation techniques), students can reduce the impact of stress on their lives.

The survey also estimated that, based on students' reporting of their height and weight, nearly 23.3% of college students are overweight and 16.3% are obese. Although heredity plays a role in determining your weight, lifestyle is also a factor in weight management.

In many studies over the past few decades, a large percentage of students have reported behaviors such as the following:

- Overeating
- Frequently eating high-fat foods
- Using alcohol and binge drinking

Clearly, eating behaviors are often a matter of choice. Although students may not see (or feel) the effects of their dietary habits today, the long-term health risks are significant. Overweight and obese persons run a higher-than-normal risk of developing diabetes, heart disease, and cancer later in life. We now know with certainty that improving one's eating habits, even a little, can lead to weight loss and improved overall health.

Other Choices, Other Problems

Students commonly make other unhealthy choices. Here are some examples from the 2015 National College Health Assessment II:

- Only 47.8% of students reported that they used a condom during vaginal intercourse in the past 30 days.
- About 18.7% of students had seven or more drinks the last time they partied.
- About 9.6% of students had smoked cigarettes at least once during the past month.

What choices do you make in these situations? Remember: It's never too late to change. The sooner you trade an unhealthy behavior for a healthy one, the longer you'll be around to enjoy the benefits.

SOURCE: American College Health Association. 2015. *American College Health Association–National College Health Assessment IIc: Reference Group Executive Summary Fall 2015.* Hanover, MD: American College Health Association. Reprinted by permission of the American College Health Association (http://www.acha-ncha.org /reports_ACHA-NCHAIIc.html).

factor. For example, breast cancer can run in families, but it also may be associated with being overweight and inactive. A woman with a family history of breast cancer is less likely to develop the disease if she controls her weight, exercises regularly, and has regular mammograms to help detect the disease in its early, most treatable stage.

Similarly, a young man with a family history of obesity can maintain a normal weight by balancing calorie intake against activities

QUICK STATS

More than two-thirds of American adults are overweight.

—National Center for Health Statistics, 2016

that burn calories. If your life is highly stressful, you can lessen the chances of heart disease and stroke by managing and coping with stress (see Chapter 2). If you live in an area with severe air pollution, you can reduce the risk of lung disease by not smoking. You can also take an active role in improving your environment. Behaviors like these can make a difference in how great an impact heredity and environment will have on your health.

REACHING WELLNESS THROUGH LIFESTYLE MANAGEMENT

As you consider the behaviors that contribute to wellness—being physically active, choosing a healthful diet, and so on—you may be doing a mental comparison with your own behaviors. If you are like most young adults, you probably have some healthy habits and some habits that place your health at risk. For example, you may be physically active and have a healthful diet but spend excessive hours playing video games. You may be careful to wear your seat belt in your car but skip meals. Moving in the direction of wellness means cultivating healthy behaviors and working to overcome unhealthy ones. This approach to lifestyle management is called **behavior change.**

As you may already know, changing an unhealthy habit (such as giving up cigarettes) can be harder than it sounds. When you embark on a behavior change plan, it may seem like too much work at first. But as you make progress, you will gain confidence in your ability to take charge of your life. You will also experience the benefits of wellness—more energy, greater vitality, deeper feelings of appreciation and curiosity, and a higher quality of life.

Getting Serious about Your Health

Before you can start changing a wellness-related behavior, you have to know that the behavior is problematic and that you *can* change it. To make good decisions, you need information about relevant topics and issues, including what resources are available to help you change.

Examine Your Current Health Habits How is your current lifestyle affecting your health today and in the future? Think about which of your current habits enhance your health and which detract from it? Begin your journey toward wellness with self-assessment: Talk with friends and family members about what they have noticed about your lifestyle and your health. Challenge any unrealistically optimistic attitudes or ideas you may hold—for example, "To protect my health, I don't need to worry about quitting smoking until I'm 40 years old" or "Being overweight won't put *me* at risk for diabetes." Health risks are very real and can become significant while you're young; health habits are important throughout life.

Many people consider changing a behavior when friends or family members express concern, when a landmark event occurs (such as turning 30), or when new information raises their awareness of risk. If you find yourself reevaluating some of your behaviors as you read this text, take advantage of the opportunity to make a change in a structured way.

---

behavior change   A lifestyle management process that involves cultivating healthy behaviors and working to overcome unhealthy ones.

target behavior   An isolated behavior selected as the object for a behavior change program.

TERMS

Choose a Target Behavior Changing any behavior can be demanding. Start small by choosing one behavior you want to change—called a **target behavior**—and working on it until you succeed. Your chances of success will be greater if your first goal is simple, such as resisting the urge to snack between classes. As you change one behavior, make your next goal a little more significant, and build on your success.

Learn about Your Target Behavior Once you've chosen a target behavior, you need to learn its risks and benefits—both now and in the future. Ask these questions:

• How is your target behavior affecting your level of wellness today?

• Which diseases or conditions does this behavior place you at risk for?

• What effect would changing your behavior have on your health?

As a starting point, use this text and the resources listed in the "For More Information" section at the end of each chapter. See the "Evaluating Sources of Health Information" box for additional guidelines.

Find Help Have you identified a particularly challenging target behavior or condition—something like overuse of alcohol, binge eating, or depression—that interferes with your ability to function or places you at a serious health risk? If so, you may need help to change a behavior or address a disorder that is deeply rooted or too serious for self-management. Don't let the problem's seriousness stop you; many resources are available to help you solve it. On campus, the student health center or campus counseling center can provide assistance. To locate community resources, consult the yellow pages, your physician, or the Internet.

Building Motivation to Change

Knowledge is necessary for behavior change, but it isn't usually enough to make people act. Millions of people have sedentary lifestyles, for example, even though they know it's bad for their health. This is particularly true of young adults, who feel healthy despite their unhealthy behaviors. To succeed at behavior change, you need strong motivation. The sections that follow address some considerations.

Examine the Pros and Cons of Change Health behaviors have short-term and long-term benefits and costs. Consider the benefits and costs of an inactive lifestyle:

• *Short-term.* Such a lifestyle allows you more time to watch TV, use social media, do your homework, and hang out with friends, but it leaves you less physically fit and less able to participate in recreational activities.

• *Long-term.* It increases the risk of heart disease, cancer, stroke, and premature death.

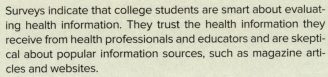

CRITICAL CONSUMER
Evaluating Sources of Health Information

Surveys indicate that college students are smart about evaluating health information. They trust the health information they receive from health professionals and educators and are skeptical about popular information sources, such as magazine articles and websites.

How good are you at evaluating health information? Here are some tips.

General Strategies

Whenever you encounter health-related information, take the following steps to make sure it is credible:

- *Go to the original source.* Media reports often simplify the results of medical research. Find out for yourself what a study really reported, and determine whether it was based on good science. What type of study was it? Was it published in a recognized medical journal? Was it an animal study, or did it involve people? Did the study include a large number of people? What did the authors of the study actually report?

- *Watch for misleading language.* Reports that tout "breakthroughs" or "dramatic proof" are probably hype. A study may state that a behavior "contributes to" or is "associated with" an outcome; this does not prove a cause-and-effect relationship.

- *Distinguish between research reports and public health advice.* Do not change your behavior based on the results of a single report or study. If an agency such as the National Cancer Institute urges a behavior change, however, follow its advice. Large, publicly funded organizations issue such advice based on many studies, not a single report.

- *Remember that anecdotes are not facts.* A friend may tell you he lost weight on some new diet, but individual success stories do not mean the plan is truly safe or effective. Check with your doctor before making any serious lifestyle changes.

- *Be skeptical.* If a report seems too good to be true, it probably is. Be wary of information contained in advertisements.

An ad's goal is to sell a product, even if there is no need for it.

- *Make choices that are right for you.* Friends and family members can be a great source of ideas and inspiration, but you need to make health-related choices that work best for you.

Internet Resources

Online sources pose special challenges; when reviewing a health-related website, ask these questions:

- *What is the source of the information?* Websites maintained by government agencies, professional associations, or established academic or medical institutions are likely to present trustworthy information. Many other groups and individuals post accurate information, but it is important to look at the qualifications of the people who are behind the site. (Check the home page or click the "About Us" link.)

- *How often is the site updated?* Look for sites that are updated frequently. Check the "last modified" date of any web page.

- *Is the site promotional?* Be wary of information from sites that sell specific products, use testimonials as evidence, appear to have a social or political agenda, or ask for money.

- *What do other sources say about a topic?* Be cautious of claims or information that appear at only one site or come from a chat room, bulletin board, newsgroup, or blog.

- *Does the site conform to any set of guidelines or criteria for quality and accuracy?* Look for sites that identify themselves as conforming to some code or set of principles, such as those established by the Health on the Net Foundation or the American Medical Association. These codes include criteria such as use of information from respected sources and disclosure of the site's sponsors.

To successfully change your behavior, you must believe that the benefits of change outweigh the costs.

Carefully examine the pros and cons of continuing your current behavior and of changing to a healthier one. Focus on the effects that are most meaningful to you, including those that are tied to your personal identity and values. For example, engaging in regular physical activity and getting adequate sleep can support an image of yourself as an active person who is a good role model for others. To complete your analysis, ask friends and family members about the effects of your behavior on them. A younger sister may say that your smoking habit influenced her decision to start smoking.

The short-term benefits of behavior change can be an important motivating force. Although some people are motivated by long-term goals, such as avoiding a disease that may hit them in 30 years, most are more likely to be moved to action by shorter-term, more personal goals. Feeling better, doing better in school, improving at a sport, reducing stress, and increasing self-esteem are common short-term benefits of health behavior change.

Boost Self-Efficacy   A big factor in your eventual success is whether you feel confident in your ability to change. **Self-efficacy** refers to your belief in your ability to successfully take action and perform a specific task. Strategies for boosting self-efficacy include developing an internal locus of control, using visualization and self-talk, and getting encouragement from supportive people.

> **self-efficacy**   The belief in your ability to take action and perform a specific task.   **TERMS**

LOCUS OF CONTROL Who do you believe is controlling your life? Is it your parents, friends, or school? Is it "fate"? Or is it you? **Locus of control** refers to the extent to which a person believes he or she has control over the events in his or her life. People who believe they are in control of their lives are said to have an *internal locus of control*. Those who believe that factors beyond their control determine the course of their lives are said to have an *external locus of control*.

For lifestyle management, an internal locus of control is an advantage because it reinforces motivation and commitment. An external locus of control can sabotage efforts to change behavior. For example, if you believe that you are destined to die of breast cancer because your mother died from the disease, you may view regular screening mammograms as a waste of time. In contrast, if you believe that you can take action to reduce your risk of breast cancer despite hereditary factors, you will be motivated to follow guidelines for early detection of the disease.

If you find yourself attributing too much influence to outside forces, gather more information about your wellness-related behaviors. List all the ways that making lifestyle changes will improve your health. If you believe you'll succeed, and if you recognize that you are in charge of your life, you're on your way to wellness.

VISUALIZATION AND SELF-TALK One of the best ways to boost your confidence and self-efficacy is to visualize yourself successfully engaging in a new, healthier behavior. Imagine yourself going for an afternoon run three days a week or no longer smoking cigarettes. Also visualize yourself enjoying all the short-term and long-term benefits that your lifestyle change will bring. Create a new self-image: What will you and your life be like when you become a regular exerciser or a nonsmoker?

You can also use *self-talk,* the internal dialogue you carry on with yourself, to increase your confidence in your ability to change. Counter any self-defeating patterns of thought with more positive or realistic thoughts: "I am a strong, capable person, and I can maintain my commitment to change." (See Chapter 3 for more about self-talk.)

ROLE MODELS AND SUPPORTIVE PEOPLE Social support can make a big difference in your level of motivation and your chances of success. Perhaps you know people who have reached the goal you are striving for. They could be role models or mentors for you, providing information and support for your efforts. Gain strength from their experiences, and tell yourself, "If they can do it, so can I." Find a partner who wants to make the same changes you do and who can take an active role in your behavior change program. For example, an exercise partner can provide companionship and encouragement when you might be tempted to skip your workout.

Identify and Overcome Barriers to Change Don't let past failures at behavior change discourage you. They can

be a great source of information you can use to boost your chances of future success. Make a list of the problems and challenges you faced in any previous behavior change attempts. To this, add the short-term costs of behavior change that you identified in your analysis of the pros and cons of change. Once you've listed these key barriers to change, develop a practical plan for overcoming each one. For example, if you are not getting enough sleep when you're with certain friends, decide in advance how you will turn down their next late-night invitation.

Enhancing Your Readiness to Change

The transtheoretical, or "stages of change," model has been shown to be an effective approach to lifestyle self-management. According to this model, you move through distinct stages of action as you achieve your target behavior. First, determine what stage you are in now so that you can choose appropriate strategies to progress through the cycle of change. This will help you enhance your readiness and intention to change. Read the following sections to determine what stage you are in. Let's use exercise as an example of changing unhealthy behavior to active, engaging behavior.

Precontemplation At this stage, you think you have no problem and don't intend to change your behavior. For example, your friends have commented that you should exercise more, but you are resistant. You have tried to exercise in the past and now think your situation is hopeless. You are unaware of risks associated with being sedentary; and you also blame external factors like other people for your condition. You believe that there are more important reasons *not* to change than there are reasons to change.

To move forward in this stage, try raising your awareness. *Research* the importance of exercise, for example. How does exercise affect the body and mind? *Look also at the mechanisms you use to resist change,* such as denial or rationalization. Find ways to counteract these mechanisms of resistance.

Seek social support. Friends and family members can help you identify target behaviors (e.g., fitting in exercise into your time schedule or encouraging you while you work out). *Other resources* might include exercise classes or stress management workshops offered by your school.

Contemplation You now know you have a problem and within six months intend to do something about it, such as invite a friend to work out with you. You realize that getting more exercise will help decrease your stress level. You acknowledge the benefits of behavior change but are also aware that the barriers to change may be difficult to overcome. You consider possible courses of action but don't know how to proceed.

To take charge, start by *keeping a journal*. Record what you have done so far and include your plan of action. *Do a cost-benefit analysis:* Identify the costs (e.g., it will cost money to take an exercise class) and benefits (e.g., I will probably stick to my goal if someone else is guiding me through the exercise). *Identify barriers to change* (e.g., I hate getting sweaty when I have no opportunity to shower). Knowing these obstacles can help you overcome them. Next, *engage your emotions*. Watch movies or read books about people with your target behavior. Imagine what your life will be like if you don't change.

Other ways to move forward in the contemplation stage include *creating a new self-image* and thinking before you act. *Imagine what you'll be like* after changing your unhealthy behavior. Try to think of yourself in those new terms right now. *Learn why you engage in the unhealthy behavior.* Determine what "sets you off" and train yourself not to act reflexively.

Preparation   At this stage, you plan to take action within a month or you may already have begun to make small changes in your behavior. You may have discovered a place to go jogging but have not yet gone regularly or consistently. You may have created a plan for change but are worried about failing.

Work on creating a plan. Include a start date, goals, rewards, and specific steps you will take to change your behavior. *Make change a priority.* Create and sign a contract with yourself. *Practice visualization and self-talk.* Say, "I see myself jogging three times a week and going to yoga on Fridays." "I know I can do it because I've met challenging goals before." *Take small steps.* Successfully practicing your new behavior for a short time—even a single day—can boost your confidence and motivation.

Action   You outwardly modify your behavior and your environment. Maybe you start riding your bike to school or work. The action stage requires the greatest commitment of time and energy, and people in this stage are at risk of relapsing into old, unhealthy patterns of behavior. *Monitor your progress.* Keep up with your journal entries. *Make changes* that will discourage the unwanted behavior—for example, park your car farther from your house or closer to the stairs. *Find alternatives* to your old behavior. Make a list of things you can do to replace the behavior.

Reward yourself. Rewards should be identified in your change plan. *Praise yourself* and focus on your success. *Involve your friends.* Tell them you want to change, and ask for their help. Don't get discouraged. Real change is difficult.

Maintenance   You have maintained your new, healthier lifestyle for at least six months by working out and riding your bike. Lapses have occurred, but you have been successful in quickly reestablishing the desired behavior. The maintenance stage can last months or years.

Keep going. Continue using the positive strategies that worked in earlier stages. And *be prepared for lapses.* If you find yourself skipping exercise class, don't give up on the whole project. Try inviting a friend to join you and then keep the date. *Be a role model.* Once you successfully change your behavior, you may be able to help someone do the same thing.

Termination   For some behaviors, you may reach the sixth and final stage of termination. At this stage, you have exited the cycle of change and are no longer tempted to lapse back into your old behavior. You have a new self-image and total control with regard to your target behavior.

Dealing with Relapse

People seldom progress through the stages of change in a straightforward, linear way. Rather, they tend to move to a certain stage and then slip back to a previous stage before resuming their forward progress. Research suggests that most people make several attempts before they successfully change a behavior, and four out of five people experience some degree of backsliding. For this reason, the stages of change are best conceptualized as a spiral in which people cycle back through previous stages but are farther along in the process each time they renew their commitment (Figure 1.5).

If you experience a lapse (a single slip) or a relapse (a return to old habits), don't give up. Relapse can be demoralizing, but it is not the same as failure; failure means stopping before you reach your goal and never changing your target behavior. During the early stages of the change process, it's a good idea to plan for relapse so that you can avoid guilt and self-blame and get back on track quickly. Forgive yourself for the

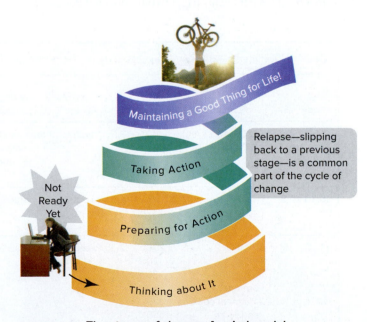

Relapse—slipping back to a previous stage—is a common part of the cycle of change

FIGURE 1.5   The stages of change: A spiral model.

SOURCE: Adapted from Centers for Disease Control and Prevention. n.d. *PEP Guide: Personal Empowerment Plan for Improving Eating and Increasing Physical Activity.* Dallas, TX: The Cooper Institute.

slip, give yourself credit for the progress you have already made, and move on.

If relapses keep occurring or you can't seem to control them, you may need to return to a previous stage of the behavior change process. If this is necessary, reevaluate your goals and strategy. A different or less stressful approach may help you avoid setbacks when you try again.

Developing Skills for Change: Creating a Personalized Plan

Once you are committed to making a change, put together a plan of action. Your key to success is a well-thought-out plan that sets goals, anticipates problems, and includes rewards.

1. Monitor Your Behavior and Gather Data   Keep a record of your target behavior and the circumstances surrounding it. Record this information for at least a week or two. Keep your notes in a health journal or notebook or on your computer (see the sample journal entries in Figure 1.6). Record each occurrence of your behavior, noting the following:

- What the activity was
- When and where it happened
- What you were doing
- How you felt at that time

For example, if your goal is to start an exercise program, track your activities to determine how to make time for workouts.

2. Analyze the Data and Identify Patterns   After you have collected data on the behavior, analyze the data to identify patterns. When are you most likely to overeat? To skip a meal? What events trigger your appetite? Perhaps you are especially hungry at midmorning or when you put off eating dinner until 9:00. Perhaps you overindulge in food and drink when you go to a particular restaurant or when you're with certain friends. Note the connections between your feelings and such external cues as time of day, location, situation, and the actions of others around you.

3. Be "SMART" about Setting Goals   If your goals are too challenging, you will have trouble making steady progress and will be more likely to give up altogether. If, for example, you are in poor physical condition, it will not make sense to set a goal of being ready to run a marathon within two months. If you set goals you can live with, it will be easier to stick with your behavior change plan and be successful.

Experts suggest that your goals meet the "SMART" criteria; that is, your behavior change goals should be

- *Specific.* Avoid vague goals like "eat more fruits and vegetables." Instead state your objectives in specific terms, such as "eat two cups of fruit and three cups of vegetables every day."

- *Measurable.* Recognize that your progress will be easier to track if your goals are quantifiable, so give your goal a number. You might measure your goal in terms of time (such as "walk briskly for 20 minutes a day"), distance ("run two miles, three days per week"), or some other amount ("drink eight glasses of water every day").

- *Attainable.* Set goals that are within your physical limits. For example, if you are a poor swimmer, you might not be able to meet a short-term fitness goal by swimming laps. Walking or biking might be better options.

- *Realistic.* Manage your expectations when you set goals. For example, a long-time smoker may not be able to quit

Date November 5					Day M TU W TH F SA SU						
Time of day	M/S	Food eaten	Cals.	H	Where did you eat?	What else were you doing?	How did someone else influence you?	What made you want to eat what you did?	Emotions and feelings?	Thoughts and concerns?
7:30	M	1 C Crispix cereal 1/2 C skim milk coffee, black 1 C orange juice	110 40 — 120	3	home	looking at news headlines on my phone	alone	I always eat cereal in the morning	a little keyed up & worried	thinking about quiz in class today
10:30	S	1 apple	90	1	hall outside classroom	studying	alone	felt tired & wanted to wake up	tired	worried about next class
12:30	M	1 C chili 1 roll 1 pat butter 1 orange 2 oatmeal cookies 1 soda	290 120 35 60 120 150	2	campus food court	talking	eating w/ friends; we decided to eat at the food court	wanted to be part of group	excited and happy	interested in hearing everyone's plans for the weekend
	M/S = Meal or snack			H = Hunger rating (0–3)						

FIGURE 1.6   Sample health journal entries.

cold turkey. A more realistic approach might be to use nicotine replacement patches or gum for several weeks while getting help from a support group.

• *Time frame–specific.* Give yourself a reasonable amount of time to reach your goal, state the time frame in your behavior change plan, and set your agenda to meet the goal within the given time frame.

Using these criteria, sedentary people who want to improve their health and build fitness might set a goal of being able to run three miles in 30 minutes, to be achieved within a time frame of six months. To work toward that goal, they might set a number of smaller, intermediate goals that are easier to achieve. For example, their list of goals might look like this:

WEEK	FREQUENCY (DAYS/WEEK)	ACTIVITY	DURATION (MINUTES)
1	3	Walk < 1 mile	10–15
2	3	Walk 1 mile	15–20
3	4	Walk 1–2 miles	20–25
4	4	Walk 2–3 miles	25–30
5–7	3–4	Walk/run 1 mile	15–20
⋮			
21–24	4–5	Run 2–3 miles	25–30

For some goals and situations, it may make more sense to focus on something other than your outcome goal. If you are in an early stage of change, for example, your goal may be to learn more about the risks associated with your target behavior or to complete a cost-benefit analysis. If your goal involves a long-term lifestyle change, such as reaching a healthy weight, focus on developing healthy habits rather than targeting a specific weight loss. Your goal in this case might be exercising for 30 minutes every day, reducing portion sizes, or eliminating late-night snacks.

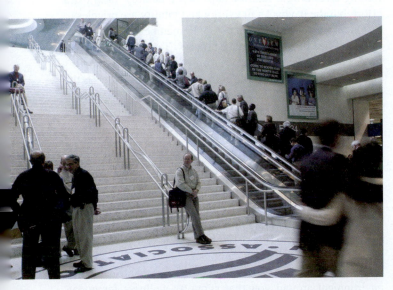

Your environment contains powerful cues for both positive and negative lifestyle choices. Identifying and using the healthier options available to you throughout the day is a key part of a successful behavior change program.

4. Devise a Plan of Action   Develop a strategy that will support your efforts to change. Your plan of action should include the following steps:

• *Get what you need.* Identify resources that can help you. For example, you can join a community walking club or sign up for a smoking cessation program. You may also need to buy some new running shoes or nicotine replacement patches. Get the items you need right away; waiting can delay your progress.

• *Modify your environment.* If you have cues in your environment that trigger your target behavior, control them. For example, if you typically have alcohol at home, getting rid of it can help prevent you from indulging. If you usually study with a group of friends in an environment that allows smoking, move to a nonsmoking area. If you always buy a snack at a certain vending machine, change your route so that you don't pass by it.

• *Control related habits.* You may have habits that contribute to your target behavior. Modifying these habits can help change the behavior. For example, if you usually plop down on the sofa while watching TV, try putting an exercise bike in front of the set so that you can burn calories while watching your favorite programs.

• *Reward yourself.* Giving yourself instant, real rewards for good behavior will reinforce your efforts. Plan your rewards; decide in advance what each one will be and how you will earn it. Tie rewards to achieving specific goals or subgoals. For example, you might treat yourself to a movie after a week of avoiding snacks. Make a list of items or events to use as rewards. They should be special to you and preferably unrelated to food or alcohol.

• *Involve the people around you.* Tell family and friends about your plan and ask them to help. To help them respond appropriately to your needs, create a specific list of dos and don'ts. For example, ask them to support you when you set aside time to exercise or avoid second helpings at dinner.

• *Plan for challenges.* Think about situations and people that might derail your program and develop ways to cope with them. For example, if you think it will be hard to stick to your usual exercise program during exams, schedule short bouts of physical activity (such as a brisk walk) as stress-reducing study breaks.

Ask Yourself

QUESTIONS FOR CRITICAL THINKING AND REFLECTION

Think about the last time you made an unhealthy choice instead of a healthy one. How could you have changed the situation, the people in the situation, or your own thoughts, feelings, or intentions to avoid making that choice? What can you do in similar situations in the future to produce a different outcome?

5. Make a Personal Contract A serious personal contract—one that commits you to your word—can result in a better chance of follow-through than a casual, offhand promise. Your contract can help prevent procrastination by specifying important dates and can also serve as a reminder of your personal commitment to change.

Your contract should include a statement of your goal and your commitment to reaching it. The contract should also include details such as the following:

- The date you will start
- The steps you will take to measure your progress
- The strategies you plan to use to promote change
- The date you expect to reach your final goal

Have someone—preferably someone who will be actively helping you with your program—sign your contract as a witness.

Figure 1.7 shows a sample behavior change contract for someone who is committing to eating more fruit every day.

You can apply the general behavior change planning framework presented in this chapter to any target behavior. Additional examples of behavior change plans appear in the Behavior Change Strategy sections at the end of many chapters in this text. In these sections, you will find specific plans for quitting smoking, starting an exercise program, and making other positive lifestyle changes.

Putting Your Plan into Action

When you're ready to put your plan into action, you need commitment—the resolve to stick with the plan no matter what temptations you encounter. Remember all the reasons you have to make the change—and remember that *you* are the boss. Use all your strategies to make your plan work. Make sure your environment is change-friendly, and get as much support and encouragement from others as possible. Keep track of your progress in your health journal and give yourself regular rewards. And don't forget to give yourself a pat on the back—congratulate yourself, notice how much better you look or feel, and feel good about how far you've come and how you've gained control of your behavior.

Ask Yourself

QUESTIONS FOR CRITICAL THINKING AND REFLECTION

Have you tried to change a behavior in the past, such as exercising more or quitting smoking? How successful were you? Do you feel the need to try again? If so, what would you do differently to improve your chances of success?

BEING HEALTHY FOR LIFE

Your first few behavior change projects may never go beyond the planning stage. Those that do may not all succeed. But as you begin to see progress and changes, you'll start to experience new and surprising positive feelings about yourself. You'll probably find that you're less likely to buckle under stress. You may accomplish things you never thought possible—running a marathon, traveling abroad, or finding a rewarding relationship. Being healthy takes extra effort, but the paybacks in energy and vitality are priceless.

Once you've started, don't stop. Remember that maintaining good health is an ongoing process. Tackle one area at a time, but make a careful inventory of your health strengths and weaknesses and lay out a long-range plan. Take on the easier problems first, and then use what you have learned to attack more difficult areas. Keep informed about the latest health news and trends; research is continually providing new information that directly affects daily choices and habits.

You can't completely control every aspect of your health. At least three other factors—heredity, health care, and environment—play important roles in your well-being. After you quit smoking, for example, you may still be inhaling smoke from other people's cigarettes. Your resolve to eat better foods may suffer a setback when you have trouble finding healthy choices on campus.

But you can make a difference—you can help create an environment around you that supports wellness for everyone. You can support nonsmoking areas in public places. You can speak up in favor of more nutritious foods and better physical fitness facilities. You can provide nonalcoholic drinks at your parties.

Behavior Change Contract

1. I, _Tammy Lau_, agree to _increase my consumption of fruit from 1 cup per week to 2 cups per day._

2. I will begin on ___10/5___ and plan to reach my goal of _2 cups of fruit per day_ by _12/7_

3. To reach my final goal, I have devised the following schedule of mini-goals. For each step in my program, I will give myself the reward listed.

I will begin to have ½ cup of fruit with breakfast	10/5	see movie
I will begin to have ½ cup of fruit with lunch	10/26	new video game
I will begin to substitute fruit juice for soda 1 time per day	11/16	concert

   My overall reward for reaching my goal will be _trip to beach_

4. I have gathered and analyzed data on my target behavior and have identified the following strategies for changing my behavior: _Keep the fridge stocked with easy-to-carry fruit. Pack fruit in my backpack every day. Buy lunch at place that serves fruit._

5. I will use the following tools to monitor my progress toward my final goal: _Chart on fridge door_ _Health journal_

   I sign this contract as an indication of my personal commitment to reach my goal: _Tammy Lau_ _9/28_

   I have recruited a helper who will witness my contract and _also increase his consumption of fruit; eat lunch with me twice a week._
   Eric March _9/28_

FIGURE 1.7 A sample behavior change contract.

You can also work on larger environmental challenges: air and water pollution, traffic congestion, overcrowding and overpopulation, global warming and climate change, toxic and nuclear waste, and many others. These difficult issues need the attention and energy of people who are informed and who care about good health. On every level, from personal to planetary, we can all take an active role in shaping our environment.

TIPS FOR TODAY AND THE FUTURE

You are in charge of your health. Many of the decisions you make every day have an impact on the quality of your life, both now and in the future. By making positive choices, large and small, you help ensure a lifetime of wellness.

RIGHT NOW YOU CAN:

- Go for a 15-minute walk.
- Have a piece of fruit for a snack.
- Call a friend and arrange a time to catch up with each other.
- Think about whether you have a health behavior you'd like to change. If you do, consider the elements of a behavior change strategy. For example, begin a mental list of the pros and cons of the behavior, or talk to someone who can support you in your attempts to change.

IN THE FUTURE YOU CAN:

- Stay current on health- and wellness-related news and issues.
- Participate in health awareness and promotion campaigns in your community—for example, support smoking restrictions at local venues.
- Be a role model for (or at least be supportive of) someone else who is working on a health behavior you have successfully changed.

SUMMARY

- Wellness is the ability to live life fully, with vitality and meaning. Wellness is dynamic and multidimensional. It incorporates physical, emotional, intellectual, interpersonal, cultural, spiritual, environmental, financial, and occupational dimensions.

- As chronic diseases have emerged as major health threats in the United States, people must recognize that they have greater control over, and greater responsibility for, their health than ever before.

- With the Affordable Care Act (ACA) and the Healthy People initiative, the U.S. government is seeking to achieve a better quality of life for all Americans. The ACA gives students several options for obtaining health insurance. The Healthy People initiative aims to eliminate preventable disease and improve Americans' quality of life at every stage.

- Health-related disparities that have implications for wellness can be described in the context of sex and gender, race and ethnicity, income and education, disability, geographic location, and sexual orientation and gender identity.

- Although heredity, environment, and health care all play roles in wellness and disease, behavior can mitigate their effects.

- To make lifestyle changes, you need information about yourself, your health habits, and resources available to help you change.

- You can increase your motivation for behavior change by examining the benefits and costs of change, boosting self-efficacy, and identifying and overcoming key barriers to change.

- The "stages of change" model describes six stages that people move through as they try to change their behavior: precontemplation, contemplation, preparation, action, maintenance, and termination.

- You can develop a specific plan for change by (1) monitoring your behavior by keeping a journal; (2) analyzing those data; (3) setting specific goals; (4) devising strategies for modifying the environment, rewarding yourself, and involving others; and (5) making a personal contract.

- To start and maintain a behavior change program, you need commitment, a well-developed plan, social support, and a system of rewards.

- Although you cannot control every aspect of your health, you can make a difference in helping create an environment that supports wellness for everyone.

FOR MORE INFORMATION

The Internet addresses listed here were accurate at the time of publication.

Centers for Disease Control and Prevention (CDC). The CDC provides a wide variety of health information for researchers and the general public.

  http://www.cdc.gov

Federal Deposit Insurance Corporation. "Money Smart for Young Adults" is a free source of information, unaffiliated with commercial interests, that includes eight modules on topics such as "borrowing basics" and "paying for college and cars."

  http://www.fdic.gov/consumers/consumer/moneysmart/young.html

Federal Trade Commission: Consumer Protection—Health. Includes online brochures about a variety of consumer health topics, including fitness equipment, generic drugs, and fraudulent health claims.

  http://www.ftc.gov/bcp/menus/consumer/health.shtm

Healthfinder. A gateway to online publications, websites, support and self-help groups, and agencies and organizations that produce reliable health information.

  http://www.healthfinder.gov

Healthy People 2020. Provides information on Healthy People objectives and priority areas.

  http://www.healthypeople.gov

MedlinePlus. Provides links to news and reliable information about health from government agencies and professional associations;

also includes a health encyclopedia and information about prescription and over-the-counter drugs.

> http://www.nlm.nih.gov/medlineplus/

National Health Information Center (NHIC). Puts consumers in touch with the organizations that are best able to provide answers to health-related questions.

> http://www.health.gov/nhic/

National Institutes of Health (NIH). Provides information about all NIH activities as well as consumer publications, hotline information, and an A-to-Z listing of health issues with links to the appropriate NIH institute.

> http://www.nih.gov

National Wellness Institute. Serves professionals and organizations that promote health and wellness.

> http://www.nationalwellness.org

Office of Minority Health. Promotes improved health among racial and ethnic minority populations.

> http://minorityhealth.hhs.gov

Office on Women's Health. Provides information and answers to frequently asked questions.

> http://www.womenshealth.gov

Surgeon General. Includes information on activities of the Surgeon General and the text of many key reports on topics such as tobacco use, physical activity, and mental health.

> http://www.surgeongeneral.gov

World Health Organization (WHO). Provides information about health topics and issues affecting people around the world.

> http://www.who.int/en

SELECTED BIBLIOGRAPHY

American Cancer Society. 2016. Cancer Facts and Figures—2016. Atlanta, GA: American Cancer Society.

American College Health Association. 2015. *American College Health Association—National College Health Assessment IIc: Reference Group Executive Summary Fall 2015.* Hanover, MD: American College Health Association.

American Heart Association. 2016. *Heart Disease and Stroke Statistics—2016 Update.* Dallas, TX: American Heart Association.

Bennett, I. M., et al. 2009. The contribution of health literacy to disparities in self-rated health status and preventive health behaviors in older adults. *Annals of Family Medicine* 7(3): 204–211.

Bleich, S. N., et al. 2012. Health inequalities: Trends, progress, and policy. *Annual Review of Public Health* 33: 7–40.

Centers for Disease Control and Prevention. 2016. *At A Glance 2016 Diabetes: Working to Reverse the U.S. Epidemic* (http://www.cdc.gov/chronicdisease/resources/publications/aag/diabetes.htm)

Everett, B. G, et al. 2013. The nonlinear relationship between education and mortality: An examination of cohort, race/ethnic, and gender differences. *Population Research and Policy Review* 32(6).

Fisher, E. G., et al. 2011. Behavior matters. *American Journal of Preventive Medicine* 40(5): e15–e30.

Flegal, K. M., et al. 2016. Trends in obesity among adults in the United States, 2005–2014. *JAMA* 315(21): 2284–2291.

Frieden, T. R. 2016. Foreword. *MMWR* 65(Suppl.) DOI: http://dx.doi.org/10.15585/mmwr.su6501a1.

Galea, S., et al. 2011. Estimated deaths attributable to social factors in the United States. *American Journal of Public Health* 101(8): 1456–1465.

Guinier, L. 2013. Identity and demography. *New York Times*, March 25 (http://www.nytimes.com/roomfordebate/2011/02/13/the-two-or-more-races-dilemma/identity-and-demography).

Herd, P., et al. 2007. Socioeconomic position and health: The differential effects of education versus income on the onset versus progression of health problems. *Journal of Health and Social Behavior* 48(3): 223–238.

Horneffer-Ginter, K. 2008. Stages of change and possible selves: Two tools for promoting college health. *Journal of American College Health* 56(4): 351–358.

Kaiser Family Foundation. (October 2013). Kaiser Health Tracking Poll, unpublished estimates.

Kohl, H. K., et al. 2011. Healthy People: A 2020 vision for the social determinants approach. *Health Education & Behavior* 38(6): 551–557.

National Center for Health Statistics. 2010. Health behaviors of adults: United States, 2005–07. *Vital and Health Statistics* 10(245).

National Center for Health Statistics. 2011. *Health, United States, 2012. With Special Feature on Socioeconomic Status and Health.* Hyattsville, MD: National Center for Health Statistics.

National Center for Health Statistics. 2016. *Health, United States, 2015: With Special Feature on Racial and Ethnic Health Disparities.* Hyattsville, MD: National Center for Health Statistics.

O'Loughlin, J., et al. 2007. Lifestyle risk factors for chronic disease across family origin among adults in multiethnic, low-income, urban neighborhoods. *Ethnicity and Disease* 17(4): 657–663.

Pinkhasov, R. M., et al. 2010. Are men shortchanged on health? Perspective on health care utilization and health risk behavior in men and women in the United States. *International Journal of Clinical Practice* 64(4): 475–487.

Printz, C. 2012. Disparities in cancer care: Are we making progress? A look at how researchers and organizations are working to reduce cancer health disparities. *Cancer* 118(4): 867–868.

Prochaska, J. O., J. C. Norcross, and C. C. DiClemente. 1995. *Changing for Good: The Revolutionary Program That Explains the Six Stages of Change and Teaches You How to Free Yourself from Bad Habits.* New York: Morrow.

Thorpe, R. J., et al. 2008. Social context as an explanation for race disparities in hypertension: findings from the Exploring Health Disparities in Integrated Communities (EHDIC) Study. *Social Science and Medicine* 67(10): 1604-1611.

University of California, Berkeley. 2011 Update. *Evaluating Web Pages: Techniques to Apply and Questions to Ask* (http://www.lib.berkeley.edu/TeachingLib/Guides/Internet/Evaluate.html).

U.S. Department of Health and Human Services. 2016. *Healthy People 2020: Lesbian, Gay, Bisexual, and Transgender Health* (https://www.healthypeople.gov/2020/topics-objectives/topic/lesbian-gay-bisexual-and-transgender-health).

Williams, D. R. 2012. Miles to go before we sleep: Racial inequities in health. *Journal of Health and Social Behavior* 53(3): 279–295.

Wojno, M. A. 2013. 12 Things college students don't need. *Kiplinger*, August 29.

Yudell, M., et al. 2016. Taking race out of human genetics. *Science* 351(6273): 564.

1. I, _____, agree to _____
_____

2. I will begin on _____ and plan to reach my goal of _____
_____ by _____

3. To reach my final goal, I have devised the following schedule of mini-goals. For each step in my program, I will give myself the reward listed.

Mini-goal	Target date	Reward
_____	_____	_____
_____	_____	_____
_____	_____	_____

My overall reward for reaching my goal will be _____

4. I have gathered and analyzed data on my target behavior and have identified the following strategies for changing my behavior:
_____
_____

5. I will use the following tools to monitor my progress toward my final goal: _____
_____
_____

I sign this contract as an indication of my personal commitment to reach my goal: _____
_____

I have recruited a helper who will witness my contract and _____
_____
_____

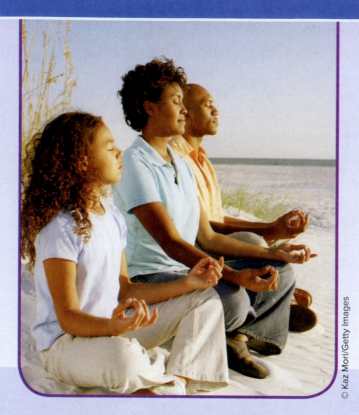

© Kaz Mori/Getty Images

CHAPTER OBJECTIVES

- Explain what stress is
- Describe the relationship between stress and health
- List common sources of stress
- Describe and apply techniques for managing stress
- Explain the health-related benefits of sleep and the consequences of disrupted sleep

CHAPTER **2**

Stress: The Constant Challenge

Like the term *wellness, stress* is a word many people use without understanding its precise meaning. Stress is popularly viewed as an uncomfortable response to a negative event, which probably describes *nervous tension* more than the cluster of physical and psychological responses that actually constitutes stress. In fact, stress is not limited to negative situations; it is also a response to pleasurable physical challenges and the achievement of personal goals.

Whether stress is experienced as pleasant or unpleasant depends largely on the situation and the individual. Learning effective responses to stress can enhance psychological health and help prevent a number of serious diseases, and stress management can be an important part of daily life.

As a college student, you may be in one of the most stressful times of your life. This chapter explains the physiological and psychological reactions that make up the stress response and describes how these reactions can put your health at risk. The chapter also presents methods of managing stress and establishing healthy sleep patterns.

WHAT IS STRESS?

In common usage, the term *stress* refers to two things: the mental states or events that trigger physical and psychological reactions (e.g., "That relationship is way too much stress"), *and* the reactions themselves (e.g., "I feel a lot of stress every time I walk into that classroom"). This text uses the more precise term **stressor** for a physical or psychological event that triggers physical and emotional reactions and the term **stress response** for the reactions themselves. Thoughts or feelings about an approaching event can be just as stressful as the event itself, such as a first date or a final exam; sweaty palms and a pounding heart are symptoms of the stress response. We'll use the term **stress** to describe the

TERMS

stressor Any physical or psychological event or condition that produces physical and psychological reactions.

stress response The physical and emotional reactions to a stressor.

stress The general physical and emotional state that the stressor produces.

general physical and emotional state that accompanies the stress response.

Each individual's experience of stress depends on many factors, including the nature of the stressor and how it is perceived. Stressors take many different forms. Like a fire in your home, some occur suddenly and neither last long nor repeat. Others, like air pollution or quarreling parents, can continue for a long time. The memory of a stressful occurrence can itself be a stressor years after the event, such as the memory of the loss of a loved one. Responses to stressors can include a wide variety of physical, emotional, and behavioral changes. A short-term response might be an upset stomach or insomnia, whereas a long-term response might be a change in your personality or social relations.

Physical Responses to Stressors

Imagine a close call: As you step off the curb, a car careens toward you. With just a fraction of a second to spare, you leap safely out of harm's way. In that split second of danger and in the moments following it, you experience a predictable series of physical reactions. Your body goes from a relaxed state to one prepared for physical action to cope with a threat to your life.

Two systems in your body are responsible for your physical response to stressors: the nervous system and the endocrine system. Through rapid chemical reactions affecting almost every part of your body, you are primed to act quickly and appropriately in time of danger.

The Nervous System   The **nervous system** consists of the brain, spinal cord, and nerves. Part of the nervous system is under voluntary control, as when you tell your arm to reach for a chocolate. The part that is *not* under conscious supervision—for example, the part that controls the digestion of the chocolate—is the **autonomic nervous system.** In addition to digestion, it controls your heart rate, breathing, blood pressure, and hundreds of other involuntary functions.

The autonomic nervous system consists of two divisions:

- The **parasympathetic division** is in control when you are relaxed. It aids in digesting food, storing energy, and promoting growth.

- The **sympathetic division** is activated when your body is stimulated, for example, by exercise, and when there is an emergency, such as severe pain, anger, or fear.

Sympathetic nerves affect nearly every organ, sweat gland, blood vessel, and muscle in order to enable your body to best handle an emergency.

Actions of the Nervous and Endocrine Systems Together   During stress, the sympathetic nervous system triggers the **endocrine system.** This system of glands, tissues, and cells helps control body functions by releasing **hormones** and other chemical messengers into the bloodstream to influence metabolism and other body processes.

The nervous system handles very short-term stress, whereas the endocrine system deals with both short-term (*acute*) and long-term (*chronic*) stress. How do both systems work together in an emergency? Higher cognitive areas in your brain decide that you are facing a threat. The nervous and endocrine systems activate adrenal glands, which are located near the top of the kidneys. These glands release the hormones **cortisol** and **epinephrine** (also called adrenaline). These hormones then trigger the physiological changes shown in Figure 2.1, including the following:

- Heart and respiration rates accelerate to speed oxygen through the body.

- Hearing and vision become more acute.

- The liver releases extra sugar into the bloodstream to boost energy.

- Perspiration increases to cool the skin.

- The brain releases **endorphins**—chemicals that can inhibit or block sensations of pain—in case you are injured.

As a group, these nearly instantaneous physiological changes are called the **fight-or-flight reaction.** These changes give you the heightened reflexes and strength you need to dodge a car or deal with other stressors. Although these physiological changes may vary in intensity, the same basic set of physiological reactions occurs in response to

TERMS

nervous system   The brain, spinal cord, and nerves.

autonomic nervous system   The part of the nervous system that controls certain basic body processes; consists of the sympathetic and parasympathetic divisions.

parasympathetic division   The part of the autonomic nervous system that moderates the excitatory effect of the sympathetic division, slowing metabolism and restoring energy supplies.

sympathetic division   Division of the autonomic nervous system that reacts to danger or other challenges by accelerating body processes.

endocrine system   The system of glands, tissues, and cells that secrete hormones into the bloodstream to influence metabolism and other body processes.

hormone   A chemical messenger produced in the body and transported in the bloodstream to target cells or organs for specific regulation of their activities.

cortisol   A steroid hormone secreted by the cortex (outer layer) of the adrenal gland; also called *hydrocortisone*.

epinephrine   A hormone secreted by the medulla (inner core) of the adrenal gland that affects the functioning of organs involved in responding to a stressor; also called *adrenaline*.

endorphins   Brain secretions that have pain-inhibiting effects.

fight-or-flight reaction   A defense reaction that prepares a person for conflict or escape by triggering hormonal, cardiovascular, metabolic, and other changes.

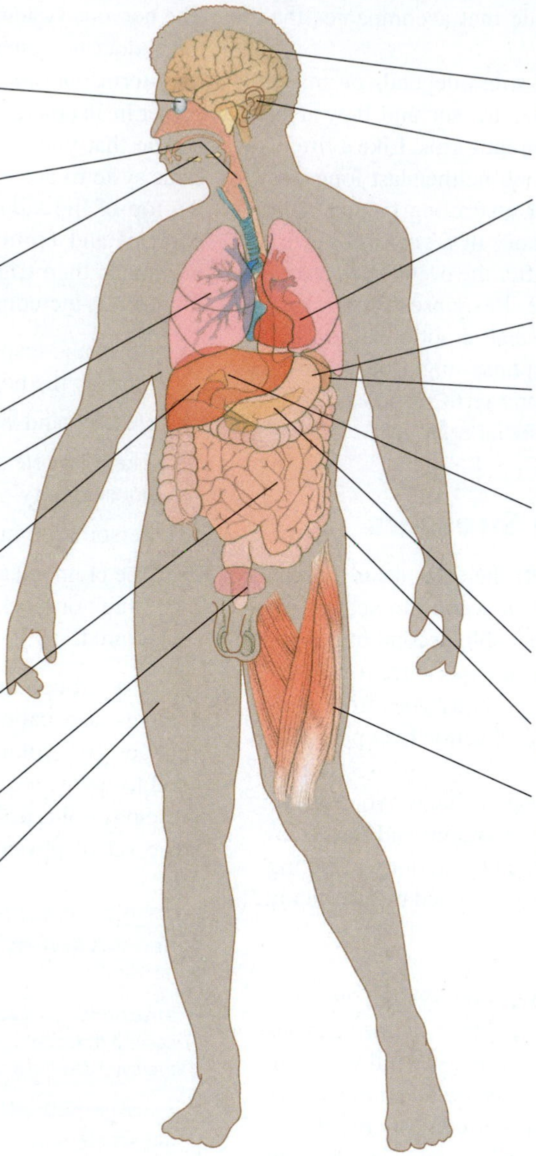

Pupils dilate to admit extra light for more sensitive vision.

Mucous membranes of nose and throat shrink, while muscles force a wider opening of air passages to allow easier airflow.

Secretion of saliva and mucus decreases; digestive activities have a low priority in an emergency.

Air passages dilate to allow more air into lungs.

Perspiration increases, especially in armpits, groin, hands, and feet, to flush out waste and cool the overheating body by evaporation.

Liver releases sugar into bloodstream to provide energy for muscles and brain.

Muscles of intestines stop contracting because digestion has halted.

Bladder relaxes. Emptying of bladder contents releases excess weight, making it easier to flee.

Blood vessels in skin and internal organs contract; those in skeletal muscles dilate. This increases blood pressure and delivery of blood to where it is most needed.

Endorphins are released to block any distracting pain.

Hearing becomes more acute.

Heart accelerates rate of beating. Strength of contraction increases to allow more blood flow where it is needed.

Digestion halts.

Spleen releases more red blood cells to meet an increased demand for oxygen and to replace any blood lost from injuries.

Adrenal glands stimulate secretion of epinephrine, increasing blood sugar, blood pressure, and heart rate; also spur increase in amount of fat in blood. These changes provide an energy boost.

Pancreas decreases secretions because digestion has halted.

Fat is removed from storage and broken down to supply extra energy.

Voluntary (skeletal) muscles contract throughout the body, readying them for action.

FIGURE 2.1   The fight-or-flight reaction. In response to a stressor, the autonomic nervous system and the endocrine system prepare the body to deal with an emergency.

any type of stressor—positive or negative, physiological or psychological.

The Return to Homeostasis   Once a stressful situation ends, the parasympathetic division of your autonomic nervous system takes command and halts the stress response. It restores **homeostasis,** a state in which blood pressure, heart rate, hormone levels, and other vital functions are maintained within a narrow range of normal. Your parasympathetic nervous system calms your body down, slowing a rapid heartbeat, drying sweaty palms, and returning breathing to normal. Gradually your body resumes its normal "housekeeping" functions, such as digestion and temperature regulation. Damage that may have been sustained during the fight-or-flight reaction is repaired. The day after you narrowly dodge the car, you wake up feeling fine. In this way, your body can grow,

repair itself, and acquire new reserves of energy. When the next crisis comes, you'll be ready to respond again instantly.

The Fight-or-Flight Reaction in Modern Life   The fight-or-flight reaction is part of our biological heritage, and it's a survival mechanism that has served humans well. In modern life, however, it is often absurdly inappropriate. Many of the stressors we face in everyday life do not require a physical response—for example, an exam, a mess left by a roommate, or a stoplight. The fight-or-flight reaction prepares the body for physical action regardless of whether a particular stressor necessitates such a response.

homeostasis   A state of stability and consistency in an individual's physiological functioning.   **TERMS**

Psychological and Behavioral Responses to Stressors

People's perceptions of potential stressors—and of their reactions to such stressors—vary greatly. For example, you may feel confident about taking exams but be nervous about talking to people you don't know, whereas your roommate may love challenging social situations but may be nervous about taking tests. Our individual ways of perceiving things play a huge role in the stress equation.

Your *cognitive* (mental) *appraisal* of a potential stressor strongly influences how you view it. Two factors that can reduce the magnitude of the stress response are successful prediction and the perception of control. For instance, receiving a course syllabus at the beginning of the term allows you to predict the timing of major deadlines and exams. Having this predictive knowledge also allows you to exert some control over your study plans and can help reduce the stress caused by exams.

Cognitive appraisal is highly individual and strongly related to emotions. The facts of a situation—Who? What? Where? When?—typically are evaluated fairly consistently from person to person. But evaluation with respect to personal outcome varies: What does this mean for me? Can I do anything about it? Will it improve or worsen?

If a person perceives a situation as exceeding her or his ability to cope, the result can be negative emotions and an inappropriate stress response. If, by contrast, a person perceives a situation as a challenge that is within her or his ability to manage, more positive and appropriate responses are likely. A certain amount of stress, if coped with appropriately, can help promote optimal performance (Figure 2.2).

FIGURE 2.2 Stress level, performance, and well-being. A moderate level of stress challenges individuals in a way that promotes optimal performance and well-being. Too little stress, and people are not challenged enough to improve; too much stress, and the challenges become stressors that can impair physical and emotional health.

© Image Source/Getty Images; © John Fedele/Getty Images; © John Lund/Drew Kelly/Blend Images LLC

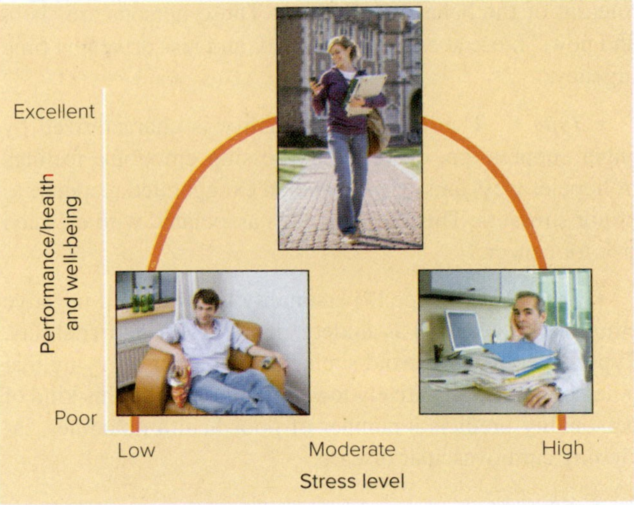

Effective and Ineffective Responses Common psychological responses to stressors include anxiety, depression, and fear. Although emotional responses are determined in part by inborn personality or temperament, we often can moderate or learn to control them. Coping techniques are discussed later in the chapter.

Unlike behavioral reactions, our behavioral responses to stressors are controlled by the **somatic nervous system,** which manages our *conscious* actions. Effective behavioral responses such as talking, laughing, exercising, meditating, learning time management skills, and becoming more assertive can promote wellness and enable us to function at our best. Ineffective behavioral responses to stressors include overeating; expressing hostility; and using tobacco, alcohol, or other drugs.

QUICK STATS

86.7% of college students reported feeling overwhelmed by their workload at least once in the past year.

—American College Health Association–National College Health Assessment II, 2015

Personality and Stress Some people seem to be nervous, irritable, and easily upset by minor annoyances. Others are calm and composed even in difficult situations. Scientists remain unsure just why this is or how the brain's complex emotional mechanisms work. But **personality**—the sum of cognitive, behavioral, and emotional tendencies—clearly affects how people perceive and react to stressors. To investigate the links among personality, stress, and wellness, researchers examine characteristic "personality types" and "personality traits."

PERSONALITY TYPES Depending on the situation, most of us display some of the behaviors characteristic of one or more of the following types.

- ***Type A.*** People with Type A personality are overly competitive, controlling, impatient, and aggressive. Type A people have a higher perceived stress level and more problems coping with stress. They react explosively to stressors and are upset by events that others would consider only annoyances. Studies indicate that certain characteristics of the Type A pattern—anger, cynicism, and hostility—increase the risk of heart disease, cancer, and other life-threatening conditions.

- ***Type B.*** The Type B personality is relaxed and contemplative. Type B people are less frustrated by daily events and more

TERMS

somatic nervous system The branch of the peripheral nervous system that governs motor functions and sensory information, largely under conscious control.

personality The sum of behavioral, cognitive, and emotional tendencies.

tolerant of the behavior of others. These persons are "here and now," more at ease in the world, and less driven by time urgency.

- *Type C.* The Type C personality is characterized by anger suppression, difficulty expressing emotions, feelings of hopelessness and despair, and an exaggerated response to minor stressors. This type has been associated with elevated risk for cancer.

- *Type D.* The Type D personality tends toward negative emotional states such as anxiety, depression, and irritability. Type D people also avoid social interactions, worrying that others will react negatively toward them. Having this kind of personality predicts a number of poor health outcomes, including cardiovascular disease.

PERSONALITY TRAITS Researchers have also looked for personality traits that enable people to deal more effectively with stress. One such trait is *hardiness,* a particular form of optimism. People with a hardy personality view potential stressors as challenges and opportunities for growth and learning, rather than as burdens. They see fewer situations as stressful and react less intensely to stress than nonhardy people might. Hardy people are committed to their activities, have a sense of inner purpose and an inner locus of control, and feel at least partly in control of their lives.

Another psychological characteristic that prompts you to behave in a certain way is motivation. Two types of motivation have been studied that relate to stress and health. *Stressed power motivation* is associated with people who are aggressive and argumentative, and who need to have power over others. One study of college students found that persons with this personality trait tend to get sick when their need for power is blocked or threatened. In contrast, people with *unstressed affiliation motivation* are drawn to others and want to be liked as friends. The same study of college students found that students with this trait reported the least illness. Another important personality trait—**resilience**—is especially associated with social and academic success in groups at risk for stress, such as people from low-income families and those with mental or physical disabilities. Resilient people tend to face adversity effectively and recover quickly after facing challenges. There are three basic types of resilience, and each one can determine how a person responds to stress:

- *Nonreactive resilience,* in which a person does not react to a stressor
- *Homeostatic resilience,* in which a person may react strongly but returns to baseline functioning quickly
- *Positive growth resilience,* in which a person learns and grows from the stress experience

Resilience is associated with emotional intelligence and violence prevention and is also a trait demonstrated to improve with mindfulness-based stress reduction.

Contemporary research repeatedly demonstrates that you can change some basic elements of your personality as well as your typical behaviors and patterns of thinking using positive stress-management techniques like those described later in the chapter.

Cultural Background Young adults from around the world come to the United States for a higher education; most students finish college with a greater appreciation for other cultures and worldviews. The clash of cultures, however, can be a big source of stress for many students—especially when it leads to disrespectful treatment, harassment, or violence. It is important to consider that our reactions to stressful events are influenced by family and cultural background. Learning to appreciate the cultural backgrounds of other people can be both a mind-opening experience and a way to avoid stress over cultural differences.

Gender Your **gender role**—the activities, abilities, and behaviors your culture expects of you based on your sex—can affect your experience of stress. Some behavioral responses to stressors, such as crying or openly expressing anger, may be deemed more appropriate for one gender than another.

Strict adherence to gender roles, however, can limit one's response to stress and can itself become a source of stress. Gender roles can also affect one's perception of a stressor. If a man derives most of his self-worth from his work, for example, retirement may be more stressful for him than for a woman whose self-image is based on several different roles.

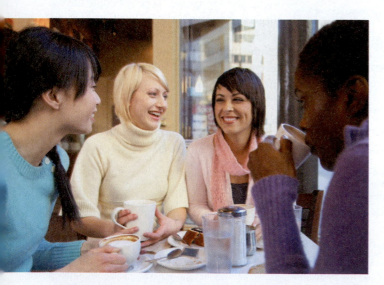

A person's emotional and behavioral responses to stressors depend on many factors, including personality, gender, and cultural background.

© Fancy/Alamy

resilience A personality trait associated with the ability to face adversity and recover quickly from difficulties.

gender role A culturally expected pattern of behavior and attitudes determined by a person's sex.

TERMS

Since the American Psychological Association began its yearly "Stress in America" survey in 2007, women have reported a higher level of stress than men. In 2015, 11.2% of female college students reported "tremendous stress," as compared to 8.1% of male college students. The survey also shows that women are more likely than men to try to reduce their stress, although a lower percentage say they were successful than the percentage of men who tried to reduce theirs. Women coped with stress through behaviors such as reading, spending time with friends, or meditating, in contrast to men, who preferred playing sports.

Experience Past experiences can profoundly influence the evaluation of a potential stressor. Consider someone who has had a bad experience giving a speech in the past. He or she is much more likely to perceive an upcoming speech as stressful than someone who has had positive public speaking experiences.

STRESS AND HEALTH

According to the American Psychological Association, 76% of the general population report suffering physical symptoms related to stress (such as tense muscles or headaches), and 71% report nonphysical symptoms (emotional or behavioral problems). The role of stress in health is complex, but evidence suggests that stress can increase vulnerability to many ailments. Several theories have been proposed to explain the relationship between stress and disease.

The General Adaptation Syndrome

Biologist Hans Selye was one of the first scientists to develop a comprehensive theory of stress and disease in the 1930s and 1940s. His theory became the foundation for subsequent research into how stress affects the human body. Selye described what he called the **general adaptation syndrome (GAS),** a universal and predictable response pattern to all stressors. This research identified an automatic self-regulation system of the mind and body that attempts to return the body to a state of homeostasis (inner balance) after being subjected to stress. As mentioned earlier, stressors can be either pleasant (attending a party) or unpleasant (getting a bad grade). According to the GAS theory, the stress resulting from a stressor perceived to be pleasant although perhaps a challenge is called **eustress;** stress brought on by a stressor perceived to be unpleasant and a hindrance is called **distress.** The sequence of physical responses associated with GAS is the same for eustress and distress and occurs in the same three stages: alarm, resistance, and exhaustion (see Figure 2.3).

- *Alarm.* The body initially experiences a stressor in a *shock phase.* This is followed by an *antishock phase,* which includes the complex sequence of events brought on by the fight-or-flight response. In these two phases, the body is more susceptible to disease or injury because it is using

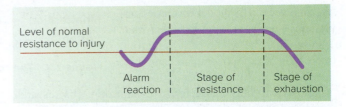

FIGURE 2.3   The general adaptation syndrome. During the alarm phase, the body's resistance to injury lowers. With continued stress, resistance to injury is enhanced. With prolonged exposure to repeated stressors, exhaustion sets in.

resources and energy to deal with a crisis. Someone in this stage may experience headaches, indigestion, anxiety, and disrupted eating or sleep patterns.

- *Resistance.* Under continued stress, the body develops a new level of homeostasis in which it is more resistant to disease and injury than usual. In this stage, a person can cope with normal life and added stress. However, at some point, the body's resources will become depleted.

- *Exhaustion.* The first two stages of GAS require a great deal of energy. If a stressor persists, or if several stressors occur in succession, general exhaustion sets in. This is not the sort of exhaustion you feel after a long, busy day. Rather, it's a life-threatening physiological exhaustion. The body's resources are depleted, and the body is unable to maintain normal function. If this stage is extended, long-term damage may result, manifesting itself in ulcers, digestive system trouble, depression, diabetes, cardiovascular problems, and/or mental illnesses.

Selye's GAS theory compelled further research into just how stress and health are connected, but at the time, scientists did not have the technology needed to study that relationship effectively. Another step in stress research was taken in the 1970s and 1980s with the advent of "biofeedback" techniques, through which researchers could use instruments to measure brain waves, skin conduction, heart rates, and muscle tone. One of these researchers was Gary Schwartz, at Yale University.

Connectedness and Health

Schwartz proposed a model that used biofeedback techniques to enable people to become more aware of their own physiological functions and to moderate these functions to better

> **TERMS**
>
> **general adaptation syndrome (GAS)** A pattern of stress responses consisting of three stages: alarm, resistance, and exhaustion.
>
> **eustress** Stress resulting from a stressor perceived to be pleasant.
>
> **distress** Stress resulting from a stressor perceived to be unpleasant.

manage stress. His model was based on systems theory, an approach that recognizes that the whole of a system is more than its component parts and that it self-regulates in ways that to this day scientists can only characterize as amazing. His research employed the premise that bodies maintain inner balance through self-regulating feedback loops among systems related to mental states, respiration, and heart rate. Furthermore, he established that self-regulation is the means through which bodies maintain stability as they adapt to life circumstances.

Schwartz used the term *disregulation* to describe what happens when a physiological system becomes imbalanced. He further proposed that disregulation is one of the consequences of inattention and disconnection between feedback loops of mind and body that progressively lead to disorder and disease. For example, finding yourself stuck in a traffic jam while already late for a midterm exam, you notice that you are clenching your teeth so tightly that your jaw aches, and you realize that your dentist was right! The ache you have been suffering in your jaw is because you *have been* clenching your teeth, and you now know you clench when you feel anxious! You now focus on an important connection between your mind and body, and you are in a better position to find relief.

Schwartz's model was further developed and modified by his student, Shauna Shapiro, a mindfulness researcher at Santa Clara University. The model she and her colleagues created from Schwartz's early research is called IAA (intention, attention, attitude), and it demonstrates the real value of intentional attention to the mind and body to restore connectedness, balance, and health in a mind–body system that has become disregulated and diseased. Shapiro's model emphasizes the cultivation of **mindfulness**—intentional cultivation of attention in a way that is nonjudging and nonstriving and therefore an ideal means of restoring natural self-regulation and health. Her research demonstrates that by mindfully attending to what is happening even in the midst of a serious disorder or disease, you can once again develop connectedness and self-regulation and gradually reverse the progression of disorder and disease.

Here is a useful way to remember this resource for self-regulation and health: Inattention leads to disconnection, disconnection leads to disregulation, disregulation leads to disorder, and disorder may lead to illness. Mindfulness practices (discussed in more detail later in this chapter) can reverse this deadly progression and promote wellness (see Figure 2.4): Attention leads to connection, which leads to regulation, which leads to order, which leads to ease. We may call this responding to stressors rather than reacting to them, and continued research repeatedly demonstrates the health benefits.

Allostatic Load

Long-term overexposure to stress hormones such as cortisol has been linked to health problems. Further, although physical stress reactions promote homeostasis, they may also have

Inattention ⟶ disconnection ⟶ disregulation ⟶ disorder ⟶ disease
Attention ⟶ connection ⟶ regulation ⟶ order ⟶ ease

FIGURE 2.4   The consequences of inattention; the benefits of attention.

negative effects. The "wear and tear" on the body that results from long-term exposure to repeated or chronic stress is known as **allostatic load.** The concept of allostatic load explains how frequent activation of the body's stress response, although essential for managing acute threats, can in fact damage the body in the long run if stress reactions are occurring when they are not really called for. For example, a person may be so afraid of snakes that just seeing a coiled up rope in the grass can trigger the fight-or-flight reaction of the autonomic nervous system. Allostatic load is generally measured through indicators of cumulative strain on several organs and tissues, especially on the cardiovascular system.

Ask Yourself

QUESTIONS FOR CRITICAL THINKING AND REFLECTION

Think of the last time you faced a significant stressor. How did you react? List the physical, emotional, and behavioral reactions you experienced. Were the reactions appropriate to the circumstances? Did these reactions help you better deal with the stress, or did they interfere with your efforts to handle it?

Psychoneuroimmunology

One of the most fruitful areas of current research into the relationship between stress and disease is **psychoneuroimmunology (PNI).** PNI is the study of the interactions among the nervous system, the endocrine system, and the immune system. The underlying premise of PNI is that stress, through the actions of the nervous and endocrine systems, impairs the immune system and thereby affects health.

A complex network of nerve and chemical connections exists among the nervous and the endocrine systems. In general, increased levels of cortisol are linked to a decreased number of immune system cells, or *lymphocytes*. Epinephrine appears to promote the release of lymphocytes but at the same time reduces their efficiency. Scientists have identified hormone-like substances called *neuropeptides* that appear to translate stressful emotions into biochemical events, some of

mindfulness   The intentional cultivation of attention in a way that is nonjudging and nonstriving. **TERMS**

allostatic load   The "wear and tear" on the body that results from long-term exposure to repeated or chronic stress.

psychoneuroimmunology (PNI)   The study of the interactions among the nervous, endocrine, and immune systems.

which affect the immune system, providing a physical link between emotions and immune function.

Different types of stress may affect immunity in different ways. For instance, during **acute stress** (typically lasting between 5 and 100 minutes), white blood cells move into the skin, where they enhance the immune response. During a stressful event sequence, such as a personal trauma and the events that follow, however, there are typically no overall significant immune changes. Chronic (ongoing) stressors such as unemployment have negative effects on almost all functional measures of immunity. **Chronic stress** may cause prolonged secretion of cortisol (sometimes called the "anti-stress hormone" because it seeks to return the nervous system to homeostasis after a stress reaction) and may accelerate the course of diseases that involve inflammation, including multiple sclerosis, heart disease, type 2 diabetes, and clinical depression. In other words, this is one way that too many stress reactions over a prolonged length of time can have a negative impact on health.

Mood, personality, behavior, and immune functioning are intertwined. For example, people who are generally pessimistic may neglect the basics of health care, become passive when ill, and fail to engage in health-promoting behaviors. People who are depressed may reduce physical activity and social interaction, which may in turn affect the immune system and the cognitive appraisal of a stressor. Optimism, successful coping, and positive problem solving, by contrast, may positively influence immunity. Although much remains to be learned, it is clear that people who have unresolved chronic stress in their lives or who handle stressors poorly are at risk for a wide range of health problems.

Cardiovascular Disease
During the stress response, heart rate increases and blood vessels constrict, causing blood pressure to rise. Chronic high blood pressure is a major cause of *atherosclerosis,* a disease in which blood vessels become damaged and caked with fatty deposits. These deposits can block arteries, causing heart attacks and strokes. The stress response can precipitate a heart attack in someone with atherosclerosis. The stress response can also cause stress cardiomyopathy ("broken heart syndrome"), a condition that mimics a heart attack but doesn't block the blood vessels supplying the heart.

Certain emotional responses may increase a person's risk of CVD. As described earlier, people who tend to react to situations with anger and hostility are more likely to have heart attacks than are people with less explosive, more trusting personalities. Inflammation has been linked to stress and is a key component of the damage to blood vessels that leads to heart attacks (see Chapter 12 for more about CVD.)

Psychological Problems
Many stressors are inherently anxiety-producing, depressing, or both. Stress has been found to contribute to psychological problems such as

depression, panic attacks, anxiety, eating disorders, and posttraumatic stress disorder (PTSD). PTSD, which afflicts war veterans, rape and child abuse survivors, and others who have suffered or witnessed severe trauma, is characterized by nightmares, flashbacks, and a diminished capacity to experience or express emotion. (For information about psychological health, see Chapter 3.)

Altered Immune Function
PNI research helps explain how stress affects the immune system. Some of the health problems linked to stress-related changes in immune function include vulnerability to colds and other infections, asthma and allergy attacks, and flare-ups of chronic sexually transmitted infections such as genital herpes and HIV infection.

Headaches
More than 45 million Americans suffer from chronic, recurrent headaches. Headaches come in various types but are often grouped into the following three categories:

• *Tension headaches.* Approximately 90% of all headaches are tension headaches, characterized by a dull, steady pain, usually on both sides of the head. It may feel as though a band of pressure is tightening around the head, and the pain may extend to the neck and shoulders. Acute tension headaches may last from hours to days, whereas chronic tension headaches may occur almost every day for months or even years. Ineffective stress management skills, poor posture, and immobility are the leading causes of tension headaches. There is no cure, but the pain can sometimes be avoided and relieved with mindfulness skills, over-the-counter painkillers, and therapies such as massage, acupuncture, relaxation, hot or cold showers, and rest.

• *Migraine headaches.* Migraines typically progress through a series of stages lasting from several minutes to several days. They may produce a variety of symptoms, including throbbing pain that starts on one side of the head and may spread; heightened sensitivity to light; visual disturbances such as flashing lights or temporary blindness; nausea; dizziness; and fatigue. Women are more than twice as likely as men to suffer from migraines. Potential triggers include menstruation, stress, fatigue, atmospheric changes, bright light, specific sounds or odors, and certain foods. The frequency of attacks varies from a few in a lifetime to

TERMS

acute stress Stress immediately following a stressor; may last only minutes or may turn into chronic stress.

chronic stress Stress that continues for days, weeks, or longer.

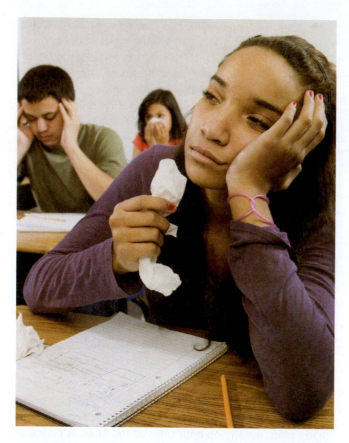

Ongoing stress has been shown to make people more vulnerable to everyday ailments, such as colds and allergies.

© Somos/Veer/Getty Images

several per week. Treatment can help reduce the frequency, severity, and duration of migraines.

• **Cluster headaches.** Cluster headaches are extremely severe headaches that cause intense pain in and around one eye. They usually occur in clusters of one to three headaches each day over a period of weeks or months, alternating with periods of remission in which no headaches occur. More than twice as many men than women suffer from cluster headaches. There is no known cause or cure for cluster headaches, but a number of treatments are available. During cluster periods, it is important to refrain from smoking cigarettes and drinking alcohol, because these activities can trigger attacks. For more information on treating headaches and when a headache may signal a serious illness, see Appendix B.

Other Health Problems Many other health problems may be caused or worsened by excessive stress, including skin disorders, asthma, cancer, and insomnia and fatigue. Additional problems include the following:

• Digestive problems such as stomachaches, diarrhea, constipation, irritable bowel syndrome, and ulcers

• Injuries, including on-the-job injuries caused by repetitive strain

• Menstrual irregularities, impotence, and pregnancy complications

Ask Yourself

QUESTIONS FOR CRITICAL THINKING AND REFLECTION
Have you ever been so stressed that you felt ill? If so, what were your symptoms? How did you handle them? Did the experience affect the way you reacted to other stressful events?

COMMON SOURCES OF STRESS

Recognizing potential sources of stress is an important step in successfully managing the stress in your life.

Major Life Changes

Any major change in your life that requires adjustment and accommodation can be a source of stress. Early adulthood and the college years are associated with many significant changes, such as moving out of the family home. Even changes typically thought of as positive—graduation, job promotion, marriage—can be stressful.

Clusters of life changes, particularly those that are perceived negatively, may be linked to health problems in some people. Personality and coping skills, however, are important moderating influences. People with strong support networks and stress-resistant personalities are less likely to become ill in response to life changes than are people with fewer resources.

Daily Hassles

Although major life changes are stressful, they seldom occur regularly. Researchers have proposed that minor problems—life's daily hassles, such as losing your keys or wallet—can be an even greater source of stress because they occur much more often.

People who perceive hassles negatively are likely to experience a moderate stress response every time they face one. Over time, this can take a significant toll on health. Studies indicate that, for some people, daily hassles contribute to a general decrease in overall wellness.

College Stressors

College is a time of major changes and minor hassles. For many students, college means being away from home and family for the first time. Nearly all students share stresses like the following:

• **Academic stress.** Exams, grades, and an endless workload await every college student but can be especially troublesome for students just out of high school.

• **Interpersonal stress.** Most students are more than just students; they are also friends, children, employees, spouses, parents, and so on. Managing relationships while juggling the rigors of college life can be daunting, especially if some friends or family members are less than supportive.

• *Time pressures.* Class schedules, assignments, and deadlines are an inescapable part of college life. But these time pressures can be compounded drastically for students who also have job or family responsibilities.

• *Financial concerns.* The majority of college students need financial aid not just to cover the cost of tuition but also to survive from day to day while in school. For many, college life isn't possible without a job, and the pressure to stay afloat financially competes with academic and other stressors.

• *Worries about anything but especially about the future.* As college comes to an end, students face the next set of decisions. This decision making means thinking about a career, choosing a place to live, and leaving the friends and routines of school behind. Students may find it helpful to go to the campus career center.

Job-Related Stressors

Americans rate their jobs as a key source of stress in their lives. Various surveys indicate that 40–50% of working Americans say they typically feel tense or stressed out while at work. Tight schedules and overtime leave less time to exercise, socialize, and engage in other stress-proofing activities. Although daily work activities can be stressful enough on their own, stress can be even worse for people who are left out of important decisions relating to their jobs. When workers are given the opportunity to shape how their jobs are performed, job satisfaction goes up and stress levels go down.

Social Stressors

Social networks can be real or virtual. Both types can help improve your ability to deal with stress, but any social network can also become a stressor in itself.

Real Social Networks   Although social support is a key buffer against stress, your interactions with others can themselves be a source of stress. The college years, in particular, can be a time of great change in interpersonal relationships. The larger community where you live can also act as a stressor.

Social stressors include prejudice and discrimination. You may feel stress as you try to relate to people of other ethnic, racial, or socioeconomic groups. You may feel pressure to assimilate into mainstream society, or to spend as much time as possible with others who share your background. If English is not your first language, you may face the added burden of conducting daily activities in a language with which you are not comfortable. All these pressures can become significant sources of stress. (See the box "Diverse Populations, Discrimination, and Stress.")

Virtual Social Networks   Technology can help you save time, but it can also increase stress. Being electronically connected to work, family, and friends all the time can impinge on your personal space, waste time, and distract you from your current real situation. If you are "always on"— that is, always available by voice or text messaging—some friends or colleagues may think it's all right to contact you anytime, even if you're in class or trying to work, and they may expect an immediate response. The convenience of staying electronically connected comes at a price.

Other Stressors

Have you tried to eat at a restaurant where the food was great, but the atmosphere was so noisy that it put you on edge? This is an example of a minor environmental stressor—a condition or event in the physical environment that causes stress. Examples of more disturbing and disruptive, even catastrophic, environmental stressors include natural disasters, acts of violence, industrial accidents, and intrusive noises or smells.

Like the noisy atmosphere of some restaurants, many environmental stressors are mere inconveniences that are easy to avoid. Others, such as pollen or construction noise, may be unavoidable daily sources of stress. For those who live in poor or violent neighborhoods, the environment can contain major stressors, and in every corner of the country today, people are exposed to disturbing news and images via the media (see the box "Coping with News of Traumatic Events").

Many stressors are found not in our environment but within ourselves, and often are created by the ways we think and look at things. Here is one useful way to think about this: Stress is 10% what's happening and 90% how you look at it. For example, we pressure ourselves to reach goals and continually judge our progress and performance. Striving to reach goals can enhance self-esteem if the goals are reasonable. Unrealistic expectations, however, can be a significant source of stress and can damage self-esteem. Other internal stressors are emotional states such as despair or hostility, and physical states, such as chronic illness and exhaustion; each can be both a cause and an effect of unmanaged stress.

Ask Yourself

QUESTIONS FOR CRITICAL THINKING AND REFLECTION

What are the top two or three stressors in your life right now? Are they new to your life—as part of your college experience— or have you experienced them in the past? Do they include both positive and negative experiences (eustress and distress)?

MANAGING STRESS

You can control the stress in your life by taking the following steps:

• Shore up your support system.
• Improve your communication skills.
• Develop healthy exercise and eating habits.

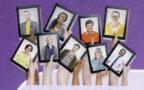

DIVERSITY MATTERS
Diverse Populations, Discrimination, and Stress

Stress is universal, but an individual's response to stress can vary depending on gender, cultural background, prior experience, and genetic factors. In diverse multiethnic and multicultural nations such as the United States, some groups face special stressors and have higher-than-average rates of stress-related physical and emotional problems. These groups include racial and ethnic minorities, the poor, those with physical or mental disabilities, and those who don't express mainstream gender roles.

Discrimination occurs when people speak or act according to their prejudices—biased, negative beliefs or attitudes toward some group. A blatant example, rising to the level of hate speech and criminal activity, is painting a swastika on a Jewish studies house or vandalizing a mosque. A more subtle example is when Middle Eastern American or African American students notice that residents in a mostly white college town tend to keep a close eye on them.

Immigrants to the United States have to learn to live in a new society. Doing so requires a balance between assimilating and changing to be like the majority, and maintaining a connection to their own culture, language, and religion. The process of acculturation is generally stressful, especially when the person's

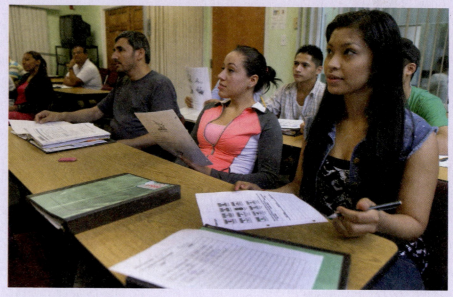

© Boston Globe/Getty Images

background is radically different from that of the people he or she is now living among, or when people in the new community are suspicious or unwelcoming, as has recently been the case with immigrants from war-torn regions of the Middle East.

Both immigrants and minorities who have lived for generations in the United States can face job- and school-related stressors because of stereotypes and discrimination. They may make less money in comparable jobs with comparable levels of education and may find it more difficult to achieve leadership positions.

On a positive note, however, many who experience hardship, disability, or prejudice develop effective goal-directed coping skills and are successful at overcoming obstacles and managing the stress they face.

- Learn to identify and moderate individual stressors.
- Learn mindfulness skills.

Adequate sleep is another key strategy for managing stress and for improving your overall wellness. Sleep is described in detail in the next section.

The effort required for stress management is well worth the time. People who manage stress effectively not only are healthier but also have more time to enjoy life and accomplish goals.

Social Support

Having the support of friends and family members contributes to the well-being of body and mind. Research supports this conclusion and demonstrates the value of affiliation or connectedness, as the following examples demonstrate:

• A study of college students living in overcrowded apartments revealed that those with a strong social support

system were less distressed by their cramped quarters than were the loners who navigated life's challenges on their own.

• Young adults who have strong relationships with their parents tend to cope with stress better than peers with poor parental relationships.

• Many studies show that married people live longer than single people (including those who are divorced, widowed, or never married) and have lower death rates from practically all causes.

Social support can provide a critical counterbalance to the stress in our lives. Give yourself time to develop and maintain a network of people you can count on for emotional support, feedback, and nurturing. If you believe you don't have enough social support, consider becoming a volunteer to help build your network of friends and to enhance your spiritual wellness.

We are continually exposed to news of tragic events: natural disasters, war, terrorism, and poverty. Both experiencing trauma and observing it can result in extreme stress, requiring time and effort to recover. Such events can weaken your sense of security and create uncertainty about how the future may unfold. People react to such news in different ways, depending on their proximity to the event and how recent it was. People far from the site may suffer emotional reactions simply from watching endless coverage on television.

Responses to trauma include disbelief, shock, fear, anger, resentment, anxiety, mood swings, irritability, sadness, depression, panic, guilt, apathy, feelings of isolation or powerlessness, and many of the symptoms of excess stress. Some people affected by such violence develop posttraumatic stress disorder (PTSD), a more serious condition.

In the case of the shooting rampages in 2015 at a workplace in San Bernardino, California, and in 2016 at a nightclub in Orlando, Florida, both of which left multiple people dead and injured, communities mobilized quickly to respond to the expected surge in behavioral health needs generated by the attacks. Information sources and support groups were established for people grieving the loss of friends, family, neighbors, or colleagues.

Unfortunately these kinds of horrific events have been repeated numerous times in recent years. If you are becoming preoccupied with some recent disastrous event, such as a school shooting or terrorist attack, take these steps:

• Be sure you have the best information about what happened and whether a continuing risk is present. That information may be available through websites or on local radio or TV stations.

• Don't expose yourself to so much media coverage that it overwhelms you.

• Take care of yourself. Use the stress-relief techniques discussed in this chapter.

• Share your feelings and concerns with others. Be a supportive listener.

• If you feel able, help others in any way you can, such as by volunteering to work with victims.

• If you feel emotionally distressed days or weeks after the event, consider asking for professional help.

Volunteering

Studies show that not all giving is the same—for example, donating money does not have the same beneficial health effects as volunteering that involves personal contact. A few simple guidelines can help you get the most out of giving:

• Choose a volunteer activity that puts you in contact with people.

• Volunteer with a group. Sharing your interests with other volunteers increases social support.

• Know your limits. Helping that goes beyond what you can handle depletes your own resources and is detrimental to your health.

Communication

Communicating in an assertive way that respects the rights of others—while protecting your own rights—can prevent stressful situations from getting out of control. Better communication skills can also help everyone form and maintain healthy relationships. Chapter 4 discusses communication techniques for building healthy relationships.

Exercise

Exercise helps maintain a healthy body and mind and even stimulates the birth of new brain cells. Regular physical

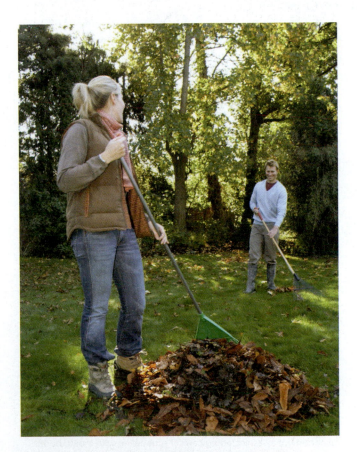

Exercise—even light activity—can be an antidote to stress.
© Nick Daly/Getty Images

activity can also reduce many of the negative effects of stress. Consider the following examples:

- Taking a long walk can decrease anxiety and blood pressure.
- A brisk 10-minute walk can leave you feeling more relaxed and energetic for up to two hours.
- People who exercise regularly react with milder physical stress responses before, during, and after exposure to stressors.
- In one study, people who took three brisk 45-minute walks each week for three months reported fewer daily hassles and an increased sense of wellness.

Nutrition

A healthful diet gives you an energy bank to draw from whenever you experience stress. Eating wisely also can enhance your feelings of self-control and self-esteem. Learning the principles of sound nutrition is easy, and sensible eating habits rapidly become second nature when practiced regularly. (For information about nutrition and healthy eating habits, see Chapter 9.)

For managing stress, limit or avoid caffeine. Although one or two cups of coffee a day probably won't hurt you, caffeine is a mildly addictive stimulant that leaves some people jittery, irritable, and unable to sleep. Consuming caffeine during stressful situations can raise blood pressure and increase levels of cortisol.

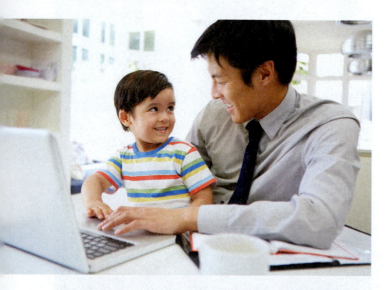

Managing the many commitments of adult life—including work, school, and parenthood—can produce a great deal of stress. Time management skills, including careful scheduling with a date book, smartphone, or tablet, can help people cope with busy days.

© Cathy Yeulet/123RF

QUICK STATS

53% of adults say they feel good about themselves after exercising, **35%** say it puts them in a good mood, and **30%** say they feel less stressed.

—American Psychological Association, 2014

Although your diet affects the way your body handles stress, the reverse is also true. Excess stress can negatively affect the way you eat. Many people, for example, respond to stress by overeating; other people skip meals or stop eating altogether during stressful periods. Not only are both responses ineffective (they don't address the causes of stress), but they are also potentially unhealthy.

Time Management

Overcommitment, procrastination, and even boredom are significant stressors for many people. Try these strategies for improving your time management skills:

- *Set priorities.* Divide your tasks into three groups: essential, important, and trivial. Focus on the first two, and ignore the third.

- *Schedule tasks for peak efficiency.* You've probably noticed you're most productive at certain times of the day (or night). Schedule as many of your tasks for those hours as you can, and stick to your schedule.

- *Set realistic goals and write them down.* Attainable goals spur you on. Impossible goals, by definition, cause frustration and failure. Fully commit yourself to achieving your goals by putting them in writing.

- *Budget enough time.* For each project you undertake, calculate how long it will take to complete. Then tack on another 10–15%, or even 25%, as a buffer.

- *Break up long-term goals into short-term ones.* Instead of waiting for large blocks of time, use short amounts of time to start a project or keep it moving.

- *Visualize the achievement of your goals.* By mentally rehearsing your performance of a task, you will be able to reach your goal more smoothly.

- *Keep track of the tasks you put off.* Analyze why you procrastinate. If the task is difficult or unpleasant, look for ways to make it easier or more fun.

- *Consider doing your least favorite tasks first.* Once you have the most unpleasant ones out of the way, you can work on the tasks you enjoy more.

- *Consolidate tasks when possible.* For example, try walking to the store so that you run your errands and exercise in the same block of time.

- *Identify quick transitional tasks.* Keep a list of 5- to 10-minute tasks you can do while waiting or between other tasks.

- *Delegate responsibility.* Ask for help when you have too much to do. Just don't delegate the jobs you know you should do yourself.

- *Say no when necessary.* If the demands made on you don't seem reasonable, say no—tactfully, but without guilt or apology.

- *Give yourself a break.* Allow time for play—free, unstructured time when you can ignore the clock. Play renews you and enables you to work more efficiently.

- *Avoid your personal "time sinks."* Identify your own time sinks—activities that consistently use up more time than you anticipate and put you behind schedule, like watching television, surfing the Internet, or talking on the phone. On particularly busy days, avoid these problematic activities altogether. For example, if you have a big paper due, don't sit down for a five-minute TV break if that's likely to turn into a two-hour break. Try a five-minute walk instead.

- *Stop thinking or talking about what you're going to do, and just do it!* Sometimes the best solution for procrastination is to stop waiting for the right moment and just get started. You will probably find that things are not as bad as you feared, and your momentum will keep you going.

Cultivating Spiritual Wellness

Spiritual wellness is associated with more effective coping skills and higher levels of overall wellness. It is a very personal wellness component, and there are many ways to develop it. Researchers have linked spiritual wellness to longer life expectancy, reduced risk of disease, faster recovery, and improved emotional health. Although spirituality is difficult to study, and researchers aren't sure how or why spirituality seems to improve health, several explanations have been offered:

- *Social support.* Attending religious services or joining a weekly meditation group as well as investing time participating in volunteer organizations helps people feel that they are part of a community with similar values and promotes social connectedness and caring.

- *Healthy habits.* Some paths to spiritual wellness encourage healthy behaviors, such as eating a vegetarian diet or consuming less meat and alcohol, while discouraging harmful habits like smoking.

- *Positive attitude.* Spirituality can give a person a sense of meaning and purpose, and these qualities create a more positive attitude, which in turn helps her or him cope with life's challenges.

- *Moments of relaxation.* When invested in practices like meditation and prayer, people can feel profound states of relaxation and are no longer caught up in thoughts and habits of mind that create distress.

Spiritual wellness does not require participation in organized religion. Many people find meaning and purpose in other ways. Spending time appreciating the marvels in nature

or working to care for the environment are powerful ways to feel continuity with the natural world. Spiritual wellness may also come through helping others in your community or by promoting human rights, peace, and harmony among people globally through art, the written word, or personal relationships.

Spiritual wellness can make you more aware of your personal values and can help clarify them. Living according to values means considering your options carefully before making a choice, choosing between options without succumbing to outside pressures that oppose your values, and making a choice and acting on it rather than doing nothing.

Confiding in Yourself through Writing

Keeping a diary is analogous to confiding in others, except that you are confiding in and becoming more attuned to yourself. This form of coping with severe stress may be especially helpful for those who find it difficult to open up to others. Although writing about traumatic and stressful events may have a short-term negative effect on mood, over the long term, stress is reduced and positive changes in health occur. A key to promoting health and well-being through journaling is to write about your emotional responses to stressful events. Set aside a special time each day or week to write down your feelings about stressful events in your life.

Cognitive Techniques

Some stressors arise in your own mind. Ideas, beliefs, perceptions, and patterns of thinking can add to your stress level. Each of the following techniques can help you change unhealthy thought patterns to ones that will help you cope with stress (also see the box "Mindfulness Meditation"). As with any skill, mastering these techniques takes practice and patience.

Think and Act Constructively Think back to the worries you had last week. How many of them were needless? By growing more aware of the ways you habitually think and feel, you can learn to recognize habits of mind that create distress and divest from them before they overwhelm you. Think about things you *can* control, particularly your way of looking at things. Try to stand aside from the problem, consider more effective steps you can take to solve it, and then carry them out. Remember that between a stimulus and a response there is a space, and in that space lies your freedom and power. In other words, if you can successfully recognize that a stressor is occurring, you can better control your response to it. In the evening, invest energy in considering how you may better promote the things you want individually or socially. This may mean reflecting on how you may better deal with an unpleasant person or stay focused in a class you find boring. By taking a constructive approach, you can prevent stressors from becoming negative events and perhaps even turn them into positive experiences.

TAKE CHARGE
Mindfulness Meditation

Mindfulness is both a mental state and the practices that cultivate this mental state. We cultivate this mental state by paying attention in a kind way to our mental, physical, and behavioral activities as they happen. By investing this kind of attention in ourselves and our lives, we soon discover that we all create most of our own stress, and that we can each do more than anyone else can to reduce that stress and take better care of ourselves. Here are two practices to use for stress reduction.

Mindful Breathing

You are always breathing, so this is a powerful and convenient way to become present wherever you go and in whatever you do. After you read these instructions, please close your eyes and invest 5–15 minutes in being present with your breath.

Sitting comfortably where you are right now, bring your body into a posture that is upright and supported, with a sense of balance and dignity. See if you can align your head, neck, and body in a way that is neither too rigid nor too relaxed, but somewhere in between. The intention is to be wakeful and alert, yet not tense; at ease, but not sleeping.

Bring attention to your breathing, wherever you feel it most prominently and notice the sensations of your breath coming and going as it will, in its own way and with its own pace. If your mind wanders from your breath, return to it by feeling the sensations of the breath as they come and go. Use these sensations as your way to be present, here and now, in each successive moment for the time you have set aside. Research has repeatedly demonstrated that extending this practice to 30 or 45 minutes on a regular basis significantly reduces stress and stress-related illnesses and conditions.

Walking Meditation

Find a place where you can walk and be uninterrupted by other people or traffic—if possible, in natural surroundings, like in a park. You can adapt this practice to fit yourself, whatever your circumstances are with mobility—for example, it can become a mindful-rolling practice if you rely on a wheelchair. Once you're ready, begin walking—slowly at first (as slowly as possible for about 10 minutes)—paying close attention to each step and using the sensations of each foot touching the ground as your way to be present. When you are ready, accelerate your pace, broadening your attention to take in more of your experience as you walk. In this mindful-movement practice, you may walk any distance, anywhere, at any speed that feels right for you. In the beginning, however, give yourself about 30 minutes.

The principal instruction is to be fully present in each moment you are walking rather than consumed with mind chatter or destination. Be open to the experience of your environment and notice, for example, the way clouds move or how the sunlight glistens in the trees and foliage around you. Turn toward whatever calls your attention and be with it as long as you like, stopping if you want to take a close look at a bug or flowers or to listen to the rustling of leaves. Remember, the overarching intention is to be mindful, to be in this experience of the now.

As you become more skilled in mindful awareness practice, you will be able to do this anywhere, even on a bustling college campus. If you want to pick up the speed or duration of your walk, you can make this walking practice part of a regular exercise program, and you will grow in strength and cardiovascular health as well as mindfulness.

Mindfulness is a lifetime engagement—not to get somewhere else, but to be where and as you are in this very moment, whether the experience is pleasant, unpleasant, or neutral. The more you invest in the practice, the more you draw forth and nourish the mental state of mindfulness with which you were born.

Take Control   A situation often feels more stressful if you feel you're not in control of it. Time may seem to be slipping away before a big exam, for example. Unexpected obstacles may appear in your path, throwing you off course. When you feel your environment is controlling you instead of the other way around, take charge! Concentrate on what you can control rather than what you cannot, and set realistic goals. Be confident of your ability to succeed.

Problem-Solve   Students with greater problem-solving abilities report easier adjustment to university life, higher motivation levels, lower stress levels, and higher grades. When you find yourself stewing over a problem, sit down with a piece of paper and try this approach:

1. Define the problem in one or two sentences.
2. Identify the causes of the problem.
3. Consider alternative solutions. Don't just stop with the most obvious one.
4. Weigh positive and negative consequences for each alternative.
5. Make a decision—choose a solution.
6. Make a list of tasks you must perform to act on your decision.
7. Carry out the tasks on your list.
8. Evaluate the outcome and revise your approach if necessary.

Modify Your Expectations   Expectations are exhausting and restricting. The fewer expectations you have, the more you can live spontaneously and joyfully. The more you expect from others, the more often you will feel let down.

And trying to meet the expectations others have of you is often futile.

Stay Positive   If you tend to beat up on yourself—"Late for class again! You can't even cope with college! How do you expect to ever hold down a real job?"—try being kind to yourself instead. Talk to yourself as you would to a child you love: "You're a smart, capable person. You've solved other problems; you'll handle this one. Tomorrow you'll simply schedule things so you get to class with a few minutes to spare."

Practice Affirmations   One way of cultivating the positive is to systematically repeat positive thoughts, or *affirmations,* to yourself. For example, if you react to stress with low self-esteem, you might repeat sentences such as "I accept myself completely" and "It doesn't matter what others say, but what I believe." Say kinder and more loving things to yourself every day to promote more responding and less reacting.

Cultivate Your Sense of Humor   When it comes to stress, laughter may be the best medicine. It is said, "He who can laugh at himself will never cease to be amused!" Even a fleeting smile produces changes in your autonomic nervous system that can lift your spirits. A few minutes of belly laughing can be as invigorating as brisk exercise. Hearty laughter elevates your heart rate, aids digestion, eases pain, and triggers the release of endorphins and other pleasurable and stimulating chemicals in the brain. After a good laugh, your muscles go slack; your pulse and blood pressure dip below normal. You are relaxed. Cultivate the ability to laugh at yourself, and you'll have a handy and instantly effective stress reliever.

Focus on What's Important   A major source of stress is trying to store too much data. Forget unimportant details (they will usually be self-evident) and organize important information. One technique you can try is to "chunk" important material into categories. If your next exam covers three chapters from your textbook, consider each chapter a chunk of information. Then break down each chunk into its three or four most important features. Create a mental outline that allows you to trace your way from the most general category down to the most specific details. This technique can be applied to managing daily responsibilities as well.

Body Awareness Techniques

Practicing mindfulness promotes stronger connections between the prefrontal cortex and the amygdala areas of the brain. This connection has been demonstrated to facilitate greater problem-solving skills, emotional self-regulation, and resilience. Practicing mindfulness has been shown to be particularly effective in devaluing bothersome thoughts and enabling presence and emotional balance to occur at their own pace.

Yoga   Hatha yoga, the most common yoga style practiced in the United States, emphasizes physical balance and breath control. It integrates components of flexibility, muscular strength and endurance, and muscle relaxation; it also sometimes serves as a preliminary to meditation. A session of yoga typically involves a series of postures, each held for a few seconds to several minutes, which involve stretching and balance and coordinated breathing. Yoga can be a powerful way to cultivate body awareness, ease, and flexibility. If you are interested in trying yoga, take a class with an experienced instructor.

Tai Chi   This martial art (in Chinese, *taijiquan*) is a system of self-defense that incorporates philosophical concepts from Taoism and Confucianism. In addition to self-defense, tai chi aims to bring the body into balance and harmony to promote health and spiritual growth. It teaches practitioners to remain calm and centered, to conserve and concentrate energy, and to manipulate force by becoming part of it—by "going with the flow." Tai chi is considered the gentlest of the martial arts. Instead of quick and powerful movements, tai chi consists of a series of slow, fluid, elegant movements, which reinforce the idea of moving *with* rather than *against* the stressors of everyday life. As with yoga, it's best to start tai chi with a class led by an experienced instructor.

Qigong   Qigong (pronounced "chee-gung") originates in China and has as its goal the restoration of energy and balance to the body. It is used to relieve stress and chronic pain through various exercises of flowing movements, visualization, and breathing while assuming postures. Although its popularity is rising, there is no scientific evidence so far that it helps relieve stress or pain.

Counterproductive Coping Strategies

College is a time when you'll learn to adapt to new and challenging situations and gain skills that will last a lifetime. It is also a time when many people develop counterproductive and unhealthy habits in response to stress. Such habits can last well beyond graduation.

Tobacco Use   Cigarettes and other tobacco products contain *nicotine,* a chemical that enhances the actions of neurotransmitters. Nicotine can make you feel relaxed and even increase your ability to concentrate, but it is highly addictive. In fact, nicotine dependence itself is considered a psychological disorder. Cigarette smoke also contains substances that cause heart disease, stroke, lung cancer, and emphysema. These negative consequences far outweigh any beneficial effects, and tobacco use should be avoided. The easiest way to avoid the habit is to not start. See Chapter 8 for more about the health effects of tobacco use and for tips on how to quit.

Use of Alcohol and Other Drugs   Like nicotine, alcohol is addictive, and many alcoholics find it hard to relax without a drink. Having a few drinks might make you feel temporarily at ease, and drinking until you're intoxicated may help you forget your current stressors. However, using alcohol to deal with stress places you at risk for all the short- and long-term problems associated with alcohol abuse. It also does nothing to address the causes of stress in your life. For more about the responsible use of alcohol, refer to Chapter 8.

Using other psychoactive drugs to cope with stress is also usually counterproductive:

- *Stimulants,* such as *amphetamines,* can activate the stress response. They also affect the same areas of the brain that are involved in regulating the stress response.

- Use of *marijuana* causes a brief period of euphoria and decreased short-term memory and attentional abilities. Physiological effects clearly show that marijuana use doesn't cause relaxation; in fact, some neurochemicals in marijuana act to enhance the stress response, and getting high on a regular basis can elicit panic attacks. To compound this, withdrawal from marijuana may also be associated with an increase in circulating stress hormones.

- *Opioids* such as morphine and heroin can mimic the effects of your body's natural painkillers and act to reduce anxiety. However, tolerance to opioids develops quickly, and many users become dependent.

- *Tranquilizers* such as Valium and Xanax mimic some of the functions of your body's parasympathetic nervous system, and as with opioids, tolerance develops quickly, causing increased dependency and toxicity.

For more information about the health effects of using psychoactive drugs, see Chapter 7.

Unhealthy Eating Habits The nutrients in the food you eat provide energy and substances needed to maintain your body. Eating is also psychologically rewarding. The feelings of satiation and sedation that follow eating produce a relaxed state. However, regular use of eating as a means of coping with stress may lead to unhealthy eating habits. In fact, a survey by the American Psychological Association revealed that about 25% of Americans use food as a means of coping with stress or anxiety. These "comfort eaters" are twice as likely to be obese as average Americans.

Many dietary supplements are marketed for stress reduction, but supplements are not required to meet the same standards as medications in terms of safety, effectiveness, and manufacturing (see Chapters 9 and 15).

Getting Help

What are the most important sources of stress in your life? Are you coping successfully with them? No single strategy or program for managing stress will work for everyone. The most important starting point for a successful stress management plan is to learn to listen to your body. When you recognize the stress response and the emotions and thoughts that accompany it, you'll be in a position to take charge of that crucial moment and handle it in a healthy way.

If the techniques discussed so far don't provide you with enough relief, you might need to look further. Excellent self-help guides can be found in bookstores or the library. Additional resources are listed in the "For More Information" section at the end of the chapter.

Your student health center or student affairs office can tell you whether your campus has a mindfulness-based stress-reduction program. If you are seeking social support, see if your campus offers a peer counseling program. Such programs are usually staffed by volunteer students with special training that emphasizes maintaining confidentiality. Peer counselors can guide you to other campus or community resources or can simply provide understanding.

Support groups are typically organized around a particular issue or problem. In your area, you might find a support group for first-year students; for reentering students; for single parents; for students of your race or ethnicity, religion, or national origin; for people with eating disorders; or for rape survivors. The number of such groups has increased in recent years as more and more people discover how therapeutic it can be to talk with others who share the same situation.

Short-term psychotherapy can also be tremendously helpful in dealing with stress-related problems. Your student health center may offer psychotherapy on a sliding-fee scale; the county mental health center in your area may do the same. If you belong to any type of religious organization, check to see whether pastoral counseling is available. Your physician can refer you to psychotherapists in your community. Not all therapists are right for all people, so be prepared to have initial sessions with several. Choose the one with whom you feel most comfortable.

SLEEP

Don't underestimate the value of a good night's sleep as a means of managing stress. Getting enough sleep isn't just good for you physically. Adequate sleep also improves mood, fosters feelings of competence and self-worth, enhances mental functioning, and supports emotional functioning.

How Sleep Works: The Physiology of Sleep

Sleep occurs in two phases: **rapid eye movement (REM) sleep** and **non–rapid eye movement (NREM) sleep.** A sleeper goes through several cycles of NREM and REM sleep each night.

TERMS

rapid eye movement (REM) sleep The portion of the sleep cycle during which dreaming occurs.

non–rapid eye movement (NREM) sleep The portion of the sleep cycle that involves deep sleep; NREM sleep includes four stages of successively deeper sleep.

NREM Sleep   NREM sleep includes four stages of successively deeper sleep (I, II, III, IV). As you move through these stages, a variety of physiological changes occur:

- Blood pressure drops.
- Respiration and heart rates slow.
- Body temperature declines.
- Growth hormone is released.
- Brain wave patterns become slow and even.

Each stage is characterized by a different pattern of electrical brain activity, measured by the electroencephalogram (EEG). When a person is awake but resting with eyes closed, the EEG shows the resting wakefulness pattern, which is called the alpha rhythm. Stage I of sleep occurs when the alpha rhythm disappears and a slower rhythm, called the theta rhythm, emerges. In Stage II, there are bursts of highly synchronized activity called K complexes and spindles that mark a brain state in which most sensory stimuli from the environment no longer can reach the higher-level brain centers. In Stages III and IV of sleep, there are large synchronized slow waves, creating a pattern that has similarities to large waves in the ocean. In slow wave sleep, it is difficult to arouse people quickly, and they may be confused when awakened.

REM Sleep   The last stage is REM sleep. During REM sleep, dreams occur. REM sleep is characterized by rapid movement of the eyes under closed eyelids, similar to when people move their eyes while awake. Blood pressure and respiration and heart rates rise, and brain activity increases to levels equal to or greater than those during waking hours. Muscles in the limbs relax completely, because the body is prevented from moving during dreaming, like a form of paralysis.

Sleep Cycles   When people fall asleep, they cycle through the four stages of NREM and then REM sleep (Figure 2.5). The sequence lasts about 90 minutes, and then the cycle repeats. During one night of sleep, a person is likely to go through four to five cycles, but the cycles differ somewhat over the course of the night: The slow-wave periods are longer in the first part of the night, and the REM periods are longer in the last part of the night. Because people have more slow wave sleep in the first part of the night, confusional awakening and sleep walking are more likely to occur then. Because people have more REM sleep in the last part of the night, that is when dreaming more often occurs.

Natural Sleep Drives

Two main natural forces drive us toward sleep—the homeostatic sleep drive and the circadian rhythm. Understanding how these work and learning how to strengthen them can have a big impact on sleep.

Homeostatic Sleep Drive   A force called the **homeostatic sleep drive** gets stronger the longer you are awake. When people are awake during the day, a neurochemical called adenosine accumulates in the brain. This is a by-product of energy used by the brain, and it promotes sleep onset. The homeostatic drive is strengthened if you get up at a reasonably early time in the morning and then remain awake until your intended bedtime at night. Naps or dozing in the afternoon will strongly reduce this sleep drive at night, as will sleeping late in the morning. People who have problems falling asleep or staying asleep can strengthen the sleep drive by avoiding naps and setting a reasonably early wake time goal every day. This allows for enough wake time during the day for the sleep drive to accumulate. Caffeine blocks the homeostatic sleep drive by blocking adenosine receptors in the brain, and if a person has problems falling asleep, reduction of caffeine can be very important.

Circadian Rhythm   The **circadian rhythm** is the sleep and wake pattern coordinated by the brain's master internal clock, the suprachiasmatic nucleus (SCN). The SCN controls the sleep-wake cycle of the brain as well as the entire body: Every cell in every organ has a sleep-wake cycle, and the SCN sends signals not only to the rest of the brain, but also to organs such as the liver, gastrointestinal tract, pancreas, heart, muscles, and even the cells in the blood and skin. Each cell has DNA machinery that produces an internal clock, but the SCN has to synchronize this clock with all the other clocks.

> **homeostatic sleep drive**   The drive to sleep that strengthens during prolonged wakefulness and lessens during sleep.
>
> **circadian rhythm**   The sleep and wake pattern coordinated by the brain's master internal clock.
>
> **TERMS**

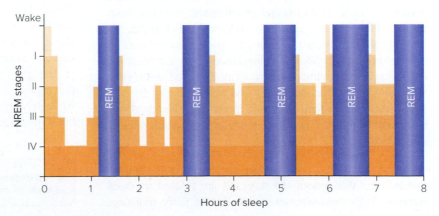

FIGURE 2.5   **Sleep stages and cycles.** During one night of sleep, the sleeper typically goes through four or five cycles of NREM sleep (four stages) followed by REM sleep.

SOURCE: Adapted from Krejcar, O., J Jirka, and D. Janckulik. 2011. Use of mobile phones as intelligent sensors for sound input analysis and sleep state detection. *Sensors* 11(6): 6037–6055.

Anyone who has traveled to another time zone is probably familiar with jet lag, which occurs when the internal body clock is set to a different time from that of a new environment. People with jet lag commonly experience nausea and loss of appetite, which is related to the gastrointestinal system's being out of sync with the new time zone. It can also be difficult to fall asleep and wake up at the appropriate times in the new location.

But jet lag is not the only disrupter of circadian rhythms. Some people have habits that cause their internal body clocks to be set at a time that is different from the time zone where they live. An example is a person who stays up regularly until four in the morning, and then sleeps until noon, a pattern called delayed sleep phase. If this person occasionally has to wake up earlier, the switch can be difficult, and the person will feel poorly, just like a person with jet lag.

The master clock can be reset by "time-givers," or *zeitgebers*. Although there are many *zeitgebers*, including activity, exercise, and eating, the strongest is light. Light has a direct connection to the SCN master clock via specific cells in the eye that instead of processing vision send impulses directly to the SCN to allow measurement of outside light. If the person is exposed to light in the morning at a certain time on a regular basis, it will indicate to the SCN that it should set the internal clock to wake around that time. Through another pathway, when light is reduced at night, as when natural dusk occurs, the SCN conveys impulses to a gland in the brain to produce melatonin, which signals systems involved in preparation for sleep. People who are blind often have problems with sleep because they do not have the usual light signals to help synchronize their circadian rhythms.

To strengthen the circadian rhythm, get good light exposure in the morning and daytime and reduce exposure to light at night. The challenge in the modern age is that we live with abundant sources of artificial light to which we can be exposed at all times of the day, allowing us to be insulated from the natural 24-hour rhythm of the sun. For information on personal electronic devices and sleep, see the box "Digital Devices: Help or Harm for a Good Night's Sleep?"

Adequate Sleep and Your Health

Poor-quality or insufficient sleep has been associated with a number of health problems and impairments, including heart disease, high blood pressure, depression, earlier death, increased risk for dementia, weight gain, poorer glucose control, increased risk for accidents, reduced motivation and attention, and increased irritability or hyperactivity. The good news is that with more knowledge about sleep, and the factors that affect it, people can improve their sleep and, in turn, their health. Along with exercise and good nutrition, good sleep is a critical pillar of good health.

Sleep and Stress   Stress hormone levels in the bloodstream vary throughout the day and are related to sleep patterns. Peak concentrations occur in the early morning,

followed by a slow decline during the day and evening. Concentrations return to peak levels during the final stages of sleep and in the early morning hours. Stress hormone levels are low during NREM sleep and increase during REM sleep. With each successive sleep cycle during the night, REM sleep lasts a little longer. This increase in REM sleep duration with each sleep cycle may underlie the progressive increase in stress hormones during the final stages of sleep.

Even though stress hormones are released during sleep, it is the *lack* of sleep that has the greatest impact on stress. In someone who is suffering from **sleep deprivation** (not getting enough sleep over time), mental and physical processes deteriorate steadily. A sleep-deprived person experiences headaches, feels irritable, cannot concentrate, and is prone to forgetfulness. Poor-quality sleep has long been associated with stress and depression.

Acute sleep deprivation slows the daytime decline in stress hormones, so evening levels are higher than normal. A decrease in total sleep time also causes an increase in the level of stress hormones. Together these changes may increase stress hormone levels throughout the day and contribute to physical and mental exhaustion. Extreme sleep deprivation can lead to hallucinations and other psychotic symptoms, as well as to a significant increase in heart attack risk.

Sleep and Driving   Researchers estimate that drowsy driving is responsible for more than 70,000 crashes, 40,000 injuries, and as many as 7500 deaths per year. In surveys, about 4% of adult drivers (1 in 25) report having fallen asleep at the wheel in the previous 30 days. Even if you don't fall completely asleep, drowsiness slows your reaction time and lessens your ability to pay attention and make good decisions. Going 24 hours without sleep can impair a driver to the same extent as a blood alcohol level of 0.10%, which is above the legal limit. Some states have laws against drowsy driving; for example, New Jersey defines driving after being awake for 24 or more hours as reckless driving, in the same class as intoxicated driving.

People who are most at risk for falling asleep while driving include young adults—aged 18–29, with men at slightly greater risk than women; parents with small children; shift workers; people who have accumulated sleep debt; and those who have other untreated sleep disorders such as sleep apnea or insomnia. The peak period for drowsiness-related accidents is between 4 a.m. and 6 a.m., though they can occur at any time. Sleepiness is worsened when people take substances such as muscle relaxants, antihistamines, cold medicines, or alcohol.

The good news is that accidents due to sleepiness are preventable. First and foremost, if you find yourself drowsy while driving, pull over. Taking a nap or short rest can help, but if drowsiness persists, let someone else do the driving.

sleep deprivation   A lack of sleep over a period of time. **TERMS**

Digital Devices: Help or Harm for a Good Night's Sleep?

Many apps are promoted as sleep aids and trackers. Can they really improve sleep? Or can using digital devices hurt the body's natural sleep cycles?

Digital Devices and Sleep

Before we look at sleep apps, let's consider how use of your digital devices can negatively affect your sleep. Tablets, smartphones, and computers emit blue light, which impedes the release of melatonin, a hormone that affects sleep and wake cycles. In one study, researchers compared the sleep of people who read an e-book on a digital device in the hours before bedtime with people who did so with a print book. Those who read the digital book took longer to fall asleep, had reduced melatonin release, and were less alert the next morning.

Does heavy texting affect sleep? Psychologist Karla Murdock reported that texting was a direct predictor of sleep problems among first-year students in a study that examined links among interpersonal stress, text-messaging behavior, and three indicators of college students' health: burnout, sleep problems, and emotional well-being.

Murdock and other sleep experts suggest turning off your screens. Use them less during the day and also when preparing to sleep at night. If you have trouble relaxing and transitioning to sleep in the evenings, shut down all your devices an hour or more before you intend to sleep.

Now that you are resting in the dark, why would you consider using a sleep app or digital tracker? Ironically, a smartphone may help you get to sleep—if you tuck it into the corner of your bed.

Digital Aids for Relaxation

Many free and low-cost apps provide aids for relaxation and to improve sleep. Some include music, white noise, or sounds of nature (e.g., wind, rain, waves, or songbirds). Others offer specific techniques, such as guided meditation or breathing exercises, to promote relaxation to aid in falling asleep. Experiment to find the aids that work best for you.

Digital Sleep Trackers

More complicated technologies attempt to track and analyze sleep. Many are based on movement detectors in smartphones.

These apps estimate the amount and type of sleep you get based on your movements during the night; they may generate detailed graphs of your sleep quality and then time your wake-up alarm to a specific sleep cycle. Some apps also include a sound recorder, which detects sleep talking, snoring, and other night noises, providing further information.

In addition to smartphone apps, specialized fitness wristbands such as those by Fitbit and Garmin include sleep trackers. Many of these are also based on movement detectors, but some incorporate heart rate data as well; preliminary research indicates that adding heart rate data to movement tracking may improve the accuracy of the results. Fitbit and other wearables, along with some apps, may combine sleep and fitness data into an overall picture of an individual's activity over the course of a day.

Apps and devices may be popular, but no consumer technology yet developed can equal the capability of a sleep lab at detecting sleep stages or diagnosing specific sleep disorders. If you enjoy the features of an app or wearable tracker, go ahead and use them, but don't rely on an app to diagnose the presence or absence of a serious sleep problem. One good effect of using a sleep tracker is simply the greater focus it places on sleep.

SOURCES: Chang, A. M., et al. 2015. Evening use of light-emitting eReaders negatively affects sleep, circadian timing, and next-morning alertness. *Proceedings of the National Academy of Sciences* 112(4): 1232–1237; Bhat, S., et al. 2015. Is there a clinical role for smartphone sleep apps? Comparison of sleep cycle detection by a smartphone application to polysomnography. *Journal of Clinical Sleep Medicine,* February 3; Gradisar, M., et al. 2013. The sleep and technology use of Americans. *Journal of Clinical Sleep Medicine* 9(12): 1291–1299; Behar, J., et al. 2013. A review of current sleep screening applications for smartphones. *Physiological Measurement* 34(7): R29–R46; Lewis, J. G. 2013. Sleep cycle app: Precise, or placebo? *Mind Read: Connecting Brain and Behavior* (http://www.nature.com/scitable/blog/mind-read/sleep_cycle_app_precise_or); Murdock, K. K. 2013. Texting while stressed: Implications for students' burnout, sleep, and well-being. *Psychology of Popular Media Culture,* DOI: 10.1037/ppm0000012.

Sleep Disorders

Although many of us can attribute the lack of sleep to long workdays and family responsibilities, as many as 70 million Americans suffer from chronic sleep disorders—medical conditions that prevent them from sleeping well. Some of the most common ones are described in the sections that follow.

Chronic Insomnia Many people have trouble falling asleep or staying asleep—a condition called **insomnia.** For most people, insomnia is brief and is due to life circumstances, such as worrying about an upcoming deadline or consuming too much caffeine or alcohol on a particular day. A person is considered to have chronic insomnia if sleep disruption occurs at least three nights per week and lasts at least three months. If you experience insomnia, try the strategies described in this chapter for promoting healthy sleep patterns and in the box "Overcoming Insomnia"; see also the Behavior Change Strategy "Taking Control of Your Sleep" at the end of the chapter.

insomnia A sleep problem involving the inability to fall or stay asleep.

TERMS

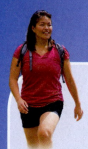

TAKE CHARGE
Overcoming Insomnia

If you're bothered by insomnia, try the following:

- Determine how much sleep you need to feel refreshed the next day, and don't sleep longer than that.

- Go to bed at the same time every night and, more important, get up at the same time every morning, seven days a week, regardless of how much sleep you got. Don't nap during the day if you can help it. If you fall asleep in the afternoon, make the nap short—less than 30 minutes.

- Exercise every day, but not too close to bedtime. Your metabolism takes up to six hours to slow down after exercise.

- Avoid caffeine late in the day and alcohol before bedtime (it causes disturbed, fragmented sleep). If you take any medications (prescription or not), ask your doctor or pharmacist if they are known to interfere with sleep.

- Do what you can to make your sleeping environment quiet, dark, and a comfortable temperature. Overhearing music or talking can make it hard to sleep.

- Have a light snack before bedtime; you'll sleep better if you're not hungry.

- Use your bed only for sleep. Don't eat, read, study, or watch television in bed.

- Relax before bedtime with a bath, a book, music, or relaxation exercises.

- If you don't fall asleep in 15–20 minutes, or if you wake up and can't fall asleep again, turn on your back and engage in a mindful breathing exercise (see guided practices, p. 38).

- If sleep problems last more than six months and interfere with daytime functioning, ask your physician for a referral to a sleep specialist. You may be a candidate for a sleep study—an overnight evaluation of your sleep pattern that can uncover many sleep-related disorders. Sleeping pills are not recommended for chronic insomnia because they can be habit-forming; they also lose their effectiveness over time.

Restless Leg Syndrome **Restless leg syndrome** (RLS) affects about 5% of the adult population and as many as 25% of pregnant women. RLS is characterized by muscle throbbing or creeping or other uncomfortable sensations in the legs, which in turn cause an uncontrollable urge to move them. Symptoms occur primarily at night or while resting. RLS can be associated with small kicking movements during the night, can interfere with falling asleep, and can make falling back to sleep more difficult. Simple measures that help RLS include getting more exercise during the day; avoiding all caffeine, tobacco, and alcohol; massaging the legs or using heating pads or a warm bath; maintaining a regular sleep pattern; and correcting any deficiencies in iron, folate, or magnesium. Medications are also available, but certain substances should be avoided: Diphenhydramine (Benadryl), which is a common ingredient in over-the-counter sleeping pills, paradoxically worsens RLS symptoms and can worsen sleep.

Sleep Apnea **Sleep apnea** occurs when a person repeatedly stops breathing for short periods while asleep. Apnea can be caused by a number of factors, but it typically results when the soft tissue at the back of the mouth (such as the tongue or soft palate) "collapses" during sleep, blocking the airway (Figure 2.6). When breathing is interrupted, so is sleep, because the sleeper awakens throughout the night to begin breathing again. In most cases, this occurs without the sleeper's even being aware of it. However, the disruption to sleep can be significant, and over time, acute sleep deprivation can result. Sleep apnea is most common among people who are overweight, but it can occur in people classified as

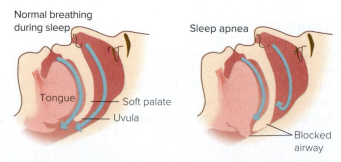

FIGURE 2.6 **Sleep apnea.** Sleep apnea occurs when soft tissues surrounding the airway relax, "collapsing" the airway and restricting airflow.

> **restless leg syndrome** A condition characterized by muscle throbbing or creeping or other uncomfortable sensations in the legs that can interfere with sleep.
>
> **sleep apnea** The interruption of normal breathing during sleep.
>
> **TERMS**

at normal weight; children with enlarged tonsils may also develop the condition. Risk increases with age, and up to 50% of adults over age 65 may have some degree of sleep apnea. Untreated, sleep apnea increases the risk of high blood pressure, heart attack, stroke, obesity, and diabetes. It also increases the risk of work-related or driving accidents.

Treatments for sleep apnea include the following:

• Lifestyle changes, including weight loss, sleeping on your side, quitting smoking, and using nasal sprays or allergy medicines to keep nasal passages open at night.

• Mouthpieces (oral appliances) that are worn at night and adjust the position of the lower jaw to help keep airways open.

• Breathing devices such as the continuous positive airway pressure (CPAP) machine, which has a mask that fits over the mouth and/or nose and gently blows air into the throat.

Improving Sleep

If you're like the average American, you get less than the recommended amount of sleep each night. The Centers for Disease Control and Prevention calls sleep deprivation a national public epidemic.

In adults, between seven and nine hours of sleep is generally sufficient, but sleep needs vary from person to person; some people need only six hours, while others need more than nine. Learning how much sleep you need for optimal function is important. Getting into bed too early can paradoxically worsen sleep, so each of us must find the appropriate sleep time goal for our individual needs.

Support Natural Sleep Rhythms and Drives Sleep is a natural physiological process, so you can't "will" yourself to sleep—meaning, don't get frustrated if you don't fall asleep. As noted, to strengthen physiological sleep drives, keep a consistent sleep schedule throughout the week. To support circadian rhythm, set a goal wake time with good light exposure, and avoid bright lights and electronic devices at night. To enhance the homeostatic drive, make your wake time sufficiently early, avoid naps, and minimize caffeine.

Create a Good Sleep Environment Your bedroom should be cool, dark, and quiet, ideally without pets. Although you'll want to be warm when you get into bed, sleep comes more easily in cool temperatures. Therefore, you may want to take a warm shower or bath before bed, to warm the body, and wear socks if you tend to have cold extremities at night. But after that, fewer blankets and a cooler temperature setting are beneficial. Generally if you tend to awaken at night, avoid activities in the bedroom that might be stimulating, such as watching television or using electronic devices.

Avoid Substances That Disrupt Sleep People vary greatly in how they are affected by caffeine, but those with poor-quality sleep, difficulty falling asleep, or nighttime awakenings need to be especially careful. Caffeine can have physiological effects for over 24 hours in susceptible people,

and even caffeine consumed in the morning can affect sleep throughout the night. Keep in mind that caffeine comes from many sources, including sodas, diet sodas, hot or iced teas, sweet teas, energy drinks, chocolate, and decaffeinated coffee. Some medications, such as Excedrin, also contain caffeine.

Alcohol is another substance that can affect sleep. Some people think that alcohol improves sleep, but it can cause poorer sleep in the second part of the night when the effects wear off and leading to increased activation and arousal. For people with poor sleep, reducing alcohol consumption can be beneficial.

Treat Conditions That Interfere with Sleep A number of readily treated medical conditions, including nasal congestion and acid reflux, can disrupt sleep. Simple interventions, such as using medications or saline spray to treat allergies or limiting foods and fluids for several hours before bedtime, can help in some cases. If symptoms are severe and continue to interfere with sleep, consult a health care provider.

Don't Equate Sleeplessness with Job or School Performance We live in a society where people work long hours, and our culture can seem to reward people who sleep less and work more. But establishing balance between sleep and life activities is important. "Cramming" all night before an exam, or staying up all night to write a paper, is something most college students have been tempted to do, but all-nighters can interfere with learning and memory. Having a full night's sleep after studying promotes long-term memory formation. Similarly, some job environments encourage longer working hours. But equating work ethic with long work hours and less sleep can lead to burnout and lower productivity.

People who work the night shift must try especially hard to protect downtime and sleep periods and refrain from adding other daytime commitments that interfere with sleep. It can be tempting in the short term to cut back on sleep, but in the longer term this is likely to backfire, resulting in increased mood problems and the health-related issues associated with sleep loss.

Avoid Sleep Pitfalls

• *Have realistic expectations.* Don't compare yourself to others: "I want to sleep like my friend Joe, who hits the pillow, falls asleep immediately, and sleeps all night." As it turns out, people like "Joe" are rare. When thinking about your own sleep, remember that everyone is different and have realistic expectations. Focusing on step-by-step sleep-health goals that are tailored to your own situation will be more productive.

• *Try not to worry about a bout of sleeplessness.* Worry can worsen sleep, and when you are having trouble sleeping, it can be easy to start worrying about the consequences for the next day. Most of the time, even if you sleep poorly, the next day's activities will be fine. The ups and down of mental and physical performance are not always correlated to the prior night's sleep.

• *Remember the value of relaxation.* Quiet relaxation has restorative value. You don't have to be sound asleep to benefit from quiet time; resting, relaxing, and dozing can also be beneficial. Consider the relaxation techniques presented earlier in this chapter.

If you find that, despite everything, you feel anxious or frustrated during the night when awake, try leaving the bedroom and engaging in a quiet activity like reading until you feel more relaxed and sleepy again.

TIPS FOR TODAY AND THE FUTURE

For the stress you can't avoid, develop a range of stress management techniques and strategies.

RIGHT NOW YOU CAN:
- Practice a mindfulness exercise for 5–45 minutes.
- Practice some aerobic exercise for 30–45 minutes.
- Get out your datebook and schedule what you'll be doing the rest of today and tomorrow. Pencil in a short walk and a conversation with a friend.
- Reflect on your sleep habits and patterns.

IN THE FUTURE YOU CAN:
- Take a class or workshop, such as mindfulness-based stress reduction or one in assertiveness training or time management, to help you overcome a source of stress.
- Find a way to build relaxing time into every day. Just 15 minutes of meditation, stretching, or yoga can induce relaxation.
- Use your knowledge of factors that improve and detract from sleep to establish healthy patterns for yourself.

SUMMARY

- When confronted with a stressor, the body undergoes a set of physical changes known as the fight-or-flight reaction. The sympathetic nervous system and endocrine system act on many targets in the body to prepare it for action.

- Emotional and behavioral responses to stressors vary among individuals. Ineffective responses increase stress but can be moderated or changed.

- Factors that influence emotional and behavioral responses to stressors include personality, cultural background, gender, and past experiences.

- The general adaptation syndrome (GAS) has three stages: alarm, resistance, and exhaustion.

- A high allostatic load characterized by prolonged or repeated exposure to stress hormones can increase a person's risk of health problems.

- Psychoneuroimmunology (PNI) looks at how the physiological changes of the stress response affect the immune system and thereby increase the risk of illness.

- Health problems linked to stress include cardiovascular disease, colds and other infections, asthma and allergies, flare-ups of chronic diseases, psychological problems, digestive problems, headaches, insomnia, and injuries.

- A cluster of major life events that require adjustment and accommodation can lead to increased stress and an increased risk of health problems. Minor daily hassles increase stress if they are perceived negatively.

- Sources of stress associated with college may be academic, interpersonal, time related, or financial pressures.

- Job-related stress is common, particularly for employees who have little control over decisions relating to their jobs. If stress is severe or prolonged, burnout may occur.

- New and changing relationships, prejudice, and discrimination are examples of interpersonal and social stressors.

- Social support systems help buffer people against the effects of stress and make illness less likely. Good communication skills foster healthy relationships.

- Exercise, nutrition, sleep, and time management are wellness behaviors that reduce stress and increase energy.

- Cognitive techniques for managing stress involve developing new and healthy patterns of thinking, such as practicing problem solving, monitoring self-talk, and cultivating a sense of humor.

- Additional help in dealing with stress is available from self-help books, peer counseling, support groups, and psychotherapy.

- Along with exercise and good nutrition, good sleep is a critical pillar of good health.

- Understanding the physiology of sleep (REM and NREM sleep) and the two sleep drives (homeostatic sleep drive and circadian rhythm) can help you understand and improve your own sleep.

- Sleep interacts with health and well-being in many ways. Stress, driving, and sleep disorders—for example, restless leg syndrome, insomnia, and sleep apnea—all can have important impacts on and relationships with sleep and health.

- Techniques for improving sleep include supporting natural sleep rhythms and drives, creating a good sleep environment, avoiding substances that interfere with sleep, and treating conditions that interfere with it.

FOR MORE INFORMATION

American Headache Society. Provides information for consumers and clinicians about different types of headaches, their causes, and their treatment.

http://www.americanheadachesociety.org

American Psychiatric Association: Healthy Minds, Healthy Lives. Provides information about mental wellness developed especially for college students.

www.psychiatry.org/news-room/apa-blogs.

American Psychological Association. Provides information about stress management and psychological disorders.

http://www.apa.org
http://www.apa.org/helpcenter

Association for Applied Psychophysiology and Biofeedback. Provides information about biofeedback and referrals to certified biofeedback practitioners.

http://www.aapb.org

Benson-Henry Institute for Mind Body Medicine. Provides information about stress management and relaxation techniques.

http://www.massgeneral.org/bhi

Center for Mindfulness in Medicine, Health Care, and Society (U Mass Medical School). Provides information about mindfulness-based stress reduction (MBSR) professional training, research, and resources.

http://www.umassmed.edu/cfm/

National Institute of Mental Health (NIMH). Publishes brochures about stress and stress management as well as other aspects of mental health.

http://www.nimh.nih.gov

National Sleep Foundation. Provides information about sleep and how to overcome sleep problems such as insomnia and jet lag.

http://sleepfoundation.org

Spirit Rock Meditation Center. A resource for meditation retreats and education in mindfulness meditation.

http://www.spiritrock.org

SELECTED BIBLIOGRAPHY

American College Health Association. 2011. *American College Health Association–National College Health Assessment II Reference Group Executive Summary, Spring 2011.* Hanover, MD: American College Health Association.

American College Health Association. 2015. *American College Health Association–National College Health Assessment IIc: Reference Group Executive Summary Fall 2015.* Hanover, MD: American College Health Association.

American Psychological Association. 2012. *Mind/Body Health: Stress* (http://www.apa.org/helpcenter/stress.aspx).

American Psychological Association. 2014. *Stress in America: Are Teens Adopting Adults' Stress Habits?* Washington, DC: American Psychological Association.

Arita, A., et al. 2015. Risk factors for automobile accidents caused by falling asleep while driving in obstructive sleep apnea syndrome. *Sleep and Breathing* 19(4): 1229–1234.

Bartolomucci, A., and R. Leopardi. 2009. Stress and depression: Preclinical research and clinical implications. *PLoS One* 4(1): e4265.

Burch, R. C., et al. 2015. The prevalence and burden of migraine and severe headache in the United States: updated statistics from government health surveillance studies. *Headache* 55(1): 21–34.

Caldwell, K., et al. 2010. Developing mindfulness in college students through movement-based courses: Effects on self-regulatory self-efficacy, mood, stress, and sleep quality. *Journal of American College Health* 58(5): 433–442.

Centers for Disease Control and Prevention. 2012. *Coping with a Disaster or Traumatic Event: Information for Individuals and Families* (http://emergency.cdc.gov/mentalhealth/general.asp).

Centers for Disease Control and Prevention. 2015. *Drowsy Driving: Asleep at the Wheel* (http://www.cdc.gov/features/dsdrowsydriving/).

Centers for Disease Control and Prevention. 2016. *Chronic Disease Overview* (http://www.cdc.gov/chronicdisease/overview/index.htm).

Colton, H. R., and B. M. Altevogt, eds. 2006. *Sleep Disorders and Sleep Deprivation: An Unmet Public Health Problem.* Institute of Medicine Committee on Sleep Medicine and Research. Washington, DC: National Academies Press.

Dallman, M. 2010. Stress-induced obesity and the emotional nervous system. *Trends in Endocrinology and Metabolism* 21(3): 159–165.

Darabaneanu, S. 2011. Aerobic exercise as a therapy option for migraine: A pilot study. *International Journal of Sports Medicine* 32(6): 455–460.

Davidson, R., and S. Begley. 2012. *The Emotional Life of Your Brain.* New York: Penguin.

Flugel Colle, K. F., et al. 2010. Measurement of quality of life and participant experience with the mindfulness-based stress reduction program. *Complementary Therapies in Clinical Practice* 16(1): 36–40.

Foureur, M., et al. 2013. Enhancing the resilience of nurses and midwives: Pilot of a mindfulness-based program for increased health, sense of coherence and decreased depression, anxiety and stress. *Contemporary Nurse* 45: 114–125.

Fox, S., and M. Duggan. 2013. *The Diagnosis Difference. Pew Research Internet Project* (http://www.pewinternet.org/2013/11/26/the-diagnosis-difference/).

Freedman, N. 2010. Treatment of obstructive sleep apnea syndrome. *Clinics in Chest Medicine* 31(2): 187–201.

Germer, C., R. Siegel, and P. Fulton. 2005. *Mindfulness and Psychotherapy.* New York: Guilford.

Hefner, J., and D. Eisenberg. 2009. Social support and mental health among college students. *American Journal of Orthopsychiatry* 79(4): 491–499.

Hölzel, B. K., et al. 2010. Stress reduction correlates with structural changes in the amygdala. *Social Cognitive and Affective Neuroscience* 5(1): 11–17.

Hook, J. N., et al. 2010. Empirically supported religious and spiritual therapies. *Journal of Clinical Psychology* 66(1): 46–72.

Inflammation and anti-inflammatories in depression. 2013. *Bipolar Network News* 17(4) 1–15.

Jayson, S. 2013. Who's feeling stressed? *USA Today,* February 7.

Kabat-Zinn, J. 2011. *Mindfulness for Beginners: Reclaiming the Present Moment—and Your Life.* Louisville, CO: Sounds True.

Kemeny, M. 2012. Contemplative/emotion training reduces negative emotional behavior and promotes prosocial responses. *Emoticon* [1528–3542] (12): 338–350.

Kim, B. 2014. *How the Body Works: Overview of the Nervous and Endocrine Systems* (http://drbenkim.com/nervous-endocrine-system.htm).

Manzoni, G. C., et al. 2016. Age of onset of episodic and chronic cluster headache—a review of a large case series from a single headache centre. *Journal of Headache Pain* 17: 44.

National Institute of Neurological Disorders and Stroke. 2015. *Restless Legs Syndrome Fact Sheet* (http://www.ninds.nih.gov/disorders/restless_legs/detail_restless_legs.htm).

National Sleep Foundation. 2011. *2011 Sleep in America Poll.* Washington, DC: National Sleep Foundation.

Nordboe, D. J., et al. 2007. Immediate behavioral health response to the Virginia Tech shootings. *Disaster Medicine and Public Health Preparedness* 1(Suppl. 1): S31–S32.

Owens, J., and Adolescent Sleep Working Group, committee on Adolescence. 2014. Insufficient sleep in adolescents and young adults: An update on causes and consequences. *Pediatrics* 134(3): e921–e932.

Ratneswaran, C., J. Mushtaq, and J. Steier. 2016. Clinical update sleep: Year in review 2015–2016. *Journal of Thoracic Disease* 8(2): 207–212

Roddenberry, A., and K. Renk. 2010. Locus of control and self-efficacy: Potential mediators of stress, illness, and utilization of health services in college students. *Child Psychiatry and Human Development* 41(4): 353–370.

Roth, H. L. 2012. Dementia and sleep. *Neurologic Clinics* 30(4): 1213–1248.

Schwartz, G. E. 1979. Biofeedback and the behavioral treatment of disorders of disregulation. *Yale Journal of Biology and Medicine* 52(6): 581–596.

Shapiro, S. L., and L. E. Carlson. 2009. *The Art and Science of Mindfulness: Integrating Mindfulness into Psychology and the Helping Professions.* Washington, DC: American Psychological Association.

Sirri, L., et al. 2012. Type A behavior: A reappraisal of its characteristics in cardiovascular disease. *International Journal of Clinical Practice* 66(9): 854–861.

Substance Abuse and Mental Health Services Administration. 2015. Behavioral health trends in the United States: Results from the 2014 National Survey on Drug Use and Health (HHS Publication No. SMA 15-4927, NSDUH Series H-50). Retrieved from http://www.samhsa.gov/data.

Telles, S., et al. 2009. Effect of a yoga practice session and a yoga theory session on state anxiety. *Perceptual and Motor Skills* 109(3): 924–930.

U.S. Department of Health and Human Services, National Institutes of Health. 2012. *Stress* (http://www.nlm.nih.gov/medlineplus/stress.html).

Wheaton, A. G., et al. 2014. Drowsy driving and risk behaviors—10 states and Puerto Rico, 2011–2012. *MMWR* 63: 557–562.

BEHAVIOR CHANGE STRATEGY
Taking Control of Your Sleep

Monitor Your Current Sleep Habits

Begin by keeping a sleep diary to track your typical sleep pattern. Record what time you went to bed, about when you fell asleep, when you woke up, and the estimated length of any periods of wakefulness during the night. You don't need to be exact; your best estimate is good enough. You may use a sleep app to inform your estimates. (Don't keep checking the time, however, as that may negatively affect your sleep.) If relevant, also record the time of day when you exercised, consumed caffeine and/or alcohol, and took any medication; these factors can help you pinpoint blockers for a good night's sleep. You may want to use the format of the two-week sleep diary from the American Academy of Sleep Medicine (http://www.sleepeducation.org).

Analyze Your Sleep Log

Use your log to answer the following questions:

- What is my current sleep schedule during the week? On the weekends?
- How many hours of sleep do I currently average per night? How much sleep do I need to function well? How do the numbers compare? Remember, the amount of sleep time varies by individual.
- Am I more of a night owl or a morning lark? What would be my ideal sleep period if I could sleep anytime I wanted? 11 p.m. to 6 a.m.? 2 a.m. to 9 a.m.? 9 p.m. to 4:30 a.m.?
- What would be the best sleep period for me to get adequate sleep, considering my obligations and preferences?
- Do I have any symptoms of sleep deprivation, such as drowsy driving or falling asleep in classes or work meetings?
- Could my consumption of caffeine or alcohol, or my use of medications, be affecting my sleep?
- Do I have any medical conditions like nasal allergies or acid reflux that could interfere with sleep? Do I have signs or a history of a sleep disorder, such as restless leg syndrome or sleep apnea?

Set Goals and Identify Strategies

Based on your analysis, identify problems with your sleep pattern or with sleep blockers. Set appropriate SMART goals and then develop strategies to achieve them.

One of the most commonly recommended techniques for insomnia is sleep restriction. Even a small restriction can increase the homeostatic sleep drive, and if you also keep the sleep period more consistent, you can reset the circadian rhythm. How does this work? There are many protocols, but all are based on reducing the time you spend in bed *not* sleeping. If you currently spend 8 hours in bed but sleep only 6 hours, you could start by limiting your time in bed to your actual sleeping time (6 hours) plus half your non-sleeping time (2 hours ÷ 2 = 1 hour), for a total of 7 hours. You might set your new sleep window for midnight to 7:00 a.m. But don't reduce it to less than 5 hours. As long as you do sleep within that restricted sleep window, the physiological sleep drives will be strengthened. Continue to monitor your sleep; make adjustments as needed to avoid excessive daytime sleepiness (add time) or to reduce non-sleeping time spent in bed (reduce time).

Once you are sleeping for at least 85–90% of your time spent in bed, extend that time in 15- to 30-minute increments. Over time, you'll increase your sleep time while maintaining your new sleep efficiency. Sleep restriction can have long-lasting benefits. Be aware, however, that you may sleep less than usual at the start of the process, so you should take necessary steps to stay safe.

Avoid the temptation to sleep in late if you get a poor night's sleep—or to go to bed early the following evening. Both these strategies weaken the sleep drives and make sleep more difficult going forward. People with healthy sleep patterns can sleep a little later on some days to compensate for sleep loss on others. But if problems with sleep emerge, keep a more regular schedule with a late enough bedtime and an early enough wake time.

The following are strategies to consider for common sleep problems.

If you have trouble falling asleep:

- Eliminate all sources of caffeine, even in the morning.
- Avoid daytime naps or limit to a total of 20 minutes before 2 p.m.
- Avoid bright lights and electronic activities in the hour prior to bedtime, and remove timepieces from the bedroom; charge cell phones in another room.
- Increase bright-light exposure in the morning.
- Avoid exercising in the evening or at night.
- Set bedtime late enough to allow for sleep drive to accumulate (an appropriate bedtime might be 11 p.m. or later for some people).
- Set wake time early enough to allow for the sleep need to develop during the day.
- Don't doze prior to bedtime; if needed, sit in a less comfortable chair or be more active in the evenings.

If you have trouble staying asleep (i.e., you wake up during the night):

- Don't eat or drink within 3 hours of bedtime.
- Treat any medical issues that interfere with sleep.
- Eliminate caffeine, and reduce alcohol consumption, especially before bed.
- Check your sleep environment and adjust it as needed (see p. 45).
- If you snore or have a family history of apnea, consider obtaining a medical evaluation.

If you have trouble waking up in the morning:

- Adjust your sleep schedule to keep your wake time consistent.
- Anchor your circadian rhythm with more light in the morning.
- Consider whether you are getting enough sleep; if not, try the strategies for those sleep problems.

SOURCES: Falloon, K., et al. 2015. Simplified sleep restriction for insomnia in general practice: A randomised controlled trial. *British Journal of General Practice* 65(637): e508–e515; National Sleep Foundation. 2016. *Sleep Tools* (https://sleepfoundation.org/sleep-tools-tips); National Heart, Lung, and Blood Institute. 2012. *Sleep Deprivation and Deficiency* (https://www.nhlbi.nih.gov/health/health-topics/topics/sdd).

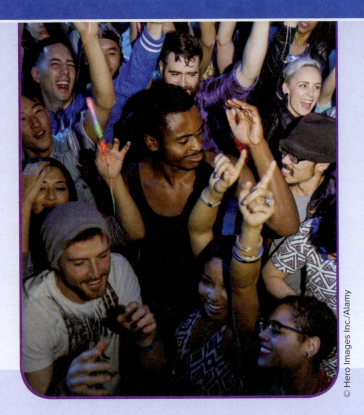

© Hero Images Inc./Alamy

CHAPTER OBJECTIVES

- Describe what it means to be psychologically healthy
- Discuss psychological approaches you can use to face life's challenges with a positive self-concept
- Describe common psychological disorders
- Recognize the warning signs, risk factors, and protective factors related to suicide
- Summarize the models of human nature on which therapies are based
- Describe the types of help available for psychological problems

CHAPTER **3**

Psychological Health

Psychological health contributes to every dimension of wellness. It can be difficult to maintain emotional, social, or even physical wellness if you are not psychologically healthy.

Psychological health, however, is a broad concept—one that is as difficult to define as it is important to understand. That is why the first section of this chapter is devoted to explaining what psychological health is. The rest of the chapter discusses a number of common psychological problems (including mental illnesses), their symptoms, and their treatments.

DEFINING PSYCHOLOGICAL HEALTH

Psychological health (or *mental health*) can be defined either negatively, as the absence of sickness, or positively, as the presence of wellness. The vast majority of people do not suffer from mental illness, yet all of us have to deal with stress, interpersonal conflicts, and difficult emotions. Psychological health refers to the extent to which we are able to

function optimally in the face of these challenges, whether or not we have a mental illness.

Positive Psychology

In his book *Toward a Psychology of Being,* psychologist Abraham Maslow adopted a perspective that he called "positive psychology." Maslow developed a *hierarchy of needs* (Figure 3.1): The most important kind is the satisfaction of physiological needs; following this is a feeling of safety, a state of being loved, maintenance of self-esteem, and finally, self-actualization.

When urgent (life-sustaining) needs—such as the need for food and water—are satisfied, less basic needs take priority. Maslow's conclusions were based on his study of a group of visibly successful people who seemed to have lived, or to be living, at their fullest. He suggested that these people had

psychological health Mental health, defined negatively as the absence of illness or positively as the presence of wellness. **TERMS**

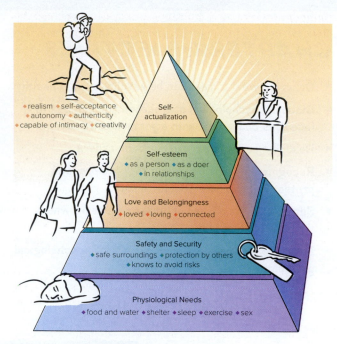

FIGURE 3.1 **Maslow's hierarchy of needs.**

SOURCE: Maslow, A. 1970. *Motivation and Personality,* 2nd ed. New York: Harper & Row.

fulfilled a good measure of their human potential and achieved **self-actualization.** Self-actualized people all share certain qualities:

• *Realism.* Self-actualized people know the difference between what is real and what they want. As a result, they can cope with the world as it exists without demanding that it be different; they know what they can and cannot change. Just as important, realistic people accept evidence that contradicts what they want to believe.

• *Acceptance.* Self-accepting people have a positive but realistic **self-concept,** or *self-image.* They typically feel satisfaction and confidence in themselves, and thus they have healthy **self-esteem.** Self-acceptance also means being tolerant of your own imperfections—an ability that makes it easier to accept the imperfections of others.

• *Autonomy.* *Autonomous* people can direct themselves, acting independently of their social environment. **Autonomy** is more than physical independence. It is social, emotional, and intellectual independence, as well.

• *Authenticity.* Self-actualized people are not afraid to be themselves. Sometimes, in fact, their capacity for being "real" may give them a certain childlike quality. They respond in a genuine, or *authentic,* spontaneous way to whatever happens, without pretense or self-consciousness.

• *Capacity for intimacy.* People capable of intimacy can share their feelings and thoughts without fear of rejection. They are open to the pleasure of physical contact and the satisfaction of being close to others—but without being afraid of the risks involved in intimacy, such as the possibility of rejection. (Chapters 4 and 5 discuss intimacy in more detail.)

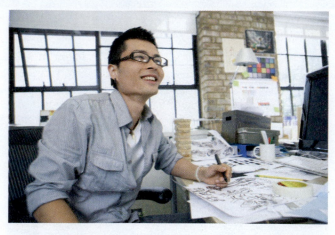

You can develop happiness in any number of ways. The keys are to focus on work and activities you enjoy and to develop a supportive network of friends and family.

© Ciaran Griffin/Getty Images RF

• *Creativity.* Creative people continually look at the world with renewed appreciation and curiosity. Such buoyancy can enhance creativity.

Self-actualization is an ideal to strive for rather than something most people can reasonably hope to achieve. Maslow himself believed it was achieved quite rarely. Still, fulfilling your own potential is a goal that everyone can work toward.

Influenced by the work of Abraham Maslow, psychologist Martin Seligman suggests that the goal of **positive psychology** is "to find and nurture genius and talent" and "to make normal life more fulfilling" rather than just to identify and treat illness. In other words, it means being able to define positive goals and identify concrete, measurable ways of achieving them.

According to Seligman, happiness can come to us through three equally valid dimensions:

• *The pleasant life.* This life is dedicated to maximizing positive **emotions** about the past, present, and future, and to minimizing pain and negative emotions.

• *The engaged life.* This life involves cultivating positive personality traits (such as courage, leadership, kindness, and integrity) and actively using your talents. "Engagement"

---

self-actualization The highest level of growth in Maslow's hierarchy of needs. **TERMS**

self-concept The ideas, feelings, and perceptions a person has about himself or herself; also called *self-image.*

self-esteem Satisfaction and confidence in yourself; the valuing of yourself as a person.

autonomy Independence; the sense of being self-directed.

positive psychology The ability to define positive goals and to identify concrete, measurable ways of achieving them.

emotion A feeling state involving some combination of thoughts, physiological changes, and an outward expression or behavior.

also involves cultivating a capacity to "live in the moment" and immerse yourself fully in your activities.

A key to being engaged and successful in life is the positive personality trait of **emotional intelligence.** An emotionally intelligent person can identify and manage his or her own emotions and respond to the emotions of others. People with higher emotional intelligence can perceive their own emotions and can also channel them to reach their intended goals. Psychologists and educators believe that emotional intelligence is not as rooted as abstract intelligence and that it can be learned.

• *The meaningful life.* Another road to happiness entails working with others toward a meaningful end. Many people find meaning in their connections with and service to families, friends, religious institutions, social causes, and/or work. The happiness to be found by following this path is strongest when meaning comes from more than one source.

Seligman and his colleagues are developing methods of assessing these ways of life and of teaching people how to become happier by adopting one or more of them. They need not be mutually exclusive.

Not everyone accepts the ideas of positive psychology—or even the concept of psychological health—because they involve value judgments that are inconsistent with psychology's scientific status. Defining psychological health requires making assumptions and value judgments about what human goals are desirable, and some people think these are matters for religion or philosophy. Positive psychology has also been criticized as promoting a shortsighted denial of reality and unwarranted optimism. In particular, therapists guided by existential philosophy believe that psychological health comes from acknowledging and accepting the painful realities of life.

What Psychological Health Is Not

We can define normal body temperature because a few degrees above or below this temperature means physical sickness, but we cannot measure psychological health this way. Your ideas and attitudes can vary tremendously without impeding your

ability to function well or causing you to feel emotional distress. Moreover, psychological diversity—the understanding, acceptance, and respect for how much individuals differ in psychological terms—is actually a valuable asset; encountering a wide range of ideas, lifestyles, and attitudes broadens our perspectives and helps us solve problems of the social world. Psychological health does not mean being "normal": What is considered healthy for one person may be quite different for someone else.

Not seeking help for personal problems does not prove you are psychologically healthy, any more than seeking help proves you are mentally ill or unhealthy. Unhappy people may avoid seeking help for many reasons, and severely disturbed people may not even realize they need help.

Further, we can't say people are "mentally ill" or "mentally healthy" based solely on the presence or absence of symptoms. Consider the symptom of anxiety, for example. Anxiety can help you face a problem and solve it before it becomes too big. Someone who shows no anxiety may be refusing to recognize problems or to do anything about them. A person who is anxious for good reason is likely to be judged more psychologically healthy in the long run than someone who is inappropriately calm.

Finally, we cannot judge psychological health from the way people look. All too often, a person who seems to be okay and even happy suddenly takes his or her own life. At an early age, we learn to conceal our feelings and even to lie about them. We may believe that our complaints put unfair demands on others. Although maintaining privacy about emotional pain may seem to be a virtue, it can also be an impediment to getting help.

MEETING LIFE'S CHALLENGES WITH A POSITIVE SELF-CONCEPT

Life is full of challenges—large and small. Everyone, regardless of heredity and family influences, must learn to cope successfully with new situations and new people.

Growing Up Psychologically

Our responses to life's challenges influence the development of our personality and identity.

Developing an Adult Identity   A primary task beginning in adolescence is the development of an adult identity: a unified sense of self, characterized by attitudes, beliefs, and ways of acting that are genuinely our own. People with

Ask Yourself

QUESTIONS FOR CRITICAL THINKING AND REFLECTION

Have you ever had a reason to feel concerned about your own psychological health? If so, what was the reason? Did your concern lead you to talk to someone about the issue, or to seek professional help? If you did, what was the outcome, and how do you feel about it now?

emotional intelligence   The capacity to identify and manage your own emotions and the emotions of others.   TERMS

adult identities know who they are, what they are capable of, what roles they play, and their place among their peers. They have a sense of their own uniqueness but also appreciate what they have in common with others. They view themselves realistically and can assess their strengths and weaknesses without relying on the opinions of others. Achieving an identity also means that we can form intimate relationships with others while maintaining a strong sense of self.

Our identities evolve as we interact with the world and make choices about what we'd like to do and whom we'd like to model ourselves after. Developing an adult identity is particularly challenging in a heterogeneous, secular, and relatively affluent society like ours, in which many roles are possible, many choices are tolerated, and ample time is allowed for experimenting and making up your mind.

This idea of a core self may seem contradictory to the idea that we are always changing. We show different sides of ourselves, not just as we pass through different ages, but also from one day to the next, depending on whom we're with or the environment we're in.

Early identities are often modeled after parents and adult caregivers—or the opposite of parents, in rebellion against what they represent. Over time, peers, rock stars, sports heroes, and religious figures are added to the list of possible role models. In high school and college, people often join cliques that assert a certain identity, such as "jocks," "nerds," or "slackers." Although much of our identity is internal—a way of viewing ourselves and the world—certain aspects of it can be external, such as styles of talking and dressing, ornaments like earrings, and hairstyles.

Early identities are rarely permanent. A hardworking student seeking approval one year can turn into a dropout devoted to sleeping all day and partying all night the next year. At some point, however, most of us adopt a more stable, individual identity that ties together the experiences of childhood and the expectations and aspirations of adulthood. Erikson's theory does not suggest that one day we suddenly assume our final identity and never change after that. Life is more interesting for people who continue evolving into more distinct individuals, rather than being rigidly controlled by their pasts. Identity reflects a lifelong process, and it changes as a person develops new relationships and roles.

Developing an adult identity is an important part of psychological wellness. Without a personal identity, we begin to feel confused about who we are. Erikson called this situation an **identity crisis**. Until we have "found ourselves," we cannot have much self-esteem because a self is not firmly in place.

Developing Intimacy People with established identities can form intimate relationships and sexual unions characterized by sharing, open communication, long-term commitment, and love. Those who lack a firm sense of self may have difficulty establishing relationships because they feel overwhelmed by closeness and the needs of another person. As a result, they experience only short-term, superficial relationships with others and may remain isolated.

Developing Values and Purpose in Your Life Erikson assigned his last two stages, *generativity versus self-absorption* and *integrity versus despair,* to middle adulthood and older adulthood, respectively. But these stages concern values that need to be addressed by young people and reexamined throughout life.

Values are criteria for judging what is good and bad, and they underlie our moral decisions and behavior. The first morality of the young child is to consider "good" to mean what brings immediate and tangible rewards, and "bad" to mean whatever results in punishment. An older child will explain right and wrong in terms of authority figures and rules. But the final stage of moral development, one that not everyone attains, is being able to conceive of right and wrong in more abstract terms such as justice and virtue.

As adults we need to assess how far we have evolved morally and what values we have adopted. Without an awareness of our personal values, our lives may be hurriedly driven forward by immediate desires and the passing demands of others. Living according to values means considering your options carefully before making a choice, choosing among options without succumbing to outside pressures that conflict with your values, and making a choice and acting on it rather than doing nothing. Your actions and how you justify them proclaim to others what you stand for.

Achieving Healthy Self-Esteem

Having a healthy level of self-esteem means regarding your self—which includes all aspects of your identity—as good,

identity crisis   Internal confusion about who you are.

values   Criteria for judging what is good and bad, which underlie an individual's moral decisions and behavior.

TERMS

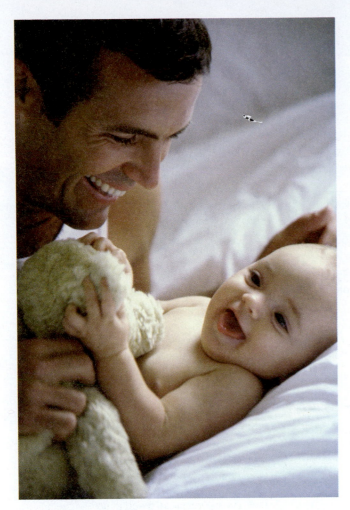

A positive self-concept begins in infancy. The knowledge that he's loved and valued by his parents gives this baby a solid basis for lifelong psychological health.

© Purestock/PunchStock RF

contradictions. People who have gotten mixed messages about themselves from parents and friends may have contradictory self-images, which defy integration and make them vulnerable to shifting levels of self-esteem. At times they regard themselves as entirely good, capable, and lovable—an ideal self—and at other times they see themselves as entirely bad, incompetent, and unworthy of love. Neither of these extreme self-concepts allows people to see themselves or others realistically, and their relationships with other people are filled with misunderstandings and ultimately with conflict.

The concepts we have about ourselves and others are an important part of our personalities. And all the components of our self-concepts profoundly influence our interpersonal relationships.

Meeting Challenges to Self-Esteem As an adult, you sometimes run into situations that challenge your self-concept. People you care about may tell you they don't love you or feel loved by you, for example, or your attempts to accomplish a goal may end in failure.

You can react to such challenges in several ways. The best approach is to acknowledge that something has gone wrong and try again, adjusting your goals to your abilities without radically revising your self-concept. Less productive responses are denying that anything went wrong and blaming someone else. These attitudes may preserve your self-concept temporarily, but in the long run they keep you from meeting the challenge.

The worst reaction is to develop a lasting negative self-concept in which you feel bad, unloved, and ineffective—in other words, to become demoralized. Instead of coping, the demoralized person gives up (at least temporarily), reinforcing the negative self-concept and setting in motion a cycle of bad self-concept and failure. In people who are genetically predisposed to depression, demoralization can progress to additional symptoms, which are discussed later in the chapter.

NOTICE YOUR PATTERNS OF THINKING One method for fighting demoralization is to recognize and test the negative thoughts and assumptions you may have about yourself and others. Note exactly when an unpleasant emotion—feeling worthless, wanting to give up, feeling depressed—occurs or gets worse, to identify the events or daydreams that trigger that emotion, and to observe whatever thoughts come into your head just before or during the emotional experience. Keep a daily journal about such events.

AVOID FOCUSING ON THE NEGATIVE Imagine that you are waiting for a friend to meet you for dinner, but he's 30 minutes late. What kinds of thoughts go through your head? You might wonder what caused the delay: Perhaps he is stuck in traffic, you think, or needs to help a roommate who has the flu. This kind of reaction is healthy.

By contrast, people who are demoralized tend to use all-or-nothing thinking. They overgeneralize from negative events. They overlook the positive and jump to negative conclusions, minimizing their own successes and magnifying the successes of others. They take responsibility for unfortunate situations that are not their fault, then jump to more negative

competent, and worthy of love. It is a critical component of wellness.

Developing a Positive Self-Concept Ideally a positive self-concept begins in childhood, based on experiences both within the family and outside it. Children need to develop a sense of being loved and being able to give love and to accomplish their goals. If they feel rejected or neglected by their parents, they may fail to develop feelings of self-worth. They may grow to have a negative concept of themselves.

Another component of self-concept is *integration*. An integrated self-concept is one that you have made for yourself—not someone else's image of you or a mask that doesn't quite fit. Important building blocks of self-concept are the personality characteristics and mannerisms of parents, which children may adopt without realizing it. Later they may be surprised to find themselves acting like one of their parents. Eventually such building blocks may be reshaped and integrated into a new, individual personality.

Another aspect of self-concept is *stability*. Stability depends on the integration of the self and its freedom from

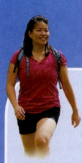

TAKE CHARGE
Realistic Self-Talk

Do your patterns of thinking make events seem worse than they truly are? Do negative beliefs you have about yourself become self-fulfilling prophecies? Substituting realistic self-talk for negative self-talk can help you build and maintain self-esteem and cope better with the challenges in your life. Here are some examples of common types of distorted, negative self-talk, along with suggestions for more accurate and rational responses:

COGNITIVE DISTORTION	NEGATIVE SELF-TALK	REALISTIC SELF-TALK
Focusing on negatives	Babysitting is such a pain in the neck; I wish I didn't need the extra money so bad.	This is a tough job, but at least the money's decent and I can study once the kids go to bed.
Expecting the worst	I know I'm going to get an F in this course. I should just drop out of school now.	I'm not doing too well in this course. I should talk to my professor to see what kind of help I can get.
Overgeneralizing	My hair is a mess and I'm gaining weight. I'm so ugly. No one would ever want to date me.	I could use a haircut and should try to exercise more. This way I'll start feeling better about myself and will be more confident when I meet people.
Minimizing	It was nice of everyone to eat the dinner I cooked, even though I ruined it. I'm such a rotten cook.	Well, the roast was a little dry, but they ate every bite. The veggies and rolls made up for it. I'm finally getting the hang of cooking!
Blaming others	Everyone I meet is such a jerk. Why aren't people friendlier?	I am going to make more of an effort to meet people who share my interests.
Expecting perfection	I cannot believe I flubbed that solo. They probably won't even let me audition for the orchestra next year.	It's a good thing I didn't stop playing when I hit that sour note. It didn't seem like anyone noticed it as much as I did.
Believing you're the cause of everything	Tom and Sara broke up, and it's my fault. I shouldn't have insisted that Tom spend so much time with me and the guys.	It's a shame Tom and Sara broke up. I wish I knew what happened between them. Maybe Tom will tell me at soccer practice. At any rate, it isn't my fault; I've been a good friend to both of them.
Thinking in black and white	I thought that Mike was really cool, but after what he said today, I realize we have nothing in common.	I was really surprised that Mike disagreed with me today. I guess there are still things I don't know about him.
Magnifying events	I stuttered when I was giving my speech today in class. I must have sounded like a complete idiot. I'm sure everyone is talking about it.	My speech went really well, except for that one stutter. I bet most people didn't even notice it, though.

conclusions and more unfounded overgeneralizations. Patterns of thinking that make events seem worse than they are in reality are called **cognitive distortions.**

DEVELOP REALISTIC SELF-TALK When you react to a situation, an important piece of that reaction is your **self-talk**—the statements you make to yourself inside your own mind.

Once you get used to noticing the way your mind works, you may be able to catch yourself thinking negatively and change the process before it goes too far. This approach to controlling your reactions is not the same as positive thinking—which means substituting a positive thought for a negative one. Instead you simply try to make your thoughts as logical and accurate as possible, based on the facts of the situation as you know them, and not on snap judgments or conclusions that may turn out to be false.

Demoralized people can be tenacious about their negative beliefs—so tenacious that they make their beliefs come true in a self-fulfilling prophecy. For example, if you conclude that you are so boring that no one will like you anyway, you may decide not to bother socializing. This behavior could make the negative belief become a reality because you limit your opportunities to meet people and develop new relationships.

For additional tips on changing distorted, negative ways of thinking, see the box "Realistic Self-Talk."

cognitive distortion A pattern of negative thinking that makes events seem worse than they are. **TERMS**

self-talk The statements a person makes to himself or herself.

Psychological Defense Mechanisms— Healthy and Unhealthy

We are always trying to manage our feelings, even if we aren't aware we are doing it. We try to manage uncomfortable feelings through what are called psychological defenses. By using defense mechanisms, we change unacceptable feelings (like shame or anger or anxiety) into ones with which we are more comfortable. Table 3.1 lists some standard **defense mechanisms.** Defense mechanisms can be healthy and adaptive—such as humor and altruism—but sometimes they are what are called maladaptive. For example, it would be maladaptive to displace your anger at your teacher by yelling at your roommates because doing so doesn't help your relationship with your teacher or your roommates. The drawback of many defenses is that they make feelings better temporarily but don't address underlying causes.

Recognizing our own defense mechanisms can be difficult because we are not aware of them, as they occur unconsciously. But we all have some inkling about how our minds operate. By remembering the details of conflict situations, a person may be able to figure out which defense mechanisms she or he used in successful or unsuccessful attempts to cope. Having insight into what strategies you typically use can lead to new, more rewarding and effective ways of coping.

Being Optimistic

Most of us have a predisposition toward optimism or pessimism. **Pessimism** is a tendency to focus on the negative and expect an unfavorable outcome; **optimism** is a tendency to emphasize the hopeful and expect a favorable outcome. Pessimists not only expect repeated failure and rejection but also accept it as deserved. They do not see themselves as capable of success and irrationally dismiss any evidence of their own accomplishments. This negative point of view is learned, typically at a young age from parents and other authority figures. Optimists, by contrast, consider bad events to be temporary and consider failure to be limited and look forward to new pursuits.

You can learn to be optimistic by recording adverse events in a diary, along with the reactions and beliefs with which you met those events. By doing so, you learn to recognize and dispute the false, negative predictions you generate about yourself.

Maintaining Honest Communication

Another important area of psychological functioning is communicating honestly with others. It can be very frustrating for us and for people around us if we cannot express what we want and feel. Others can hardly respond to our needs if they

---

TERMS

defense mechanism A mental mechanism for coping with conflict or anxiety.

pessimism The tendency to expect an unfavorable outcome.

optimism The tendency to expect a favorable outcome.

Table 3.1	Defense and Coping Mechanisms	
MECHANISM	**DESCRIPTION**	**EXAMPLE**
Projection	Reacting to unacceptable impulses by denying their existence in yourself and attributing them to others	A student who dislikes his roommate feels that the roommate dislikes him.
Repression	Keeping an unpleasant feeling, idea, or memory out of awareness	The child of an alcoholic, neglectful father remembers only when her father showed consideration and love.
Denial	Refusing to acknowledge to yourself what you really know to be true	A person believes that smoking cigarettes won't harm her because she's young and healthy.
Displacement	Shifting your feelings about a person to another person	A student who is angry with one of his professors returns home and yells at one of his housemates.
Dissociation	Detaching from a current experience to avoid emotional distress	Rather than listen to his angry father, Beethoven composes a piece in his mind.
Rationalization	Giving a false, acceptable reason when the real reason is unacceptable	A shy young man decides not to attend a dorm party, telling himself he'd be bored.
Reaction formation	Concealing emotions or impulses by exaggerating the opposite ones	A person who dislikes children frequently buys expensive gifts for, and speaks with enthusiasm about, the children of her friends.
Substitution	Replacing an unacceptable or unobtainable goal with an acceptable one	A man in love with an unavailable partner throws himself into training for a marathon.
Acting out	Engaging in an action that makes an unacceptable feeling go away	A person who feels disrespected and devalued gets into a fight at a bar with a stranger.
Humor	Finding something funny in unpleasant situations	A student whose bicycle has been stolen thinks how surprised the thief will be when he or she starts downhill and discovers the brakes don't work.
Altruism	Serving others without expecting anything in return	A person who grew up in an upper-class neighborhood volunteers at a foundation that helps people get out of poverty.

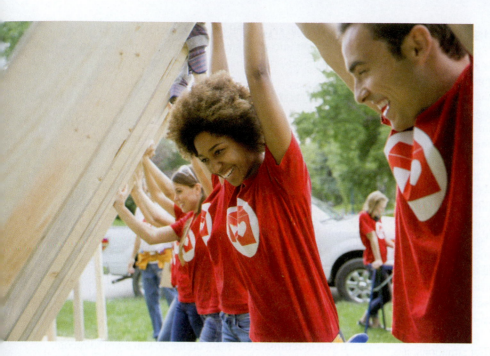
College offers many antidotes to loneliness in the forms of clubs, organized activities, sports, and just hanging out with friends.

© Hero Images/Getty Images

Dealing with Anger

Anger is a part of the array of normal emotions, yet it is often confusing and difficult to deal with. Some people feel that expressing anger is beneficial for psychological and physical health. However, if angry words or actions damage relationships or produce feelings of guilt or loss of control, they do not contribute to psychological wellness. It is important to distinguish between a destructive expression of anger and a reasonable level of self-assertiveness.

At one extreme are people who never express anger or any opinion that might offend others, even when their own rights and needs are being jeopardized. They may be trapped in unhealthy relationships or chronically deprived of satisfaction at work and at home. If you have trouble expressing your anger, consider training in assertiveness and appropriate expressions of anger to help you learn to express yourself constructively.

At the other extreme are people whose anger is explosive or misdirected—such expression of anger can signal a condition called *intermittent explosive disorder (IED)*. It may also be a symptom of a more serious problem—angry outbursts, for instance, are associated with posttraumatic stress disorder. Explosive anger may also happen during periods of intoxication with alcohol or drugs such as amphetamines or cocaine. Explosive anger or rage, like a child's tantrum, renders an individual temporarily unable to think straight or to act in his or her own best interest. During an IED episode, a person may lash out uncontrollably, hurting someone else physically or verbally, or destroying property. Anyone who expresses anger this way should seek professional help. Some studies have suggested that overtly hostile people seem to be at higher risk for heart attacks.

Managing Your Anger If you feel explosive anger coming on, consider the following two strategies to head it off. First, try to *reframe* what you're thinking at that moment. You'll be less angry at another person if there is a possibility that his or her behavior was not intentionally directed against you. Imagine that another driver suddenly cuts in front of you. You would certainly be angry if you knew the other driver did it on purpose, but you probably would be less angry if you knew he simply did not see you. If you're angry because you've just been criticized, avoid mentally replaying scenes from the past when you received other unjust criticisms. Think about what is happening now, and try to act differently than you would have in the past—less defensively and more analytically.

don't know what those needs are. We must recognize what we want to communicate and then express it clearly.

Some people know what they want others to do but don't state it clearly because they fear denial of the request, which they interpret as personal rejection. Such people might benefit from assertiveness training: learning to insist on their rights and to bargain for what they want. **Assertiveness** includes being able to say no or yes depending on the situation.

Dealing with Loneliness

It can be hard to strike the right balance between being alone and being with others. Some people are motivated to socialize from fear of being alone. If you discover how to enjoy being by yourself, you'll be better able to cope with periods when you're forced to be alone—for example, when you are no longer in a romantic relationship or when your usual friends are away on vacation.

Unhappiness with being alone may come from interpreting it as a sign of rejection—that others are not interested in spending time with you. Before you reach such a conclusion, be sure that you give others a real chance to get to know you.

Examine your patterns of thinking: You may harbor unrealistic expectations about other people—for example, that everyone you meet must like you and, if they don't, you must be flawed.

Loneliness is a passive feeling state. If you decide that you're not spending enough time with people, change the situation. College life provides many opportunities to meet people. If you're shy or introverted, you may have to push yourself to join a group. Look for something you've enjoyed in the past or in which you have a genuine interest.

assertiveness Expression that is forceful but not hostile. **TERMS**

Second, until you're able to change your thinking, try to *distract* yourself. Use the old trick of counting to 10 before you respond, or start concentrating on your breathing. If necessary, cool off by leaving the situation until your anger has subsided. This does not mean that you should permanently avoid the sensitive topics. Return to the matter after you've had a chance to think clearly about it.

Dealing with Anger in Other People

Anger can be infectious, and it disrupts cooperation and communication. If someone you're with becomes very angry, respond "asymmetrically" by reacting not with anger but with calm. Try to validate the other person by acknowledging that he or she has some reason to be angry: "I totally get that this is making you mad," or "If I were you, I'd be upset, too." This does not mean apologizing if you don't think you're to blame, or accepting verbal abuse. It means that you have considered the other's perspective and that you understand why she might be angry. Finally, if the person cannot be calmed, it may be best to disengage, at least temporarily. After a time-out, you may have better luck trying to solve the problem rationally.

Ask Yourself

QUESTIONS FOR CRITICAL THINKING AND REFLECTION

Think about the last time you were truly angry. What triggered your anger? How did you express it? Do you typically handle your anger in the same manner? How appropriate does your anger-management technique seem?

PSYCHOLOGICAL DISORDERS

All of us feel anxious at times. In dealing with anxiety, we may avoid doing something we want to do or should do. Most of us have periods of feeling down when we become pessimistic, less energetic, and less able to enjoy life. Many of us are bothered at times by irrational thoughts or odd feelings. Such feelings and thoughts can be normal responses to the ordinary challenges of life, but when emotions or irrational thoughts interfere with daily activities and rob us of peace of mind, they can be considered symptoms of a psychological disorder.

Psychological disorders are generally the result of many factors. Genetic differences, which underlie differences in how the brain processes information and experiences, are known to play an important role, especially in certain disorders such as autism, schizophrenia, and bipolar disorder. However, exactly which genes are involved, and how they alter the structure and chemistry of the brain, is still under study. A dysfunctional interaction between neurotransmitters and their receptors is associated with some psychiatric disorders (Figure 3.2). The trouble begins when neurotransmitters (chemicals that transmit messages between nerve cells) misfire and the nerve cells do not communicate properly.

Learning and life events are important, too: Although one identical twin is often at higher risk of having a disorder if the other has it, the two don't necessarily have the same psychological disorders despite having identical genes. Some people have been exposed to more traumatic events than others, leading either to greater vulnerability to future traumas or, conversely, to the development of better coping skills. Further, what your

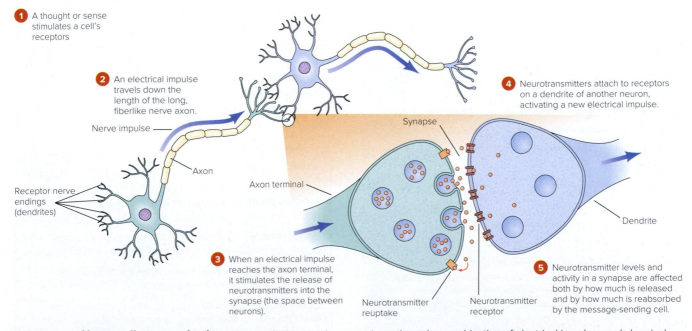

FIGURE 3.2 **Nerve cell communication.** Nerve cells (neurons) communicate through a combination of electrical impulses and chemical messages. Neurotransmitters such as serotonin and norepinephrine alter the overall responsiveness of the brain and are responsible for mood, levels of attentiveness, and other psychological states. Many psychological issues are related to problems with neurotransmitters and their receptors, and drug treatments frequently target them. For example, some antidepressant drugs increase levels of serotonin by slowing the resorption (reuptake) of serotonin.

parents, peers, and others have taught you strongly influences your level of self-esteem and how you deal with frightening or depressing life events (see the box "Ethnicity, Culture, and Psychological Health").

This section examines some of the more common psychological disorders, including anxiety disorders, mood disorders, and schizophrenia. Table 3.2 shows the likelihood of these disorders occurring during a lifetime.

Anxiety Disorders

Fear is a basic and useful emotion. Its value for our ancestors' survival cannot be overestimated. For modern humans, fear motivates us to protect ourselves and to learn how to cope with new or potentially dangerous situations. We consider fear to be a problem only when it is out of proportion to real danger. **Anxiety** is another word for fear, in particular, fear that is not in response to any definite threat. It becomes a disorder when it occurs almost daily or in life situations that recur and cannot be avoided, interfering with your relationships and the ability to function in social and professional situations.

In 2014, an estimated **43.6 million** adults age 18 and older in the United States had a mental illness. This number represented **18.1%** of all U.S. adults.

—National Institute of Mental Health, 2015

Specific Phobia The most common and understandable anxiety disorder, called **specific phobia,** is a fear of something definite like lightning, a particular type of animal, or a place. Snakes, spiders, and dogs are commonly feared animals; high or enclosed spaces are often frightening places. Sometimes, but not always, these fears originate in bad experiences, such as being bitten by a snake.

Social Phobia The 15 million Americans with **social phobia** fear humiliation or embarrassment. Fear of speaking in public is perhaps the most common phobia of this kind. Extremely shy people can have social fears in almost all social situations. People with these kinds of fears may not continue in school as far as they could and may restrict themselves to lower-paying jobs in which they do not have to come into contact with new people.

Panic Disorder People with **panic disorder** experience sudden unexpected surges in anxiety, accompanied by symptoms such as rapid and strong heartbeat, shortness of breath, loss of physical equilibrium, and a feeling of losing mental control. Such attacks usually begin in a person's early twenties and can lead to a fear of being in crowds or closed places or of driving or flying. Sufferers fear that a panic attack will occur in a situation from which escape is difficult (in an elevator), where the attack could be incapacitating and result in a dangerous or embarrassing loss of control (driving a car or shopping), or where no medical help would be available if needed (alone away from home). Fears such as these lead to avoidance of situations that might cause trouble. The fears and avoidance may spread to a large variety of situations until a person is virtually housebound, a condition called **agoraphobia.** People with panic disorder can often function normally in feared situations if with someone they trust. Panic disorder is different from an occasional **panic attack,**

VITAL STATISTICS

Table 3.2	Lifetime Prevalence of Selected Psychological Disorders among Americans	
DISORDER	MEN %	WOMEN %
Anxiety Disorders		
Specific Phobia	6.7	15.7
Social phobia	11.1	15.5
Panic disorder	2.0	5.0
Generalized anxiety disorder	3.6	6.6
Obsessive-compulsive disorder	1.7	2.8
Posttraumatic stress disorder	5.0	10.4
Mood disorders		
Major depressive episode	11.2	20.7
Manic episode	1.4	1.9
Schizophrenia and related disorders	0.8	0.4

SOURCES: Centers for Disease Control and Prevention. 2011. Mental illness surveillance among adults in the United States. *MMWR* 60 (Suppl.): 1–29; Kessler, R. C., et al. 2005. Prevalence, severity, and comorbidity of twelve-month DSM-IV disorders in the National Comorbidity Survey Replication (NCSR). *Archives of General Psychiatry* 62(6): 617–627; Kessler, R. C., et al. 1994. Lifetime and 12-month prevalence of DSM-III-R psychiatric disorders in the United States. *Archives of General Psychiatry* 51(1): 8–19; Kessler, R. C., et al. 1995. Posttraumatic stress disorder in the National Comorbidity Survey. *Archives of General Psychiatry* 52(12): 1048–1060.

TERMS

anxiety Fear that is not a response to any definite threat.

specific phobia A persistent and excessive fear of a specific object, activity, or situation.

social phobia An excessive fear of being observed by others; speaking in public is the most common example.

panic disorder A syndrome of severe anxiety attacks accompanied by physical symptoms.

agoraphobia An anxiety disorder characterized by fear of being alone away from help and by avoidance of many different places and situations; in extreme cases, a fear of leaving home.

panic attack A brief surge of overwhelming anxiety that usually resolves in an hour or less.

58 CHAPTER 3 PSYCHOLOGICAL HEALTH

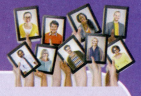

Cultures develop unique ideas about mental health—about what is normal and what is problematic, how symptoms should be interpreted and communicated, whether treatment should be sought, and whether a social stigma is attached to a particular symptom or disorder. Based on their various environmental, cultural, and socioeconomic backgrounds, cultures perceive—categorize and interpret—psychological disorders differently. Climate and geography, as well as other environmental factors, such as diet, contribute to a group's health.

These culturally distinct ideas change as the group comes into contact with other groups. For example, Asian immigrants to the United States have often come from *collectivist* cultures that anticipate and care for the needs of each other, so that individuals don't need to request support. In U.S. cultures, usually no group is expected to look after the needs of an individual; rather, individuals or their close families are responsible for seeking help for themselves. For this reason Asian immigrants appear to have more trouble than European Americans asking for explicit social support.

The process by which individuals and groups adapt to each other's cultures, called *acculturation,* is an important influence on health. This adaptation ideally represents an exchange between both cultures, so that they learn how to do things a new way. Acculturation, however, often applies only to immigrants' adopting influences from a dominant culture. When a dominant group takes over the resources of a minority group—for example, a government enforces an English-only policy on bilingual speakers, thereby increasing the difficulties of the immigrants seeking help—then the socioeconomic status of the adapting group often decreases. As the following examples show, this status change may then further affect the psychological health of the group.

Arctic Native Populations

Studies of native populations around the Arctic (e.g., in northern Canada, Greenland, and Scandinavia) reveal many cases of elevated and chronic stress, accompanied by high blood pressure and cardiovascular risk. This chronic stress is linked to 50 years of rapid socioeconomic change: The population has experienced long-term unemployment, contamination of food, and a multitude of other acculturation problems. As they have acculturated, indigenous people have suffered discrimination, loss of traditional values, and lack of control over their resources. Because they live in climates with less light during winter months, they also experience seasonal affective disorder, a form of depression.

Cultural expressions of their high levels of anxiety and depression include increased incidence of suicide and violence. Adolescents, in particular, among Alaska Natives and Greenland Inuit, have recently had a high number of suicides. In these populations, levels of injury and violence reach two to four times as high as national averages.

Latinos in the United States

Latinos in the United States generally are healthier than other U.S. racial and ethnic groups, for example, in mortality rates for adults and newborn babies. Still, mortality rates, incidence of chronic illness, and some mental health conditions such as depression vary within the U.S. Latino population, depending on Latino origin or cultural heritage (e.g., Mexican, Puerto Rican, or Cuban).

One of the largest immigrant groups in the United States is from Mexico. Surprisingly, surveys show that these immigrants are psychologically healthier than their own children born in the United States. The children, who have acculturated into the dominant society—or acquired some knowledge of its language, food choice, dress, music, sports, etc.—are more likely to suffer from problems with depression, substance abuse, poor diet, and birth outcomes (e.g., prematurity, low birthweight, and teen pregnancy). Reasons for the negative effects of acculturation may be the stresses of cultural conflicts around ideas of individuality, interpersonal relationships, and what it means to succeed. Access to processed American foods high in simple sugars and excess fat may also prevail over the diets of their parents, which tend to be higher in fiber, protein, and vegetables and fruits.

Despite these problems, second-generation Americans nevertheless tend to have higher rates of insurance coverage and access to health care. Their greater facility with English is correlated with higher frequencies of general physical, vision, and dental check-ups. Regardless of one's generation, other factors affect immigrants' health outcomes living in the U.S.: education, wealth, occupational and language skills all influence their lifestyles, as well as the policies of the government and attitudes of Americans already here.

SOURCES: Fisher, E. B. 2014. Peer support in health care and prevention: Cultural, organizational, and dissemination issues. *Annual Review of Public Health* 35: 363–383; Leyse-Wallace, R. 2013. *Nutrition and Mental Health*. Boca Raton, FL: CRC Press; Snodgrass, J. J. 2013. Health of indigenous circumpolar populations. *Annual Review of Anthropology* 42: 69–87; Brick, K., et al. 2011. *Mexican and Central American immigrants in the United States.* Washington, D.C: Migration Policy Institute; Lara, M., et al. 2005. Acculturation and Latino health in the United States: A review of the literature and its sociopolitical context. *Annual Review of Public Health* 26: 367–397.

which affects about 40 million American adults age 18 and older every year. This occasional attack of overwhelming anxiety may have no obvious antecedent and usually resolves in an hour or less.

Generalized Anxiety Disorder A basic reaction to future threats is to worry about them. **Generalized anxiety** disorder **(GAD)** is a diagnosis given to people whose worries about multiple issues linger more than six months.

> **generalized anxiety disorder (GAD)** An anxiety disorder characterized by excessive, uncontrollable worry about all kinds of things and anxiety in many situations.   **TERMS**

Worries may involve family, other relationships, work, school, money, and health.

The GAD sufferer's worrying is not completely unjustified—after all, thinking about problems can result in solving them. But this kind of thinking seems to just go around in circles, and the more you try to stop it, the more you feel at its mercy. The end result is a persistent feeling of nervousness, often accompanied by depression.

Obsessive-Compulsive Disorder

Someone diagnosed with **obsessive-compulsive disorder (OCD)** struggles with obsessions, compulsions, or both. **Obsessions** are recurrent, unwanted thoughts or impulses. Unlike the worries of GAD, they are not ordinary concerns but improbable fears such as of suddenly committing an antisocial act or of having been contaminated by germs.

Compulsions are repetitive, difficult-to-resist actions usually associated with obsessions. A common compulsion is hand washing, associated with an obsessive fear of contamination by dirt. Other compulsions are counting and repeatedly checking whether something has been done—for example, whether a door has been locked or a stove turned off.

People with OCD feel anxious, out of control, and embarrassed. Their rituals can occupy much of their time and make them inefficient at work and difficult to live with.

Posttraumatic Stress Disorder (PTSD)

People who suffer from **posttraumatic stress disorder** are reacting to severely traumatic events (events that produce a sense of terror and helplessness) such as physical violence to themselves or their loved ones. Trauma occurs in personal assaults (rape, military combat), natural disasters (floods, hurricanes), and tragedies (fires, airplane or car crashes).

Symptoms include reexperiencing the trauma in dreams and in intrusive memories, trying to avoid anything associated with the trauma, and numbing of feelings. Hyperarousal (being on edge or easily startled), sleep disturbances, and other symptoms of anxiety and depression also commonly occur. Such symptoms can last months or even years. The symptoms of PTSD must last at least a month for the diagnosis to be made. Those whose symptoms have lasted only a month before resolving are considered to have **acute stress disorder.** PTSD symptoms often decrease over time, but up to one-third of PTSD sufferers do not fully recover. Recovery may be slower in those who have previously experienced trauma or who suffer from ongoing psychological problems.

A study by the U.S. Department of Veterans Affairs National Center for PTSD found that, as a result of the Boston Marathon bombing in April 2013, many Boston-area military veterans diagnosed with PTSD experienced flashbacks, unwanted memories, and other psychological effects. The study raised awareness of the effects that tragic events such as terror attacks

and mass shootings have on people directly involved but also on those with PTSD and other preexisting psychological conditions. The researchers urged health care systems to be prepared in the future to provide treatment for individuals either directly or indirectly affected by such tragedies.

Treating Anxiety Disorders Therapies for anxiety disorders range from medication to psychological interventions concentrating on a person's thoughts and behavior. Both drug treatments and cognitive-behavioral therapies are effective in panic disorder, OCD, and GAD. Specific phobias are best treated without drugs.

Attention-Deficit/Hyperactivity Disorder

Attention-deficit/hyperactivity disorder (ADHD) is one of the most common disorders of childhood and adolescence. The main features of ADHD are inattention, hyperactivity, and/or impulsivity. A diagnosis of ADHD is made only if the individual exhibits a persistent pattern of these behaviors; the behaviors must also interfere with the individual's functioning or development, as well as negatively affect school performance, peer relationships, or behavior at home. To be diagnosed, a person must have symptoms of ADHD before age 12 (even if an adult at first diagnosis). There must also be evidence that the ADHD behaviors are present in two or more settings—for example, at home, school or work; with friends and family; and in other activities. Someone who can pay attention at work but is inattentive only at home usually wouldn't qualify for a diagnosis of ADHD.

ADHD has no cure, and scientists are still working on treatments. They are using tools such as brain imaging to find ways to prevent it. The use of medications is controversial. At best it can relieve some symptoms of the disorder. Other treatments include psychotherapy, education and training, and a combination of treatments.

Mood Disorders

We've all experienced sadness and feeling "down" or elated or irritable, but sometimes these feelings can be persistent or severe and interfere with life functioning. The two main types of **mood disorder,** major depressive disorder and bipolar disorder (what used to be called manic-depression) are together the most common mental disorders in the United States.

Depression   Depression differs from person to person but includes the following symptoms that persist most of the day and last more than two consecutive weeks:

- A feeling of sadness and hopelessness or loss of pleasure in doing usual activities (anhedonia)
- Poor appetite and weight loss or, alternatively, increased eating compared to usual
- Insomnia or disturbed sleep, including waking up and being unable to fall back to sleep or sleeping more than normal
- Decreased energy
- Restlessness or, alternatively, slowed thinking or activity
- Thoughts of worthlessness and guilt
- Trouble concentrating or making decisions
- Thoughts of death or suicide

A person experiencing depression may not have all of these symptoms but must have depressed mood or anhedonia and at least four other symptoms. Sometimes instead of poor appetite and insomnia, the opposite occurs—eating too much and sleeping too long. Thus depression may contribute to weight gain in young women. People can have multiple symptoms of depression without feeling depressed, although they usually experience a loss of interest or pleasure.

In some cases, depression is a clear-cut reaction to a specific event, such as the loss of a loved one or a failure in school or work, whereas in other cases no trigger event is obvious. Regardless of the reason, severe symptoms should be taken seriously. Someone who has symptoms of major depression for more than two weeks, even if it is in reaction to a specific event, should consider treatment. One danger of severe depression is suicide, which is discussed later in this chapter, but the overall impact of depression on general health and ability to function, with or without suicidal thoughts, can be devastating.

The National Institutes of Health estimates that **depression** strikes nearly 6.7% of Americans annually—20% of people have it in their lifetime—making depression the most common mood disorder. Depression affects the young as well as adults; about 3% of adolescents aged 13–18 suffer a major depressive episode each year, and nearly 50% of college students report depression severe enough to hinder their daily functioning. Depression tends to be more severe and persistent in blacks than in people of other races. Despite this, only about 60% of blacks affected by depression receive treatment for it. Almost twice as many women as men have serious depression. Overall, about three times as many women as men attempt suicide, but women's attempts are less likely to be lethal.

Why women have more depression than do men is a matter of debate. Some experts think much of the difference is the result of reporting bias: Women are more willing to admit experiencing negative emotions, being stressed, or having difficulty coping. Women may also be more likely to seek treatment. Other experts point to biologically based sex differences, particularly in the level and action of hormones. It may also be that men are more likely than women to have symptoms such as anger or irritability when they are depressed, leading them to be misdiagnosed or for the diagnosis to be missed. In addition, women's social roles and expectations often differ from those of men. Women may put more emphasis on relationships in determining self-esteem, so the deterioration of a relationship is a cause of depression that can hit women harder than men. Culturally determined gender roles are more likely to place women in situations where they have less control over key life decisions, and lack of autonomy is associated with depression.

Although treatments are highly effective, only about 35% of people who suffer from depression currently seek treatment. Treatment for depression depends on its severity and on whether the depressed person is suicidal.

The best initial treatment for moderate to severe depression is probably a combination of drug therapy and psychotherapy. Newer prescription antidepressants work well, although they may need several weeks to take effect, and patients may need to try multiple medications before finding one that works well. If someone is severely depressed and at risk of suicide, hospitalization for more intensive treatment to ensure the patient's safety is sometimes necessary.

mood disorder   An emotional disturbance that is **TERMS** intense and persistent enough to affect normal function; two common mood disorders are depression and bipolar disorder.

depression   A mood disorder characterized by loss of interest, sadness, hopelessness, loss of appetite, disturbed sleep, and other physical symptoms.

Antidepressants work by targeting key neurotransmitters in the brain, including serotonin. When you take an antidepressant, your levels of serotonin increase. This increase has been revealed to help depression and other bodily conditions that serotonin influences, including mood, sexual desire and function, appetite, sleep, memory and learning, temperature regulation, and some social behavior.

When women take antidepressants, they may need a lower dose than men; at the same dosage, blood levels of medication tend to be higher in women. An issue for women who may become pregnant is whether antidepressants can harm a fetus or newborn. The best evidence indicates that the most frequently prescribed types of antidepressants do not cause birth defects, although some studies have reported withdrawal symptoms in some newborns whose mothers used certain antidepressants.

Electroconvulsive therapy (ECT) is effective for severe depression when other approaches have failed, including medications and other electronic therapies. In ECT, an epileptic-like seizure is induced by an electrical impulse transmitted through electrodes placed on the head. Patients are given an anesthetic and a muscle relaxant to reduce anxiety and prevent injuries associated with seizures. ECT usually includes three treatments per week for two to four weeks.

For patients with **seasonal affective disorder (SAD)**—a type of depression—the treatment involves sitting with eyes open in front of a bright light source every morning. For patients with SAD, depression worsens during winter months as daylight hours diminish. Light therapy may work by extending the perceived length of the day and thus convincing the brain that it is summertime even during the winter months. The American Psychiatric Association estimates that 10–20% of Americans suffer symptoms that may be linked to SAD. SAD is more common among people who live at higher latitudes, where there are fewer hours of light in winter.

Bipolar Disorder People who experience **mania,** characteristic of a severe mood disorder called **bipolar disorder,** undergo discrete periods of time when they may be restless, have excess energy or activity, feel rested with less sleep than usual, and speak rapidly. They may feel elevated (that is, much better than normal) or abnormally irritable. These feelings are often accompanied by impulsive behavior without regard for the consequences—for example, spending too much money or engaging in risky sexual activity. When such episodes are severe (requiring hospitalization, for example, or producing severe consequences), they are known as manic episodes, and the person who experiences them has what is known as *bipolar I disorder.* If such episodes of elevation or irritability are not so severe as to significantly impair

functioning, they are known as *hypomanic episodes.* If hypomania alternates with periods of depression, that person is diagnosed with what is known as *bipolar II disorder.*

People with bipolar disorder typically have periods of both mania or hypomania and depression, and the periods of depression can be persistent and severe. Bipolar disorder typically begins in the late teens through the twenties. Many people with bipolar disorder also struggle with substance and alcohol use disorders and anxiety. Suicide rates are high in bipolar disorders, especially early in life. This syndrome affects men and women equally.

Antimanic drugs include lithium (a salt that calms manic episodes), mood stabilizers, and antipsychotic medications. For people who have recurrent episodes of mania or depression, continued, lifelong medication treatment is recommended. Specific medications to treat bipolar depression may also be prescribed.

Schizophrenia

Schizophrenia is a devastating mental disorder that affects a person's thinking and perceptions of reality. People with schizophrenia frequently develop paranoid ideas and false beliefs (delusions), or may have auditory hallucinations (hearing "voices"). People with schizophrenia are often convinced that the voices they hear are "real." The disease can be severe and debilitating or so mild that it's hardly noticeable. Although people are capable of diagnosing their own depression, they usually don't diagnose their own schizophrenia because they often can't see that anything is wrong. This disorder is not rare; in fact, 1 in every 100 people has schizophrenia, most commonly starting in adolescence, which is perhaps what is most tragic and disturbing about the disease—that it starts to affect people in the prime of their lives.

Schizophrenia is likely caused by a combination of genes and environmental factors that occur during pregnancy

TERMS

electroconvulsive therapy (ECT) The use of electric shock to induce brief, generalized seizures; used in the treatment of selected psychological disorders.

seasonal affective disorder (SAD) A mood disorder characterized by seasonal depression, usually occurring in winter, when there is less daylight.

mania A mood disorder characterized by excessive elation, irritability, talkativeness, inflated self-esteem, and expansiveness.

bipolar disorder A mental illness characterized by alternating periods of depression and mania.

schizophrenia A psychological disorder that involves a disturbance in thinking and in perceiving reality.

and development. For example, children born to older fathers have higher rates of schizophrenia, as do children with prenatal exposure to certain infections or medications. Some general characteristics of schizophrenia include the following:

- **Disorganized thoughts.** Thoughts may be expressed in a vague or confusing way.

- **Inappropriate emotions.** Emotions may be either absent or strong but inappropriate.

- **Delusions.** People with delusions—firmly held false beliefs—may think that their minds are controlled by outside forces, that people can read their minds, that they are great personages like Jesus Christ or the president of the United States, or that they are being persecuted by a group such as the CIA. Paranoid delusions can give people the feeling that they are in grave danger of being harmed.

- **Auditory hallucinations.** People with schizophrenia may hear voices when no one is present. Sometimes these voices tell them to do things (like harm themselves or others), belittle and criticize them, or give individuals a running commentary on someone's thoughts and behaviors. These voices can seem very real to the person hearing them and therefore are quite terrifying.

- **Deteriorating social and work functioning.** Social withdrawal and increasingly poor performance at school or work may be so gradual that they are hardly noticed at first, but over time people suffering from the disease fall far behind their peers—and far behind others' earlier expectations.

None of these characteristics is invariably present. Some schizophrenic people are quite logical except on the subject of their delusions. Others show disorganized thoughts but no delusions or hallucinations.

A schizophrenic person needs help from a mental health professional. Suicide is a risk in schizophrenia, and expert treatment can reduce that risk and minimize the social consequences of the illness by shortening the period when symptoms are active. The key element in treatment is regular medication. At times medication is like insulin for diabetes—it makes the difference between being able to function or not. Sometimes hospitalization is required temporarily to relieve family and friends.

SUICIDE

In the United States, suicide is the second leading cause of death for young people aged 15–24 and the 10th leading cause for people of all ages. In 2013, among adults age 18 and over, 1.1% made suicide plans, and 0.6% went ahead and attempted it. (see Figure 3.3 for data on suicidal thoughts). Suicide rates vary by race or ethnicity: Among adolescents and young adults, the suicide rate is highest among American Indians or Alaska Natives; among adults, non-Hispanic whites have the highest suicide rate. The suicide rate among men is still more than three times higher than that among women, but the gap has narrowed in recent years. Overall, non-Hispanic white men aged 45–54 have the highest suicide rate.

Suicide rarely occurs without warning signs (see Table 3.3). About 60% of people who kill themselves are depressed. The more symptoms of depression a person has, the greater the risk. A threat of suicide should not be taken as only a cry for help but also as a possible future occurrence. Here are specific warning signs:

- Any mention of dying, disappearing, jumping, shooting oneself, or other types of self-harm.

- Changes in personality, including sadness, withdrawal, irritability, anxiety, fatigue, indecisiveness, or apathy.

- A sudden, inexplicable brightening of mood (which can mean the person has decided to attempt suicide).

- A sudden move to give away important possessions, accompanied by statements such as, "I won't be needing these anymore."

- An increase in reckless behaviors.

In addition to warning signs, certain risk factors increase the likelihood that someone will attempt suicide

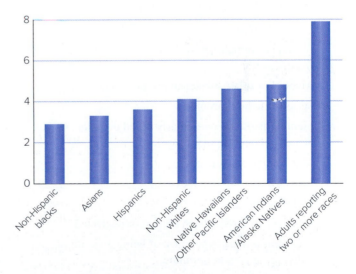

FIGURE 3.3 **Percentages of Americans age 18 and over having suicidal thoughts in the past year.**

SOURCE: Centers for Disease Control and Prevention. 2015. *Suicide. Facts at a Glance.* National Center for Injury Prevention and Control. Atlanta, GA (http://www.cdc.gov/violenceprevention/pdf/suicide-datasheet-a.pdf).

Table 3.3 — Myths about Suicide: Don't Be Misled

MYTH	FACT
People who really intend to kill themselves do not let anyone know about it.	This belief can be an excuse for doing nothing when someone says he or she might attempt suicide. In fact, most people who eventually follow through with suicide *have* talked about doing it.
People who made a suicide attempt but survived did not really intend to die.	This belief may be true for certain people, but people who seriously want to end their lives may fail because they misjudge what it takes. Even a pharmacist may misjudge the lethal dose of a drug.
People who succeed in suicide really wanted to die.	We cannot be sure of that either. Some people are only trying to make a dramatic gesture or plea for help but miscalculate.
People who really want to kill themselves will do it regardless of any attempts to prevent them.	Few people are single-minded about suicide even at the moment of attempting it. People who are quite determined to take their lives today may completely change their minds tomorrow.
Suicide is proof of mental illness.	Many suicides are carried out by people who do not meet ordinary criteria for mental illness, although people with depression, schizophrenia, and other psychological disorders have a much higher than average suicide rate.
People inherit suicidal tendencies.	Certain kinds of depression that lead to suicide do have a genetic component. But many examples of suicide running in a family can be explained by factors such as psychologically identifying with a family member who kill themselves, often a parent.
All suicides are irrational.	By some standards, all suicides may seem "irrational." But many people find it at least understandable that someone might want to attempt suicide—for example, when approaching the end of a terminal illness or when facing a long prison term.

(see the box "Deliberate Self-Harm"). Protective factors decrease the likelihood. Risk factors and protective factors can be *intrapersonal, social/situational,* or *cultural.*

The following are key risk factors:

- A history of previous attempts
- A sense of hopelessness, helplessness, guilt, or worthlessness
- Alcohol or other substance use disorders
- Serious medical problems
- Mental disorders, particularly mood disorders such as depression and bipolar disorder
- Availability of a weapon
- Family history of suicide
- Social isolation
- A history of having been abused or neglected
- A current or past experience of being a victim of bullying, in person or online

The following are key protective factors:

- Strong religious faith or other cultural prohibition on suicide
- Connection to other people, including family that is supportive
- Engagement in treatment in which the person is getting help
- Connection with one's own children (or even pets)
- Lack of access to lethal means (guns, pills, railroad tracks)

If you are severely depressed or know someone who is, expert help from a mental health professional is essential. Don't be afraid to discuss the possibility of suicide with someone you fear is suicidal. You won't give them an idea they haven't already thought of. Ask direct questions to determine whether someone seriously intends to kill themselves. Encourage your friend to talk and to take positive steps to improve his or her situation.

You can call the National Suicide Prevention Lifeline at 800-273-TALK (8255). Trained crisis workers are available to talk 24 hours a day, 7 days a week. If you think someone is in immediate danger, do not leave him or her alone. Call for help or take him or her to an emergency room.

Most communities have emergency help available, often in the form of a hotline telephone counseling service run by a suicide prevention agency.

Firearms are used in more suicides than homicides. Among gun-related deaths in the home, 83% are the result of suicide, often by someone other than the gun owner. If you learn someone at high risk for suicide has access to a gun, try to convince him or her to put it in safekeeping.

Deliberate Self-Harm

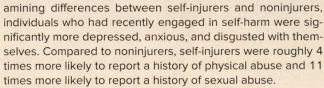

In general, people want to be well and healthy and to protect themselves from harm. But many individuals—predominantly in their teens and adolescence—do deliberately harm themselves, although in a nonfatal way. A common method of self-harm involves people cutting or burning their own skin, leaving scars that they hide beneath their clothes.

Self-cutting and other self-injurious behaviors are not aesthetically motivated. Many people who engage in these behaviors report seeking the physical sensations (including pain) produced by a self-inflected injury, which may temporarily relieve feelings of tension, perhaps through a release of endorphins.

In 2011, a research group led by Alicia Meuret, an associate professor of psychology at Southern Methodist University, conducted surveys on more than 550 college students and found that over 20% had engaged in self-injury at some point,

which is consistent with prevalence estimates in other studies on college populations. In examining differences between self-injurers and noninjurers, individuals who had recently engaged in self-harm were significantly more depressed, anxious, and disgusted with themselves. Compared to noninjurers, self-injurers were roughly 4 times more likely to report a history of physical abuse and 11 times more likely to report a history of sexual abuse.

Self-injury is not the same as a suicide attempt, but individuals who repeatedly hurt themselves are more likely than the general population to kill themselves. In any case, self-injury should be taken seriously. Treatment usually includes group therapy, individual therapy, medication (e.g., antidepressants), or stress reduction and management skills.

MODELS OF HUMAN NATURE AND THERAPEUTIC CHANGE

Human problems such as the psychological disorders discussed in this chapter can be evaluated from at least four perspectives: biological, behavioral, cognitive, and psychodynamic. Each perspective has a distinct view of human nature, and from those views of human nature come distinct therapeutic approaches.

The Biological Model

The *biological model* emphasizes that the mind's activity depends entirely on an organic structure, the brain, whose composition is genetically determined. The activity of neurons, mediated by complex chemical reactions, gives rise to our most complex thoughts, our most ardent desires, and our most pathological behaviors. As an organ, the brain responds well to healthy lifestyle behaviors such as maintaining a nutritious diet and exercising. When true mental health issues arise, however, drug therapies can help.

Pharmacological Therapy   The most important kind of therapy inspired by the biological model is pharmacological, or medication treatment. All medications require a prescription from a psychiatrist or other medical doctor. All have received U.S. Food and Drug Administration approval as being safe and more effective than a placebo. However, a patient may have to try several drugs before finding one that is effective and has acceptable side effects.

Issues in Drug Therapy   The discovery that many psychological disorders have a biological basis in disordered brain chemistry has led to a revolution in the treatment of many disorders, particularly depression. The new view of depression as based in brain chemistry has also lessened the stigma attached to the condition, leading more people to seek treatment. Antidepressants are now among the most widely prescribed drugs in the United States. The development of effective drugs has provided relief for many people, but the wide use of antidepressants has also raised many questions. Critics of drug therapy ask whether the new drugs are really better than the old ones or are just being marketed by drug companies because their patents on old drugs have run out. Critics also say that the efficacy of antidepressants has been exaggerated by drug company–sponsored research and that psychological treatments of depression are usually just as good.

Research indicates that, for mild cases of depression, psychotherapy and antidepressants are about equally effective. For major depression, combined therapy is significantly more effective than either type of treatment alone. Therapy can help provide insight into factors that precipitated the depression, such as high levels of stress or a history of abuse. A therapist can also provide guidance in changing patterns of thinking and behavior that contribute to the problem.

The Behavioral Model

The *behavioral model* focuses on what people do—their overt behavior—rather than on brain structures and chemistry or on thoughts and consciousness. This model regards psychological problems as "maladaptive behavior" or bad habits. When and how a person learned maladaptive behavior is less important than what makes it continue in the present.

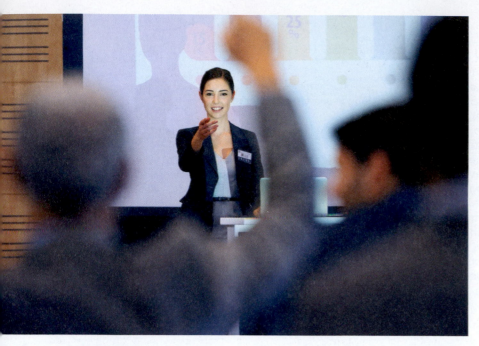

Behavioral therapy can help people overcome many kinds of fears, including that of public speaking.

© Yuri Arcurs/Getty Images

Cognitive therapy tries to expose and identify false ideas that produce feelings such as anxiety and depression. For example, a student afraid of speaking in class may harbor thoughts such as "If I begin to speak, I'll say something stupid; if I say something stupid, the teacher and my classmates will lose respect for me; then I'll get a low grade, my classmates will avoid me, and life will be hell." In cognitive therapy, these ideas will be examined critically. If the student prepares, will he or she really sound stupid? Does every sentence said have to be exactly correct and beautifully delivered, or is that an unrealistic expectation? Will classmates' opinions be completely transformed by one presentation? Do classmates even care that much? And why does the student care so much about what *they* think? People in cognitive therapy are taught to notice their unrealistic thoughts and to substitute more realistic ones, and they are advised to repeatedly test their assumptions.

Behaviorists analyze behavior in terms of **stimulus, response,** and **reinforcement.** The essence of behavior therapy is to discover what reinforcements keep an undesirable behavior going and then to try to alter those reinforcements. For example, if people who fear speaking in class (the stimulus) remove themselves from that situation (the response), they experience immediate relief, which acts as reinforcement for future avoidance and escape.

To change their behavior, fearful people are taught to practice **exposure**—to deliberately and repeatedly enter the feared situation and remain in it until their fear begins to abate. A student who is afraid to speak in class might begin his behavioral therapy program by keeping a diary listing each time he makes a contribution to a classroom discussion, how long he speaks, and his anxiety levels before, during, and after speaking. He would then develop concrete but realistic goals for increasing his speaking frequency and contract with himself to reward his successes by spending more time in activities he finds enjoyable.

Although exposure to the real situation works best, exposure in your imagination or through the virtual reality of computer simulation can also be effective. For example, in the case of someone who is afraid of flying, a simulated scenario would likely be vivid enough to elicit the fear necessary to practice exposure techniques.

The Cognitive Model

The *cognitive model* emphasizes the effect of ideas on behavior and feeling. According to this model, behavior results from complicated attitudes, expectations, and motives rather than from simple, immediate reinforcements.

The Psychodynamic Model

The *psychodynamic model* also emphasizes thoughts. Proponents of this model, however, do not believe thoughts can be changed directly because they are fed by other unconscious ideas and impulses. Symptoms are not isolated pieces of behavior but the result of a complex set of wishes and emotions hidden by active defenses (see Table 3.1). In psychodynamic therapy, patients speak as freely as possible in front of the therapist and try to gain an understanding of the basis of their feelings toward the therapist and others. Through this process, patients gain insights that help them overcome their maladaptive patterns. Current therapies of this type tend to focus more on the present (the here and now) than on the past, and the therapist tries to facilitate self-exploration rather than providing explanations.

Evaluating the Models

Ignoring theoretical conflicts among psychological models, therapists have recently developed pragmatic *cognitive-behavioral therapies* (CBTs) that combine effective elements of both models in a single package. For example, the package for treating social anxiety emphasizes exposure as

stimulus Anything that causes a response.	**TERMS**

response A reaction to a stimulus.

reinforcement Increasing the future probability of a response by following it with a reward.

exposure A therapeutic technique for treating fear; the subject learns to come into direct contact with a feared situation.

well as changing problematic patterns of thinking (see the Behavior Change Strategy "Dealing with Social Anxiety" at the end of the chapter). Combined therapies have also been developed for panic disorder, obsessive-compulsive disorder, generalized anxiety disorder, and depression. These packages, involving 10 or more individual or group sessions with a therapist and homework between sessions, have been shown to produce significant improvement.

Drug therapy and CBTs are also sometimes combined, especially in the case of depression. For anxiety disorders, both kinds of therapy are equally effective, but the effects of drug therapy last only as long as the drug is being taken, whereas CBTs produce longer-term improvement. For schizophrenia, drug therapy is a must, but a continuing relationship with therapists who give support and advice is also indispensable.

Psychodynamic therapies have been attacked as ineffective and endless. Of course, effectiveness is hard to demonstrate for therapies that do not focus on specific symptoms. But common sense tells us that being able to open yourself up and discuss your problems with a supportive but objective person who focuses on you and lets you speak freely can enhance your sense of self and reduce feelings of confusion and despair.

Other Psychotherapies

In addition to existing forms of treatment, newer psychotherapies such as *dialectical behavior therapy* (DBT) have become available. Developed by Marsha Linehan, DBT is used to treat borderline personality disorder and chronic suicidal behavior, but it has since been expanded to treat other disorders, such as drug addiction and eating disorders. This therapy uses the principles of standard CBT by encouraging distress tolerance and acceptance of painful feelings and emotions through **mindfulness** (mindful awareness, discussed in Chapter 2), originally derived from Buddhist meditation and other Eastern practices. Mindfulness aims to allow a person to be aware of feelings rather than react to them, and to learn techniques to regulate emotions, by decreasing the intensity of emotional reactions. Mindfulness is practiced in group and individual therapy, often involving the use of workbooks and homework between sessions.

Another newer therapy called *acceptance and commitment therapy (ACT)* is a scientifically studied psychological intervention that uses acceptance and mindfulness strategies, together with commitment and behavior change strategies, to increase psychological flexibility. **Psychological flexibility** is the process of embracing the present moment fully as a conscious human being, and then changing or continuing your behavior in the service of your own chosen values. It was developed in the 1980s by psychologists Steven C. Hayes, Kelly G. Wilson, and Kirk D. Strosahl.

GETTING HELP

Knowing when you need help dealing with a mental health problem is usually not as difficult as deciding which self-help method or which mental health professional to choose.

Self-Help

A smart way to begin helping yourself is by finding out what you can do on your own. For example, certain behavioral and cognitive approaches can be effective because they all involve becoming more aware of self-defeating actions and ideas and combating them in some way: being more assertive; communicating honestly; raising your self-esteem by counteracting the negative thoughts, people, and actions that undermine it; and confronting, rather than avoiding, the things you fear. Although information from books in the psychology or self-help sections of libraries and bookstores can be helpful, you should avoid any that make fantastic claims or deviate from mainstream approaches.

Some people find it helpful to express their feelings in a journal. Grappling with a painful experience in this way provides an emotional release and can help you develop more constructive ways of dealing with similar situations in the future. Research indicates that using a journal in this way can improve physical as well as emotional wellness.

For some people, religious belief and practice may promote psychological health. Religious organizations provide a social network and a supportive community, and religious practices, such as prayer and meditation, offer a path for personal change and transformation.

Peer Counseling and Support Groups

Sharing your concerns with others is another helpful way of dealing with psychological health challenges. Just being able to share what's troubling you with an accepting, empathetic

---

TERMS

mindfulness   Attention to physical sensations, perceptions, thoughts, and imagery.

psychological flexibility   The process of embracing the present moment fully as a conscious human being, and then changing or continuing your behavior in the service of your own chosen values.

Ask Yourself

QUESTIONS FOR CRITICAL THINKING AND REFLECTION

Are you open to discussing the intimate details of your life, your emotions, your fears, your deepest thoughts? Have you ever truly opened up to another person in this manner? Would you be open to this kind of sharing if it meant getting help for a psychological disorder?

Mental health workers belong to various professions and have different roles. Psychiatrists are medical doctors. They are experts in deciding whether a medical disease lies behind psychological symptoms, and they are usually involved in treatment if medication or hospitalization is required. Clinical psychologists typically hold a doctoral degree (PhD); they are often experts in behavioral and cognitive therapies. Other mental health workers include social workers, licensed counselors, and clergy with special training in pastoral counseling. In hospitals and clinics, various mental health professionals may join together in treatment teams.

In choosing a mental health professional, financial considerations are important. Research the costs and what your health insurance will cover. City, county, and state governments may support mental health clinics for those with few financial resources. Some on-campus services may be free or offered at very little cost.

The cost of treatment is linked to how many therapy sessions will be needed, which in turn depends on the type of therapy and the nature of the problem. Getting this information before you start treatment is important. Many mental health professionals do not accept health insurance payments and only accept direct payments from patients. Psychological therapies focusing on specific problems may require weekly visits for a period of 8–24 sessions, depending on the type of therapy. Therapies based on CBT, DBT, and ACT are often time limited, and your therapist can tell you how many sessions to expect. Therapies aiming for psychological awareness and personality change, such as psychodynamic therapies, can last months or years.

Deciding whether a therapist is right for you will require meeting the therapist in person. Before or during your first meeting, find out about the therapist's background and training:

- Does she or he have a degree from an appropriate professional school and a state license to practice?

- Has she or he had experience treating problems similar to yours?

- How much will therapy cost?

You have a right to know the answers to these questions and should not hesitate to ask them. After your initial meeting, evaluate your impressions:

- Does the therapist seem like a warm, intelligent person who would be able to help you and seems interested in doing so?

- Are you comfortable with the therapist's personality, values, and beliefs?

- Is he or she willing to talk about the techniques in use? Do these techniques make sense to you?

If you answer yes to these questions, this therapist may be satisfactory for you. If you feel uncomfortable—and you're not in need of emergency care—it's worthwhile to set up one-time consultations with one or two others before you make up your mind. Take the time to find someone who feels right for you.

Later in your treatment, evaluate your progress:

- Are you being helped by the treatment?

- If you are displeased, is it because you aren't making progress, or because therapy is raising difficult, painful issues you don't want to deal with?

- Can you express dissatisfaction to your therapist? Such feedback can improve your treatment.

The most important predictor of whether your therapy will be helpful is how much rapport you feel with your therapist *at the first session*. This has been shown to be true no matter what model of psychotherapy the therapist is practicing. You have to like your therapist and feel that she or he will be able to help you—if you do, there's a good chance that it will be helpful. If you sense that your therapy isn't working or is actually harmful, thank your therapist for her or his efforts, and find another. It's extra work for you, but it's important for your health.

person can bring relief. Comparing notes with people who have problems similar to yours can give you new ideas about coping.

Many colleges offer peer counseling through a health center or through the psychology or education department. Volunteer students specially trained in maintaining confidentiality are usually those who offer counsel. They may steer you toward an appropriate campus or community resource or simply offer a sympathetic ear.

Many self-help groups work on the principle of bringing together people with similar problems to share their experiences and support one another. Support groups are typically organized around a specific problem, such as eating disorders or substance abuse. Self-help groups may be listed online or in the campus newspaper.

Professional Help

Sometimes trying self-help or talking to nonprofessionals is not enough, especially if you might have a mental illness. Overcoming the stigma about seeking help is a first step. In many communities and cultures, great shame and stigma are associated with talking to a mental health professional; in others, there is much less. You may someday find yourself having to overcome your own reluctance, or that of a friend, about seeking help.

A person has many options when seeking professional help (see the box "Choosing and Evaluating Mental Health Professionals"). For students, the student health center is a great start. The professionals there have extensive experience evaluating and working with people who have all sorts of needs, from the stress of adjusting to college life and dealing with relationships, to severe mental illnesses. Pediatricians and primary care providers can also make referrals.

Many kinds of professionals are trained to evaluate people's psychological and psychiatric needs and to provide treatment. Psychotherapists, for example, come from a variety of backgrounds and include licensed social workers or family and marital therapists (with master's degrees); specially trained nurses with advanced degrees; psychologists (with doctorates); and psychiatrists, who have medical degrees and thus can prescribe medication.

Many national organizations have websites that may be useful in finding help. Here are some examples:

Anxiety and Depression Association of America—adaa.org

Depression and Bipolar Support Alliance—dbsalliance.org

National Alliance on Mental Illness—nami.org

National Association of Social Workers—socialworkers.org

American Psychological Association—apa.org

American Psychiatric Association—psychiatry.org

Professional help is appropriate in any of the following situations:

- Depression, anxiety, or other emotional problems interfere seriously with school or work performance or in getting along with others.

TIPS FOR TODAY AND THE FUTURE

Most of life's psychological challenges can be met with self-help and everyday skills. You can take many steps to maintain your mental health.

RIGHT NOW YOU CAN:

- Take a serious look at how you've felt recently. If you have any feelings that are especially hard to handle, consider how you can get help with them.
- Think of the way in which you are most creative (an important part of self-actualization), whether it's in music, art, or whatever you enjoy. Try to focus at least an hour each week on this activity.
- Review the list of defense mechanisms in Table 3.1. Have you used any of them recently or consistently over time? Think of a situation in which you used one of those mechanisms and determine how you could have coped with it differently.

IN THE FUTURE YOU CAN:

- Write 100 positive adjectives that describe you. This exercise may take several days to complete. Post your list in a place where you will see it often.
- Record your reactions to upsetting events in your life. Are your reactions and self-talk typically negative or neutral? Decide whether you are satisfied with your reactions and if they are healthy.

- Suicide is attempted or is seriously considered (see the warning signs listed earlier in the chapter).
- Symptoms such as hallucinations, delusions, incoherent speech, or loss of memory occur.
- Alcohol or drugs are used to the extent that they impair normal functioning during much of the week, that finding or taking drugs occupies much of the week, or that reducing their dosage leads to psychological or physiological withdrawal symptoms.

SUMMARY

- Psychological health refers to the extent to which we are able to function optimally in the face of challenges, whether we have a mental illness or not.

- Maslow's definition of psychological health centers on self-actualization, the highest level in his hierarchy of needs. Self-actualized people have high self-esteem and are realistic, inner directed, authentic, capable of emotional intimacy, and creative.

- Psychological health encompasses more than a single particular state of normality. Psychological diversity—the understanding, acceptance, and respect for how much individuals differ in psychological terms—is valuable among groups of people.

- Crucial parts of psychological wellness include developing an adult identity, establishing intimate relationships, and developing values and purpose in life.

- A sense of self-esteem develops during childhood as a result of giving and receiving love and learning to accomplish goals. Self-concept is challenged every day; healthy people adjust their goals to their abilities.

- Using defense mechanisms to cope with problems can make finding solutions harder. Analyzing thoughts and behavior can help people develop less defensive and more effective ways of coping.

- A pessimistic outlook can be damaging; it can be overcome by developing more realistic self-talk.

- Honest communication requires recognizing what needs to be said and saying it clearly. Assertiveness enables people to insist on their rights and to participate in the give-and-take of good communication.

- People may be lonely if they haven't developed ways to be happy on their own or if they interpret being alone as a sign of rejection. Lonely people can take action to expand their social contacts.

- Dealing successfully with anger involves distinguishing between a reasonable level of assertiveness and gratuitous expressions of anger; heading off rage by reframing thoughts and distracting yourself; and responding to the anger of others with an asymmetrical, problem-solving orientation.

- Some people with psychological disorders have symptoms severe enough to interfere with daily living.

- Anxiety is a fear that is not directed toward any definite threat. Anxiety disorders include simple phobias, social phobias, panic disorder, generalized anxiety disorder, obsessive-compulsive disorder, and posttraumatic stress disorder.

- Depression is a common mood disorder in which a person experiences loss of interest or pleasure in things (anhedonia) in combination with at least four other symptoms. Severe depression carries a high risk of suicide, and suicidal depressed people need professional help.

- Symptoms of mania include abnormally elevated moods or abnormal irritability with unrealistically high self-esteem, little need for sleep, and rapid speech. Mood swings between mania and depression characterize bipolar disorder.

- Schizophrenia is characterized by disorganized thoughts, inappropriate emotions, delusions, auditory hallucinations, and deteriorating social and work performance.

- The biological model emphasizes that the mind's activity depends on the brain, whose composition is genetically determined. Therapy based on the biological model is primarily pharmacological.

- The behavioral model focuses on overt behavior and treats psychological problems as bad habits. Behavior change is the focus of therapy.

- The cognitive model considers how ideas affect behavior and feelings; behavior results from complicated attitudes, expectations, and motives, not just from simple reinforcements. Cognitive therapy focuses on changing a person's thinking.

- The psychodynamic model asserts that false ideas are fed by unconscious ideas and cannot be addressed directly. In psychodynamic therapy, patients speak as freely as possible in front of the therapist and try to gain an understanding of the basis of their feelings toward the therapist and others.

- Help is available in a variety of forms, including self-help, peer counseling, support groups, and therapy with a mental health professional.

FOR MORE INFORMATION

American Association of Suicidology. Provides information about suicide and resources for people in crisis.

http://www.suicidology.org

Anxiety and Depression Association of America (ADAA). Provides information and resources related to anxiety disorders and depression.

http://www.adaa.org

Cope, Care, Deal. Offers information on mental health issues specifically for teens.

http://www.annenbergpublicpolicycenter.org/ahrci/
     copecaredeal-org/

Depression and Bipolar Support Alliance (DBSA). Provides educational materials and information about support groups.

http://www.dbsalliance.org

Mental Health America. Provides consumer information on a variety of issues, including how to find help.

http://www.mentalhealthamerica.net

NAMI (National Alliance on Mental Illness). Provides information and support for people affected by mental illness.

800-950-NAMI (help line)

http://www.nami.org

National Hopeline Network. 24-hour hotline for people who are thinking about suicide or know someone who is; calls are routed to local crisis centers.

800-442-HOPE

800-SUICIDE

http://www.hopeline.com

National Institute of Mental Health (NIMH). Provides helpful information about anxiety, depression, eating disorders, and other challenges to psychological health.

http://www.nimh.nih.gov

Substance Abuse and Mental Health Services Administration. A one-stop source for information and resources relating to mental health.

http://samhsa.gov

U.S. Food and Drug Administration. Provides access to Medication Guides, which are paper handouts that come with many prescription drugs.

http://www.fda.gov/Drugs/DrugSafety/ucm085729.htm

SELECTED BIBLIOGRAPHY

Ahmedani, Brian K. 2015. "Racial/Ethnic Differences in Health Care Visits Made Before Suicide Attempt across the United States." *Medical Care* 53(5): 430–435.

American Psychiatric Association. 2013. *Diagnostic and Statistical Manual of Mental Disorders (DSM-5),* 5th ed. Washington, DC: American Psychiatric Publishing.

American Psychiatric Association. 2015. *Mental Health* (http://www.psychiatry.org/patients-families/what-is-mental-illness).

Asselmann, E., et al. 2016. Risk factors for fearful spells, panic attacks and panic disorder in a community cohort of adolescents and young adults. *Journal of Affective Disorders* 193: 305–308.

Banks, M. V., and K. Salmon. 2013. Reasoning about the self in positive and negative ways: Relationship to psychological functioning in young adulthood. *Memory* 21(1): 10–26.

Beard, C., et al. 2010. Health-related quality of life across the anxiety disorders: Findings from a sample of primary care patients. *Journal of Anxiety Disorders* 24(6): 559–564.

Bureau of Labor Statistics, U.S. Department of Labor, Occupational Outlook Handbook, 2016–17 Edition (http://www.bls.gov/ooh).

Carver, C. S., M. F. Scheier, and S. C. Segerstrom. 2010. Optimism. *Clinical Psychology Review* 30(7): 879–889.

Cawood, C. D., and S. K. Huprich. 2011. Late adolescent nonsuicidal self-injury: The roles of coping style, self-esteem, and personality pathology. *Journal of Personality Disorders* 25(6): 765–781.

Centers for Disease Control and Prevention. 2010. Attitudes toward Mental Illness—35 States, District of Columbia, and Puerto Rico, 2007. *Morbidity and Mortality Weekly Report* 59(20): 619–625.

Ferrier-Auerback, A. G., et al. 2010. Predictors of emotional distress reported by soldiers in the combat zone. *Journal of Psychiatric Research* 44(7): 470–476.

Greenhoot, A. F., et al. 2013. Making sense of traumatic memories: Memory qualities and psychological symptoms in emerging adults with and without abuse histories. *Memory* 21(1): 125–142.

Hayes, Steven. n.d. *Acceptance & Commitment Therapy (ACT).* (http://contextualscience.org/about_act).

Kirov, G. G., et al. 2016. Evaluation of cumulative cognitive deficits from electroconvulsive therapy. *British Journal of Psychiatry* 208(3): 266–270.

Klein, D. N., et al. 2013. Predictors of first lifetime onset of major depressive disorder in young adulthood. *Journal of Abnormal Psychology* 122(1): 1–6.

Kochanek, K. D., et al. 2016. Deaths: Final data for 2014. *National Vital Statistics Reports* 65(4).

Lin, Y. R., et al. 2008. Evaluation of assertiveness training for psychiatric patients. *Journal of Clinical Nursing* 17(21): 2875–2883.

National Institute of Mental Health. 2016. *Social Phobia (Social Anxiety Disorder)* (http://www.nimh.nih.gov/health/topics/social-phobia-social-anxiety-disorder/index.shtml).

National Institute of Mental Health. 2015. Prevalence: Any Mental Illness (AMI) Among U.S. Adults (http://www.nimh.nih.gov/health/statistics/prevalence/any-mental-illness-ami-among-us-adults.shtml).

National Institute of Mental Health. 2014. *Depression* (http://www.nimh.nih.gov/health/topics/depression/index.shtml?utm_source=BrainLine.orgutm_medium=Twitter).

Oldis, M., et al. 2016. Trajectory and predictors of quality of life in first episode psychotic mania. *Journal of Affective Disorders* 195: 148–155.

Penn State Center for Collegiate Mental Health. 2016. *2015 Annual Report on Student Counseling Centers.* (Publication No. STA 15–108).

Pozzi, M., et al. 2016. Antidepressants and, suicide and self-injury: Causal or casual association? *International Journal of Psychiatry in Clinical Practice* 20(1): 47–51.

Rickwood, D., and S. Bradford. 2012. The role of self-help in the treatment of mild anxiety disorders in young people: An evidence-based review. *Psychology Research and Behavior Management* 5: 25–36.

Rosenthal, B. S., and W. C. Wilson. 2012. Race/ethnicity and mental health in the first decade of the 21st century. *Psychological Reports* 110(2): 645–662.

Seligman, M. E. P. 2008. Positive health. *Applied Psychology: An International Review* 57, 3–18.

Simon, G. 2009. Collaborative care for mood disorders. *Current Opinion in Psychiatry* 22(1): 37–41.

Singh, N. N., et al. 2007. Individuals with mental illness can control their aggressive behavior through mindfulness training. *Behavior Modification* 31(3): 313–328.

Soeteman, D., M. Miller, and J. J. Kim. 2012. Modeling the risks and benefits of depression treatment for children and young adults. *Value in Health* 15(5): 724–729.

Thurber, C. A., and E. A. Walton. 2012. Homesickness and adjustment in university students. *Journal of American College Health* 60(5): 415–419.

Turner, B. J., A. L. Chapman, and B. K. Layden. 2012. Intrapersonal and interpersonal functions of nonsuicidal self-injury: Associations with emotional and social functioning. *Suicide & Life-Threatening Behavior* 42(1): 36–55.

U.S. Department of Health and Human Services. 2014. Results from the 2013 National Survey on Drug Use and Health: Mental Health Findings. Substance Abuse and Mental Health Services Administration. Rockville, MD: Center for Behavioral Health Statistics and Quality.

U.S. Department of Veterans Affairs. 2015. How Common Is PTSD? (http://www.ptsd.va.gov/public/PTSD-overview/basics/how-common-is-ptsd.asp).

Williams, D., et al. 2007. Prevalence and distribution of major depressive disorder in African Americans, Caribbean blacks, and non-Hispanic whites. *Archives of General Psychiatry* 64: 305–315.

BEHAVIOR CHANGE STRATEGY
Dealing with Social Anxiety

Shyness is often the result of both high anxiety levels and lack of key social skills. To help overcome shyness, you need to learn to manage your fear of social situations and to develop social skills such as making appropriate eye contact, initiating topics in conversations, and maintaining the flow of conversations by asking questions and making appropriate responses.

As described in the chapter, repeated *exposure* to the source of your fear—in this case, social situations—is the best method for reducing anxiety. When you practice new behaviors, they gradually become easier and you experience less anxiety.

A counterproductive strategy is avoiding situations that make you anxious. Although this approach works in the short term—you eliminate your anxiety because you escape the situation—it keeps you from meeting new people and having new experiences. Another counterproductive strategy is to self-medicate with alcohol or drugs. Being under their influence actually prevents you from learning new social skills and new ways to handle your anxiety.

To reduce your anxiety in social situations, try some of the following strategies:

- Remember that physical stress reactions are short-term responses to fear. Don't dwell on them. Remind yourself that they will pass, and they will.

- Refocus your attention away from the stress reaction you're experiencing and toward the social task at hand. Your nervousness is much less visible than you think.

- Allow a warm-up period for new situations. Realize that you will feel more nervous at first, and take steps to relax and become more comfortable. Refer to the suggestions for deep breathing and other relaxation techniques in Chapter 2.

- If possible, take breaks during anxiety-producing situations. For example, if you're at a party, take a moment to visit the restroom or step outside. Alternate between speaking with good friends and striking up conversations with new acquaintances.

- Watch your interpretations. Having a stress reaction doesn't mean that you don't belong in the group, that you're unattractive or unworthy, or that the situation is too much for you. Think of yourself as excited or highly alert instead of anxious.

- Avoid cognitive distortions and practice realistic self-talk. Replace your self-critical thoughts with more supportive ones, such as "No one else is perfect, and I don't have to be either" or "It would have been good if I had a funny story to tell, but the conversation was interesting anyway."

- Give yourself a reality check: Ask if you're really in a life-threatening situation (or just at a party), if the outcome you're imagining is really likely (or the worst thing that could possibly happen), or if you're the only one who feels nervous (or if many other people might feel the same way).

- Don't think of conversations as evaluations. Remind yourself that you don't have to prove yourself with every social interaction. And remember that most people are thinking more about themselves than they are about you.

Starting and maintaining conversations can be difficult for shy people, who may feel overwhelmed by their physical stress reactions. If small talk is a problem for you, try the following strategies:

- Introduce yourself early in the conversation. If you tend to forget names, repeat your new acquaintance's name to help fix it in your mind ("Nice to meet you, Amelia").

- Ask questions and look for shared topics of interest. Simple, open-ended questions like "How's your presentation coming along?" or "How do you know our host?" encourage others to carry the conversation for a while and help bring up a variety of subjects.

- Take turns talking, and elaborate on your answers. Simple yes and no answers don't move the conversation along. Try to relate something in your life—a course you're taking or a hobby you have—to something in the other person's life. Match self-disclosure with self-disclosure.

- Have something to say. Expand your mind and become knowledgeable about current events and local or campus news. If you have specialized knowledge about a topic, practice discussing it in ways that both beginners and experts can understand and appreciate.

- If you get stuck for something to say, try giving a compliment ("Great presentation!" or "I love your earrings.") or performing a social grace (pass the chips or get someone a drink).

- Be an attentive listener. Reward the other person with your full attention and with regular responses. Make frequent eye contact and maintain a relaxed but alert posture. (See Chapter 4 for more on being an effective listener.)

- At first, your new behaviors will likely make you anxious. Don't give up—things *will* get easier.

SOURCES: Aron, E. 2010. *The Undervalued Self.* New York: Little, Brown; Brown, B. 2010. *The Gifts of Imperfection: Let Go of Who You Think You're Supposed to Be and Embrace Who You Are. Your Guide to a Wholehearted Life.* Center City, MN: Hazelden.

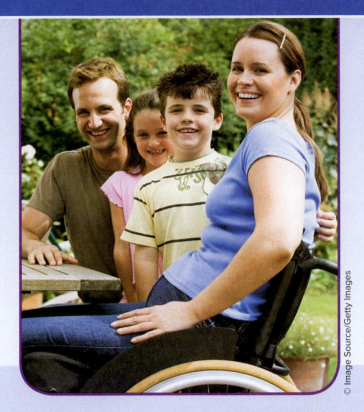

© Image Source/Getty Images

CHAPTER 4

Intimate Relationships and Communication

CHAPTER OBJECTIVES

- Explain the qualities that help people develop intimate relationships
- Explain elements of healthy and productive communication
- Describe types of love relationships as well as singlehood
- Discuss the benefits and challenges of marriage
- Describe challenges and rewards of family life

Human beings need social relationships; we cannot thrive as solitary creatures. Our survival as a species relies on our ability to cherish and support each other, form strong mutual attachments with each other, and create families in which to raise children. Simply put, people need people.

Although we are held together in relationships by a variety of factors, the foundation of many relationships is the ability to both give and receive love. Love in its many forms—romantic, passionate, platonic, parental—is the wellspring from which much of life's meaning and delight flows. In our human culture, love binds us together as partners, parents, children, and friends.

DEVELOPING INTIMATE RELATIONSHIPS

Successful intimate relationships depend on a belief in ourselves and the people around us. We must be willing to share our ideas, feelings, time, and needs and to accept what others want to give us in return. Just as important is the relationship we develop with ourselves—that is, how we generally feel about ourselves, which is the principal element that we bring to all our relationships. What does it mean to have a healthy relationship with oneself?

Self-Concept, Self-Esteem, and Self-Acceptance

To have successful relationships, we must first accept and feel good about ourselves. Having a healthy relationship with yourself means being able to self-soothe, regulate your emotions, and feel comfortable with your own company. The factors that contribute to a healthy sense of self include a positive *self-concept* (how you perceive your self), a healthy level of *self-esteem* (how you feel about your self), and an affirmative *self-acceptance* (how you value your self). Each of these factors allows us to love and respect others.

As discussed in Chapter 3, the roots of our identity and sense of self can be found in childhood, in the relationships we had with our caregivers. As adults, we are more likely to have a sense that we are basically lovable, and to view ourselves as worthwhile people who can trust others, if we had the following experiences as babies and children:

- We felt loved, valued, accepted, and respected.
- Adults responded to our needs in appropriate ways.
- Adults gave us the freedom to play, explore, and develop a sense of being separate individuals.

These conditions not only encourage us to develop a positive self-concept and healthy self-acceptance, but they also contribute to a basic self-confidence that helps us navigate life's inevitable challenges.

Gender Role and Communication   We also learn in early childhood how to take on a **gender role**—the activities, abilities, and characteristics deemed culturally appropriate for us based on our sex. From almost day one of our lives, we receive messages about how a boy versus a girl, or a man versus a woman, should act. As will be discussed in detail in Chapter 5, sex and gender are not the same thing, and the gender and gender role assigned by one's culture may not match one's own internal sense of being male or female—that is, one's gender identity.

Cultural expectations associated with traditional gender roles for men prescribed that they provide for their families; assume aggressive, competitive, and power-oriented behaviors; and solve problems logically. Women were expected to take care of home and children; be cooperative, supportive, and nurturing; and approach life emotionally and intuitively.

As transgender and feminist movements have progressed, and women have entered more positions of power, expectations have also changed. It is now common for women to work outside the home and for men to participate more actively in parenting. Studies have shown that girls do not necessarily play cooperatively, and that gender behaviors that previously seemed so ingrained can be changed depending on the messages children receive from caregivers, mass media, and other institutions.

You may have heard that men and women speak different languages, and that this difference lies behind many conflicts. But do men speak in a more logical way and women in a more emotional way? Although we can find differing patterns in the language of some men and some women, this observation does not fit the data of many studies on gendered communication. There is no gene for gendered language. We learn how to speak just as we learn how to become men and women, and we can decide how we want to communicate based on any particular situation.

Still, don't we observe differences in the way men and women communicate? Yes, there are some patterns among certain *groups* of women, men, girls, and boys, and not because of hardwiring but because we (sometimes unconsciously) follow cultural norms. For example, sociolinguist Penny Eckert finds that in early adolescence, girls start using their voices so that in one moment they speak in a very low pitch and in the next a very high one. Boys, by contrast, decrease their range in pitch, sounding relatively monotone.

These changes represent ways that girls and boys differentiate themselves, preparing to participate in what Eckert calls a heterosexual market. They speak differently so as to fit in socially and to anticipate finding a mate.

Attachment   Another thing we learn in childhood is how to relate to others. Psychologists have suggested that our adult styles of loving may be based on the type of **attachment** we established in infancy with our mother, father, siblings, or other primary caregivers. According to this view, people who are secure in their intimate relationships as adults probably had a secure, trusting, mutually satisfying attachment to their mother, father, or other parenting figure. Securely attached people find it relatively easy to get close to others, and don't worry excessively about being abandoned or having someone get too close to them. They feel that other people accept them and are generally well intentioned.

People who run from relationships may have experienced an "anxious/avoidant" attachment as children. In this type of attachment, a parent's responses were either engulfing or abandoning. Anxious/avoidant adults feel uncomfortable being close to others and seek escape from another's control. They're distrustful and fearful of becoming dependent on and intimate with their partners.

Individuals who endured distant and aloof attachments as children can still establish satisfying relationships later in life. In fact, relationships established during adolescence and adulthood give us the opportunity to work through unresolved issues and conflicts. Human beings can be resilient and flexible. We have the capacity to change our ideas, beliefs, and behaviors. We can learn ways to raise our self-esteem and become more trusting, accepting, and appreciative of others and ourselves. We can acquire the communication and conflict resolution skills needed to maintain successful relationships. Although it helps to have a good start in life, it may be even more important to begin again, right from where you are.

Friendship

Friendships are the first relationships we form outside the family. The friendships we form in childhood are an important part of our growth. Through them, we learn about tolerance, sharing, and trust. Friendships usually include the following characteristics:

- *Companionship is the good feeling you have when you're with someone else.* Friends are usually relaxed and

> **TERMS**
>
> **gender role**   The activities, abilities, and characteristics deemed culturally appropriate for us based on our sex.
>
> **attachment**   The emotional tie between an infant and his or her caregiver or between two people in an intimate relationship.

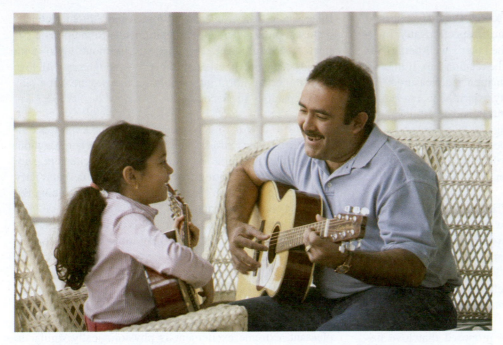

The type and strength of our attachment to our caregivers can affect other relationships throughout our lives.
© Ariel Skelley/Blend Images LLC RF

• **Reciprocity.** Friendships are reciprocal. There is give-and-take between friends and the feeling that both share joys and burdens more or less equally.

Intimate partnerships are like friendships in many ways, but they have additional characteristics. These relationships usually include sexual desire and expression, a greater demand for exclusiveness, and deeper levels of caring. Friendships may be more stable and longer lasting than intimate partnerships. Friends are often more accepting and less critical than lovers, perhaps because their expectations differ. Like love relationships, friendships bind society together, providing people with emotional support and buffering them from stress.

happy when they're together. They typically share common values and interests and plan to spend time together. Real friends can also be tense and unhappy with each other. Even on bad days, we support our friends as we would want them to support us.

• **Respect.** Friends have a basic respect for each other's individuality. Good friends respect each other's feelings and opinions and work to resolve their differences without demeaning or insulting each other. They also show their respect by expressing honest feelings.

• **Acceptance.** Friends accept each other "warts and all." They feel free to be themselves and express their feelings without fear of ridicule or criticism.

• **Help.** Friends know they can rely on each other in times of need. Help may include sharing time, energy, and even material goods.

• **Trust.** Friends are secure in the knowledge that they will not intentionally hurt each other. They feel safe confiding in one another.

• **Loyalty.** Friends can count on one another. In moments of challenge, a friend will stand up for his or her partner rather than join the opposition.

• **Mutuality.** Friends retain their individual identities, but close friendships are characterized by a sense of mutuality—"what affects you affects me." Friends share the ups and downs in each other's lives.

Love, Sex, and Intimacy

Love is one of the most basic and profound human emotions. It is a powerful force in all our intimate relationships. Love encompasses opposites: affection and anger, excitement and boredom, stability and change, bonds and freedom. Love does not give us perfect happiness, but it can give us more meaning in our lives.

In many kinds of adult relationships, love is closely affected by sexuality. In the past, marriage was considered the only acceptable context for sexual activities, but for many people today, sex is legitimized by love. According to Gallup and other surveys, the proportion of adults who view sex between an unmarried man and woman as morally acceptable increased from 29% in 1972 to 67% in 2016. Many couples, gay and straight, live together in committed relationships, and many Americans now use personal standards rather than social norms to make decisions about sex. Shifts in cultural attitudes related to sex and marriage can happen slowly or quickly. The most rapid recent change, according to Gallup surveys, has been in Americans' attitudes toward same-sex marriage: between 2005 and 2016, acceptance rose from 37% to 61%.

Many people, however, worry about this trend and the bypassing of traditional norms and values. They fear that the prevailing attitude about sexuality has resulted in a greater emphasis on sex over love and a permissiveness that has undermined the commitment needed to make a loving relationship work.

For most people, love, sex, and commitment are closely linked. Love reflects the

QUICK STATS

The number of people aged 18–29 who are single and not living with a partner rose from 52% in 2004 to 64% in 2014.
—Gallup surveys, 2015

positive factors that draw people together and sustain their relationship. It includes trust, caring, respect, loyalty, interest in the other, and concern for the other's well-being. Sex brings excitement and passion to the relationship. It intensifies the relationship and adds fascination and pleasure.

Commitment contributes stability, which helps maintain a relationship. Responsibility, reliability, and faithfulness are characteristics of commitment. Although love, sex, and commitment are related, they are not necessarily connected. One can exist without the others. Despite the various "faces" of love, sex, and commitment, many of us long for a special relationship that contains them all.

Other elements can be identified as features of love, such as euphoria, preoccupation with the loved one, idealization or devaluation of the loved one, and so on, but these elements tend to be temporary. These characteristics may include **infatuation,** which will fade or deepen into something more substantial. As relationships progress, the central aspects of love and commitment take on more importance.

Psychologist Robert Sternberg proposed that love has three dimensions: intimacy, passion, and a commitment component (Figure 4.1). *Intimacy* refers to feelings of attachment, closeness, connectedness, and bondedness. *Passion* encompasses motivational drives and sexual attraction. *Commitment* relates to the decision to remain together with the ultimate goal of making long-term plans with that person. The amount of love one experiences depends on the absolute strength of each of the three components and on the strengths relative to each other.

Different stages and types of love can be understood as different combinations of the three dimensions. Ultimately a relationship based on a single element is less likely to survive than is one based on two or three dimensions.

Researchers suggest that gender plays a role in the relationship between love (intimacy) and sex (passion). Although many men report that their most erotic sexual experiences occur in the context of a love relationship, many studies have found that men separate love from sex more easily than women do. Women more often view sex from the point of view of a relationship. Some people believe you can have satisfying sex without love—with friends, acquaintances, or strangers. Although sex with love is an important norm in our culture, the two are often pursued separately in practice.

The Pleasure and Pain of Love   The experience of intense love has confused and tormented lovers throughout history. They live in a tumultuous state of excitement, subject to wildly fluctuating feelings of joy and despair. They lose their appetite, can't sleep, and can think of nothing but the loved one. Is this happiness? Misery? Both?

The contradictory nature of passionate love can be understood by recognizing that human emotions have two components: physiological arousal and an emotional explanation for the arousal. Love is just one of many emotions accompanied by physiological arousal. Many unpleasant emotions can also generate arousal, such as fear, rejection, and frustration. Although experiences like attraction and sexual desire are pleasant, extreme excitement is physiologically similar to fear and can be unpleasant. For this reason, passionate love may be too intense for some people to enjoy. Over time, the physical intensity and excitement tend to diminish. When this happens, pleasure may actually increase.

The Transformation of Love   Human relationships change over time, and love relationships are no exception. At first, love is likely to be characterized by high levels of passion and rapidly increasing intimacy. After a while, passion decreases as we become habituated to it and to the person. The diminishing of romance or passionate love can be experienced as a crisis in a relationship. If a more lasting love fails to emerge, the relationship will likely break up.

Unlike passion, however, commitment does not necessarily diminish over time. When intensity diminishes, partners often discover a more enduring love. They can now move from absorption in each other to a relationship that includes external goals and projects, friends, and family. In this kind of intimate, more secure love, satisfaction comes not just from the relationship itself but also from achieving other creative goals, such as work or child rearing. The key to successful relationships is in transforming passion into an intimate love based on closeness, caring, and the promise of a shared future.

Challenges in Relationships

Many people believe that love naturally makes an intimate relationship easy to begin and maintain, but in fact obstacles arise and challenges occur. Even in the best of circumstances, a loving relationship will be tested. Partners enter a relationship

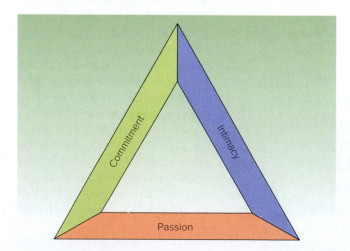

FIGURE 4.1   The triangular theory of love.

infatuation   An idealizing, obsessive attraction, characterized by a high degree of physical arousal.   **TERMS**

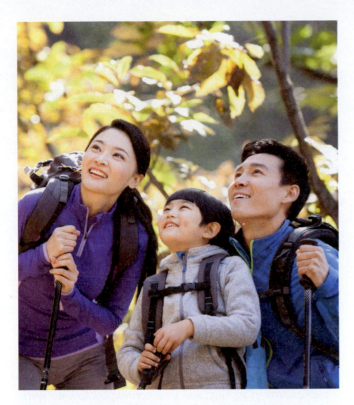

Although passion and physical intimacy often decline with time, other aspects of a relationship—such as commitment—tend to grow as the relationship matures.

© Lane Oatey/Blue Jean Images/Getty Images

with diverse needs and desires, some of which emerge only at times of change or stress. Common relationship challenges relate to self-disclosure, commitment, expectations, competitiveness, and jealousy.

Honesty and Openness   At the beginning of a relationship most of us prefer to present ourselves in the most favorable light. Although sharing thoughts and feelings can be emotionally risky, honesty is necessary to achieve the freedom for the next step of the relationship. Over time, you and your partner will learn more about each other and feel more comfortable sharing. In fact, intimate familiarity with your partner's life is a key characteristic of successful long-term relationships.

Emotional Intelligence   In his book *Emotional Intelligence—Why It Can Matter More Than IQ,* Daniel Goleman argues that classical IQ is *not* destiny and that our traditional view of intelligence is too narrow. He asserts that the traditional view ignores a range of abilities vital to how well we function in life. Goleman illuminates the factors at work when people with high IQs flounder and those with modest IQs do remarkably well. These factors include self-awareness, self-discipline, and empathy, and they add up to a different way of being intelligent, known as "emotionally intelligent."

Psychologists Peter Salovey and John D. Mayer define emotional intelligence as "the subset of social intelligence that involves the ability to monitor one's own and others' feelings and emotions, to discriminate among them and to use this information to guide one's thinking and actions." The key to developing emotional intelligence lies in cultivating the overarching skill of mindfulness—the ability to dispassionately observe thoughts and feelings as they occur (see Chapter 2). When we are able to note and observe emotions without judging them or immediately acting on them, we can make more measured, wise, and skillful responses. These skills can be particularly helpful when we are involved in an argument or a conflict with someone with whom we have a close relationship.

Mindfulness can be cultivated by paying more attention to the operation of our minds, slowing down our lives enough to make more detailed observations, and staying in the moment as we go about our day-to-day activities. Although we often have limited control over external events, we have a great deal of ability to discipline, focus, and train our minds. Practicing mindfulness and developing emotional intelligence will improve your sense of self and the quality of your relationships, and may even result in the peace of mind that many people find so elusive.

Unequal or Premature Commitment   When one person in an intimate partnership becomes more serious about the relationship than the other, it can be difficult to maintain it without someone feeling hurt. Sometimes a couple makes a premature commitment, and then one of the partners has second thoughts and wants to break off the relationship. Eventually both partners recognize that something is wrong, but each is afraid to tell the other. It may be painful but necessary to resolve this conflict by stepping up and saying, "We have a problem. Can we have an honest talk about it?" Such problems usually can be resolved only by honest and sensitive communication.

Unrealistic Expectations   Each partner brings hopes and expectations to a relationship, some of which may be unrealistic, unfair, and ultimately damaging to the relationship. These include the following:

• Expecting your partner to change.

• Assuming that your partner has all the same opinions, priorities, interests, and goals as you.

• Believing that a relationship will fulfill all of your personal, financial, intellectual, and social needs.

Competitiveness   Games and competitive sports add flavor to the bonding process—as long as the focus is on fun. If one partner always feels compelled to compete and win, it can detract from the sense of connectedness, interdependence, equality, and mutuality between partners. The same can be said for a perfectionistic need to be right in every instance—to "win" every argument.

If competitiveness is a problem for you, ask yourself if your need to win is more important than your partner's feelings or

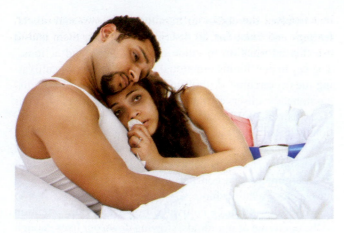

Supportiveness is a sign of commitment and compassion and is an important part of any healthy relationship.

© Justin Horrocks/Getty Images

the future of your relationship. Try noncompetitive activities or an activity where you are a beginner and your partner excels. Accept that your partner's views may be just as valid and important to your partner as your own views are to you.

Balancing Time Together and Apart   You may enjoy time together with your partner, but you may also want to spend time alone or with other friends. If you or your partner interpret time apart as rejection or lack of commitment, it can damage the relationship. Talk with your partner about what time apart means and share your feelings about what you expect from the relationship in terms of time together. Consider your partner's feelings carefully, and try to reach a compromise that satisfies both of you.

Differences in expectations about time spent together can mirror differences in ideas about emotional closeness. Any romantic relationship involves giving up some degree of autonomy in order to develop an identity as a couple. But remember that every person is unique and has different needs for distance and closeness in a relationship.

Jealousy   Jealousy is the angry, painful response to a partner's real, imagined, or possible involvement with a third person. Some people think that the existence of jealousy proves the existence of love, but jealousy is actually a sign of insecurity or possessiveness.

In its irrational and extreme forms, jealousy can destroy a relationship by its insistent demands and attempts at control. Jealousy is a factor in precipitating violence in dating relationships among both high school and college students, and abusive spouses often use jealousy to justify their violence. (Problems with control and violence in relationships are discussed in Chapter 16.)

People with a healthy level of self-esteem are less likely to feel jealous. When jealousy occurs in a relationship, it's important for the partners to communicate clearly with each other about their feelings. In this sense, jealousy can offer partners the chance to look closely at issues like possessiveness,

insecurity, and low self-esteem and thereby strengthen the relationship by working through jealousy.

Supportiveness   Another key to successful relationships is the ability to ask for and give support. Partners need to know that they can count on each other during difficult times.

Unhealthy Relationships

Everyone should be able to recognize when a relationship is unhealthy. Relatively extreme examples of unhealthy relationships are those that are physically or emotionally abusive or that involve codependency.

Even relationships that are not abusive or codependent can still be unhealthy. If your relationship lacks love and respect and places little value on the time you and your partner have spent together, it may be time to get professional help or to end the partnership. Further, if your relationship is characterized by communication styles that include criticism, contempt, defensiveness, and withdrawal—despite real efforts to repair these destructive patterns—the relationship may not be salvageable.

Spiritual leaders suggest that relationships are unhealthy when you feel that your sense of spontaneity, your potential for inner growth and joy, and your connection to your spiritual life are deadened. There are negative physical and mental consequences of being in an unhappy relationship. Although breaking up is painful and difficult, it is ultimately better than living in a toxic relationship.

Ending a Relationship

Even when a couple starts out with the best of intentions, an intimate relationship may not last. Some breakups occur quickly following direct action by one or both partners, but many occur over an extended period as the couple goes through a cycle of separating and reconciling.

Ending an intimate relationship is usually difficult and painful. Both partners may feel attacked and abandoned, but feelings of distress are likely to be more acute for the rejected partner. If you are involved in a breakup, the following suggestions may help make the ending easier:

• Give the relationship a fair chance before breaking up.

• Be fair and honest.

• Be tactful and compassionate.

• If you are the rejected person, give yourself time to resolve your anger and pain.

• Recognize the value in the experience.

Use the recovery period following a breakup for self-renewal. Redirect more of your attention to yourself, and reconnect with people and areas of your life that may have been neglected as a result of the relationship. Time will help heal the pain of the loss of the relationship.

Finally, be aware of the tendency or impulse to "rebound" quickly into another relationship. Although a new relationship may mute the pain of a breakup, forming a relationship in order to avoid feeling pain is not a good strategy. Too often, rebound relationships fail because they were designed to be "lifeboats" or because one or both of the partners is not truly ready to be close to someone else again.

COMMUNICATION

The key to developing and maintaining any type of intimate relationship is good communication. Most of the time we don't think about communicating; we simply talk and behave naturally. But when problems arise—when we feel others don't understand us or when someone accuses us of not listening—we become aware of our limitations or, more commonly, what we think are other people's limitations. Miscommunication creates frustration and distances us from our friends and partners.

Nonverbal Communication

Even when we're silent, we're communicating. We send messages when we look at someone or look away, lean forward or sit back, smile or frown. Especially important forms of nonverbal communication are touch, eye contact, and proximity. If someone we're talking to touches our hand or arm, looks into our eyes, and leans toward us when we talk, we get the message that the person is interested in us and cares about what we're saying. If a person keeps looking around the room while we're talking or takes a step backward, we get the impression the person is uninterested or wants to end the conversation.

The ability to interpret nonverbal messages correctly is important to the success of relationships. It's also important, when sending messages, to make sure our body language agrees with our words. When our verbal and nonverbal messages don't correspond, we send a mixed message.

Attunement, or tuning in to each other's tone of voice, is important. More than any other cue, tone of voice conveys most accurately a person's emotional state. Our effectiveness at connecting or reconnecting emotionally with another depends on the accuracy of our attunement. Effective attunement recreates a healthy child-caregiver connection, or it provides a connection that was lacking during childhood.

How we feel when communicating with another can give the listener important data about the speaker. If "out of nowhere" we begin to feel sad, anxious, or angry, these may be emotional states the other person is communicating. An example would be feeling sad when communicating with a grieving friend.

Digital Communication and Our Social Networks

Social media enable us to communicate more rapidly, but some experts question whether this capability is undermining interpersonal relations generally and, specifically, our ability to relate to others in person. Some evidence suggests just the opposite is true: Surveys by the Pew Internet and American Life Project found that technology users had larger and more diverse discussion networks and were just as involved in their communities as people who communicate face-to-face. Many young adults (aged 18–29 years) who were in a serious relationship reported feeling closer to their spouse or partner due to online or text-message conversations. Some said they were able to resolve arguments that they couldn't face-to-face.

Social media tools afford wide-ranging types of communication. For example, the brief immediacy of a tweet is very different from an extended conversation over Skype. However, people often overlook these distinctions, and some observers worry about the effect of the technologies because they change the nature of the social environment and the size and makeup of social networks. Facebook, for example, facilitates relationships with people we have shared interests with but may never meet in person. These relationships are *achieved,* rather than *ascribed* to us, like the relationships with relatives and neighbors. Some people view these achieved relationships as weaker or less valuable than the ascribed ones, but these relationships do not necessarily take away from stronger ones.

The bottom line is that social media can be an advantage or a disadvantage, depending on how one uses them. For instance, social media allow for instant and easy communication with others across the globe. But such ease of communication also makes it easier to communicate impulsively, such as sending drunk or angry texts or messages, "Facebook-stalking" one's ex when feeling lonely, or sending flirtatious messages to someone new despite being in a monogamous relationship.

Using social media while avoiding their pitfalls means being mindful of how these technologies can influence communication and relationships. In addition to the capacity for impulsive communication, here are some other problem areas online:

• *Missing nonverbal cues such as body language and tone of voice.* A comment or joke intended as playful may instead come off as critical or harsh.

• *Promoting an idealized version of oneself.* Since we have control of our online image (to a degree), many of us promote a version that involves only the most flattering photos and happiest moments. Doing so can have a serious

Ask Yourself

QUESTIONS FOR CRITICAL THINKING AND REFLECTION

Have you ever ended an intimate relationship? If so, how did you handle it? How did you feel after the breakup? How do you think the breakup affected your former partner? Did the experience help you in other relationships?

downside if the gap between one's "real" and online lives becomes too large, or the pull to maintain this image becomes too consuming.

- **Spying.** In the past, people who suspected their partners of cheating had to follow them or hire detectives to see what they were doing. These days, it is as easy as checking statuses and messages, which makes it more tempting to invade a partner's privacy when feeling suspicious or insecure.

- **Checking one's phone rather than staying present.** How often have you seen a couple out at a nice restaurant, and both of them are checking their phones rather than engaging in conversation? Social media can be a great tool, but only when it doesn't replace experiencing life in the moment.

- **Publicizing more areas of one's life.** Messages, photos, and status updates are often accessible to large numbers of people, making it important to think carefully about what information to share on social media. Sometimes people in a relationship differ dramatically in their ideas about what should be public versus private, so this is an important topic for discussion.

Communication Skills

Three skills essential to good communication in relationships are self-disclosure, listening, and feedback:

- **Self-disclosure** involves revealing personal information that we ordinarily wouldn't reveal due to the risk involved. It usually increases feelings of closeness and moves the relationship to a deeper level of intimacy. Friends often disclose the most to each other, sharing feelings, experiences, hopes, and disappointments. Married couples sometimes share less and may make unwarranted assumptions because they think they already know everything about each other.

- **Listening** requires that we spend more time and energy trying to fully understand another person's "story" and less time judging, evaluating, blaming, advising, analyzing, or trying to control. Empathy, warmth, respect, and genuineness are qualities of skillful listeners. Attentive listening encourages friends or partners to share more and, in turn, to be attentive listeners. To connect with other people and develop real emotional intimacy, listening is essential.

- **Feedback,** a constructive response to another's self-disclosure, is the third key to good communication. Giving positive feedback means acknowledging that the friend's or partner's feelings are valid—no matter how upsetting or troubling—and offering self-disclosure in response. If, for example, your partner discloses unhappiness about your relationship, it is more constructive to say that you're concerned or saddened by that and want to hear more about it than to get angry,

blame, try to inflict pain, or withdraw. Self-disclosure and feedback can open the door to change, whereas other responses block communication and change. (For tips on improving your skills, see the box "Guidelines for Effective Communication.")

Conflict and Conflict Resolution

Conflict is natural in intimate relationships. No matter how close two people become, they still remain separate individuals with their own needs, desires, past experiences, and ways of seeing the world. In fact, the closer the relationship, the more differences and the more opportunities for conflict.

Conflict itself isn't dangerous to a relationship. In fact, it may indicate that the relationship is growing. But if it isn't handled constructively, conflict can damage—and ultimately destroy—the relationship. Consider the guidelines discussed here, but remember that different couples communicate in different ways around conflict.

Conflict is often accompanied by anger—a natural emotion—but one that can be difficult to handle. If we express anger aggressively, we risk creating distrust, fear, and distance. If we act out our anger without thinking things through, we can cause the conflict to escalate. If we suppress anger, it turns into resentment and hostility. The best way to handle anger in a relationship is to recognize it as a symptom of something that requires attention and needs to be addressed. When angry, partners should exercise restraint so as not to become abusive. It is important to express anger skillfully and not in a way that is out of proportion to the issue at hand. The best time to express yourself is almost certainly when you are not boiling over with strong emotions.

The sources of conflict for couples change over time but revolve primarily around these issues: finances, sex, children, in-laws, and housework. Although there are numerous

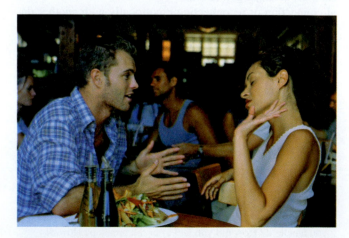

Conflict is an inevitable part of any intimate relationship. How can we resolve our conflicts in constructive ways?
© Photodisc/Getty Images RF

Getting Started

• When you want to have a serious discussion with your partner, choose a private place and a time when you won't be interrupted or rushed. Avoid having important conversations via text or other media.

• Face your partner and maintain eye contact. Use nonverbal feedback to show that you are interested and involved.

Being an Effective Speaker

• State your concern or issue as clearly as you can.

• Use "I" statements rather than statements beginning with "you." When you use "I" statements, you take responsibility for your feelings. "You" statements are often blaming or accusatory and will probably get a defensive or resentful response. The statement "I feel unloved," for example, sends a clearer, less blaming message than the statement "You don't love me."

• Focus on a behavior, not the whole person. Be specific about the behavior you like or don't like. Avoid generalizations beginning with "you always" or "you never." Such statements make people feel defensive.

• Make constructive requests. Opening your request with "I would like" keeps the focus on your needs rather than your partner's supposed deficiencies.

• Avoid blaming, accusing, and belittling. Even if you are right, you have little to gain by putting your partner down. When people feel criticized or attacked, they are less able to think rationally or solve problems constructively.

• Set up your partner for success. Tell your partner what you would like to have happen in the future; don't wait for him or her to blow it and then express anger or disappointment.

Being an Effective Listener

• Provide appropriate nonverbal feedback (nodding, smiling, making eye contact, and so on).

• Don't interrupt.

• Listen reflectively. Don't judge, evaluate, analyze, or offer solutions (unless asked to do so). Your partner may just need to sort out his or her feelings. By jumping in to "fix" the problem, you may cut off communication.

• Don't offer unsolicited advice. Giving advice implies that you know more about what a person needs to do than she or he does; therefore, it often evokes anger or resentment.

• Clarify your understanding of what your partner is saying by restating it in your own words and asking if your understanding is correct. "I think you're saying that you would feel uncomfortable having dinner with my parents and that you'd prefer to meet them in a more casual setting. Is that right?" This type of specific feedback prevents misunderstandings and helps validate the speaker's feelings and message.

• Be sure you are really listening, not off somewhere in your mind rehearsing your reply. Try to tune in to your partner's feelings and needs as well as the words. Accurately reflecting the other person's feelings and needs is often a more powerful way of connecting than just reframing his or her thoughts.

• Let your partner know that you value what he or she is saying and want to understand. Respect for the other person is the cornerstone of effective communication.

---

theories on and approaches to conflict resolution, the following strategies can be helpful:

1. *Clarify the issue.* Take responsibility for thinking through your feelings and discovering what's really bothering you. Agree that one partner will speak first and have the chance to speak fully while the other listens. Then reverse the roles. Try to understand your partner's position fully by repeating what you've heard and asking questions to clarify or elicit more information. Agree to talk only about the topic at hand and not get distracted by other issues. Sum up what your partner has said.

2. *Find out what each person wants.* Ask your partner to express his or her desires. Don't assume you know what your partner wants, and don't speak for him or her.

3. *Determine how you both can get what you want.* Brainstorm to come up with a variety of options.

4. *Decide how to negotiate.* Work out a plan for change. For example, one partner will do one task and the other will do another task. Be willing to compromise, and avoid trying to "win."

5. *Solidify the agreements.* If necessary, go over the plan and write it down, to ensure that you both understand and agree to it.

6. *Review and renegotiate.* Decide on a time frame for trying out your plan, and set a time to discuss how it's working. Make adjustments as needed.

To resolve conflicts, partners have to feel safe in voicing disagreements. They have to trust that the discussion won't get out of control, that they won't be abandoned, and that the partner won't take advantage of their vulnerability. Partners should follow some basic ground rules when they argue, such as avoiding ultimatums, resisting the urge to give the silent treatment, refusing to "hit below the belt," and not using sex to smooth over disagreements.

When you argue, maintain a spirit of goodwill and avoid being harshly critical or contemptuous. Remember—you care about your partner and want things to work out. See the disagreement as a difficulty that the two of you have together rather than as something your partner does to you. Finish serious discussions on a positive note by expressing your respect and affection for your partner and your appreciation for having been listened to. If you and your partner find that you argue again and again over the same issue, it may be better to stop trying to resolve that problem and instead come to accept the differences between you.

PAIRING AND SINGLEHOOD

Although most people eventually marry or commit to a partner, everyone spends some time as a single person, and nearly all people make some attempt, consciously or unconsciously, to find a partner. Intimate relationships are as important for singles as for couples.

Choosing a Partner

Most people select partners for long-term relationships through a fairly predictable process, although they may not be consciously aware of it. First attraction is based on easily observable characteristics: looks, dress, social status, and reciprocated interest. Studies have shown that most people pair with someone who lives in the same geographic area, comes from a similar racial, ethnic, and socioeconomic background, has a similar educational status, leads a lifestyle like theirs, has (what they think is) the same level of physical attractiveness as themselves.

Once the euphoria of romantic love winds down, personality traits and behaviors become more significant factors in how partners view each other. The emphasis shifts to basic values and future aspirations regarding career, family, and children. At some point, they decide whether the relationship feels viable and is worthy of their continued commitment.

Perhaps the most important question for potential mates to ask is, "How much do we have in common?" Although differences add interest to a relationship, similarities increase the chances of a relationship's success. Differences can affect a relationship in the areas of values, religion, race, ethnicity, attitudes toward sexuality and gender roles, socioeconomic status, familiarity with each other's culture, and interactions with the extended family. But acceptance and communication skills go a long way toward making a relationship work, no matter how different the partners.

Dating

Every culture has certain rituals for pairing and finding mates. Parent-arranged marriages, still the norm in many cultures, are often stable and permanent. Although the American cultural norm is personal choice in courtship and mate selection, the popularity of dating services and online matchmaking suggests that many people want help finding a suitable partner.

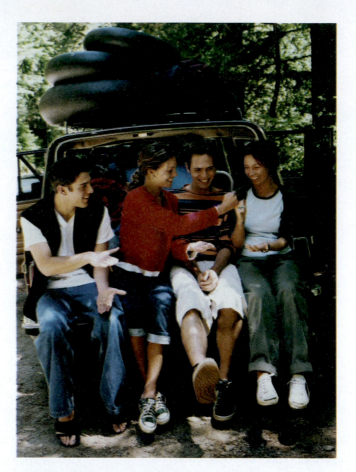

For many college students today, group activities have replaced dating as a way to meet and get to know potential partners.
© Brook Slezak/Stone/Getty Images

Many people find romantic partners through some form of dating. They narrow the field through a process of getting to know each other. Dating often revolves around a mutually enjoyable activity, such as seeing a movie or having dinner. Casual dating may then evolve into steady or exclusive dating, then engagement, and finally marriage.

In recent years, traditional dating has given way to a more casual form of getting together in groups. Two people may begin to spend more time together, but often with other couples or groups. If sexual involvement develops, it is more likely to be based on friendship, respect, and common interests than on expectations related to gender roles. In this model, mate selection may progress from getting together to living together to marriage.

Among some teenagers and young adults, dating has been supplanted by *hooking up*—casual sexual activity without any relationship commitment. For more about this trend, see the box "Hooking Up."

Online Dating and Relationships

Connecting with people online has advantages and drawbacks. It allows people to communicate in a relaxed way, try out different personas, and share things they might not share when face-to-face with family or friends. It's easier to put

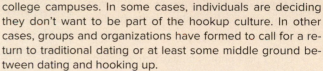

Hooking up—having casual sexual encounters with acquaintances or strangers with no commitment or investment in an emotionally intimate relationship—is said to be a current trend among teenagers and young adults. Although casual sex is not new, the difference today is that hooking up is said to be the main form of sexual activity for many people, as opposed to sexual activity within a relationship. Some data indicate that more than 80% of college students have had at least one hookup experience. If dating occurs at all, it happens after people have had sex and become a couple.

Hooking up is said to have its roots in the changing social and sexual patterns of the 1960s. Since then, changes in college policies have contributed to the shift, such as the move away from colleges acting *in loco parentis* (in the place of parents), the trend toward coed dorms, a trend toward getting married at a later age, and the availability of dating apps such as Tinder. Hooking up addresses the desire for "instant intimacy" but also protects the participants from the risk or responsibility of emotional involvement.

Because hooking up is often fueled by alcohol, it is associated with sexual risk taking and negative health effects, including the risk of acquiring a sexually transmitted infection. According to the Centers for Disease Control and Prevention (CDC), in 2014, young adults aged 15–24 had rates of chlamydia that were almost five times the overall incidence rate for the general population. Hooking up can also have adverse emotional and mental health consequences, including sexual regret and psychological distress.

Due to these and other concerns, a backlash against hooking up has taken place on some college campuses. In some cases, individuals are deciding they don't want to be part of the hookup culture. In other cases, groups and organizations have formed to call for a return to traditional dating or at least some middle ground between dating and hooking up.

However, recent studies question whether hookup culture is actually anything new. Results from the General Social Survey, which explores attitudes and behaviors around a wide variety of issues, suggest that millennials are actually less promiscuous than previous generations. If that's true, then how did the idea of hookup culture become so widespread? First, we tend to look at the past with rose-colored glasses and thus imagine the "good old days" when people had sex only in the context of committed relationships. Second, young people have a tendency to assume (incorrectly) that all their peers are having sex—that everyone around them is hooking up, except for them. Third, people who aren't the norm (that is, outliers who are having outrageous amounts of sex) are the ones who tend to get media attention, since they provide a more titillating story.

SOURCES: Carpenter, L., and J. DeLamater, eds. 2012. *Sex for Life: From Virginity to Viagra, How Sexuality Changes Throughout Our Lives.* New York: New York University Press, pp. 128–144; Garcia, J. R., et al. 2013. Sexual hook-up culture. *Monitor on Psychology* 44(2): 60.

yourself out there without too much investment; you can get to know someone from the comfort of your own home, set your own pace, and start and end relationships at any time. With millions of singles using dating sites that let them describe exactly what they are seeking, the Internet can increase a person's chance of finding a good match.

However, participants sometimes misrepresent themselves, pretending to be very different—older or younger or even of a different sex—than they really are. Investing time and emotional resources in such relationships can be painful. In rare cases, online romances become dangerous or even deadly (see Chapter 16 for information on cyberstalking).

Because people have greater freedom to reveal only what they want to, users should also be aware of a greater tendency to idealize online partners. If your online friend seems perfect, take that as a warning sign. You may search for perfection, find fault quickly, and not give people a chance; conversely, you may act on impulse with insufficient information.

QUICK STATS

About **15%** of all American adults, and **27%** of those age 18–24, have used an online dating site or mobile dating app.
—Pew Research Center, 2016

Relationship sites also remove an important and powerful source of information from the process: chemistry and in-person intuition. Much of our communication is transmitted through body language and tone, which aren't obvious in text messages and can't be captured fully even by web cams and microphones. Consider these questions. Are you comfortable in disclosing personal information about yourself? Is there a balance in the amount of time spent talking by each of you? Is the other person respecting your boundaries? Just as in face-to-face dating, online relationships require you to use common sense and to trust your instincts.

If you pursue an online relationship, the following guidelines may help you have a positive experience and stay safe:

• Choose a site that fits with your own relationship goals. Some sites are primarily geared for hookups—that is, arranging meetings for casual sex—whereas others aim to facilitate classic dating relationships. Inspect each site thoroughly before registering or providing any information about yourself.

If you aren't comfortable with a site's content or purpose, close your web browser and clear out its cache and its store of cookies. (If you don't know how to do this, check your browser's help section for instructions.)

• Know what you are looking for as well as what you can offer someone else. If you are looking for a relationship, make that fact clear. Find out the other person's intentions.

• Don't post photos unless you are completely comfortable with potential consequences (e.g., they might be downloaded by others).

• Don't give out personal information, including your real full name, school, or place of employment, until you feel sure that you are giving the information to someone who is trustworthy.

• Set up a second e-mail account for sending and receiving dating-related e-mails.

• If someone does not respond to a message, don't take it personally. There are many reasons why a person may not pursue the connection. Don't continue to send messages to an unresponsive person; doing so could lead to an accusation of stalking.

• Before deciding whether to meet an online contact in person, consider talking over the phone.

• Don't agree to meet someone face-to-face unless you feel comfortable about it. Always meet initially in a public place—a museum, a coffee shop, or a restaurant. Consider bringing along a friend to increase your safety, and let others know where you will be.

If you pursue online relationships, don't let them interfere with your other personal relationships and social activities. To support your emotional and personal wellness, use the Internet to widen your circle of friends, not shrink it.

Living Together

According to the U.S. Census Bureau, about 5.4 million opposite-sex couples and 700,000 same-sex couples live together in the United States. The Human Rights Campaign, however, estimates that the number of same-sex couples in the United States is closer to 1.6 million. Living together, or cohabitation, is one of the most rapid and dramatic social changes that has occurred in our society. By age 30, about half of all adults will have cohabited. Several factors are involved in this change, including greater acceptance of sex outside of marriage, increased availability of contraceptives, the tendency for people to wait longer before getting married, and a larger pool of single and divorced individuals.

Cohabitation is more popular among younger people than older, although a significant number of older couples live

together without marrying. Cohabitation provides many of the benefits of marriage: companionship; a setting for an enjoyable and meaningful relationship; a chance to develop greater intimacy through learning, compromising, and sharing; a satisfying sex life; and a way to save on living costs.

Are there advantages to living together over marriage? For one thing, it may give the partners a greater sense of autonomy. Not bound by the social rules and expectations that are part of marriage, partners may find it easier to keep their identities and more of their independence. Cohabitation doesn't incur the same obligations as marriage. If things don't work out, the partners may find it easier to leave a relationship that hasn't been legally sanctioned. Researchers previously believed that cohabiting before marriage led to higher divorce rates, but a 2014 study by the Council on Contemporary Families found that the age at which couples first cohabit or marry has a greater impact on relationship longevity. Those who wait until at least age 23 have the best relationship outcomes.

Of course, living together has drawbacks as well. In many cases, the legal protections of marriage are absent, such as health insurance benefits and property and inheritance rights. These considerations can be particularly serious if the couple has children. Couples may feel social or family pressure to marry or otherwise change their living arrangements, especially if they have young children. The general trend, however, is toward legitimizing nonmarital partnerships; for example, some employers, communities, and states now extend benefits to unmarried domestic partners.

Sexual Orientation and Gender Identity in Relationships

People demonstrate great diversity in their emotional and sexual attractions (see Chapter 5). **Sexual orientation** refers to a consistent pattern of emotional and sexual attraction to persons of the same sex or gender, a different sex or gender, or more than one sex or gender. A word that has come into use to describe sexual orientations other than heterosexual/straight is **queer.** People who prefer to self-identify as queer do so because it is an umbrella term, meaning it does not require one to specify between categories such as gay and bisexual.

TERMS

sexual orientation A consistent pattern of emotional and sexual attraction based on biological sex; it exists along a continuum that ranges from exclusive heterosexuality (attraction to people of the other sex) through bisexuality (attraction to people of both sexes) to exclusive homosexuality (attraction to people of one's own sex).

heterosexual/straight Attraction to people of the other sex.

queer Sexual orientations other than heterosexual/straight.

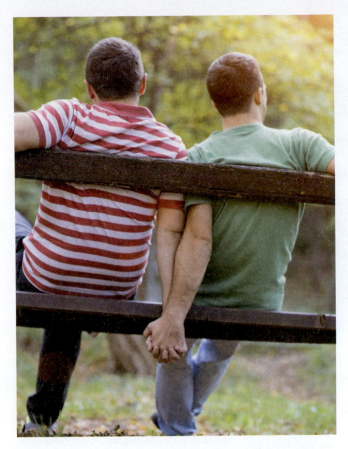

Although they constitute a minority of the population, same-sex partnerships are more visible than they used to be.

© Pekic/iStock/360/Getty Images RF

Rejecting categorization can feel like a relief to those who are still exploring their sexual orientation, or who experience it as fluid. Since *queer* is a pejorative term that has been reclaimed, never use it to label other people without their permission. In other words, respect the identity people choose for themselves rather than applying your own label to them.

Regardless of sexual orientation, most people look for love in a committed relationship. In this sense, queer couples have more similarities than differences from straight couples. Like any intimate relationship, queer partnerships provide intimacy, passion, and security. However, there are also some significant differences between these partnerships. Same-sex partnerships tend to be more egalitarian (equal) and less organized around traditional gender roles. Same-sex couples put greater emphasis on partnership than on role assignment. Domestic tasks are shared or split, and both partners usually support themselves financially.

Although many challenges for queer partnerships are common to all relationships, some issues are unique. Sexual minorities often have to deal with societal hostility or ambivalence toward their relationships, in contrast to the societal approval and rights given to heterosexual couples (see the box "Marriage Equality"). **Homophobia,** which is fear

| homophobia | Fear or hatred of homosexuals. | **TERMS** |

or hatred of homosexuals, can be obvious, as in the case of violence or discrimination. Or it can be subtler—for example, if same-sex couples are portrayed in a stereotypical way in the media. Additional stress can arise if a sexual minority individual belongs to a family, cultural group, or religion that doesn't accept her or his sexual orientation. Because of the rejection these individuals experience by society at large, community resources and support are often more important for queer-identified individuals than for heterosexuals. Many communities offer support groups for same-sex partners and families to help them build social networks.

See Chapter 5 for more information about sexual orientation, gender identity, and sexual behavior.

Singlehood

Despite the popularity of marriage, a significant and growing number of adults in our society never marry. Currently more than 116 million single individuals—the largest group of unmarried adults—have never been married (Figure 4.2).

Several factors contribute to the growing number of single people. One is the changing view of singlehood, which is increasingly being viewed as a legitimate alternative to marriage. Education and careers are delaying the age at which young people are marrying. The median age for marriage is now 29 years for men and 27 years for women. More young people are living with their parents as they complete their education, seek jobs, or strive for financial independence. Many other single people live together without being married. High divorce rates mean more singles, and people who have

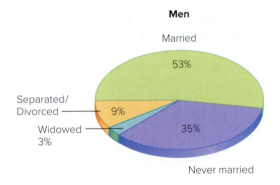

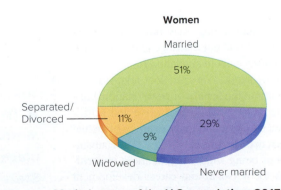

FIGURE 4.2   **Marital status of the U.S. population, 2015.**

SOURCE: U.S. Census Bureau. 2016. *Families and Living Arrangements: 2015* (https://www.census.gov/hhes/families/data/marital.html).

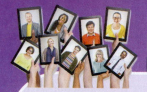

DIVERSITY MATTERS
Marriage Equality

In its legal definitions, marriage is an institution in which couples derive legal and economic rights and responsibilities from state and federal statutes. The U.S. Government Accountability Office says more than 1000 federal laws make distinctions based on marriage. Marital status affects many aspects of life, such as Social Security benefits, federal tax status, inheritance, and medical decision making.

The push for legal recognition of same-sex partnerships has gone on for decades. Supporters of same-sex marriage rights have met opposition at the local, state, and federal levels, in both the public and private sectors. However, support for marriage equality has increased rapidly in the past several years. In 2001, Americans opposed marriage equality by a 57% to 35% margin, but in 2016, a majority of Americans (61%) supported marriage equality, compared with 37% who opposed it. In 2013, the U.S. Supreme Court ruled that the federal government must recognize same-sex marriages performed by states that allow them, and in 2015, it declared all state bans on same-sex marriage unconstitutional.

Couples in which one or both partners are transgender are affected by this ruling as well, but only if their legal gender classifies them as a same-sex couple at the time of their marriage. Heterosexual transgender couples were generally able to marry previous to this ruling, so long as they were legally man-and-woman at the time of the marriage.

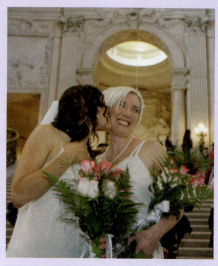
© Eric Risberg/AP Images

What are benefits of marriage for same-sex couples?

• Health insurance and retirement benefits for employees' spouses

• Social Security benefits for spouses, widows, and widowers

• Support and benefits for military spouses, widows, and widowers

• Joint income tax filing and exemption from federal estate taxes

• Immigration protections for binational couples

• Rights to creative and intellectual property

• Protection from some types of employment discrimination (e.g., getting fired for marrying a same-sex spouse)

Marriage also matters in terms of child rearing. Children who grow up with married parents benefit because their parents' relationship is recognized by law and receives legal protections. Additionally, spouses are generally entitled to joint child custody and visitation should the marriage end in divorce. They also bear an obligation to pay child support.

Finally, marriage can have an impact on emotional well-being. Research shows that married people tend to live longer, have higher incomes, engage less frequently in risky behaviors, have a healthier diet, and have fewer psychological problems than unmarried people. Overall, unmarried couples have lower levels of happiness and well-being than married couples. Finally, studies show that denying same-sex couples the right to marry has a negative impact on their mental health. The long-term impact of marriage equality is not yet known, but it is likely to benefit the legal, economic, and emotional well-being of millions of Americans.

SOURCES: Shah, Dayna K. 2004. Letter to Senator Bill Frist. (http://www.gao.gov/new.items/d04353r.pdf); Marriage Equality FAQ: Frequently Asked Questions about the Supreme Court's Marriage Ruling (https://marriageequalityfacts.org/); Gonzales, G. 2014. Same-sex marriage—A prescription for better health. *New England Journal of Medicine* 370: 1373–1376; Wight, R. G. 2013. Same-sex legal marriage and psychological well-being: Findings from the California Health Interview Survey. *American Journal of Public Health* 103(2): 339–346.

---

experienced divorce may have more negative attitudes about marriage and more positive attitudes about singlehood.

Being single, however, does not mean living without the benefit of close relationships. Single people date, enjoy active and fulfilling social lives, and have a variety of sexual experiences and relationships. Other advantages of being single include more opportunities for personal and career development without concern for family obligations and more freedom and control in making life choices. Disadvantages include loneliness

QUICK STATS

Just over 2 million marriages took place in the United States in 2014.
—National Center for Health Statistics (CDC), 2014

and a lack of companionship, as well as economic hardships (particularly for single women, who on average earn less than men). Single men and women alike experience some discrimination and often are pressured to get married.

Nearly every adult has at least one episode of being single, whether prior to marriage, between marriages, following divorce or the death of a spouse, or for his or her entire life. How enjoyable and valuable this single time is depends on several factors, including how deliberately the person has chosen it; how satisfied the person is with his or her social relationships, standard of living, and job; how comfortable the person feels when alone; and how resourceful and energetic the person is about creating an interesting and fulfilling life.

MARRIAGE

The majority of Americans marry at some time in their lives. Marriage continues to remain popular because it satisfies several basic needs. There are many important social, moral, economic, and political aspects of marriage, all of which have changed over the years. In the past people married mainly for practical reasons, such as raising children or forming an economic unit. Today people marry more for personal, emotional reasons.

The Benefits of Marriage

The primary functions and benefits of marriage are those of any intimate relationship: affection, personal affirmation, companionship, sexual fulfillment, and emotional growth. Marriage also provides a setting in which to raise children, although an increasing number of couples choose to remain childless, and people can also choose to raise children without being married. Marriage is also important for providing for the future. By committing themselves to the relationship, people hope to establish themselves with lifelong companions as well as some insurance for their later years. Research shows that good marriages have myriad positive effects on individuals' health.

Issues and Trends in Marriage

Marital roles and responsibilities have undergone profound changes over time. Many couples no longer accept traditional role assumptions, such as that the husband is solely responsible for supporting the family and the wife is solely responsible for domestic work. Many husbands share domestic tasks, and many wives work outside the home. About 60% of married women are in the labor force, including women with babies under one year of age. Although women still take most of the responsibility for home and children even when they work and although men still suffer more job-related stress and health problems than women do, the trend is toward an equalization of responsibilities in the home.

Other recent trends include couples choosing not to marry, couples marrying later—after a lengthy cohabitation, and couples marrying without a formal marriage certificate. A second, later-life union (cohabitation or marriage) is also common. A recent study reports that both women and men experienced health benefits from second unions; from first unions, men in particular had reduced emotional distress from getting married without first living together.

What about love? Although we might like to believe otherwise, love is not enough to make a successful marriage. Relationship problems can become magnified rather than

solved by marriage. The following relationship characteristics appear to be the best predictors of a happy marriage:

- The partners have realistic expectations about their relationship.
- Each feels good about the personality of the other.
- Partners develop friendships with other couples.
- They communicate well.
- They have effective ways of resolving conflicts.
- They agree on religious/ethical values.
- They have an egalitarian role relationship.
- They have a good balance of individual versus joint interests and leisure activities.

Once married, couples must provide each other with emotional support, negotiate and establish marital roles, establish domestic and career priorities, handle their finances, make sexual adjustments, manage boundaries and relationships with their extended family, and participate in the larger community.

The Role of Commitment

Studies show that commitment not only brings stability to a relationship but also is essential to overcoming the inevitable ups and downs experienced in relationships. Commitment is based on conscious choice rather than on feelings, which, by their very nature, are transitory. Commitment is a promise of a shared future—a promise to be together, come what may. No matter how they feel, committed partners put effort and energy into the relationship. They take time to attend to their partners, give compliments, and deal with conflict when necessary. Commitment has become an important concept in recent years. To many people, commitment is the most important part of a relationship.

Separation and Divorce

Although the rates have dropped by about 20% since the year 2000, divorce is still fairly common in the United States. Those who have never experienced divorce personally—either their own or that of their parents—almost certainly have friends or relatives who have. The high rate of divorce in the United States may reflect our extremely high expectations for emotional fulfillment and satisfaction in marriage.

It may also indicate that our culture no longer embraces the concept of marriage as permanent.

The process of divorce usually begins with an emotional separation. Often one partner is unhappy and looks for a more satisfying relationship. Dissatisfaction increases until the unhappy partner decides he or she can no longer stay. Physical separation follows, although it may take some time for the relationship to be over emotionally.

Except for the death of a spouse or family member, divorce may be the greatest stress-producing event in life. Studies show that divorced women are more likely to develop heart disease than married, remarried, or widowed women. Both men and women experience turmoil, depression, and lowered self-esteem during and after divorce. People experience separation distress and loneliness for about a year and then begin a recovery period of one to three years. During this time they gradually construct a postdivorce identity, along with a new pattern of life. Most people are surprised how long it takes to recover from divorce.

Children are especially vulnerable to the trauma of divorce, and sometimes counseling is appropriate to help them adjust to the change. However, recent research has found that children who spend substantial time with both parents are usually better adjusted than those in sole custody and are as well-adjusted as their peers from intact families. Coping with divorce has been found to be difficult for children at any age, including adult children.

Despite the distress of separation and divorce, the negative effects are usually balanced sooner or later by the possibility of finding a more suitable partner, constructing a new life, and developing new aspects of the self. About 75% of all people who divorce remarry, often within five years. One result of the high divorce and remarriage rate is a growing number of stepfamilies.

FAMILY LIFE

American families are very different today than they were even a few decades ago. In 1960, 73% of children under the age of 18 lived with both parents in their first marriage; in 2014, it was 46%. Over the same time period, the proportion of children living with a single parent grew from 9% to 26%.

Becoming a Parent

Few new parents are prepared for the job of parenting, yet they literally must assume the role overnight. They must quickly learn how to hold and feed a baby, change diapers, and differentiate a cry of hunger from a cry of pain or fear. No wonder the birth of the first child is one of the most stressful transitions for any couple.

Even couples with an egalitarian relationship before their first child is born find that their marital roles become more traditional with the arrival of the new baby. In heterosexual couples, the father typically becomes the primary provider and protector, and the mother typically becomes the primary nurturer. Most research indicates that mothers have to make greater changes in their lives than fathers do. Although men today spend more time caring for their infants than ever before, women still take the ultimate responsibility for the baby. Women are usually the ones who make job changes, either quitting work or reducing work hours in order to stay home with the baby for several months or more. Many mothers juggle the multiple roles of mother, homemaker, and employer/employee and feel guilty that they never have enough time to do justice to any of these roles.

Parenting

Parents may wonder about the long-term impact of each decision they make on their child's well-being and personality. According to parenting experts, no one action or decision (within limits) will determine a child's personality or development. Instead the *parenting style,* or overall approach to parenting, is most important. Parenting styles vary according to the levels of two characteristics of the parents:

• *Demandingness* encompasses the use of discipline and supervision, the expectation that children act responsibly and maturely, and the direct reaction to disobedience.

• *Responsiveness* refers to a parent's warmth and intent to facilitate independence and self-confidence in a child by being supportive, connected, and understanding of the child's needs.

Several parenting styles have been identified. Each style emerges according to the parents' balance of demandingness and responsiveness. Here are some examples:

• *Authoritarian* parents are high in demandingness and low in responsiveness. They give orders and expect obedience, giving very little warmth or consideration to their children's special needs.

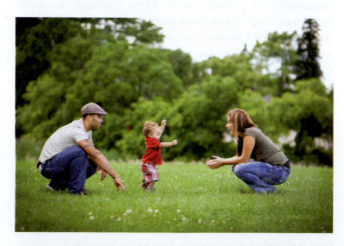

Setting clear boundaries, holding children to high expectations, and responding with warmth to children's needs are all positive parenting strategies.

© Rosemarie Gearhart/Getty Images

• *Authoritative* parents are high in both demandingness and responsiveness. They set clear boundaries and expectations, but they are also loving, supportive, and attuned to their children's needs.

• *Permissive* parents are high in responsiveness and low in demandingness. They do not expect their children to act maturely but instead allow them to follow their own impulses. They are very warm, patient, and accepting, and they are focused on not stifling their child's innate creativity.

• *Uninvolved* parents are low in both demandingness and responsiveness. They require little from their children and respond with little attention, frequency, or effort. In extreme cases, this style of parenting might reach the level of child neglect.

At each stage of the family life cycle, the relationship between parents and children changes. And with those changes come new challenges. The parents' primary responsibility to a baby is to ensure its physical well-being around the clock. As babies grow into toddlers and begin to walk and talk, they begin to be able to take care of some of their own physical needs. For parents, the challenge at this stage is to strike a balance between giving children the freedom to explore and setting limits that will keep the children safe and secure. As children grow toward adolescence, parents need to give them increasing independence and gradually be willing to let them risk success or failure on their own.

Marital satisfaction for most couples tends to decline while the children are in school. Reasons include the financial and emotional pressures of a growing family and the increased job and community responsibilities of parents in their thirties, forties, and fifties. Once the last child has left home, marital satisfaction can increase because the parents have more time to focus on each other.

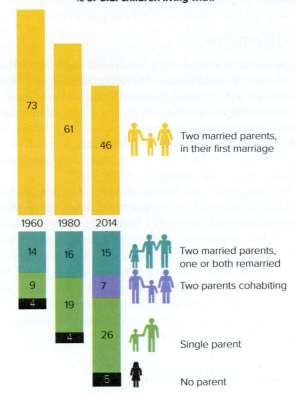

Growing Diversity in Family Living Arrangements
% of U.S. children living with:

73 1960 / 61 1980 / 46 2014 — Two married parents, in their first marriage

14 / 16 / 15 — Two married parents, one or both remarried

9 / — / 7 — Two parents cohabiting

4 / 19 / 26 — Single parent

— / 4 / 5 — No parent

FIGURE 4.4 **Family living arrangements for American families with children under age 18.**

NOTE: Data regarding cohabitation are not available for 1960 and 1980; in those years, children with cohabiting parents are included in "single parent." For 2014, the total share of children living with two married parents is 62% after rounding. "Married parents" refer to those in a heterosexual marriage only. Figures do not add up to 100% due to rounding.

SOURCE: Pew Research Center. 2015. Parenting in America: Outlook, Worries, Aspirations Are Strongly Linked to Financial Situation (http://www .pewsocialtrends.org/2015/12/17/parenting-in-america)

Single Parents

Today the family life cycle for many adults is marriage, parenthood, divorce, single parenthood, remarriage, and potentially widow- or widower-hood. According to Pew Research Institute, about 26% of children today are living with a single parent (Figure 4.4). In some single-parent families, the traditional family life cycle is reversed and the baby comes before the marriage. In these families, the single parent is often (but not always) a teenage mother.

Even if both parents work after a divorce, their combined incomes must support two households, straining finances. Economic difficulties are the primary problem for single mothers, especially for unmarried mothers who have not finished high school and have difficulty finding work. Divorced mothers usually experience a sharp drop in income the first few years on their own, but if they have job skills or education they usually can eventually support themselves and their children. Other problems for single

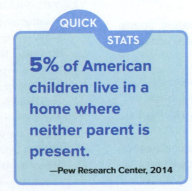

QUICK STATS

5% of American children live in a home where neither parent is present.

—Pew Research Center, 2014

mothers are the often-conflicting demands of being both father and mother and the difficulty of satisfying their own needs for adult companionship and affection.

Financial pressures are also a complaint of single fathers, but due to higher incomes among men, they do not experience them to the extent that single mothers do. Because they are likely to have less practice than mothers in juggling parental and professional roles, they may worry that they do not spend enough time with their children.

Research about the effect on children of growing up in a single-parent family is inconclusive. Evidence seems to indicate that these children tend to have less success in school and in their careers than children from two-parent families, but these effects may be associated more strongly with lower educational attainment and fewer financial resources of the single parent than with the absence of the second parent. Two-parent families are not necessarily better if one of the parents spends little time relating to the children or is physically or emotionally abusive.

Stepfamilies

Single parenthood is usually a transitional stage: About three out of four divorced women and about four out of five divorced men will ultimately remarry. Rates are lower for widowed men and women, but overall almost half the marriages in the United States are remarriages for the husband, the wife, or both. If either partner brings children from a previous marriage into the new family unit, a stepfamily (or "blended family") is formed.

Stepfamilies are significantly different from primary families and should not be expected to duplicate the emotions and relationships of a primary family. Research has shown that healthy stepfamilies are less cohesive and more adaptable than healthy primary families; they have a greater capacity to allow for individual differences and accept that biologically related family members will have emotionally closer relationships. Stepfamilies gradually gain more of a sense of being a family as they build a history of shared daily experiences and major life events.

Successful Families

Family life can be extremely challenging. A strong family is not a family without problems; it's a family that copes successfully with stress and crisis. Successful families are intentionally connected—members share experiences and meanings.

An excellent way to build strong family ties is to develop family rituals and routines—organized, repeated activities that have meaning for family members. Families with regular routines and rituals have healthier children, more satisfying marriages, and stronger family relationships. Some of the most common routines identified in research studies are dinnertime, a regular bedtime, and household chores; common rituals include birthdays, holidays, and weekend activities. Family routines may even serve as protective factors, balancing out potential risk factors associated with single-parent families and families with divorce and remarriage. Incorporating a regular family mealtime into a family's routine allows parents and children to develop closer relationships and leads to better parenting, healthier children, and better school performance.

Although you can find tremendous variation among American families, experts have proposed that seven major qualities or themes appear in strong families:

1. *Commitment.* The family is very important to its members, and members take their responsibilities seriously. Everyone knows they are loved, valued, and special to each other.

2. *Appreciation.* Family members care about one another and express their appreciation. They don't wait for special occasions to celebrate each other.

3. *Communication.* Family members spend time listening to one another and enjoying one another's company. They talk through disagreements and attempt to solve problems.

4. *Time together.* Family members do things together—often simple activities that don't cost money. They put down their devices and their work, and they focus on each other.

5. *Spiritual wellness.* The family promotes sharing, love, and compassion for other human beings.

6. *Stress and crisis management.* When faced with illness, death, marital conflict, or other crises, family members pull together, seek help, and use other coping strategies to meet the challenge.

7. *Affectionate physical contact.* People of all ages need hugs, cuddles, and caresses for their emotional health and to demonstrate caring and love for one another.

It may surprise some people that members of strong families are often seen at counseling centers. They know that the smartest thing to do in some situations is to get help.

Ask Yourself

QUESTIONS FOR CRITICAL THINKING AND REFLECTION

Do you think of your own family as successful? Why or why not? Either way, what could you do to make your relationships in your family more successful? Are you comfortable talking to your family about these issues?

TIPS FOR TODAY AND THE FUTURE

A balanced life includes ample time for nourishing relationships with friends, family, and intimate partners.

RIGHT NOW YOU CAN:
- Seek out an acquaintance or a new friend and arrange a coffee date to get to know the person better.
- Call someone you love and tell him or her how important the relationship is to you. Don't wait for a crisis.

IN THE FUTURE YOU CAN:
- Think about the conflicts you have had in the past with your close friends or loved ones and consider how you handled them. Decide whether your conflict management methods were helpful. Using the suggestions in this chapter and Chapter 3, determine how you could better handle similar conflicts in the future.
- Think about your prospects as a parent. What kind of example have your parents set? How do you feel about having children in the future (if you don't have children already)? What can you do to prepare yourself to be a good parent?

SUMMARY

- Healthy intimate relationships are an important component of the well-being of both individuals and society. Many intimate relationships are held together by love.

- Successful relationships begin with a positive sense of self and reasonably high self-esteem. Personal identity, gender roles, and attachment styles, all rooted in childhood experiences, contribute to this sense of self.

- Characteristics of friendship include companionship, respect, acceptance, help, trust, loyalty, mutuality, and reciprocity.

- Love, sex, and commitment are closely linked ideals in intimate relationships. Love includes trust, caring, respect, and loyalty. Sex brings excitement, fascination, and passion to the relationship. Commitment contributes stability, which helps maintain a relationship.

- Common challenges in relationships relate to issues of self-disclosure, commitment, expectations, competitiveness, balance of time together and apart, and jealousy.

- Partners in successful relationships have strong communication skills and support each other during difficult times. Social media can ease communication but they can also undermine relationships.

- The keys to good communication in relationships are self-disclosure, listening, and feedback.

- Conflict is inevitable in intimate relationships; partners need to find ways to negotiate their differences. Conflict is often accompanied by anger, and the best way to handle anger in a relationship is to recognize it as a symptom of something that needs to be addressed.

- People usually choose partners like themselves. If partners are very different, acceptance and good communication skills are especially necessary to maintain the relationship.

- Most Americans find partners through dating or getting together in groups. Internet sites that match people can expand dating options and create positive experiences as long as safety precautions are taken. Cohabitation is a growing social pattern that allows partners to get to know each other intimately without being married.

- Same-sex partnerships are similar to heterosexual partnerships, with some differences. Compared with heterosexual partners, same-sex couples put greater emphasis on partnership than on role assignment, and they may experience societal hostility or ambivalence rather than approval of their partnerships.

- Singlehood is a growing lifestyle decision in our society. Advantages include greater variety in sex partners and more freedom in making life decisions; disadvantages include loneliness and possible economic hardship, especially for single women.

- Marriage fulfills many functions for individuals and society. It can provide people with affection, affirmation, and sexual fulfillment; a context for child rearing; and the promise of lifelong companionship.

- Love isn't enough to ensure a successful marriage. Partners must be realistic, feel good about each other, have communication and conflict resolution skills, share values, and balance their individual and joint interests.

- When problems can't be worked out, people often separate and divorce. Divorce is traumatic for all involved, especially children, but the negative effects are usually balanced in time by positive ones.

- At each stage of the family life cycle, relationships change. Marital satisfaction may be lower during the child-rearing years and higher later.

- Many families today are single-parent families. The primary problem for single parents is economic difficulties.

- Stepfamilies are formed when single, divorced, or widowed people remarry and create new family units. Stepfamilies gradually gain more of a sense of being a family as they build a history of shared experiences.

- Important qualities of successful families include commitment to the family, appreciation of family members, communication, physical affection, time spent together, spiritual wellness, and effective methods of dealing with stress.

FOR MORE INFORMATION

For resources in your area, check your campus directory for a counseling center or peer counseling program, or search online.

American Association for Marriage and Family Therapy. Provides information about a variety of relationship issues and referrals to therapists.

http://www.aamft.org

Association for Couples in Marriage Enrichment (ACME). Promotes activities to strengthen marriage; a resource for books, tapes, and other materials.

http://www.bettermarriages.org

Conflict Resolution Information Source. Provides links to a broad range of Internet resources for conflict resolution. Information covers interpersonal, marital, family, and other types of conflicts.

http://www.crinfo.org

Family Education Network. Provides information about education, safety, health, and other family-related issues.

http://www.familyeducation.com

The Gottman Institute. Includes tips and suggestions for relationships and parenting, including an online relationships quiz.

http://www.gottman.com

Parents Without Partners (PWP). Provides educational programs, literature, and support groups for single parents and their children. Search the online directory for a referral to a local chapter.

http://www.parentswithoutpartners.org

Pew Research Center. Surveys Americans about issues and attitudes and analyzes publications in mass media and social science research.

http://www.pewresearch.org

U.S. Census Bureau. Provides current statistics on births, marriages, and living arrangements.

http://www.census.gov

U.S. Government Accountability Office. Acts like a "congressional watchdog," investigating how the federal government spends taxpayer money.

http://www.gao.gov

SELECTED BIBLIOGRAPHY

American College Health Association. 2015. *American College Health Association–National College Health Assessment II Reference Group Executive Summary, Spring 2015.* Hanover, MD: American College Health Association.

Centers for Disease Control and Prevention. 2015. Summary health statistics for U.S. adults: National Health Interview Survey, 2014. *Vital and Health Statistics* (http://www.cdc.gov/nchs/nhis/SHS/tables.htm)

Centers for Disease Control and Prevention, National Center for Health Statistics. 2015. Births, marriages, divorces, and deaths. Final data for 2014. *National Vital Statistics Reports* (http://www.cdc.gov/nchs/nvss.htm)

Council on Contemporary Families. 2014. *Does Premarital Cohabitation Raise Your Risk of Divorce?* (https://contemporaryfamilies.org/cohabitation-divorce-brief-report/)

Eckert, P., and S. McConnell-Ginet. 2013. *Language and Gender,* 2nd ed. New York: Cambridge University Press.

Federal Interagency Forum on Child and Family Statistics. 2015. *America's Children: Key National Indicators of Well-Being, 2015.* Washington, DC: U.S. Government Printing Office.

Gallup. 2015. Fewer Young People Say I Do—to Any Relationship (http://www.gallup.com/poll/183515/fewer-young-people-say-relationship.aspx).

Gallup. 2016. Marriage. (http://www.gallup.com/poll/117328/marriage.aspx)

Goleman, D. 1995. *Emotional Intelligence: Why It Can Matter More Than IQ.* New York: Bantam Books.

Goodwin, M. H. 2006. *The Hidden Life of Girls: Games of Stance, Status, and Exclusion.* Oxford, UK: Blackwell.

Kirschenbaum, H., and V. Henderson. 1989. *The Carl Rogers Reader.* Boston: Houghton Mifflin.

McPherson, M., L. Smith-Lovin, and M. Brashears. 2006. Social isolation in America: Changes in core discussion networks over two decades. *American Sociological Review* 71: 353–375.

Mernitz, S. E., and C. Kamp Dush. 2016. Emotional health across the transition to first and second unions among emerging adults. *Journal of Family Psychology* 30(2): 233–244.

National Conference of State Legislatures. 2015. *Same-Sex Marriage Laws.* (http://www.ncsl.org/research/human-services/same-sex-marriage-laws.aspx)

Pew Research Center. 2016. Report: 15% of American Adults Have Used Online Dating Sites or Mobile Dating Apps (http://www.pewinternet.org/2016/02/11/15-percent-of-american-adults-have-used-online-dating-sites-or-mobile-dating-apps).

Roisman, G. I., et al. 2008. Adult romantic relationships as contexts of human development: A multimethod comparison of same-sex couples with opposite-sex dating, engaged, and married dyads. *Developmental Psychology* 44(1): 91–101.

Salovey, P., et al., eds. 2004. *Emotional Intelligence: Key Readings on the Mayer and Salovey Model.* Port Chester, NY: Dude Publishing.

Schoen, R., et al. 2007. Family transitions in young adulthood. *Demography* 44(4): 807–820.

Tufekci, Z. 2014. The social Internet: Frustrating, enriching, but not lonely. *Public Culture* 26(1): 13–23.

Turkle, S. 2012. *Alone Together: Why We Expect More from Technology and Less from Each Other.* New York: Basic Books.

Twenge, J. M., R. A. Sherman, and B. E. Wells. 2015. Changes in American adults' sexual behavior and attitudes. *Archives of Sexual Behavior* 44: 2273.

U.S. Bureau of Labor Statistics. 2015. Women in the labor force: a databook. *BLS Reports,* December 2015, Report 1059.

U.S. Census Bureau. 2016. *Families and Living Arrangements: Marital Status* (https://www.census.gov/hhes/families/data/marital.html).

Wang, W. and K. Parker. 2014. Record share of Americans have never married: As values, economics and gender patterns change. Washington, D.C.: Pew Research Center's Social & Demographic Trends Project.

Yarber, W., B. Sayad, and B. Strong. 2012. *Human Sexuality: Diversity in Contemporary America,* 8th ed. New York: McGraw-Hill.

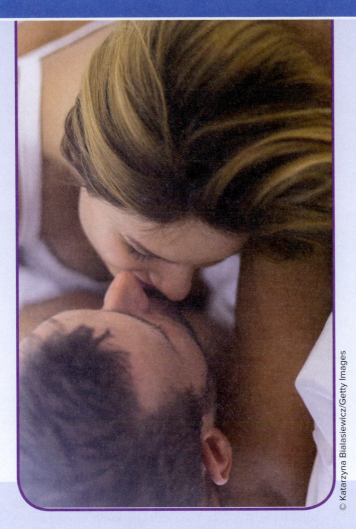

© Katarzyna Bialasiewicz/Getty Images

CHAPTER OBJECTIVES

- Describe the structure and function of human sexual anatomy
- Explain the reproductive life cycle and the role hormones play in it
- Describe how the sex organs function during sexual activity
- Explain the range of gender roles and sexual orientations
- Explain the varieties of sexual behavior
- Explain the principles of fertility and infertility
- Describe the physical and emotional changes related to pregnancy
- Identify the stages of fetal development
- Explain the importance of good prenatal care
- Understand potential complications of pregnancy
- Describe the choices and processes related to childbirth

CHAPTER **5**

Sexuality, Pregnancy, and Childbirth

The term **sexuality** refers to far more than sexual behavior. It is a complex, interacting group of biological characteristics and acquired behaviors people learn while growing up in a particular family, community, and society. Sexuality includes one's biological sex (which includes being male, female, or intersex, a term we will explain later in this chapter), gender (masculine, feminine, genderqueer, and transgender identities—also to be explored more fully later), sexual anatomy and physiology, sexual functioning and practices, and social and sexual interactions with others. An individual's sense of identity is powerfully influenced by sexuality, and because sexuality is so variable and multifaceted, it should be thought of as a spectrum of identities rather than as a binary system of either/or.

Basic information about the body, sexual functioning, sexual identity, and sexual behavior is vital to sexual wellness. Those who understand the facts have a better basis for evaluating the messages they get and for making informed, responsible choices about their sexual activities.

SEXUAL ANATOMY

Despite their different appearances, male and female sex organs arise from the same structures and fulfill many of the same functions. **Gonads** (ovaries in females and testes in

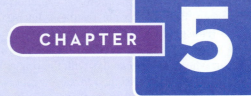

sexuality   A dimension of personality shaped by biological, psychosocial, and cultural forces and concerning all aspects of sexual behavior and feelings.

gonads   The primary organs that produce germ cells and sex hormones; the ovaries and testes.

TERMS

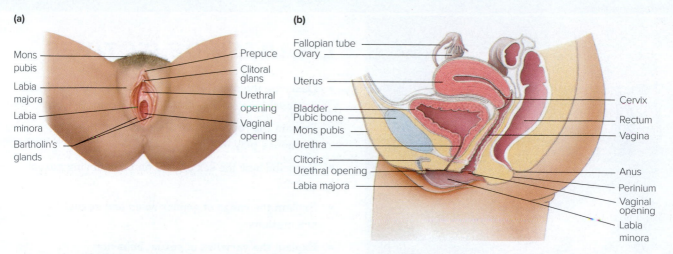

FIGURE 5.1   **The female sex organs.** (a) An external view of the vulva. (b) An internal view of the female pelvis.

males) produce **germ cells** and sex hormones. Germ cells are called **ova** (eggs) in females and **sperm** in males. Ova and sperm are the basic units of reproduction.

According to the American Psychological Association, experts estimate that as many as 1 in 1500 infants, due to genetic or hormonal abnormalities, is born with genitals that cannot easily be assigned to the category of male or female, a condition known as **intersex.** Parents and doctors of intersex infants sometimes use surgery to assign these children to a particular sex, but many adults who have undergone such procedures are now calling for an end to these surgeries so that people with intersex conditions can choose for themselves when the time is right for them. Intersex is not the same as **transgender,** which is the word used to describe a person whose genitals align with the category male or female, but who does not identify with the gender (masculine or feminine) typically assigned to those genitals. Transgender will be discussed more fully later in this chapter.

Female Sex Organs

The external sex organs, or genitals, of the female are called the **vulva** (Figure 5.1). The vulva, commonly confused with the vagina, includes the *mons pubis*, *labia majora* and *minora*, clitoris, and urethral and vaginal openings. The *mons pubis,* a rounded mass of fatty tissue over the pubic bone, becomes covered with hair during puberty (biological maturation). Below it are two paired folds of skin called the *labia majora* (outer lips) and the *labia minora* (inner lips). Enclosed within these folds are the *clitoris*, the opening of the urethra, and the opening of the vagina. Despite a rise in surgeries designed to reduce them, the *labia majora* vary widely in size, color, shape, and overall appearance, and they often play a significant role in sexual sensation and pleasure.

The **clitoris** is highly sensitive to stimulation and also plays an important role in female sexual arousal, orgasm, and pleasure. The clitoris consists of 8000 nerve endings concentrated in the glans, or head. The clitoris may be externally visible between the labia. It then extends internally into

the anterior wall of the vagina (Figure 5.1b). Inside the clitoris, spongy, erectile tissue fills with blood during sexual excitement, creating engorgement of the genitals. The clitoral hood, or **prepuce,** covers the glans and is formed from the upper portion of the inner lips.

The female **urethra** is a duct that leads directly from the urinary bladder to its opening between the clitoris and the opening of the vagina. The urethra conducts urine from the bladder. Women have a much shorter urethra than men and as a result are more likely to suffer from urinary tract infections, or UTIs. Both males and females should urinate after sexual activity to cleanse this tube.

Some women are able to expel fluid or ejaculate during sexual activity. If so, the fluid exits the urethra, not the vagina. This fluid has been tested and is typically not urine, although some remnants of urine have been found simply because urine travels out of the same tube. This fluid is similar to prostatic fluid in men.

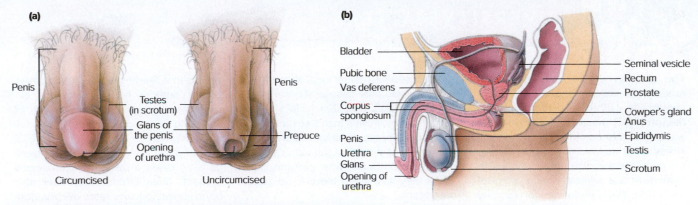

(a)

Penis

Testes
(in scrotum)

Glans of
the penis

Opening
of urethra

Circumcised

Penis

Prepuce

Uncircumcised

(b)

Bladder

Pubic bone

Vas deferens

Corpus
spongiosum

Penis

Urethra

Glans

Opening of
urethra

Seminal vesicle

Rectum

Prostate

Cowper's gland

Anus

Epididymis

Testis

Scrotum

FIGURE 5.2 **The male sex organs.** (a) An external view. (b) An internal view.

The **vagina** is the passage that leads to the internal sexual organs and can be used for **sexual intercourse** and penetration. It is a potential birth canal and allows menstrual fluid to be expelled from the uterus. Located about 1–2 inches internally in the vagina, is the Gräfenberg- or *G-spot*. This spot—or more accurately, region—is the root of the clitoris and can be highly sensitive in some women. Projecting into the upper part of the vagina is the **cervix,** which is the opening of the **uterus**—or *womb*—where a fertilized egg is implanted and develops into a *fetus*.

A pair of **fallopian tubes** (or *oviducts*) extends from the top of the uterus. The end of each oviduct surrounds an **ovary** and guides the mature ovum down into the uterus after the egg exits the ovary.

Male Sex Organs

Male external sex organs, or genitals, are the penis and the scrotum (Figure 5.2). The **penis** consists of the glans, often referred to as the head, which is typically the most sensitive part of the penis. The shaft extends from the head to the body of the penis and is made up of spongy tissue that becomes engorged with blood during sexual excitement, causing the organ to enlarge and become erect.

The **scrotum** is a pouch that contains a pair of sperm-producing male gonads, called **testes.** The scrotum maintains the testes at a temperature approximately 5°F below that of the rest of the body—that is, at about 93.6°F. The process of sperm production is extremely heat sensitive. In hot temperatures, the muscles in the scrotum relax and the testes move away from the heat of the body. This ability to regulate the temperature of the testes is important because elevated testicular temperature can interfere with normal sperm production. Men should regularly perform testicular exams and examine the testes for any unusual growths. The best place to do this is in the shower because it is warm and the scrotal sac will hang farther away from the body.

The male urethra is a tube that runs through the entire length of the penis. The urethra carries both urine and

QUICK STATS

20 million or more sperm per milliliter of semen is considered a normal sperm count.

—National Library of Medicine, 2014

semen (sperm-carrying fluid) to the opening at the tip of the penis. The **Cowper's glands** are two small structures flanking the urethra. During sexual arousal, these glands excrete a clear, mucus-like fluid that appears at the tip of the penis. This preejaculatory fluid is thought to help lubricate the urethra to facilitate the passage of sperm and flush out any remaining urine in the tube. The release of preejaculatory fluid is an involuntary reflex and may contain sperm, so withdrawal of the penis before

TERMS

vagina The canal leading from the female genitals to the internal reproductive organs. Sometimes referred to as the birth canal.

sexual intercourse Sexual relations involving penetration of the genitals or anus; also called coitus; also known as making love.

cervix The opening of the uterus in the upper part of the vagina.

uterus The hollow, thick-walled, muscular organ in which the fertilized egg develops and where menstrual blood collects each month. Sometimes called the *womb*.

fallopian tube A duct that guides a mature ovum from the ovary to the uterus; also called an *oviduct*.

ovaries Paired glands that produce ova (eggs) and sex hormones; ovaries are the female gonads.

penis The male genital structure consisting of the glans and shaft, spongy tissue that often becomes engorged with blood during sexual excitement.

scrotum The loose sac of skin and muscle fibers that contains the testes.

testis One of two male gonads, the site of sperm production; plural, *testes*. Also called *testicle*.

semen The fluid that carries sperm out of the penis during ejaculation.

Cowper's gland In the male reproductive system, a small organ that produces preejaculatory fluid.

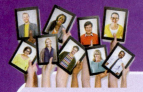

The alteration of the appearance and function of children's genitalia, either shortly after birth or as part of a puberty rite, provokes much controversy worldwide. The most common form of genital alteration is male circumcision—the removal of the foreskin of the penis. Circumcision is a relatively minor surgical procedure that is performed for a variety of cultural, religious, aesthetic, and medical reasons. Worldwide an estimated one-third of males are circumcised. In the United States a little more than one-half of male newborns are circumcised (from a high of nearly 90% in the 1960s); over time, fewer American parents are having their sons circumcised.

The procedure, though minor, carries some medical risks, including bleeding, infection, damage to the penis, and even death. Circumcision causes pain to the infant, although most pain can be alleviated with appropriate use of local anesthetic. Circumcision may change the sensitivity of the penis, and some critics claim that it can diminish a man's sexual pleasure. Opponents of circumcision point to the fact that most of the world's men are uncircumcised; why perform surgery, they ask, when there is no clear need for it?

On the other side of the debate, a number of health benefits are claimed to be associated with circumcision. Proponents of the procedure argue that it promotes cleanliness and reduces the risk of urinary tract infections in newborns and sexually transmitted infections in later life. The American Academy of Pediatrics states that the "preventive health benefits of elective circumcision of male newborns outweigh the risks of the procedure," so that families who choose the procedure should have access to it. Studies conducted in developing countries have shown that circumcision can reduce a man's risk of acquiring human immunodeficiency virus (HIV), herpes simplex virus type 2, human papillomavirus (HPV), and genital ulcer disease through heterosexual contact. Male circumcision has also been shown to lower rates of HPV, genital ulcer disease, bacterial vaginosis, and trichomoniasis among female partners, although one study in Uganda showed increased rates of HIV infection for women whose male partners were circumcised. Ultimately education about STIs, the practice of abstinence or low-risk sexual behaviors, and the use of barrier methods such as condoms have a far greater impact on the transmission of STIs than does circumcision.

Far more controversial is the practice of female genital cutting (FGC), also

---

ejaculation is not a reliable form of contraception. It is also possible to contract a sexually transmitted infection (STI) from preejaculatory fluid.

Starting at about age 14, males begin producing sperm, around 400 million per day. The sperm take the following journey:

1. Sperm are produced inside a maze of tiny, tightly packed tubules within the testes. As they begin to mature, sperm flow into a single storage tube called the **epididymis**, which lies on the surface of each testis.

2. Sperm move from each epididymis into another tube—called the **vas deferens.**

3. The two *vasa deferentia* eventually merge into a pair of **seminal vesicles,** whose secretions provide nutrients for the sperm. The sperm then pass through an organ called the **prostate gland,** where they pick up a milky fluid and become semen.

4. On the final stage of their journey, sperm flow into the **ejaculatory ducts.** Although urine and semen share a common passage, they are prevented from mixing together by muscles that control their entry into the urethra.

The smooth, rounded tip of the penis is the highly sensitive **glans,** an important component in sexual arousal (Figure 5.2a shows a frontal view; Figure 5.2b shows a side view). The glans is partially covered by the foreskin, or prepuce, a retractable fold of skin that is removed by **circumcision** in about 55% of newborn males in the United States. Circumcision is performed for cultural, religious, and medical reasons. Rates of circumcision vary widely among groups (see the box "Genital Alteration").

Ask Yourself

QUESTIONS FOR CRITICAL THINKING AND REFLECTION

What are your personal views on circumcision? What are your views about other forms of genital cutting? Who or what has influenced those opinions? Are the bases of your views primarily cultural, moral, or medical? If you had a son or daughter, would you have their genitals altered?

called female genital mutilation or modification. FGC ranges from removal of the external genitalia (including the clitoris and labia) to sewing up the labia but leaving a small opening through which urine and menstrual fluid can pass. A common explanation for the practice is that FGC controls a woman's sexuality and ensures she remains a virgin before marriage. Other explanations refer to empowerment for girls: Through the bonding and educational experiences surrounding the ceremonies, girls attain a status similar to cohorts of boys the same age who are undergoing circumcision. These explanations are cultural rather than medical.

Each year about 3 million female children undergo FGC, usually between infancy and age 15, and about 140 million women worldwide are estimated to have had some form of genital cutting. FGC is often performed under unsterile conditions and without adequate anesthesia. Serious complications are common and include severe pain, infection, bleeding, and death. Common long-term health issues include infertility, difficulties with childbirth, and problems with urinary and sexual function.

The World Health Organization has come out strongly against FGC, declaring it a violation of the human rights of girls and women. FGC is now illegal in many countries, including the United States, but it is still performed on large numbers of girls where the cultural tradition persists. In a parallel move, the American Congress of Obstetricians and Gynecologists has spoken out against the practice of cosmetic genital surgeries in the United States and elsewhere, calling the procedures "not medically necessary." Though these cosmetic surgeries are performed under sterile and voluntary conditions, it is worth noting that all forms of cutting mentioned here are related to cultural beliefs regarding the purpose and appearance of female genitals.

SOURCES: Boyle, E. H., and A. C. Corl. 2010. Law and culture in a global context: Interventions to eradicate female genital cutting. *Annual Review of Law and Social Science* 6: 195–215; Centers for Disease Control and Prevention. 2011. Trends in in-hospital newborn male circumcision—United States, 1999–2010. *MMWR* 60(34): 1167–1168; World Health Organization. 2012. *Female Genital Mutilation* (http://www.who.int/topics/female_genital_mutilation/en/); Tobian, A. A. R., et al. 2014. Male circumcision: A globally relevant but under-utilized method for the prevention of HIV and other sexually transmitted infections. *Annual Review of Medicine* 65: 293–306.

HORMONES AND THE REPRODUCTIVE LIFE CYCLE

The sex hormones produced by the ovaries or testes have a major influence on the development and function of the sexual organs throughout life. In addition to their effects on these organs, sex hormones influence many other parts of the body, including the brain.

Both males and females produce testosterone, estrogens, and progestogens; however, the quantities differ in male and female bodies. The male sex hormones, made by the testes, are called **androgens,** the most important of which is *testosterone*. Males will produce lower levels of estrogen and progesterone. The female sex hormones, produced by the ovaries, belong to two groups: **estrogens** and **progestogens.** The ovaries also produce a small amount of testosterone. The **adrenal glands** also produce sex hormones in both males and females.

Sex hormones are regulated by the hormones of the **pituitary gland,** located at the base of the brain. This gland in turn is controlled by hormones produced by the **hypothalamus** in the brain.

In Chapter 14, we examine endocrine-disrupting chemicals (EDCs), an example of a substance from the environment that acts like hormones and disrupts normal endocrine activity, particularly activity related to reproduction and development. The most studied EDCs are environmental estrogens, which mimic the female sex hormone estrogen and can duplicate or exaggerate its effects. Other EDCs can block estrogen, mimic or block androgens (male sex hormones), or otherwise alter hormonal responses in the body.

Differentiation of the Embryo

How do we become what might eventually be called a girl or a boy? All human cells typically contain 23 pairs of chromosomes. In 22 of the pairs, the two partner chromosomes match. But in the 23rd pair, one comes from the mother and one from the father; these are called the **sex chromosomes.** Mothers contribute an X and fathers an X or a Y, making the Y chromosome the primary determinant of a child's sex. Females are XX and males are XY, and this genetic fact occurs at the moment of conception.

TERMS

androgens   Male sex hormones, produced by the testes.

estrogens   A class of female sex hormones, produced by the ovaries, that bring about sexual maturation at puberty and maintain reproductive and other sexual functions.

progestogens   A class of female sex hormones, produced by the ovaries, that sustain reproductive and other sexual functions.

adrenal glands   Endocrine glands, located over the kidneys, that produce sex hormones.

pituitary gland   An endocrine gland at the base of the brain that produces hormones and regulates the release of hormones—including sex hormones—by other glands.

hypothalamus   A region of the brain above the pituitary gland whose hormones control the secretions of the pituitary; also involved in the control of many bodily functions, including hunger, thirst, temperature regulation, and sexual functions.

sex chromosomes   The X and Y chromosomes, which determine an individual's biological sex.

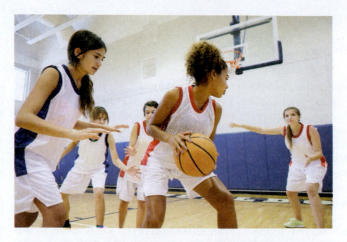

Once they reach puberty, adolescents are biologically adults, but it will take several more years for them to become adults in social and psychological terms.

© Cathy Yeulet/123RF

Abnormalities sometimes occur in the sex chromosomes; the two most common disorders of sex chromosomes—also known as intersex conditions—are Klinefelter syndrome and Turner syndrome. Klinefelter syndrome, a condition in which a male carries two or more X chromosomes in addition to the Y chromosome, occurs in about 1 in 1000 males and causes infertility and underdeveloped genitalia. Turner syndrome occurs in about 1 in 2500 females. Women with Turner have only a single complete X chromosome. People with this condition will need technological assistance to have children and can sometimes have other medical problems.

Genetic sex dictates whether the undifferentiated gonads become ovaries or testes. If a Y chromosome is present, the gonads become testes and produce the male hormone **testosterone.** Testosterone circulates throughout the body and causes the undifferentiated reproductive structures to develop into male sex organs (e.g., penis and scrotum). If the chromosomal arrangement is XX, the gonads become ovaries and the genital structures develop into a vagina, clitoris, and labia.

Female Sexual Maturation

Although humans are typically sexually differentiated at birth, the differences between males and females are accentuated at **puberty,** the period during which the reproductive system matures, secondary sex characteristics develop, and the bodies of males and females begin to appear more distinctive (while still overlapping in many ways). The changes of puberty are induced by testosterone in the male and estrogen and **progesterone** in the female.

Puberty in Females   The first sign of puberty in girls is often breast development, followed by a rounding of the hips and buttocks. As the breasts develop, hair appears in the pubic region and later in the underarms. Shortly after the onset of breast development, girls show an increase in growth rate. Breast development usually begins between ages 8 and 13, and the time of rapid body growth occurs between ages 9 and 15.

The Menstrual Cycle   A major landmark of puberty for most young women is the onset of the **menstrual cycle,** the monthly ovarian cycle that leads to menstruation (loss of blood and tissue lining the uterus) in the absence of pregnancy. The timing of **menarche** (the first *menstrual period*) varies with several factors, including race/ethnicity, genetics, and nutritional status. The "normal" range for the onset of menstruation is wide; some girls experience menarche as young as 9 or 10, and others when they are 16 or 17 years old. The current average age of menarche in the United States is around 12½ years of age.

The day of the onset of bleeding is considered to be day 1 of the menstrual cycle. For the purposes of our discussion, a cycle of 28 days will be used; however, normal cycles vary in length from 21 to 35 days. The menstrual cycle consists of the following four phases:

1. *Menses.* During **menses,** characterized by the menstrual flow, blood levels of hormones from the ovaries and the pituitary gland are relatively low. This phase of the cycle usually lasts from day 1 to about day 5.

2. *Estrogenic phase.* The estrogenic phase begins when the menstrual flow ceases and the pituitary gland begins to produce increasing amounts of follicle-stimulating hormone (FSH) and luteinizing hormone (LH). Under the influence of FSH, an egg-containing ovarian **follicle** begins to mature, producing increasingly higher amounts of estrogen. Stimulated by estrogen, the **endometrium** (the uterine lining) thickens with large numbers of blood vessels and uterine glands.

3. *Ovulation.* A surge of a potent estrogen called *estradiol* from the follicle causes the pituitary gland to release a large burst of LH and a smaller amount of FSH. The high concentration of LH stimulates the developing follicle to release its ovum. This event is known as

TERMS

testosterone   The hormone responsible for the development of male sex organs and secondary sex characteristics at puberty, such as deepened voice and growth of facial and body hair.

puberty   The period of biological maturation during adolescence; in this stage of development, the individual becomes capable of sexual reproduction.

progesterone   The most important female sex hormone for pregnancy; regulates the menstrual cycle and sustains pregnancy.

menstrual cycle   The monthly ovarian cycle, regulated by hormones; in the absence of pregnancy, menstruation occurs.

menarche   The first menstrual period, experienced by most young women at some point during adolescence

menses   The portion of the menstrual cycle characterized by menstrual flow.

follicle   A saclike structure within the ovary, in which an egg (ovum) matures.

endometrium   The lining of the uterus.

ovulation. After ovulation, the follicle is transformed into the **corpus luteum,** which produces progesterone and estrogen. Ovulation theoretically occurs about 14 days prior to the onset of menstrual flow, with the window of greatest fertility occurring from a few days before ovulation to about one day after. This information has been used to attempt to predict the most fertile time during the menstrual cycle for fertility treatments and natural family planning methods (see Chapter 6). However, a recent study showed that even women with regular menstrual cycles often have unpredictable ovulation, and can actually be fertile on any day of the month, including during menstruation. The "window of fertility" is especially unpredictable in teenagers and women who are approaching menopause.

4. *Progestational phase.* During the progestational phase of the cycle, the amount of progesterone secreted from the corpus luteum increases and remains high until the onset of the next menses. Under the influence of estrogen and progesterone, the endometrium continues to develop, readying itself to receive and nourish a fertilized ovum. If pregnancy occurs, the fertilized egg produces the hormone human chorionic gonadotropin (hCG), which maintains the corpus luteum. Thus levels of ovarian hormones remain high and the uterine lining is preserved, preventing menses. hCG is the hormone detected by pregnancy tests.

If pregnancy does not occur, the corpus luteum degenerates, and estrogen and progesterone levels gradually fall. Below certain hormonal levels, the endometrium can no longer be maintained, and it begins to slough off, initiating menses. As the levels of ovarian hormones fall, a slight rise in LH and FSH occurs, and a new menstrual cycle begins.

Menstrual Problems   Menstruation is a normal biological process, and physical or emotional symptoms associated with the menstrual cycle are common. Many women experience menstrual cramps, the severity of which tends to vary from cycle to cycle. **Dysmenorrhea,** discomfort associated with menstruation, can include any combination of the following symptoms: lower abdominal cramps, backache, vomiting, nausea, bloating, diarrhea, headache, and fatigue. Many of these symptoms can be attributed to uterine muscular contractions caused by chemicals called *prostaglandins.* Nonsteroidal anti-inflammatory drugs (NSAIDs) such as ibuprofen often relieve dysmenorrhea by blocking the effects of prostaglandins. Oral contraceptives are also effective in reducing dysmenorrheal symptoms in most women.

Many women experience transient emotional symptoms prior to the onset of their menstrual flow. Depending on their severity, these symptoms may be categorized along a continuum: **premenstrual tension, premenstrual syndrome (PMS),** and **premenstrual dysphoric disorder (PMDD).** Premenstrual tension symptoms are mild and may include negative mood changes and physical symptoms such as abdominal cramping and backache. More severe symptoms are classified as PMS; very severe symptoms that impair normal daily and social functioning are classified as PMDD. All three conditions share a definite pattern. Symptoms appear prior to the onset of menses and disappear within a few days after the start of menstruation. Premenstrual tension is quite common, PMS affects about 1 in 5 women, and PMDD affects fewer than 1 in 10 women.

Symptoms associated with PMS and PMDD can include breast tenderness, water retention (bloating), headache, fatigue, insomnia or excessive sleep, appetite changes, food cravings, irritability, anger, increased interpersonal conflict, depression, anxiety, tearfulness, inability to concentrate, social withdrawal, and the sense of being out of control or overwhelmed. Despite many research studies, the causes of PMS and PMDD are still unknown, and it is unclear why some women are more vulnerable than others. Most researchers agree that PMS is probably caused by a combination of hormonal, neurological, genetic, dietary, and psychological factors.

The following strategies provide relief for many women with premenstrual symptoms, and all of them can contribute to a healthy lifestyle at any time:

- *Limit salt intake.* Salt promotes water retention and bloating.
- *Exercise.* Women who exercise may experience fewer symptoms before and after menstrual periods.
- *Don't use alcohol or tobacco.* Alcohol and tobacco may aggravate certain symptoms of PMS and PMDD.

TERMS

ovulation   The release of a mature egg (ovum) from an ovary.

corpus luteum   The part of the ovarian follicle left after ovulation; secretes estrogen and progesterone during the second half of the menstrual cycle.

dysmenorrhea   Painful or problematic menstruation.

premenstrual tension   Mild physical and emotional changes associated with the time before the onset of menses.

premenstrual syndrome (PMS)   A disorder characterized by physical discomfort, psychological distress, and behavioral changes that begin after ovulation and cease when menstruation begins.

premenstrual dysphoric disorder (PMDD)   A severe form of PMS, characterized by symptoms serious enough to interfere with daily activities and relationships.

- *Eat a nutritious diet.* Choose a low-fat diet rich in complex carbohydrates from vegetables; fruits; and whole-grain breads, cereals, and pasta. Get enough calcium from calcium-rich foods and, if needed, supplements. Minimize your intake of sugar and caffeine, and avoid chocolate, which is rich in both.
- *Relax.* Stress reduction is always beneficial, and stressful events can trigger PMS symptoms. Try relaxation techniques during the premenstrual time. Orgasms, including those from **masturbation,** can also help reduce stress and relieve cramping.

If you suffer persistent premenstrual symptoms, keep a daily diary to track the types of symptoms, their severity, and their correlation with your menstrual cycle. Some women find help after being evaluated by a health care provider. Selective serotonin reuptake inhibitors (SSRIs), such as Prozac and Zoloft, are sometimes used to treat PMS and PMDD. Until recently, women using SSRIs took the medication throughout the entire menstrual cycle, but taking the medication during just the progestational phase of the cycle is effective in some women. However, these medications are not without side effects and may negatively affect sexual functioning—specifically causing low desire as well as difficulty with arousal and attaining orgasm.

Other drug treatments for PMS and PMDD include certain oral contraceptives, diuretics to minimize water retention, and NSAIDs such as ibuprofen. A number of vitamins, minerals, and other dietary supplements have also been studied for PMS relief. Only one supplement, calcium, has been shown to provide relief in rigorous clinical studies; several others show promise, but more research is needed.

Male Sexual Maturation

Reproductive maturation of boys occurs about two years later than that of girls; it usually begins at about age 10 or 11. Testicular growth is usually the first obvious sign of sexual maturity in boys. The penis also grows at this time, reaching adult size by about age 18. Pubic hair starts to develop after the genitals begin increasing in size, with underarm and facial hair gradually appearing. Hair on the chest, back, and abdomen increases later in development. Facial hair often continues to get thicker and darker for several years after puberty. The voice deepens as a result of the lengthening and thickening of the vocal cords. A small amount of breast development occurs in many boys during puberty. This is called *gynecomastia,* and it usually decreases after puberty. Excessive breast growth can occur in some boys, especially if they are overweight.

Boys grow taller for about six years after the first signs of puberty, with a rapid period of growth about two years after puberty starts. Largely because of the influence of testosterone, muscle development and bone density are much greater in males than in females. By adulthood, men, as a group, have one and a half times the lean body mass of women as a group, and nearly half the body fat. However, many individual men and women fall outside these averages.

Aging and Human Sexuality

Hormone production and sexual functioning change as we age. Although sexual functioning may diminish as one ages, sexuality and sensuality can continue to be a source of great pleasure and satisfaction. A recent study of sexuality in older Americans found that three-fourths of 57- to 64-year-olds were sexually active (defined as having had at least one sexual partner in the past year). Half of those people aged 65–74, and about one-fourth of people aged 75–85, remained sexually active. People who remain healthy and active are much more likely to continue to be sexually active in their older years.

Menopause   As a woman approaches age 50, her ovaries gradually cease to function and she enters **menopause,** the cessation of menstruation (Table 5.1). For some women, the associated drop in hormone production causes troublesome symptoms. The most common physical symptom of menopause is the hot flash, a sensation of warmth rising to the face from the upper chest, with or without perspiration and chills. During a hot flash, skin temperature can rise by more than 10 degrees. Other menopausal symptoms can include vaginal dryness, low libido, painful intercourse, night sweats, insomnia, thinning of head hair, and mood changes. Osteoporosis—decreasing bone density—can develop, making older women more vulnerable to fractures.

As a result of decreased estrogen production during menopause, the vaginal walls become thin, and lubrication in response to sexual arousal can diminish. Sexual intercourse may become painful. Hormonal treatment or the use of lubricants during intercourse can minimize these problems.

Cross-cultural studies comparing Japanese with North American women dispel the idea that hot flashes and other menopausal reactions are universal. A diet of fish and vegetables; an exercise regimen of cycling, walking, or farming; and cultural ideas about the meaning of bodily changes positively affected the Japanese experience of menopause among the women studied.

In Western medicine, doctors once regularly prescribed estrogen for postmenopausal women to relieve hot flashes,

masturbation   Self-stimulation for the purpose of sexual arousal and orgasm.

menopause   The cessation of menstruation, occurring gradually around age 50.

TERMS

Table 5.1 — Reproductive Aging in Women

AGE*	SIGNS & SYMPTOMS—WHAT'S HAPPENING	STAGE OF REPRODUCTION
9–15	First period; variable menstrual cycles	Menarche; beginning reproductive years
16–30	Regular menstrual cycle; fertility peaking	Reproductive years
31–42	Regular menstrual cycle; fertility progressively declining	Reproductive years
Early 40s	Lengths of menstrual cycle vary increasingly	Menopausal transition
Late 40s–early 50s	Two or more skipped periods; hot flashes, irritability, and sleep disturbance; bone loss begins	Menopausal transition
45–55	Final period (i.e., no period for 12 months)	Menopause
50s and beyond	Vaginal dryness, bone loss. Hot flashes can persist (for a few women, into their 60s and 70s).	Postmenopause

*Women vary a great deal in the ages at which they go through these stages. The average length of menopause and the transition leading up to it is four years, but for some women symptoms may last only a few months, and for others, 10 years.

SOURCE: American Society for Reproductive Medicine. 2012. *Reproductive Aging in Women* (http://www.reproductivefacts.org).

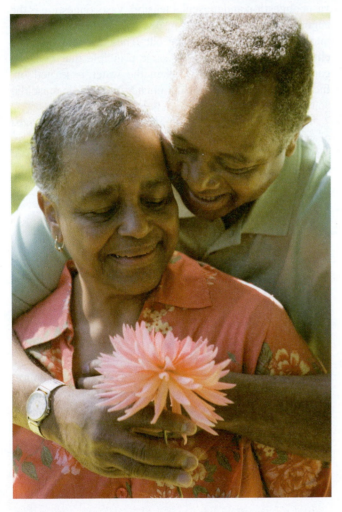

Although sexual physiology changes as people get older, many men and women readily adjust to these alterations.

© Big Cheese Photo/360/Getty Images RF

vaginal dryness, bone loss, and a host of other symptoms in a regimen called hormone replacement therapy, or HRT. However, in the past several years, reanalysis of the data on potential side effects, which include cardiovascular disease, blood clots, and breast cancer, has resulted in more individualized approaches—including, for example, low-dose estrogen, sometimes in the form of a patch, cream, or vaginal ring, designed to treat specific symptoms of menopause and with a reduced risk of side effects. (See Chapters 9, 12, and 17 for more information about osteoporosis and heart disease.)

Aging Male Syndrome Between the ages of 35 and 65, men experience a gradual decline in testosterone production, resulting in the aging male syndrome, sometimes referred to as *male menopause* or *andropause*. Some experts prefer the term *aging male syndrome* because the process is much more gradual than female menopause. Symptoms vary widely, but most men experience at least some of the following symptoms as they age: loss of muscle mass, increased fat mass, decreased sex drive, erectile problems, depressed mood, irritability, difficulties with concentration, increased urination, loss of bone mineral density, and sleep difficulties. In some cases, men who have low testosterone may benefit from carefully prescribed testosterone replacement therapy.

As men get older, they depend more on direct physical stimulation for sexual arousal. They take longer to achieve an erection and find it more difficult to maintain; orgasmic contractions are less intense. Older men with erectile dysfunction often use prescription medications that increase blood flow to the penis, resulting in a firmer erection.

Unlike women, who are born with all the eggs they will ever have and stop being fertile at menopause, men continue to produce sperm throughout their lives and can sometimes father children well into their eighties and even nineties. Starting at about age 30, however, men become gradually less fertile. The pregnancy rate drops to 50% for couples with a man over age 35, regardless of the woman's age. Men over age 40 are more likely to produce children with health problems such as autism, schizophrenia, and Down syndrome.

HOW SEX ORGANS FUNCTION DURING SEXUAL ACTIVITY

In this section, we discuss sexual physiology—how the sex organs function during sexual activity—and problems that can occur with sexual functioning. Sexual activity is based on stimulus and response. Erotic stimulation leads to sexual arousal (excitement), which may culminate in the intensely pleasurable experience of orgasm. Pleasure comes from engaging the genitals, and it also comes from engaging the entire body and mind.

Sexual Stimulation

Physical stimuli excite us directly; some people believe psychological stimuli—thoughts, fantasies, desires, perceptions—excite us even more. Regardless of the source of eroticism, all stimulation has a physical basis, to which the brain gives meaning.

Physical Stimulation Physical stimulation comes through the senses: We are aroused by things we see, hear, taste, smell, and feel. Most often, sexual stimuli come from other people, but they may also come from books, photographs, paintings, songs, films, or even ourselves through fantasy.

The most obvious and effective physical stimulation is touching. Even though culturally defined practices vary and different people have different preferences, most sexual encounters eventually involve some form of touching with hands, lips, and body surfaces. Kissing, caressing, fondling, and hugging are as much a part of sexual encounters as they are a part of expressing affection.

The most intense form of stimulation typically involves the genitals. The clitoris and the glans of the penis are particularly sensitive to such stimulation. Other highly responsive areas include the vaginal opening, nipples, breasts, insides of the thighs, buttocks, anal region, scrotum, lips, armpits, and earlobes. Such sexually sensitive areas, or erogenous zones, are especially susceptible to sexual arousal for most people, most of the time. Often, though, what determines the response is not *what* is touched but how, for how long, and by whom. Under the right circumstances, touching any part of the body can cause sexual arousal and even orgasm.

Psychological Stimulation Sexual arousal also has an important psychological component, regardless of the nature of the physical stimulation. Fantasies, ideas, memories of past experiences, and mood can all generate sexual excitement. Erotic thoughts may be linked to an imagined person or situation or to a sexual experience from the past. Fantasies may involve activities a person may not wish to experience in reality, usually because they're dangerous, frightening, or forbidden.

Arousal is also powerfully influenced by emotions and attitudes about sex. How you feel about sex and the person you are with, and how the person feels about you, matter tremendously in how sexually responsive you are likely to be. Even the most direct forms of physical stimulation carry emotional overtones. Kissing, caressing, and fondling express affection and caring. The emotional charge they give to a sexual interaction plays a significant role in sexual arousal—for some, as significant as the purely physical stimulation achieved by touching.

The Sexual Response Cycle

Men and women respond physiologically with a predictable set of reactions, regardless of the nature of the stimulation. Researchers disagree about whether male and female sexual response cycles are more different than similar, and some note that the gender roles of men and women affect their patterns of arousal and excitement. Two physiological mechanisms explain most genital and bodily reactions during sexual arousal and orgasm. These mechanisms are **vasocongestion** and muscular tension. Vasocongestion is the engorgement of tissues that results when more blood flows into an organ than is flowing out. Thus the penis and the clitoris become erect on the same principle that makes a garden hose become stiff when the water is turned on. Increased muscular tension culminates in rhythmic muscular contractions during orgasm.

There are several models of human sexual response, most of which are variations on the one described here. Some researchers include the feeling of desire as an integral part of the model, and others describe differences between men and women. In this model, developed by Masters and Johnson in 1966, four phases characterize the sexual response cycle:

1. *The excitement phase.* In men, the penis becomes erect as its tissues become engorged with blood. The testes expand and are pulled upward within the scrotum. In women, the clitoris, labia, and vaginal walls are similarly engorged with blood. Tension increases in the vaginal muscles, and the vaginal walls become moist with lubricating fluid.

2. *The plateau phase.* This is an extension of the excitement phase. Reactions become more marked. In men, the penis becomes harder, and the testes become larger. In women, the uterus rises, causing the inner one-third of the vaginal canal to lengthen and "tent" open near the cervix while the outer one-third of the vagina swells, and vaginal lubrication increases.

3. *The orgasmic phase.* In this phase, sometimes called **orgasm,** rhythmic contractions occur along the man's penis, urethra, prostate gland, seminal vesicles, and

> **TERMS**
>
> **vasocongestion** The accumulation of blood in tissues and organs by more blood flowing into an area than flowing out.
>
> **orgasm** The discharge of accumulated sexual tension with characteristic genital and bodily manifestations and a subjective sensation of intense pleasure; may include ejaculation for men and women.

muscles in the pelvic and anal regions. These involuntary muscular contractions lead to the ejaculation of semen, which consists of sperm cells from the testes and secretions from the prostate gland and seminal vesicles. In women, contractions occur in the lower part of the vagina and in the uterus, as well as in the pelvic region and the anus. Some women may also expel fluid from the urethra, known as female ejaculation.

4. *The resolution phase.* All changes initiated during the excitement phase are reversed. Excess blood drains from tissues, the muscles in the region relax, and the genital structures return to their unstimulated states. Males experience a *refractory period,* or period of time following orgasm in which more stimulation will not lead to physiological arousal.

More general physical reactions accompany the genital changes in both men and women. Beginning with the excitement phase, nipples become erect, the woman's breasts begin to swell, and in both sexes the skin of the chest becomes flushed (this is more visible in people with lighter skin); these changes are more marked in women. The heart rate doubles by the plateau phase, and respiration becomes faster. During orgasm, breathing becomes irregular and the person may moan or cry out. A feeling of warmth leads to increased sweating during the resolution phase. Deep relaxation and a sense of well-being pervade the body and the mind as the brain chemicals dopamine and oxytocin are released during the response cycle.

Male and female reactions during the sexual response cycle differ somewhat. For instance, the female excitement phase may lead directly to orgasm, or orgasmic and plateau phases may be fused. Male orgasm is marked by the ejaculation of semen. After ejaculation, men enter a refractory period. Women do not have this period and may immediately experience one or more orgasms.

Sexual Problems

Both physiological and psychological factors can interfere with sexual functioning. Many diseases specifically affect the sex organs. Any illness that affects your general health is likely to also affect your ability to function sexually. These problems may be due to physical problems, psychological issues, or a combination of both.

Common Sexual Health Problems   Medical conditions that affect women's sexual organs include the following:

• *Vaginitis* (inflammation of the vagina) is a common problem that can be caused by a variety of organisms: *Candida* (yeast infection), *Trichomonas* (trichomoniasis), and the overgrowth of a variety of bacteria (bacterial vaginosis). Symptoms include vaginal discharge, vaginal irritation, and pain during intercourse. Vaginitis is treated with a variety of topical and oral medications. (See Chapters 17 and 18 for more information about infection and sexually transmitted infections.)

• *Vulvodynia,* or chronic and unexplained vulvar pain, affects 15–18% of women in the United States. Patients describe their pain as "burning," "knifelike," and "raw." Because the condition presents diagnostic challenges, it's not uncommon for women and their sexual partners to wait five to seven years for a diagnosis and appropriate treatment.

• *Endometriosis* is the growth of endometrial-like tissue outside the uterus. It occurs most often in women of child-bearing age. Pain in the lower abdomen and pelvis is the most common symptom. Painful premenstrual intercourse may occur. Endometriosis can cause serious problems if left untreated because endometrial tissue can scar and partially or completely block the oviducts, causing infertility (difficulty conceiving) or sterility (the inability to conceive). Endometriosis is treated with medication and/or surgery.

• *Pelvic inflammatory disease (PID)* is an infection of the uterus, oviducts, or ovaries caused when microorganisms spread to these areas from the vagina. Approximately 50–75% of PID cases are caused by sexually transmitted organisms associated with diseases such as gonorrhea and chlamydia. PID can cause scarring of the oviducts, resulting in infertility or sterility. Symptoms include abdominal and pelvic pain, fever, and possibly pain during intercourse. (Chapter 18 discusses sexually transmitted infections in detail.)

• *Dyspareunia* (painful intercourse) is a common symptom in women, and it has many possible causes. Infection, lack of lubrication, endometriosis, past sexual trauma, fear of penetration, menopause, and scarring due to childbirth are a few common reasons for pain during intercourse. In some women, *vaginismus* (the involuntary contractions of pelvic muscles) makes sexual penetration difficult to impossible. This condition may also include discomfort with inserting a tampon or finger or discomfort during a pelvic exam.

Dyspareunia and vaginismus are treated first by diagnosing and treating any underlying physical cause of the problem. The use of generous amounts of lubricant during sexual activity is important. Sexual therapy for vaginismus often involves gradual desensitization techniques including the use of dilators. Dilators range in size and are inserted into the vagina in order to relax the vaginal muscles, to stop the involuntary spasms, and for the vagina to gradually stretch. The U.S. Food and Drug Administration (FDA) recently approved a procedure that uses injections of botulinum toxin, a chemical that paralyzes muscles and that has been successful in relaxing the pelvic muscles in some women with vaginismus.

Sexual health problems affecting men include the following:

• *Prostatitis* is an inflammation or infection of the prostate gland. Prostatitis can be acute (sudden) or chronic (gradual and long lasting). The symptoms of *acute bacterial prostatitis* usually appear suddenly and may include fever, chills, flu-like symptoms, pain in the lower back or groin, problems with urination, and painful ejaculation. Acute prostatitis is treated with antibiotics. It is potentially serious, so any man with these symptoms needs to seek immediate medical attention.

Chronic prostatitis is more common in men over age 40. It can be caused by infection or inflammation of the prostate and is sometimes difficult to diagnose and treat.

• *Prostate cancer* is the second most common cancer in men, especially older men. Men over 40 should have routine prostate exams done by a physician.

• *Testicular cancer* occurs most commonly in men in their twenties and thirties. A rare cancer, it has a very high cure rate if detected early. Every man should perform testicular self-exams regularly (see Chapter 16).

• *Epididymitis* is an inflammation of the epididymis (the coiled tube located on the top and back of each testicle). The most common cause of epididymitis is infection, often sexually transmitted. Symptoms include tenderness over the testicle, swelling, fever, and pain with ejaculation. The treatment is antibiotics.

• *Testicular torsion* occurs when the spermatic cord, which supplies blood to the testicle, becomes twisted. Decreased blood flow to the testicle causes severe, sudden pain, and if not treated quickly, it can cause permanent damage to the testicle. Testicular torsion is most common in adolescents and young men. It can be associated with trauma to the testicle, but it can occur spontaneously. Testicular pain should be evaluated by a medical professional promptly; sudden, severe pain is a medical emergency.

Sexual health problems affecting both women and men include *systemic diseases*—illnesses that affect organs throughout the body. A common example is diabetes (see Chapter 11), which causes a variety of problems, including neuropathy (damage to nerves), atherosclerosis (thickening and damage to the walls of the arteries), and poor immune function (making people with diabetes more prone to infection). Diabetes often results in sexual dysfunction because of poor blood flow to the sexual organs, along with impaired sensation and nerve function.

Sexual Dysfunctions

The term **sexual dysfunction** encompasses disturbances in sexual desire, performance, or satisfaction. Many physical conditions and drugs can interfere with sexual functioning. Psychological causes and relationship problems can be important factors as well. Sexual satisfaction is highly individual, so no one should feel that it is necessary to live up to a particular standard of sexual performance or "normalcy." Only you can determine if some aspect of your sexuality is creating a problem for you or your partner.

COMMON SEXUAL DYSFUNCTIONS Common sexual difficulties that men may experience are low desire, erectile dysfunction, premature ejaculation, and delayed ejaculation. **Erectile dysfunction** (previously called *impotence*) is the inability to achieve or maintain an erection sufficient for sexual activity. Erectile dysfunction occurs in men of all ages but becomes much more common as men age. **Premature**

ejaculation (ejaculation before or just after penetration) is also common, especially among younger men. If the problem is persistent and bothersome to the man and his partner, there are numerous treatments. **Delayed ejaculation** is the inability to ejaculate after an erection is achieved. Many men experience occasional difficulty achieving an erection or ejaculating because of excessive alcohol consumption, legal or illicit drugs, fatigue, or stress.

Female sexual problems can involve a lack of desire to have sex, the failure to become physically aroused and lubricated even when sex is desired, the inability to have an orgasm (**orgasmic dysfunction**), or pain during sexual penetration. All these problems can have physical and psychological components. Many medical problems can influence a woman's desire and ability to respond sexually. Factors such as hormonal birth control, menopause, and antidepressants can negatively affect sexual functioning. Psychological and social issues such as relationship difficulties, family stresses, depression, shame, guilt, and past sexual trauma are all frequent causes of sexual dysfunction for both women and men.

Orgasmic dysfunction has been the subject of a great deal of discussion over the years, as people debated the nature of the female orgasm and what constitutes dysfunction in women. Women are more likely to achieve orgasm from stimulation to the clitoris, through self-stimulation, manual stimulation with a partner, oral sex, or use of a vibrator than through sexual intercourse. Because many heterosexual couples do not engage in the practices that lead to female orgasm (cunnilingus, for example), and because women are sometimes discouraged from masturbating, many women believe they have an orgasmic dysfunction when all they need is a change in their behavior.

In general, the inability to experience orgasm is a problem only if a person considers it so.

CAUSES OF SEXUAL DYSFUNCTION For even an inkling of what might be causing a specific sexual dysfunction, the first step is to have a physical examination. This exam should evaluate an individual's overall health and explore a possible medical cause for the dysfunction. Heart disease and diabetes, for example, reduce blood flow and therefore

> **TERMS**
>
> **sexual dysfunction** A disturbance in sexual desire, performance, or satisfaction that causes distress.
>
> **erectile dysfunction** The inability to achieve or maintain an erection sufficient for sexual activity.
>
> **premature ejaculation** Involuntary orgasm before or shortly after the penis enters the vagina, mouth, or anus; ejaculation that takes place sooner than desired.
>
> **delayed ejaculation** The inability to ejaculate when you wish to during sexual activity.
>
> **orgasmic dysfunction** The inability to experience orgasm.

have a negative effect on arousal for both men and women. In men, this may cause erectile dysfunction; in fact, erectile dysfunction is often the first sign of a serious medical condition. This is one reason why men who buy drugs online to treat their erectile dysfunction without first getting a good medical evaluation may be missing out on the opportunity to diagnose and treat a potentially life-threatening disease. Up to 80% of all erectile problems are thought to be due to physical factors, particularly vascular problems involving restriction of blood flow. Smoking affects blood flow in the genitals (and throughout the body in both men and women) and is an independent risk factor for erectile dysfunction. Obesity is also a common cause of erectile dysfunction. Being overweight makes a man more vulnerable to cardiovascular problems, and it also can affect his hormonal balance.

Alcohol and many prescription and nonprescription drugs can inhibit sexual response. In particular, antidepressant drugs (especially SSRIs) are believed to cause sexual dysfunction in up to 50% of people. Sometimes drugs are used to counteract the side effects of antidepressants. Other common medications that can inhibit sexual response include certain drugs that treat high blood pressure.

TREATING SEXUAL DYSFUNCTION Most forms of sexual dysfunction are treatable. For erectile dysfunction in particular, many treatments are available. Viagra (sildenafil citrate), Cialis (tadalafil), and Levitra (vardenafil) work by enhancing the effects of nitric oxide, a chemical that relaxes smooth muscles in the penis. The relaxed muscles increase blood flow and allow a natural erection to occur in response to sexual stimulation. The medications are generally safe for healthy men, but they should not be used by men who have a high risk of heart attack or stroke. They are effective in about 70% of users, but there are potential side effects, including headaches, indigestion, facial flushing, back pain, visual and hearing disturbances, and changes in blood pressure.

The use of erectile dysfunction drugs by men between the ages of 18 and 45 has risen dramatically—possibly for recreational purposes. The drugs may cut the refractory period in men who do not have erectile dysfunction; younger men may also be using them to cope with performance anxiety or the effects of other drugs, such as antidepressants.

Although these drugs are not approved by the FDA for use by women, a growing number of women are trying them to help increase blood flow to the genitals, which is necessary for arousal and orgasm. Recent studies have shown that these drugs can sometimes help women with sexual dysfunction caused by the use of antidepressants.

Other treatments for erectile dysfunction in men are available. Prostaglandin E1 (Alprostadil) dilates blood vessels. It can be injected into the penis or placed into the tip of the penis as a tiny suppository about the size of a grain of rice. It works by relaxing the smooth muscles lining the blood vessels in the penis. Alprostadil in a cream form that can be applied to the penis is currently awaiting FDA approval. There are also vacuum devices that pull blood into the penis, and in cases where other treatments are unsuccessful, penile implants can be used. Exercise may also help improve erectile function, especially exercises that target the muscles of the pelvic floor.

For some men experiencing erectile dysfunction and low testosterone, hormone replacement therapy is an option. Testosterone replacement is a typical course of treatment when men have lower than normal levels of testosterone in the body. Symptoms of low testosterone include low libido, fatigue, anemia, increased body fat, reduced muscle mass, and mild depression.

Even when there is a physical reason for sexual dysfunction, emotional and social factors frequently compound the problem. Many people with no obvious physical disorder have sexual problems because of psychological and social issues.

Too often sexual difficulties are treated with drugs when nondrug strategies may be more appropriate. Psychosocial causes of dysfunction include troubled relationships, a lack of sexual skills, ineffective stimulation, irrational attitudes and beliefs, anxiety, prior learning and experiences, and psychosexual trauma such as sexual abuse or rape. Some sexual problems are the result of rigid gender roles that can lead men to believe they need to be the sexual "aggressor" and women to believe they should remain passive. Many of these problems can be addressed through sex therapy or counseling. A therapist may recommend books or films to help counter sexual myths and teach sexual skills. A therapist can also promote open discussion between partners and suggest specific techniques.

Premature ejaculation is an example of a common sexual problem that often responds well to nondrug therapy. On average, men typically ejaculate between 2 and 10 minutes after intercourse begins, but most men periodically ejaculate more quickly. Several nondrug techniques are frequently helpful for men who habitually ejaculate sooner than they would like. Kegel exercises, which strengthen and improve control of the pelvic muscles, as well as practicing masturbation to extend arousal, are often helpful. Certain antidepressants delay ejaculation and are sometimes prescribed for this purpose.

Women who seek treatment for orgasmic dysfunction often have not learned what types of stimulation will excite them and bring them to orgasm. Most sex therapists treat this problem with masturbation. Women are taught about their own anatomy and sexual responses and then are encouraged to experiment with masturbation, focusing on the clitoris, until they experience orgasm. Vibrators, once taboo, are becoming more common and are helpful devices during masturbation or intercourse. Once women can masturbate to orgasm, they can transfer this learning to other sexual behaviors including those with a partner. Because women are less encouraged to masturbate than are men, women sometimes have a difficult time learning this set of behaviors.

Substances being tested for the treatment of female sexual dysfunction include prostaglandin creams and testosterone patches. Testosterone replacement is currently being used "off-label" to treat low desire in women, because there has not been an FDA testosterone approved for women. A prostaglandin cream that improves blood flow to the clitoris is currently being developed and may be available to treat female sexual arousal disorder in the future. Other options are a vibrator and a device that creates suction over the clitoris to increase blood flow and sensitivity.

In 2015, a drug called Addyi (flibanserin) was introduced as a treatment for female hypoactive sexual desire disorder. The FDA approved the drug after two previous rejections and a lot of controversy. Some women were eager to have access to a "pink Viagra," but opponents argued that it had more risks than benefits. Unlike erectile dysfunction drugs, flibanserin must be taken every day, cannot be mixed with alcohol, and can lead to dizziness and even unconsciousness in users. Detractors further argue that a decreased desire for sex is a more complicated problem than erectile dysfunction (which is a matter of restoring blood flow to the penis) and that a pill will provide false reassurance to women who might benefit more from education, behavioral changes, or therapy. Clinical studies showed that the drug helped 10–12% of users, who averaged 0.5 more "sexual events" per month than nonusers. Like many medications designed to treat sexual problems, time will tell us more about flibanserin's usefulness in a general population.

GENDER ROLES AND SEXUAL ORIENTATION

As discussed in Chapters 2 and 4, your *gender role* is everything you do in your daily life that expresses your gender—your masculinity, femininity, or queerness—to others, including dress, speech patterns, and mannerisms. Parents often choose gender-specific names, clothes, and toys for their children, and children may model their own behavior after their same-gender parent. Family and friends create an environment that teaches the child how to act appropriately as a girl or a boy. Teachers, television, books, and even strangers model these gender roles. The concept of gender roles is intertwined with that of sexual orientation, a topic we also explore in this section.

Gender Roles

In general, **gender** is distinct from sex in that it refers to how people identify and feel about themselves, rather than the body parts and sexual organs they have. For example, a person who was born with a penis—and therefore assigned a male sex—may feel more like a girl or a woman than a man. They may also feel like neither, and identify as **queer** or **genderqueer.** As discussed earlier, some people who feel masculine or feminine but whose sex does not match their gender refer to themselves as transgender; people who identify as neither gender sometimes use the term **gender nonconforming.** Transgender individuals may be heterosexual, homosexual, bisexual, or asexual, or they may have any combination of sexual orientations. They are more likely to identify around the ways they do or don't feel like a woman, man, both, or neither than around who they feel attracted to, love, or want to have sex with.

Some people use the term **androgyny** to describe the state of being neither overtly male or female. Androgynous adults are less gender stereotyped in their thinking; in how they look, dress, and act; in how they divide work in the home; in how they think about jobs and careers; and in how they express themselves sexually.

The term **cisgender** describes people who do not feel transgender but who instead feel that the sex they were assigned at birth (usually male or female), and the gender they were raised with as a result, aligns with the way they feel about themselves. A cisgender woman, for example, would likely have been born with female sexual organs and genitals, would have been raised as a girl, and experiences herself as a woman.

Transsexual is a term that describes transgender people who seek sex reassignment, which involves hormonal treatments to induce secondary sex characteristics such as breasts or facial hair, and/or surgery to change the appearance of the genitals or breasts. People who were born male and use surgery and other

TERMS

gender How people identify and feel about themselves, rather than the body parts and sexual organs they have.

queer or **genderqueer** A term describing people who question gender categories and who do not dress or identify as either male or female.

gender nonconforming An alternative term describing people who question gender categories and who do not dress or identify as either male or female.

androgyny The state of being neither overtly male or female.

cisgender A term that describes individuals whose bodily sex and initial gender assignment align with their own gender identity.

transsexual A term that describes transgender people who seek sex reassignment, which involves hormonal treatments to induce secondary sex characteristics such as breasts or facial hair, and/or surgery to change the appearance of the genitals or breasts.

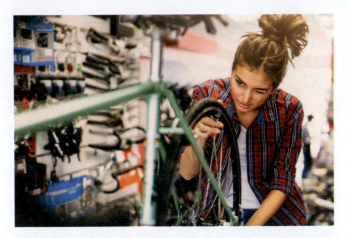

Our sense of gender is shaped by cultural factors. Gender stereotypes can limit career aspirations, but awareness can help counter stereotypes, broaden occupational choices, and provide opportunities for everyone to pursue individual goals.

© Todor Tsvetkov/Getty Images

procedures to fully transition to being a woman are sometimes called male-to-female transsexuals. People born female who undergo surgery and procedures to become men are called female-to-male transsexuals.

Not all transgender people desire surgical or hormonal treatment but still wish to live in another gender. These people might also use the terms trans woman (male-to-female transition) or trans man (female-to-male transition).

In contrast, the term **transvestite** refers to a person, usually a man, who enjoys wearing clothing identified with another gender. Cross-dressing covers a broad range of behaviors, from wearing one article of clothing associated with another sex in a private location to wearing an entire outfit in public. Though once thought to be gay men, the majority of transvestites are heterosexual, married men.

Transgender children may, from an early age, show intense and persistent distress about their sex and may behave and view themselves as another sex. Some of these children may be diagnosed with gender incongruence, and some may be given medications to slow or delay the potentially distressing bodily changes associated with puberty.

Sexual Orientation

Sexual orientation refers to the person or people you are emotionally connected to (love), romantically attached to (relationship), sexually attracted to (desire), and behaviorally

intimate with (sex). For many people, the pattern is consistent, exclusively heterosexual or exclusively homosexual for all categories: love, relationship, desire, and sex. For others, there may be more variation. As indicated, sexual orientation exists along a continuum that ranges from exclusive heterosexuality (attraction to people of the other sex) through bisexuality (attraction to people of both sexes) to exclusive homosexuality (attraction to people of your own sex) to asexuality (lack of sexual attraction to others). The terms *straight* and *gay* are often used to refer to heterosexuals and homosexuals, respectively, and female homosexuals are also referred to as *lesbians*. As mentioned earlier, in recent years the term *queer* has been reclaimed as a self-identifier by some elements of the gay community as well as by people who do not identify with conventional gender categories or with the gender they were assigned as children.

Sexual orientation involves feelings and self-concept, and individuals may or may not express their sexual orientation in their behavior. In national surveys, about 2–6% of men identify themselves as homosexuals and about 2% of women identify themselves as lesbians. Gauging the accuracy of these estimates is difficult because people may not tell the truth in surveys that probe sensitive and private aspects of their lives. In addition, people's expressed sexual orientations may be quite different from their actual sexual practices. For example, some people identify as heterosexual, but most of their sexual partners may be of their own sex.

Heterosexuality   A majority of people are heterosexual. Heterosexual relationships usually include all of the behavior and relationship patterns described in Chapter 4: dating, engagement, living together, and marriage.

Homosexuality   Though homosexuality exists in all cultures, attitudes toward homosexuality vary tremendously. In some cultures, homosexual behavior is fully accepted; in others, it is tolerated but not encouraged. In some societies, homosexuality is illegal and can be punished severely, even by death. Homosexual individuals are as varied and different from one another as heterosexuals are. Just like heterosexuals, lesbians and gay men may be in long-term, committed relationships, or they may date different people. And, as of 2016, same-sex couples can marry in more than 20 countries, including the United States.

Bisexuality   Because many experts believe that human sexuality exists on a spectrum, they also believe that many of us are potentially bisexual. However, only a relatively small number of people are more or less equally attracted to both men and women. In the United States, fewer than 5% of men and women identify themselves as bisexual. Some observers think bisexuals

> **QUICK STATS**
>
> Almost three times as many women **(17.4%)** as men **(6.2%)** aged 18–44 reported any same-sex contact in their lifetime.
>
> —National Health Statistics Report, 2016

TERMS

transvestite   A term for people, usually men, who enjoy wearing clothing identified with another gender.

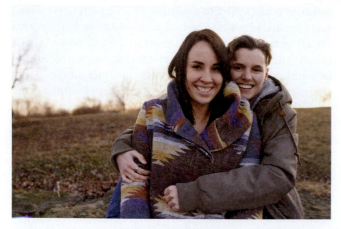

This couple's physical experiences together will be powerfully affected by their emotions, ideas, values, and the quality of their relationship.

© jeffbergen/Getty Images

are confused and do not know if they like men or women; however, most bisexuals are clear they like *both* men and women.

The Origins of Sexual Orientation   Many theories try to account for the development of sexual orientation. At this time, most experts agree that sexual orientation results from multiple genetic, hormonal, cultural, social, and psychological factors. Many people report being aware of their gender identity and sexual orientation early in life, long before they became sexually active, and most do not feel they had a choice in their sexual orientation. The majority of experts agree that conscious choice is not usually a factor in whether someone is gay, straight, or queer.

Some scientists, however, continue to look for genetic markers associated with sexual orientation in males. Current research provides evidence that our genes, while not wholly responsible for our sexual orientation, may contribute to it. And exposure to hormones before birth may also have an impact on sexual orientation.

Many psychological theories have been proposed to explain the development of heterosexual or homosexual sexual orientation. However, the significant growth of single-parent families over the past 40 years has not been accompanied by large shifts in sexual orientation among Americans, so it is unlikely that family dynamics or early learning experiences are strong factors in determining sexual orientation. In addition, parents' sexual orientation seems to have little impact on children's sexual orientation. Studies of children raised by gay or lesbian parents show that these children's ultimate sexual orientation is similar to that of children raised by heterosexual parents. In addition, most people who identify as gay or lesbian had heterosexual parents.

So far, most studies on the origin of sexual orientation have focused on males. The factors that determine sexual orientation in women may be even more complex. Although genes appear to be one likely determinant of sexual orientation, further research is required to fully understand the complex interactions that exist.

SEXUAL BEHAVIOR

A wide variety of behaviors stem from sexual impulses, and sexual expression takes a variety of forms. For some people, the most basic aspect of sexuality is reproduction; for others, sex is more about fun and pleasure than having children. In general, sexual excitement and satisfaction are aspects of sexual behavior separate from reproduction, and the intensely pleasurable sensations of arousal and orgasm are some of the strongest motivators for human sexual behavior. People are infinitely varied in the ways they seek to experience erotic pleasure.

Not all people experience sexual pleasure in the same way. **Asexual** is the term used to describe people who do not experience sexual desire but who may still enjoy being in romantic and other close relationships. Some asexual people, called demisexuals, experience sexual attraction only to people with whom they feel an intimate or loving bond.

Ask Yourself

QUESTIONS FOR CRITICAL THINKING AND REFLECTION
Whether you are straight, gay, lesbian, or asexual, how and when did you become aware of your sexual orientation?

?

Varieties of Human Sexual Behavior

Some sexual behaviors are aimed at self-stimulation only, whereas other practices involve interaction with one or more partners (see the box "Questions to Ask Before Engaging in a Sexual Relationship"). Some people feel sexual but choose not to express it, and some people do not feel any form of sexual desire.

Celibacy   Continuous abstention from sexual activities, called **celibacy,** can be a conscious and deliberate choice, or it can be necessitated by circumstances. Health considerations and religious and moral beliefs may lead some people to celibacy, particularly until marriage or until an acceptable partner appears.

Many people use the related term *abstinence* to refer to avoidance of just one sexual activity—intercourse. Celibacy and abstinence are not the same thing as asexuality because many people who identify as asexual engage in sexual activity with the people they love and feel close to. Asexuality refers to a lack of sexual desire, but not an avoidance of sexual behavior.

TERMS

asexual   The term used to describe people who do not experience sexual desire but who may still enjoy being in romantic and other close relationships.

celibacy   Continuous abstention from sexual activity.

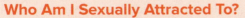

Who Am I Sexually Attracted To?

• What are the characteristics that usually attract me to someone in a physical way?

• How comfortable am I with the people I find sexually attractive? What would I change if I could? Do I feel safe when I am with them?

• Are the people I am usually sexually attracted to the same types of people with whom I could envision having a long-term, stable relationship? Why or why not?

What Sexual Behaviors are Comfortable for Me Right Now?

• What has influenced my comfort level with these behaviors?

• What am I not entirely comfortable with, but would be willing to experiment with in order to please a partner? What level of trust would I need to establish with that partner in order to proceed? What would we need to talk about ahead of time?

• What exactly do I say in order to make my comfort level clear to my partner? What do I do if my partner tries to push me beyond my comfort level?

How Can I Express My Sexual Needs, Desires, and Concerns To a Potential Sexual Partner?

• When would be the best time to talk about these needs, desires, and concerns?

• How do I start the conversation?

• What will I do if my needs are not being met or my concerns are not taken seriously?

What Preparations Do I Need To Make in Order To Engage in the Safest Sex Possible?

• If I am engaging in heterosexual sexual activity, and I do not wish to reproduce, I need to obtain birth control. Have I consulted a health professional to figure out the best method of birth control for myself and my partner? Do I know how to employ this method correctly? Have we discussed what we plan to do if a pregnancy occurs?

• If I am engaging in any type of sexual activity with a partner, I need protection from sexually transmitted infections. Have I consulted a health professional to figure out the best method of STI protection for myself and my partner? Do I know how to employ this method correctly? Have I discussed with my partner his or her sexual history, including information about risky behavior and STIs? Do I understand the ways that sexual behaviors transmit these infections?

• What do I need from my partner in order to ensure that I feel emotionally safe before, during, and after our sexual behavior together?

• Do I engage in any behaviors that cause me to participate in sexual activity that I wouldn't otherwise be comfortable with, such as excessive drinking or drug use? What do I need to do in order to reduce or eliminate these behaviors?

• Do I make sure that the people with whom I am being sexual are actively consenting to the behaviors? Do I understand what constitutes sexual consent? Do I understand that I need to stop what I'm doing if the other person asks me to or is not communicating active and willing consent?

Autoeroticism The most common sexual behavior for humans is masturbation. Masturbation is one form of **autoeroticism;** another is **erotic fantasy,** or creating imaginary experiences that range from fleeting thoughts to elaborate scenarios. Orgasms originate in our brain as it gives meaning to stimulation and pleasure. Using functional MRI (fMRI) scans to map orgasms in the brain, researchers at Rutgers University found that at the time of orgasm every part of our brain lights up and is engaged. No other activity produces the same brain response.

Touching and Foreplay For many people, touching is integral to sexual experiences, whether in the form of massage, kissing, fondling, or holding. The entire body surface is a sensory organ, and touching almost anywhere can enhance intimacy and sexual arousal. Touching can convey a variety of messages, including affection, comfort, and a desire for further sexual contact.

During arousal, many partners manually and orally stimulate each other by touching, stroking, and caressing their partner's genitals. People vary greatly in their preferences for the type, pace, and vigor of such **foreplay.** Working out the details to accommodate each other's pleasure is a key to enjoying these activities. Direct communication about preferences can enhance sexual pleasure and protect both partners from physical and psychological discomfort. There is no correct order in which to engage in sexual activity, and these behaviors can also be engaged in instead of or after penetrative intercourse.

> **TERMS**
>
> **autoeroticism** Behavior aimed at sexual self-stimulation.
>
> **erotic fantasy** Sexually arousing thoughts and daydreams.
>
> **foreplay** Kissing, touching, and any form of oral or genital contact.

Oral-Genital Stimulation **Cunnilingus** (the stimulation of the female genitals with the lips and tongue) and **fellatio** (the stimulation of the penis with the mouth) are common practices. Oral sex may be practiced either as part of foreplay or as a sex act culminating in orgasm. Although prevalence varies in different populations, 90% of men, 88% of women, and more than 50% of teens report that they have engaged in oral sex. A recent study showed that more teens aged 15–19 had engaged in oral sex than had engaged in vaginal intercourse. Some studies show that people who report having oral sex are usually talking about fellatio and not cunnilingus, and many women report that male partners are reluctant to orally stimulate their genitals. This is one reason why many women find it difficult to have regular orgasms during heterosexual encounters.

Like all acts of sexual expression between two people, oral sex requires the cooperation and consent of both partners. If they disagree about its acceptability, they need to discuss their feelings and try to reach a mutually pleasing solution.

Anal Intercourse About 36% of males and 31% of women, heterosexual and homosexual, report having engaged in anal sex. Some men and women find they are able to achieve orgasm through anal sex. Males who are being penetrated, either by a penis, finger, or sex toy, may find this induces orgasm because stimulation to the prostate may cause an ejaculation. This stimulation is often referred to as "milking the prostate" or prostate massage.

Because the anus is composed of delicate tissues that tear easily with friction, anal intercourse can be one of the riskiest of sexual behaviors for the transmission of HIV and all other STIs. If people are monogamous, up to date with their STI status, or use barrier devices such as condoms, the risk becomes lower. The use of condoms is highly recommended for anyone engaging in anal sex.

Sexual Intercourse Men and women engage in vaginal intercourse for a variety of reasons, including to fulfill sexual and psychological needs and to reproduce. Among adults aged 18–44, 92% of men and 94% of women report having had vaginal intercourse. The most common heterosexual practice involves the man inserting his erect penis into the woman's lubricated vagina after sufficient arousal.

Much has been written on how to enhance pleasure through various coital techniques, positions, and practices.

For a woman, the key factor in physical readiness for coitus is adequate vaginal lubrication, and in psychological readiness, being aroused and receptive. For a man, the setting and the partner must arouse him to attain and maintain an erection. For many people, psychological factors and the quality of the relationship are more important to overall sexual satisfaction than sophisticated or exotic sexual techniques.

The use of force and coercion in sexual relationships is one of the most serious problems in human interactions. The most extreme manifestation of **sexual coercion**—forcing a person to submit to another's sexual desires—is rape, but sexual coercion occurs in many subtler forms, such as sexual harassment.

Commercial Sex

Conflicting feelings about sexuality are apparent in the attitudes of Americans toward commercial sex: prostitution and sexually oriented materials in a variety of formats. Prostitution is illegal in most of the United States, but penalties and general social disapproval have failed to eliminate it. Pornography is readily available and widely viewed in our society, although many people are concerned about its ubiquitous nature and the blurring of pornography with popular culture.

Pornography Derived from the Greek word meaning "the writing of prostitutes," **pornography** (*porn*) is now often defined as obscene literature, art, or movies. A major problem in identifying pornographic material is that people and communities differ about what is obscene, as obscenity is typically a judgment by someone who finds it offensive. Differing definitions of obscenity have led to many legal battles over potentially pornographic materials. Currently the sale and rental of pornographic materials is restricted so that only adults can legally obtain them; however, the Internet is difficult to regulate, and many minors may have access to pornographic materials online. Child pornography—showing children who are not 18 years old naked and/or in sexual acts—is illegal.

Much of the debate about pornography focuses on whether it is harmful. Some people argue that adults who want to view pornographic materials in the privacy of their own homes should be allowed to do so. Others feel that the exposure to explicit sexual material can lead to delinquent or criminal behavior, such as rape or the sexual abuse of children. Currently there is no reliable evidence that pornography by itself leads to violence or rape, and debate is likely to continue.

TERMS

cunnilingus Oral stimulation of the female genitals.

fellatio Oral stimulation of the penis.

sexual coercion The use of physical or psychological force or intimidation to make a person submit to sexual demands.

pornography The depiction of sexual activities in pictures, writing, or other material with the intent to arouse.

Ask Yourself

QUESTIONS FOR CRITICAL THINKING AND REFLECTION

What do you consider to be appropriate, moral sexual behavior? What behaviors do you think are inappropriate or immoral? What experiences have shaped your views of such behaviors? Have they changed in the past five years? What do you think they will be like five years from now?

Online Porn and Cybersex The appearance of thousands of sexually oriented websites has expanded the number of people with access to pornography, and it has made it more difficult for authorities to enforce laws regarding porn. People who might have hesitated to buy magazines or rent videos in person can now access sexually explicit materials online. Of special concern is the increased availability of child pornography, which previously could be acquired only with great difficulty and at great legal risk. Online porn is now a multibillion-dollar industry.

In addition to (or instead of) viewing porn online, hundreds of thousands of people also use the Internet to engage in **cybersex,** or *virtual sex.* Cybersex is erotic interaction between people who are communicating over the Internet. People can engage in cybersex in many ways, such as by visiting sexually oriented websites, joining cybersex chat rooms, participating in videoconferences via web cams, or even exchanging e-mail messages. Participants may have sexually explicit discussions, share private photographs, or engage in fantasy role-playing online. Many cybersex participants report feeling some degree of sexual excitement; some masturbate while viewing erotic images online or engaging in sexual chat. Online sex is an excellent way for people who have difficulty meeting partners, for economic, psychological, or physical reasons, to meet others and maintain relationships. It is also, for many people, a fun and novel way of expressing their sexuality.

"Sexting," sending provocative photos from cell phone to cell phone, has become popular, sometimes with serious consequences. Images can end up traveling from person to person by cell phone and from there onto social networking websites. These images can haunt individuals years later when they are viewed by potential employers or partners. Some teens have found themselves charged with child pornography and have even faced jail time as a result of forwarding a sexually explicit photo of an underage person to a friend. Teens who have found pictures of themselves engaging in sexual activity posted or shared online have faced adverse effects. Some have even committed suicide.

Prostitution The exchange of sexual services for money is **prostitution,** also called **sex work.** Sex workers may be men, women (including trans men and women), or children, and the buyer of their services is nearly always a man, most of whom are white, middle class, middle aged, and married. Except in parts of Nevada, prostitution is illegal in the United States.

Purchasing sex can offer someone physical release without having to confront some of the more complicated aspects of sex: commitment, an expectation of intimacy, or a fear of rejection. Some people patronize prostitutes in order to have sex with a different type of partner than usual or to engage in a type of sex in which their usual partner is uninterested.

Sex workers come from a variety of backgrounds, and, like everyone who participates in the labor force, they are economically (rather than sexually) motivated. Many people who have sex for money lack the skills and education to engage in other forms of work, and they view their bodies as their most marketable asset. Many, though not all, report having been sexually abused as children; some begin as runaways who are escaping abusive homes and turn to prostitution as a way to survive. Queer and transgender people who have had to leave homes that do not accept their identities sometimes engage in sex work for these reasons.

Although many sex workers routinely use condoms with their clients, HIV infection and other STIs are still a concern. Some sex workers are injection drug users, and some have customers who are, contributing to a rate of HIV infection among this population that can be as high as 25–50%.

Responsible Sexual Behavior

Healthy sexuality is an important part of adult life. It can be a source of pleasurable experiences and emotions and an important part of intimate partnerships. But sexual behavior also carries many responsibilities, as well as potential consequences such as pregnancy, STIs, and emotional changes in the relationship. Consider the following with your partners:

Open, Honest Communication Each partner needs to clearly indicate what sexual involvement means to them. Does it mean love, fun, a permanent commitment, or something else? The intentions of both partners should be clear. For strategies on talking about sexual issues with your partner, see the box "Communicating about Sexuality."

Agreed-On Sexual Activities No one should pressure or coerce a partner. Sexual behaviors should be consistent with the sexual values, preferences, and comfort level of all partners. Everyone has the right to refuse sexual activity at any time, including married couples.

Sexual Privacy Intimate relationships involving sexual activity are based on trust, and that trust can be violated if partners reveal private information about the relationship to others. Sexual privacy also involves respecting other people—not engaging in activities in the presence of others that would make them uncomfortable.

Safe Sex Sexual partners should be aware of and practice safe sex to guard against STIs. Many sexual behaviors carry the risk of STIs, including HIV infection. Partners should be honest about their health and any medical conditions and work out a plan for protection.

---

cybersex Erotic interaction between people who are not in physical contact, conducted over a network such as the Internet; also called *virtual sex.*

prostitution/sex work The exchange of sexual services for money or goods.

TERMS

To talk with your partner about sexuality, follow the general suggestions for effective communication in Chapter 4. Getting started may be the most difficult part. Some people feel more comfortable if they begin by talking about talking—that is, initiating a discussion about why people are so uncomfortable talking about sexuality. Talking about sexual histories—how partners first learned about sex or how family and cultural background influenced sexual values and attitudes—is another way to get started. Reading about sex can also be a good beginning: Partners can read an article or book and then discuss their reactions.

Be honest about what you feel and what you want from your partner. Cultural and personal obstacles to discussing sexual subjects can be difficult to overcome, but self-disclosure is important for successful relationships. Research indicates that when one partner openly discusses attitudes and feelings, the other partner is more likely to do the same. If your partner seems hesitant to open up, try asking open-ended or either/or questions: "Where do you like to be touched?" or "Would you like to talk about this now or wait until later?"

If something is bothering you about your sexual relationship, choose a good time to initiate a discussion with your partner. Be specific and direct but also tactful. Focus on what you actually observe rather than on what you think the behavior means. "You didn't touch or hug me when your friends were around" is an observation. "You're ashamed of me around your friends" is an inference about your partner's feelings. Try focusing on a specific behavior that concerns you rather than on the person as a whole—your partner can change behaviors but not his or her entire personality. For example, you could say, "I'd like you to take a few minutes away from studying to kiss me" instead of "You're so caught up in your work, you never have time for me."

If you are going to make a statement that your partner may interpret as criticism, try mixing it with something positive: "I love being with you, but I feel annoyed when you. . . ." Similarly, if your partner says something that upsets you, don't lash back. An aggressive response may make you feel better in the short run, but it will not help the communication process or the quality of the relationship.

If you want to say no to some sexual activity, say no unequivocally. Don't send mixed messages. If you are afraid of hurting your partner's feelings, offer an alternative if it's appropriate: "I am uncomfortable with that. How about . . .?"

If you're in love, you may think that the sexual aspects of a relationship will work out magically without discussion. However, partners who never talk about sex deny themselves the opportunity to increase their closeness and improve their relationship.

Contraception Use   If pregnancy is not desired, contraception should be used during sexual intercourse. Both partners need to take responsibility for protecting against unwanted pregnancy. Partners should discuss contraception before sexual involvement begins.

Sober Sex   The use of alcohol or drugs in sexual situations increases the risk of unplanned, unprotected sexual activity. Such consequences are particularly true for young adults, many of whom binge-drink during social events. The link between intoxication and unsafe sex is illustrated by a recent study that found states with higher drinking ages and higher beer taxes to have lower rates of STIs.

Binge drinking also increases the risk of sexual assault. About 20% of women in college experience sexual assault. Unfortunately, a cycle then ensues for some of these women: those with a history of sexual assault are then more likely to drink heavily. Approximately 30% of underage college women engage in such heavy episodic drinking, and women under age 21 also bear the highest risk for sexual assault in college. Alcohol and drugs impair judgment and should not be used in association with sexual activity. Be honest with yourself; if you need to drink in order to engage in sexual activities, maybe it's time to rethink your social life and relationships. As noted earlier, someone who is intoxicated cannot legally consent to sex.

Ask Yourself
QUESTIONS FOR CRITICAL THINKING AND REFLECTION
If you are sexually active or plan to become active soon, how open have you been in communicating with your partner? Are you aware of your partner's feelings about sex and about their comfort level with certain activities? Do you and your partner share the same views on contraception, STI prevention, and ethical issues about sex?

UNDERSTANDING FERTILITY AND INFERTILITY

Conception is a complex process. Although many couples conceive easily, others face a variety of difficulties.

Conception

The process of conception begins with the union of the nucleus of a woman's egg cell (ovum) and the nucleus of a man's sperm cell—a process called **fertilization.** Every month during a woman's fertile years, her body prepares itself for conception and pregnancy. In one of her ovaries, an egg matures and is released from its follicle. The egg, about the size of a fine grain of sand, travels through an oviduct, or fallopian tube, to the uterus in three to four days. The endometrium, which is the lining of the uterus, has already thickened for the implantation of a **fertilized egg,** that is, a *zygote*. If the egg is not fertilized, it lasts about 24 hours and then disintegrates. The woman's body then sheds the uterine lining during menstruation.

Fertilization Sperm cells are produced in the man's testes and ejaculated from his penis into the woman's vagina during sexual intercourse (except in cases of artificial insemination or assisted reproduction; see the section "Treating Infertility"). Sperm cells are much smaller than eggs. The typical ejaculate contains millions of sperm, but only a few complete the journey through the uterus and up the fallopian tube to the egg. Many sperm cells do not survive the vagina's acidic environment.

Of those that reach the egg, only one will penetrate its hard outer layer. As sperm approach the egg, they release enzymes that soften this outer layer. Enzymes from hundreds of sperm must be released in order for the egg's outer layer to soften enough to allow one sperm cell to penetrate. The first sperm cell that bumps into a spot that is soft enough can swim into the egg cell. It then fuses with the nucleus of the egg, and fertilization occurs. The sperm's tail, its means of locomotion, is left behind on the egg's outer membrane, while the sperm's head is inside the egg. The egg then undergoes chemical change that makes it impenetrable to other sperm.

The ovum carries the hereditary characteristics of the mother and her ancestors; sperm cells carry the hereditary characteristics of the father and his ancestors. Each parent cell—egg or sperm—contains 23 chromosomes, each of which contains **genes,** which are packages of biochemical instructions for the developing baby. Genes provide the blueprint for a unique individual based on the functional and health characteristics of his or her ancestors.

Twins In the usual course of events, one egg and one sperm unite to produce one fertilized egg and one baby. But if the ovaries release two eggs during ovulation and both eggs are fertilized, twins develop. These twins will be no more alike than siblings from different pregnancies because each will have come from a different fertilized egg. Twins who develop this way are referred to as **fraternal (dizygotic) twins;** they may be the same sex or different sexes. About 70% of twins are fraternal.

Twins can also develop from the early division of a single fertilized egg into two cells that develop separately. Because these babies share all genetic material, they will be **identical (monozygotic) twins.**

The most serious complication of multiple births is preterm delivery (delivery before the fetuses are adequately mature). The higher the number of fetuses a woman carries, the earlier in gestation she will deliver. This leads to higher rates of complications due to prematurity.

Infertility

About 2 million American couples have difficulty conceiving. **Infertility** is defined as the inability to conceive after trying for a year or more. Infertility affected about 6.1% of American women of reproductive age (15–44 years) in the United States in 2013. Over 1 million women seek treatment for infertility each year. Although the focus is often on women, one-fourth (26%) of the factors contributing to infertility are male, and in one-third (35%) of infertile couples, both partners have problems. Therefore, it is important that both partners be evaluated.

Female Infertility One-third of cases of female infertility usually result from one of two key causes—tubal blockage (14%) or failure to ovulate (21%). An additional one-third (37%) of cases of female infertility are due to anatomical abnormalities, benign growths in the uterus, thyroid disease, and other uncommon conditions; the remaining 28% of cases are unexplained.

Blocked oviducts are most commonly the result of *pelvic inflammatory disease (PID)*, a serious complication of several STIs. One study found that of 100,000 women aged 20–24 who were diagnosed with PID, 16,800 (one of every six) went on to have problems with infertility. Most cases of PID are associated with untreated cases of chlamydia or gonorrhea, both of which can occur without symptoms. Tubal blockages can also be caused by prior surgery or by *endometriosis,* a condition in which endometrial (uterine) tissue grows outside the uterus. This tissue responds to hormones and can cause pelvic pain, bleeding, scarring, and adhesions (scar tissue). Endometriosis is typically treated with hormonal therapy and surgery.

TERMS

fertilization The initiation of biological reproduction; the union of the nucleus of an egg cell with the nucleus of a sperm cell.

fertilized egg The egg after penetration by a sperm; a *zygote*.

gene The basic unit of heredity; a section of a chromosome containing biochemical instructions for making a particular protein.

fraternal (dizygotic) twins Twins who develop from separate fertilized eggs; such twins are not genetically identical.

identical (monozygotic) twins Twins who develop from the division of a single zygote; such twins are genetically identical.

infertility The inability to conceive after trying for a year or more.

Age also affects fertility. Beginning at around age 30, a woman's fertility naturally begins to wane. Age is probably the main factor in ovulation failure. Exposure to toxic chemicals, cigarette smoke, or radiation also appears to reduce fertility, as do genetic factors identifiable in your family history.

Male Infertility

Male infertility accounts for about one-fourth (26%) of infertile couples. The leading causes of male infertility can be divided into four main categories: hypothalamic pituitary disease (1–2%), testicular disease (30–40%), disorders of sperm transport or posttesticular disorders (10–20%), and unexplained (40–50%). Some acquired disorders of the testes can lead to infertility, such as damage from drug use (including marijuana), smoking, infection, or environmental toxins.

Treating Infertility

The cause of infertility can be determined for about 72–85% of infertile couples. Most cases of infertility are treated with conventional medical therapies. Surgery can repair oviducts, remove endometriosis, and correct anatomical problems in men and women. Fertility drugs can help women ovulate but may cause multiple births. If these conventional treatments don't work, couples can turn to **assisted reproductive technology (ART)** techniques, as described in the following sections. According to 2016 estimates from the CDC, about 1.6% of births in the United States are the result of ART treatments.

Most infertility treatments are expensive and emotionally draining, with a live birth occurring in about a third of cases. Some infertile couples choose not to try to have children, whereas others turn to adoption. One measure you can take to avoid infertility is to follow the CDC recommendation of STI screening every year for all sexually active women younger than 25 years. Couples will need to balance the risks of age-related infertility with the competing demands of careers and academics.

INTRAUTERINE INSEMINATION Male infertility can sometimes be overcome by collecting and concentrating the man's sperm and introducing the semen by syringe into a woman's vagina or uterus, a procedure known as **artificial (intrauterine) insemination.** To increase the probability of success, the woman is often given fertility drugs to induce ovulation prior to the insemination procedure. The sperm can be provided by the woman's partner or a donor. Donor sperm are also used by single women and lesbian couples who want to conceive using artificial insemination. The success rate is about 5–20%. The wide range is due to age-related influences.

IVF A surgical technique used to overcome infertility, **in vitro fertilization (IVF)** involves surgically removing mature eggs from a woman's ovary and pairing the harvested eggs with sperm outside the woman's body (*in vitro*), in a laboratory dish. If eggs are successfully fertilized, one or more of the resulting embryos are inserted into the woman's uterus. The remaining embryos can then be frozen for future use.

Success rates determined by live birth rates vary from about 4% to 40% depending on the woman's age. It costs more than $10,000 per procedure and may require five or more attempts to produce one live birth. IVF also increases the chance of twins or triplets, which in turn increases the risk of premature birth and maternal complications, including pregnancy-related hypertension and diabetes.

GESTATIONAL CARRIER A *gestational carrier* is a fertile woman who agrees to carry a fetus for an infertile couple. The gestational carrier agrees to be artificially inseminated by the father's sperm or to undergo IVF with the couple's embryo, to carry the baby to term, and to give it to the couple at birth. In return, the couple pays her for her services and medical costs (typically around $50,000). As of 2013, less than 1% of all ART in the United States is performed through gestational carriers.

> ## Ask Yourself
>
> **?**
>
> **QUESTIONS FOR CRITICAL THINKING AND REFLECTION**
> What are your views on infertility treatments? Do you feel treatment is appropriate, or do you think infertile couples should adopt children? If you were faced with a diagnosis of infertility, what would you consider doing?

PREGNANCY

Pregnancy is usually discussed in terms of **trimesters**—three periods of about three months (or 13 weeks) each. During the first trimester, the mother experiences a few physical changes and some fairly common symptoms. During the second trimester, often the most peaceful time of pregnancy, the mother gains weight, looks noticeably pregnant, and may experience a general sense of well-being if she is happy about having a child. The third trimester is the hardest for the mother because she must breathe, digest, excrete, and circulate blood for herself and the growing fetus.

> **TERMS**
>
> **assisted reproductive technology (ART)** Advanced medical techniques used to treat infertility.
>
> **artificial (intrauterine) insemination** The introduction of semen into the vagina by artificial means.
>
> **in vitro fertilization (IVF)** Combining eggs and sperm outside the body and inserting one or more fertilized eggs into the uterus.
>
> **trimester** One of the three 3-month periods of pregnancy.

Women have access to a variety of over-the-counter home pregnancy tests today, but generally speaking, these tests all work in the same way to determine whether a woman is pregnant. Pregnancy tests are designed to detect the presence of the hormone **human chorionic gonadotropin (hCG)**, a hormone produced by the implanted fertilized egg, which is discussed in this chapter. Because the placenta releases hCG, the hormone can be detected in a woman's urine or blood when she is pregnant.

Although home pregnancy tests have become extremely accurate since their introduction in 1975, not all tests behave equally. A sensitive test will give a "positive" result with very low levels of hCG and can identify pregnancies earlier. A less sensitive test may not give an accurate result until hCG levels are much higher. Most kits will reliably detect 97% of pregnancies one week after a missed period. In 85% of normal pregnancies, the hCG levels should double every two to three days, and many women won't have a positive test result until the first day of a missed period or even a few days later.

Two types of home pregnancy tests are available—those that require the test strip to be dipped into urine, and those that require the user to urinate directly onto the test strip. Different tests use different mechanisms to display test results. Some use symbols such as a + or - sign, some spell out the words "pregnant" and "not pregnant," and others utilize a color scheme.

A clinical blood test is more accurate but not necessarily more sensitive than a home pregnancy test. A quantitative blood test, usually called a *beta hCG test*, measures the exact number of units of hCG in the blood. This type of test can detect even the most minimal level. Labs vary in what is considered a positive pregnancy test. Common cutoffs for positive are 5, 10, and 25 units. A level under 5 is considered negative.

Women need to use home pregnancy test kits with a clear understanding of their limitations. If you're comfortable waiting, a sensitive test taken a week after your period is due will almost certainly give you accurate results. If you elect to take the test as early as the day after you've missed your period, remember that a negative result isn't 100% certain. A positive result may mean either a viable pregnancy or a pregnancy destined to end shortly after it began. With either of those results, you should plan to test again a week later, just to be sure. For that reason, it's a good idea to buy tests in pairs; 15 of the 18 commercially available home testing products come as multiple-test kits.

Changes in the Woman's Body

Hormonal changes begin as soon as an egg is fertilized, and for the next nine months the woman's body nourishes the fetus and adjusts to its growth (Figure 5.3).

Early Signs and Symptoms Early recognition of pregnancy is important, especially for women with medical conditions or nutritional deficiencies. The following symptoms are not absolute indications of pregnancy, but they are reasons to visit a gynecologist, and maybe take a home pregnancy test (see the box "Home Pregnancy Tests"):

• *A missed menstrual period.* When a fertilized egg implants in the uterine wall, the endometrium is retained to nourish the embryo. A woman who misses a period after having intercourse may be pregnant.

• *Slight bleeding.* Following implantation of the fertilized egg into the endometrial lining, a slight bleed occurs in about 14% of pregnant women. Because this happens about when a period is expected, about two weeks after ovulation, the bleeding is sometimes mistaken for menstrual flow. It usually lasts only a few days.

• *Nausea.* Between 50 and 90% of pregnant women feel increased nausea, probably in reaction to surging levels of progesterone and other pregnancy hormones. Although this nausea is often called *morning sickness,* some women have it all day long. It frequently begins during the 6th week and disappears by the 12th week. In some cases it continues throughout the pregnancy.

• *Breast tenderness.* Some women experience breast tenderness, swelling, and tingling, usually described as different from the tenderness experienced before menstruation.

• *Increased urination.* Increased frequency of urination can occur soon after the missed period.

• *Sleepiness, fatigue, and emotional upset.* These symptoms result from hormonal changes. Fatigue can be surprisingly overwhelming in the first trimester but usually improves significantly around the third month of pregnancy.

The first reliable physical signs of pregnancy can be distinguished about four weeks after a woman misses her menstrual period. Increased uterine growth and blood flow contribute to softening of the uterus just above the cervix, called *Hegar's sign,* and a bluish discoloration to the cervix and labia minora, termed *Chadwick's sign.*

> **human chorionic gonadotropin (hCG)** A hormone produced by a fertilized egg that can be detected in the urine or blood of the mother shortly after conception.
>
> **TERMS**

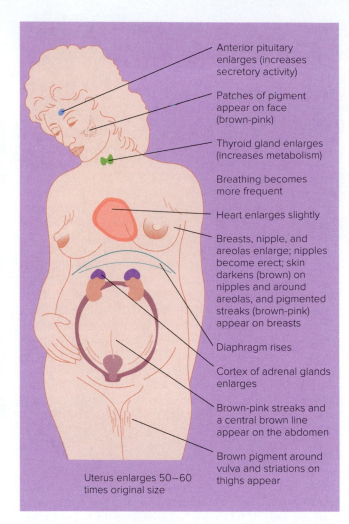

- Anterior pituitary enlarges (increases secretory activity)
- Patches of pigment appear on face (brown-pink)
- Thyroid gland enlarges (increases metabolism)
- Breathing becomes more frequent
- Heart enlarges slightly
- Breasts, nipple, and areolas enlarge; nipples become erect; skin darkens (brown) on nipples and around areolas, and pigmented streaks (brown-pink) appear on breasts
- Diaphragm rises
- Cortex of adrenal glands enlarges
- Brown-pink streaks and a central brown line appear on the abdomen
- Brown pigment around vulva and striations on thighs appear

Uterus enlarges 50–60 times original size

FIGURE 5.3 **Physiological changes during pregnancy.**

Table 5.2	Recommended Weight Gain during Pregnancy

STATUS (BMI)*	WEIGHT GAIN (POUNDS)
Underweight (<18.5)	28–40
Normal (18.5–24.9)	25–35
Overweight (25–29.9)	15–25
Obese (>30)	11–20

*BMI, or body mass index, allows comparison of body weight across different heights. (See Chapter 11 to calculate BMI.)

Continuing Changes in the Woman's Body

The most obvious changes during pregnancy occur in the reproductive organs. During the first three months, the uterus enlarges to about three times its nonpregnant size, but it still cannot be felt in the abdomen. By the fourth month, it is large enough to make the abdomen protrude. By the seventh or eighth month, the uterus pushes up under the rib cage, which makes breathing slightly more difficult. The breasts enlarge and are sensitive; by week 8, they may tingle or throb. The pigmented area around the nipple, called the *areola,* darkens and broadens. The hormones of pregnancy also contribute to hyperpigmentation and broadening of the nipple, and for some women, hyperpigmentation may show in the face or the midline of the abdomen.

Other changes are going on as well. Early in pregnancy, the muscles and ligaments attached to bones begin to soften and stretch. The joints between the pelvic bones loosen and spread, making it easier to have a baby but harder to walk. The circulatory system becomes more efficient to accommodate higher blood volume, which increases by 50%, and the heart pumps more rapidly. Much of the increased blood flow goes to the uterus and placenta (the organ that exchanges nutrients

and waste between mother and fetus). The mother's lungs also become more efficient, and her rib cage widens to permit her to inhale up to 40% more air.

The average weight gain during a healthy pregnancy is 27.5 pounds, although actual weight change varies with the individual. Table 5.2 shows the weight gains recommended by the Institute of Medicine based on a woman's prepregnancy weight status. About half of the weight gain is directly related to the baby (such as the fetus and placenta); the rest accumulates over the woman's body as fluid and fat.

Changes during the Later Stages of Pregnancy

By the end of the sixth month, the increased needs of the fetus place a burden on the mother's lungs, heart, and kidneys. Her back may ache from the pressure of the baby's weight and from having to throw her shoulders back to keep her balance while standing. Her body retains more water, perhaps up to three extra quarts of fluid. Her hands, legs, ankles, or feet may swell, and she may be bothered by leg cramps, heartburn, or constipation. Despite discomfort, both her digestion and her metabolism are working at top efficiency.

Near term, the uterus prepares for childbirth with a series of preliminary contractions, called **Braxton Hicks contractions.** Unlike true labor contractions, Braxton Hicks contractions are irregular with short duration; they are also often painless. To the mother, a contraction may initially feel only as though her abdomen is hard to the touch. As the delivery date approaches, true labor contractions become more frequent, regular, and intense, ultimately resulting in labor.

In the ninth month, increased joint laxity coupled by a softening cervix allows the baby to settle deeper into the pelvis. This process, called **lightening,** produces a visible change in the mother's abdominal profile. Pelvic pressure

Braxton Hicks contractions A pattern of late-pregnancy uterine contractions that are irregular in timing, short in duration, and painless and do not result in labor.   **TERMS**

lightening A process in which the uterus sinks down because the baby's head settles into the pelvic area.

FIGURE 5.4 **A chronology of milestones in prenatal development.**

increases, and pressure on the diaphragm lightens. Breathing becomes easier; urination becomes more frequent. Sometimes, after a first pregnancy, lightening does not occur until labor begins.

Emotional Responses to Pregnancy

Rapid changes in hormone levels can cause a pregnant woman to experience unpredictable emotions. During the first trimester, the pregnant woman may fear that she may miscarry or that the child will not be normal. During the second trimester, the pregnant woman can feel early fetal movements, and worries about miscarriages usually begin to diminish. The third trimester is the time of greatest physical stress during the pregnancy. A woman may find that her physical abilities are limited by her size. Because some women feel physically awkward and sexually unattractive, they may experience periods of depression. But many also feel a great deal of happy excitement and anticipation.

FETAL DEVELOPMENT

Now that we've seen what happens to the mother's body during pregnancy, let's consider the development of the fetus (Figure 5.4).

The First Trimester

About 30 hours after an egg is first fertilized, the cell divides, and this process of cell division repeats many times. As the cluster of cells drifts along the oviduct, several different kinds of cells emerge. The entire set of genetic instructions is passed to every cell, but each cell follows only a specific subset of the instructions; if this were not the case, there would be no different organs or body parts. For example, all cells carry genes for hair color and eye color, but only the cells of the hair follicles and irises (of the eye) respond to that information.

On about the fourth day after fertilization, the cluster of rapidly developing cells arrives in the uterus as a **blastocyst,** or a mostly hollow sphere of between 32 and 128 cells. The blastocyst attaches to the uterine wall on the sixth or seventh day, allowing for implantation into the nourishing uterine lining.

The blastocyst becomes an **embryo** by about the end of the second week after fertilization. The inner cells of the

blastocyst The stage of embryonic development, days 4–7, before the cell cluster becomes the embryo and placenta.

embryo The stage of development between blastocyst and fetus; about weeks 2–8.

TERMS

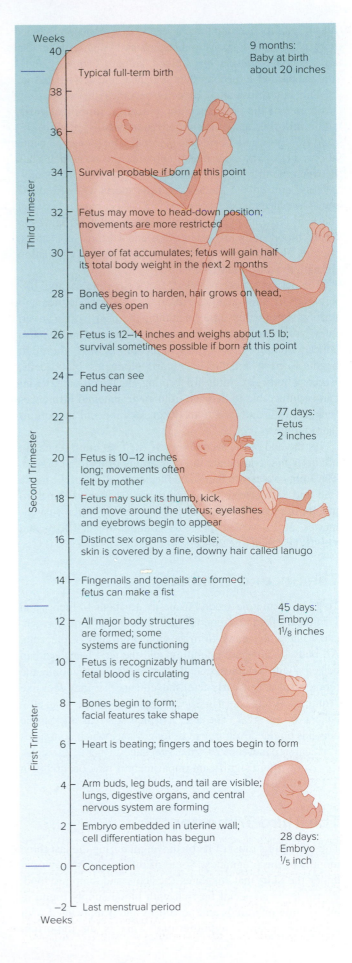

Weeks
40

— Typical full-term birth

9 months:
Baby at birth
about 20 inches

38

36

Third Trimester

34 — Survival probable if born at this point

32 — Fetus may move to head-down position; movements are more restricted

30 — Layer of fat accumulates; fetus will gain half its total body weight in the next 2 months

28 — Bones begin to harden, hair grows on head, and eyes open

26 — Fetus is 12–14 inches and weighs about 1.5 lb; survival sometimes possible if born at this point

24 — Fetus can see and hear

22

Second Trimester

77 days:
Fetus
2 inches

20 — Fetus is 10–12 inches long; movements often felt by mother

18 — Fetus may suck its thumb, kick, and move around the uterus; eyelashes and eyebrows begin to appear

16 — Distinct sex organs are visible; skin is covered by a fine, downy hair called lanugo

14 — Fingernails and toenails are formed; fetus can make a fist

45 days:
Embryo
1 1/8 inches

12 — All major body structures are formed; some systems are functioning

10 — Fetus is recognizably human; fetal blood is circulating

First Trimester

8 — Bones begin to form; facial features take shape

6 — Heart is beating; fingers and toes begin to form

4 — Arm buds, leg buds, and tail are visible; lungs, digestive organs, and central nervous system are forming

2 — Embryo embedded in uterine wall; cell differentiation has begun

28 days:
Embryo
1/5 inch

0 — Conception

−2 — Last menstrual period
Weeks

blastocyst separate into three layers. One layer becomes inner body parts—the digestive and respiratory systems; the middle layer becomes muscle, bone, blood, kidneys, and sex glands; and the third layer becomes the skin, hair, and nervous tissue.

The outermost shell of cells becomes the supporting structures of the pregnancy: the **placenta, umbilical cord,** and **amniotic sac.** A network of blood vessels called *chorionic villi* eventually forms the placenta. The human placenta allows a two-way exchange of nutrients and waste materials between the mother and the fetus. The placenta brings oxygen and nutrients to the fetus and transports waste products out. The placenta does not provide a perfect barrier between the fetal circulation and the maternal circulation, however. Some blood cells are exchanged, and certain substances, such as alcohol, pass freely from the maternal circulation through the placenta to the fetus.

The period between weeks 2 and 9 is a time of rapid differentiation and change. All major body structures are formed during this time, including the heart, brain, liver, lungs, and sex organs. Eyes, nose, ears, arms, and legs also appear. Some organs begin to function, as well; the heart begins to beat, and the liver starts producing blood cells. Because body structures are forming, the developing organism is vulnerable to damage from environmental influences such as drugs and infections (discussed in detail in sections that follow).

By the end of the second month, the fetal brain sends out impulses that coordinate the functioning of its other organs. The embryo is now a fetus, and further changes will be in the size and refinement of working body parts. In the third month, the fetus becomes active. By the end of the first trimester, at 13 weeks, the fetus is about an inch long and weighs less than one ounce.

The Second Trimester

To grow during the second trimester, to about 14 inches and 1.5 pounds, the fetus requires large amounts of food, oxygen, and water, which come from the mother through the placenta. All body systems are operating, and the fetal heartbeat can be heard with a stethoscope. By the fourth or fifth month, the mother can detect early fetal movements that may feel like "flutters." A fetus born at 24–26 weeks has a better than 50% chance of survival. The age at which survival is possible depends on the development of lung tissue, which completes a critical step in weeks 24–26 of pregnancy. Prior to 23 weeks, survival without significant impairment is rare, occurring in 3–15% of cases.

The Third Trimester

The fetus gains most of its birth weight during the last three months of the pregnancy. Some of the weight is brown fat under the skin that insulates the fetus and supplies food. *Brown fat* is a special fat rich with blood supply found in hibernating mammals and newborns and is associated with protection against hypothermia. This is an important

consideration because babies are often too small to generate much of their own heat and are too weak to move away from cold areas. The fetus also takes in other nutrients; about 85% of the calcium and iron the mother consumes goes into the fetal bloodstream.

The fetus may live if it is born during the seventh month, but it needs the fat layer acquired in the eighth month and time for organs—especially the respiratory and digestive organs—to develop. It also needs the immunity supplied by antibodies in the mother's blood during the final three months. The antibodies protect the fetus against many of the diseases to which the mother has acquired immunity.

Diagnosing Fetal Abnormalities

About 3% of babies are born with a major birth defect. Information about the health and sex of a fetus can be obtained prior to birth through prenatal testing.

Noninvasive Screening Tests   Maternal blood testing can be used to help identify fetuses with neural tube defects, Down syndrome, and other anomalies. Traditionally, blood is taken from the mother at 16–19 weeks of pregnancy and analyzed for four hormone levels—human chorionic gonadotropin (hCG), unconjugated estriol, alpha-fetoprotein (AFP), and inhibin-A. These four hormones levels, the **quadruple marker screen (QMS)**, can be compared to appropriate standards, and the results are used to estimate the probability that the fetus has particular anomalies. This type of test is a screening test rather than a diagnostic test; in the case of abnormal QMS results, parents may choose further testing such as an amniocentesis or ultrasonography.

A newer noninvasive screening test, **cell-free DNA**, uses small fragments of fetal DNA identified in the maternal serum typically after 10 weeks of pregnancy. Currently, this DNA is used primarily to identify chromosomal disorders, such as Down syndrome, in women with elevated risk for *aneuploidy* (an abnormal number of chromosomes in the fetus) such as pregnant women over age 35, or in cases where the fetus is known to be at risk for a particular chromosomal or genetic defect.

TERMS

placenta   The organ through which the fetus receives nourishment and empties waste via the mother's circulatory system; after birth, the placenta is expelled from the uterus.

umbilical cord   The cord connecting the placenta and fetus, through which nutrients pass.

amniotic sac   A membranous pouch enclosing and protecting the fetus; also holds amniotic fluid.

quadruple marker screen (QMS)   A measurement of four hormones, used to assess the risk of fetal abnormalities.

cell-free DNA   Fetal genetic material in the maternal blood supply, used to assess the risk of fetal genetic conditions, especially for fetuses already identified as having elevated risk.

Invasive Diagnostic Tests **Chorionic villus sampling (CVS)** is a diagnostic test that can be performed in weeks 10 through 12 of pregnancy for high-risk women or women with abnormal screening results. This procedure involves removing a tiny section of the chorionic villi, which contain fetal cells that can be analyzed. For later diagnosis, **amniocentesis** is typically performed between 16 and 22 weeks and removes fluid from around the developing fetus. The fluid contains fetal skin cells that can be cultured for analysis. This analysis can include genetic analyses for chromosomal disorders but also for some genetic diseases, like Tay-Sachs disease. Because the genetics are known, the sex of the fetus can also be determined.

Ultrasonography **Ultrasonography** (also called *ultrasound*) uses high-frequency sound waves to create a **sonogram,** or visual image, of the fetus in the uterus. Sonograms show the fetus's position, size, and gestational age, and identify the presence of certain anatomical problems. Sonograms can sometimes be used to determine the sex of the fetus. Sonograms are considered safe for a pregnant woman and the fetus, but the U.S. Food and Drug Administration (FDA) advises against "keepsake" sonograms performed for no medical purpose.

First-trimester screening for Down syndrome combines ultrasound evaluation of nuchal translucency (the thickness of the back of the fetus's neck) with maternal blood testing. This test can be done between the 10th and 14th weeks of pregnancy. This can be combined with serum testing at 16 weeks for a sequential screen to improve the sensitivity of noninvasive screening tests. If results indicate an increased risk of abnormality, further diagnostic studies such as amniocentesis can be done for confirmation.

Fetal Programming

Prenatal testing techniques look for chromosomal, genetic, and other anomalies that typically cause immediate problems. A new area of study known as *fetal programming theory* focuses on how conditions in the womb may influence the risk of adult diseases. For example, researchers have linked low birth weight to an increased risk of heart disease, high blood pressure, obesity, diabetes, and schizophrenia. High birth weight in female infants, however, has been linked to an increased risk of hypertension, diabetes, and some cancers in later life.

Although not all scientists embrace fetal programming theory, these studies emphasize that everything that occurs during pregnancy can have an impact on the developing fetus. In the future, people may be able to use information about their birth weight and other indicators of gestational conditions just as they now can use family history and genetic information—to alert them to special health risks and to help them improve their health.

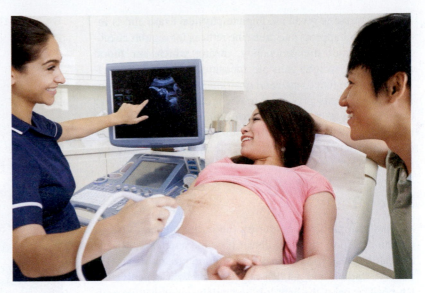

Ultrasonography provides information about the position, size, and physical condition of a fetus in the uterus.

© Monkey Business Images/Shutterstock

THE IMPORTANCE OF PRENATAL CARE

Adequate prenatal care—as described in the following sections—is essential to the health of both mother and baby. All physicians recommend that women start getting regular prenatal checkups as soon as they become pregnant. Typically this means one checkup per month during the first eight months and then one checkup per week during the final month. About 84% of pregnant women begin receiving adequate prenatal care during the first trimester; about 3.5% wait until the last trimester or receive no prenatal care at all.

Regular Checkups

In the woman's first visit to her obstetrician, she will be asked for a detailed medical history of herself and her family. Her obstetrician will note any hereditary conditions that may assume increased significance during pregnancy. The tendency to develop gestational diabetes (diabetes during pregnancy only), for example, can be inherited; appropriate treatment during pregnancy reduces the risk of serious harm.

> **TERMS**
>
> **chorionic villus sampling (CVS)** Surgical removal of a tiny section of placental villi to be analyzed for genetic defects.
>
> **amniocentesis** A process in which amniotic fluid is removed and analyzed to detect possible birth defects.
>
> **ultrasonography** The use of high-frequency sound waves to view the fetus in the uterus; also known as *ultrasound*.
>
> **sonogram** The visual image of the fetus produced by ultrasonography.

The woman is given a complete physical exam and is informed about appropriate diet. She returns for regular checkups throughout the pregnancy, during which her blood pressure and weight gain are measured, her urine is analyzed, and the fetus's size and position are monitored. Regular prenatal visits give the mother a chance to discuss her concerns and be assured that everything is proceeding normally. Physicians, midwives, health educators, and teachers of childbirth classes can provide the mother with valuable information.

Blood Tests

A blood sample is taken during the initial prenatal visit to determine blood type and detect possible anemia or Rh incompatibilities. The **Rh factor** is a blood protein. If an Rh-positive father and an Rh-negative mother conceive an Rh-positive baby, the baby's blood will be incompatible with the mother's blood. This condition is completely preventable with a serum called *Rh-immune globulin,* which coats Rh-positive cells as they enter the mother's body and prevents her immune system from recognizing them and forming antibodies. Blood may also be tested for evidence of hepatitis B, syphilis, rubella immunity, thyroid problems, and, with the mother's permission, HIV infection.

Prenatal Nutrition

A nutritious diet throughout pregnancy is essential for both the mother and her unborn baby. Not only does the baby get all its nutrients from the mother, but it also competes with her for nutrients not sufficiently available to meet both their needs. When a woman's diet is low in iron or calcium, the fetus receives most of it, and the mother may become deficient in the mineral. To meet the increased nutritional demands of her body, a pregnant woman shouldn't just eat more; she should make sure that her diet is nutritionally adequate.

To maintain her own health and help the fetus grow, a pregnant woman typically needs to consume about 250–500 extra calories per day. Breastfeeding an infant requires even more energy—about 500 or more calories per day. To ensure that she's getting enough calories and nutrients, a pregnant woman should talk to her physician or a registered dietician about her dietary habits and determine what changes she should make.

Some physicians prescribe high-potency vitamin and mineral supplements to pregnant and lactating women. Supplements can help boost the levels of nutrients available to mother and child, helping with fetal development while ensuring that the mother doesn't become nutrient-deficient. Pregnant and lactating women, however, should not take supplements without the advice of their physicians because some vitamins, such as vitamin A, can be harmful if taken in excess. Pregnant women also should not take herbal dietary supplements without consulting a physician.

Two vitamins—vitamin D and the B vitamin folate—are particularly important to pregnant women. Pregnant women who do not get enough vitamin D are more likely

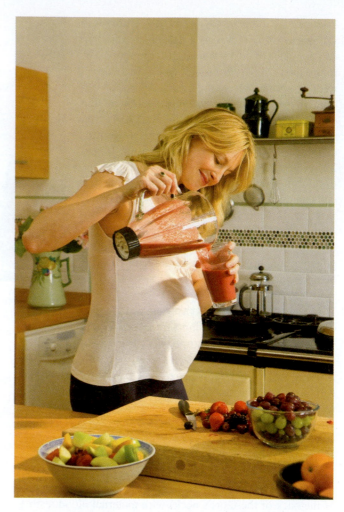

A woman's dietary needs change during pregnancy, so it's important to eat a nutritionally sound diet.

© Tim Platt/Getty Images

to deliver low-birth-weight babies. Chronic vitamin D deficiency has been linked to other health problems, including heart disease.

If a woman does not get the recommended daily amount of folate, both before and during pregnancy, her child has an increased risk of neural tube defects, including spina bifida. Any woman capable of becoming pregnant should get at least 400 micrograms (0.4 milligrams) of folic acid (the synthetic form of folate) daily from fortified foods and/or supplements, in addition to folate from a varied diet. Pregnant women should get 1000 micrograms (1 milligram) every day.

Food safety is another special dietary concern for pregnant women because foodborne pathogens can be especially dangerous to them and their unborn children. Germs

> **Rh factor** A protein found in blood; Rh incompatibility between a mother and fetus can jeopardize the fetus's health.
>
> **TERMS**

and parasites such as *Listeria monocytogenes* and *Toxoplasma gondii* are both particularly worrisome. To avoid them, pregnant women should avoid eating undercooked and ready-to-eat meats (such as hot dogs and pre-packaged deli meats) and should wash produce thoroughly before eating it. Pregnant women should also follow the FDA's recommendations for consumption of fish and seafood. For complete information about nutrition and food safety, see Chapter 9.

Avoiding Drugs and Other Environmental Hazards

Everything the mother ingests may eventually reach the fetus in some proportion. In addition to the food the mother eats, the drugs she takes and the chemicals she is exposed to affect the fetus. Some drugs harm the fetus but not the mother because the fetus is in the process of developing and because the proper dose for the mother is a proportionately massive dose for the fetus.

During the first trimester, when the major body structures are forming rapidly, the fetus is extremely vulnerable to environmental factors such as viral infections, radiation, drugs, and other **teratogens,** any of which can cause **congenital malformations,** or birth defects. As most organs are developing during the first trimester, exposures are of special concern during this critical window. The rubella (German measles) virus, for example, can cause congenital malformation of nerves supplying the eyes and ears in the first trimester, leading to blindness or deafness, but exposure to it later in the pregnancy does no damage. Similarly, excess retinoic acid (Vitamin A) exposure in the first trimester can lead to spontaneous abortion and fetal malformations such as microcephaly and cardiac anomalies. Another example is the class of medications known as anti-epileptics (such as valproic acid), which is associated with cleft palate and neural tube defect. The most common congenital malformations identified are open neural tube, cardiac defects, urinary tract defects, skeletal abnormalities, and cleft palates. Women who are taking medications known to cause birth defects must take care to avoid pregnancy (see Chapter 6 on contraception).

Alcohol Alcohol is a potent teratogen. Although 1 in 10 pregnant women reports an alcohol exposure at some point, getting drunk just one time during pregnancy may be enough to cause damage in a fetus. A high level of alcohol consumption during pregnancy is associated with spontaneous miscarriage and stillbirth. Fetuses born to mothers who have consumed alcohol are at risk for **fetal alcohol syndrome (FAS).** A baby born with FAS is likely to be characterized by mental impairment, a small head and body size, unusual facial features, congenital heart defects, defective joints, impaired vision, and abnormal behavior

patterns. Researchers doubt that any level of alcohol consumption is safe, and they recommend total abstinence during pregnancy (see Chapter 8).

Tobacco Smoking is a preventable risk factor associated with miscarriage, low birth weight, preterm birth, infant death, and other pregnancy complications that may occur via direct damage to genetic material. Nicotine, the active ingredient in cigarette smoke, impairs oxygen delivery to the fetus and leads to faster fetal heart rates and reduced fetal breathing.

Caffeine Caffeine, a powerful stimulant, puts both mother and fetus under stress by raising the level of the hormone epinephrine. Caffeine also reduces the blood supply to the uterus. A pregnant woman should limit her caffeine intake to no more than the equivalent of two cups of coffee per day.

Drugs Some prescription drugs, such as some blood pressure medications, can harm the fetus, so they should be used only under medical supervision. Antidepressant use in pregnancy can lead to withdrawal symptoms in newborns after delivery. Newborns may become fussy, with high-pitched, irritable cries, and develop difficulty feeding.

Recreational drugs, such as cocaine, are thought to increase the risk of miscarriage, stillbirth, growth abnormalities, major birth defects, and placental bleeding. Marijuana is associated with preterm birth and stillbirth. Methamphetamine use is associated with underweight babies.

STIs and Other Infections Infections, including those that are sexually transmitted, are another serious problem for the fetus. Rubella, syphilis, gonorrhea, hepatitis B, herpes, and HIV are among the most dangerous infections for the fetus. Treatment of the mother or immunization of the baby just after birth can help prevent problems from many infections. The most common cause of life-threatening infections in newborns is group B streptococcus (GBS), a bacterium that can cause pneumonia, meningitis, and blood infections. A carrier or a woman who develops a fever during labor will be given intravenous antibiotics at the time of labor to reduce the risk of passing GBS to her baby.

> **QUICK STATS**
>
> About **1%** of school-aged children in the United States have symptoms of fetal alcohol syndrome.
>
> —Centers for Disease Control and Prevention, 2015

> **TERMS**
>
> **teratogen** An agent or influence that causes physical defects in a developing fetus.
>
> **congenital malformation** A physical defect existing at the time of birth, either inherited or caused during gestation.
>
> **fetal alcohol syndrome (FAS)** A combination of birth defects caused by excessive alcohol consumption by the mother during pregnancy.

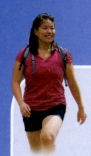

TAKE CHARGE
Physical Activity during Pregnancy

According to the U.S. Department of Health and Human Services's Physical Activity Guidelines Committee, more research is needed to fully assess the effects of regular physical activity on pregnant women. Most studies conclude that a well-managed routine of physical activity should result in no significant negative outcomes, such as low birth weight or early labor.

Maintaining a regular routine of physical activity throughout pregnancy can help a mother-to-be stay healthy and feel her best. Regular exercise can improve posture and decrease common pregnancy-related discomforts, such as backaches and fatigue. There is also evidence that physical activity may prevent gestational diabetes, relieve stress, and build stamina that can be helpful during labor and delivery.

A woman who was physically active before pregnancy should be able to continue her favorite activities in moderation, except for those that carry a risk of trauma, or unless there is a medical reason to reduce or stop exercise.

The American Congress of Obstetricians and Gynecologists (ACOG) offers advice regarding exercise during pregnancy. For example, downhill skiing or contact sports such as ice hockey, boxing, or soccer place pregnant women at risk for falls or abdominal trauma and should be avoided. Hot yoga and hot Pilates place the fetus at risk for overheating and are not recommended. In general, experts encourage low-impact aerobic activities such as walking or swimming over high-impact exercise. Physicians and pregnant women alike have concerns about exercise intensity. A good rule of thumb is never to exercise more than allows you to comfortably talk with a friend. If a pregnant woman is out of breath while exercising, she should slow down! Experts also recommend proper hydration and dressing to avoid overheating.

A woman who has never exercised regularly can safely start an exercise program during pregnancy after consulting with her health care provider. A routine of regular walking is considered safe. ACOG recommends that any pregnant woman who exercises should stop if she experiences any of the following warning signs: vaginal bleeding, increased shortness of breath, dizziness, headache, pain in the chest or calves, regular painful contractions, decreased fetal movement, and leakage of amniotic fluid. For detailed information about physical activity, see Chapter 10.

SOURCES: American College of Obstetricians and Gynecologists. 2015. Committee Opinion No. 650: Physical activity and exercise during pregnancy and the postpartum period. *Obstetrics and Gynecology* 126(6): 1326–1327; Physical Activity Guidelines Advisory Committee. 2008. Physical Activity Guidelines Advisory Committee Report, 2008. Washington, DC: U.S. Department of Health and Human Services.

Nationwide, nearly 11,000 children under age 13 have been diagnosed with human immunodeficiency virus (HIV), the virus that causes AIDS. Of those, nearly 90% acquired the infection in utero during pregnancy, at birth, or during breastfeeding. The CDC therefore recommends routine testing for all pregnant women. Antiviral drugs, given to an HIV-infected mother during pregnancy and delivery and to her newborn immediately following birth, reduce the rate of HIV transmission from mother to infant from 25% to 2%. (See Chapter 13 for more about HIV and other STIs.)

In 2015, reports emerged about an outbreak of Zika virus among pregnant women in northern Brazil. Infection was associated with poor head growth in newborns (microcephaly). Since then, the mosquito-transmitted virus has spread throughout much of South America and Central America. In the United States, the Gulf Coast states, Puerto Rico, and Hawaii are at risk as well because they share similar mosquito habitats with the affected areas; as of September 2016, cases of locally acquired Zika (not related to travel) had been reported in Florida, Puerto Rico, and the U.S. Virgin Islands.

Important concerns have surfaced regarding this new outbreak, especially because the CDC has established that the Zika virus causes birth defects, in particular, newborn microcephaly. Thus, CDC guidelines recommend preventive measures such as wearing long-sleeve shirts, using mosquito repellant, and, for all pregnant women, avoiding travel to areas with current outbreaks. Because Zika can be transmitted sexually, the CDC also suggests that couples use condoms or abstain from sexual activity if the man might have been exposed to Zika and if his sex partner is pregnant or could become pregnant. For more information, visit the CDC Zika website (www.cdc.gov/Zika).

Prenatal Activity and Exercise

Physical activity during pregnancy contributes to mental and physical wellness (see the box "Physical Activity during Pregnancy"). Women can continue working at their jobs until late in their pregnancy, provided the work isn't so physically demanding that it jeopardizes their health. At the same time, pregnant women need more rest and sleep to maintain their own well-being and that of the fetus.

Kegel exercises, to strengthen the pelvic floor muscles, are recommended for pregnant women. These exercises are performed by alternately contracting and releasing the muscles used to stop the flow of urine. Each contraction should be held for about five seconds. Kegel exercises should be done several times a day for a total of about 50 repetitions daily.

Preparing for Birth

Childbirth classes are almost a routine part of the prenatal experience for both mothers and fathers today. These classes typically teach the details of the birth process as well as relaxation techniques to help deal with the discomfort of labor and delivery. The mother learns and practices a variety of techniques so that she will be able to choose what works best for her during labor when the time comes. The father or her partner typically acts as a coach, supporting her emotionally and helping her with her breathing and relaxing. He or she remains with the mother throughout labor and delivery, even when a cesarean section is performed.

COMPLICATIONS OF PREGNANCY AND PREGNANCY LOSS

Complications can arise in pregnancy for myriad reasons: *maternal diseases and exposures* such as diabetes, hypertension, or tobacco use; *placental factors,* including abruption or placenta previa; or *fetal conditions* such as genetic conditions like Down syndrome or cystic fibrosis. Each complication benefits from early diagnosis, counseling, and, if possible, corrective action.

Ectopic Pregnancy

In an **ectopic pregnancy,** the fertilized egg implants and begins to develop outside the uterus, usually in an oviduct (Figure 5.5). As the limited space of the oviduct cannot accommodate the rapid growth of a fertilized egg, ectopic pregnancies pose high risk of emergent bleeding through tubal rupture. Although ectopic pregnancies account for only 2% of all pregnancies, they contribute to 6% of all maternal deaths.

Ectopic pregnancies usually occur because of occlusion (blockage) of the fallopian tube, most often as a result of

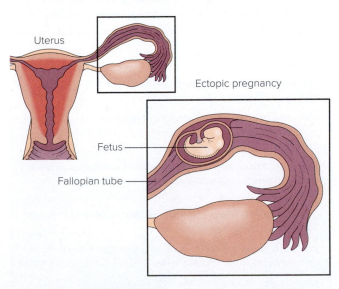

Uterus

Ectopic pregnancy

Fetus

Fallopian tube

FIGURE 5.5 Ectopic pregnancy in a fallopian tube.

pelvic inflammatory disease, although smoking also increases a woman's risk for ectopic pregnancy. The embryo may spontaneously abort, or the embryo and placenta may continue to expand until they rupture the oviduct. Sharp pain on one side of the abdomen or in the lower back, usually in about the seventh or eighth week of pregnancy, may signal an ectopic pregnancy, and there may be irregular bleeding.

Surgical removal of the embryo and the oviduct may be necessary to save the mother's life, although microsurgery can sometimes be used to repair the damaged oviduct. If diagnosed early, before the oviduct ruptures, ectopic pregnancy can often be treated successfully without surgery with the chemotherapeutic agent methotrexate.

Spontaneous Abortion

A spontaneous abortion, or miscarriage, is the termination of pregnancy before the 20th week. Most miscarriages— about 60%—are due to chromosomal abnormalities in the fetus. Certain occupations that involve exposure to chemicals or radiation may increase the likelihood of a spontaneous abortion. One miscarriage doesn't mean that later pregnancies will be unsuccessful, and about 70–90% of women who miscarry eventually become pregnant again.

Stillbirth

The terms *fetal death, fetal demise, stillbirth,* and *stillborn* all refer to the delivery of a fetus that shows no signs of life. Each year over 3 million stillbirths occur worldwide. In the United States, the stillbirth rate is a little more than 6 in 1000. Risk factors for stillbirth include smoking, advanced maternal age, obesity, multiple gestations, and chronic disease. Race is also a factor; black women have twice as many stillbirths as white women. Although some observers attribute the increased risk for stillbirth among black women to the corresponding increased risk of preterm delivery, other reasons for race-based health care disparities may include poor access to care, infection, and the combined effects of racism and poverty.

Preeclampsia

A disease unique to pregnancy, **preeclampsia** is characterized by elevated blood pressure and the appearance of protein in the urine. Left untreated, preeclampsia will worsen over time, resulting in symptoms including headache, right upper-quadrant abdominal pain, vision changes (referred to as *scotomata*), and notable increased swelling and weight gain. One of the most severe outcomes of untreated preeclampsia

---

ectopic pregnancy   A pregnancy in which the embryo develops outside the uterus, usually in an oviduct.

TERMS

preeclampsia   A condition of pregnancy characterized by high blood pressure and protein in the urine.

is the onset of seizures, a condition called **eclampsia.** Other potential complications of preeclampsia are liver and kidney damage, bleeding, fetal growth restriction, and even fetal death.

Women with preeclampsia without severe features may be monitored closely as outpatients. More severe cases may require hospitalization for close medical management and early delivery.

Placenta Previa

In **placenta previa,** the placenta either completely or partially covers the cervical opening, preventing the mother from delivering the baby vaginally. As a result, the baby must be delivered by cesarean section. This condition occurs in 1 in 250 live births. Risk factors include prior cesarean delivery, multiple pregnancies, intrauterine surgery, smoking, multiple gestations, and advanced maternal age.

Placental Abruption

In **placental abruption,** a normally implanted placenta separates prematurely from the uterine wall. Patients experience abdominal pain, vaginal bleeding, and uterine tenderness. This causes 30% of all bleeding in the third trimester. The condition also increases the risk of fetal death. The risk factors for developing a placental abruption are maternal age, smoking, cocaine use, multiple gestation, trauma, preeclampsia, hypertension, and premature rupture of membranes.

Gestational Diabetes

During gestation, about 7–18% of all pregnant women develop **gestational diabetes mellitus (GDM),** in which the body loses its ability to use insulin properly. In these women, diabetes occurs only during pregnancy. Women diagnosed with GDM have an increased risk of developing type 2 diabetes later in life. It is important to accurately diagnose and treat GDM because it can lead to preeclampsia, polyhydramnios (increased levels of amniotic fluid), large fetuses, birth trauma, operative deliveries, perinatal mortality, and neonatal metabolic complications. All women in pregnancy are therefore advised to test for GDM, which is a simple and straightforward procedure. When a diagnosis of GDM is made, treatment can be in the form of diet and exercise modification, or medication.

Preterm Labor and Birth

When a pregnant woman goes into labor before the 37th week of gestation, she is said to experience *preterm labor.* Preterm labor is one of the most common reasons for hospitalizing pregnant women, but verifying true preterm labor can be difficult, and stopping it is even harder. About 30–50% of preterm labors resolve themselves, with the pregnancy continuing to full term.

Around the world, an estimated 13 million babies are born prematurely—before 37 completed weeks of gestation—each year. In 2014, 9.6% of babies were born prematurely in the United States. The rate has declined 8% since a high in 2007. Preterm birth rates vary widely among racial and ethnic groups.

Preterm birth is the leading direct cause of newborn death, accounting for about one-third of all infant deaths. Preterm birth is also the main risk factor for newborn illness and death from other causes, particularly infection. Babies born prematurely appear to be at a higher risk of long-term health and developmental problems, including delayed development and learning problems.

Risk factors for preterm birth include lack of prenatal care, smoking, drug use, stress, personal health history, infections or illness during pregnancy, obesity, exposure to environmental toxins, a previous preterm birth, and the carrying of multiple fetuses. However, only about half the women who give birth prematurely have any known risk factors.

Labor Induction

If pregnancy continues well beyond the baby's due date, it may be necessary to induce labor artificially. This is one of the most common obstetrical procedures and is typically offered to pregnant women who have not delivered and are 7–14 days past their due dates.

Low Birth Weight and Premature Birth

A **low-birth-weight (LBW)** baby is one that weighs less than 5.5 pounds at birth. LBW babies may be **premature** (born before the 37th week of pregnancy) or full-term. Babies who are born small even though they're full-term are referred to as *small-for-dates* or *small-for-gestational-age* babies. Low birth weight affected 8.1% of babies born in the United States in 2015. About half of all cases are related to teenage pregnancy, cigarette smoking, poor nutrition, and poor maternal health. Other maternal factors include drug use, stress, depression, and anxiety. Adequate prenatal care

TERMS

eclampsia   A severe, potentially life-threatening form of preeclampsia, characterized by seizures.

placenta previa   A complication of pregnancy in which the placenta covers the cervical opening, preventing the mother from delivering the baby vaginally.

placental abruption   A complication of pregnancy in which a normally implanted placenta separates prematurely from the uterine wall.

gestational diabetes mellitus (GDM)   A form of diabetes that occurs during pregnancy.

low birth weight (LBW)   Weighing less than 5.5 pounds at birth, often the result of prematurity.

premature   Born before the 37th week of pregnancy.

Ask Yourself

QUESTIONS FOR CRITICAL THINKING AND REFLECTION

Do you know anyone who has lost a child to miscarriage, stillbirth, or a birth defect? If so, how did they cope with their loss? What would you do to help someone in this situation?

is the best way to prevent LBW. Full-term LBW babies tend to have fewer problems than premature infants.

Infant Mortality

The U.S. rate of **infant mortality,** the death of a child at less than 1 year of age, is near its lowest point ever—5.8 deaths for every 1000 live births as of 2014; however, that number remains far higher than rates in most of the developed world.

Forty-six percent of infant deaths are due to one of three leading factors: congenital abnormalities, prematurity/low birth weight, or **sudden infant death syndrome (SIDS).** SIDS is defined by a sudden and unexpected death of a child less than 1 year of age not explained by thorough investigation including autopsy. More than 1500 babies died of SIDS in 2014, the latest year for which statistics are available.

Research suggests that abnormalities in the brain stem, the part of the brain that regulates breathing, heart rate, and other basic functions, underlie the risk for SIDS. Risk is increased greatly for infants with these innate differences if they are exposed to environmental risks such as tobacco smoke, alcohol, substance use, and, most important, sleeping stomach-side down. Because infants developmentally change how they sleep between 2 and 4 months of age, this is a time period of particular risk. Additionally, suffocation risk increases with the presence of many items common to cribs: fluffy pillows, mattresses, or plush toys. Therefore, current recommendations are to place babies to sleep back down, on a firm sleep surface, without soft bedding, plush toys, or additional clothing that might cause overheating. Parental avoidance of tobacco smoke, alcohol, and illicit drugs is important. Several studies have found that the use of a pacifier significantly reduces the risk of SIDS.

CHILDBIRTH

By the end of the ninth month of pregnancy, most women are tired of being pregnant; both parents are eager to start a new phase of their lives. Most couples find the actual process of birth to be an exciting and positive experience.

Choices in Childbirth

Many parents-to-be today can choose the type of practitioner and the environment they want for the birth of their child. A high-risk pregnancy is best handled by a specialist physician, but for low-risk pregnancies, many options are available.

In 2014, 98.5% of babies in the United States were delivered in hospitals. Physicians performed 91.4% of all deliveries, and certified nurse-midwives performed about 8% of them. Although physicians typically deliver in hospital settings, nurse-midwives may attend deliveries in freestanding birth centers where the environment may feel more comfortable while still remaining close to the medical resources of a hospital.

In 2014, 1.5% of American women elected to give birth at home or in birth facilities that offer low-technology care. In 2011, ACOG recommended against homebirth. The American Academy of Pediatrics notes that, although hospital or freestanding accredited birth centers are the safest place to give birth, every infant should have access to the birth setting that is best for him or her. However, the American College of Nurse-Midwives supports out-of-hospital births for low-risk, healthy women.

Health care providers will need to assess maternal and fetal health and make decisions together with prospective parents about appropriate care providers and location. Prospective parents should discuss all aspects of labor and delivery with their provider beforehand so that they can learn what to expect and can state their preferences.

Labor and Delivery

The birth process occurs in three stages (Figure 5.6). **Labor** begins when hormonal changes in both the mother and the baby cause strong, rhythmic uterine **contractions** to begin. These contractions exert pressure on the cervix and cause the lengthwise muscles of the uterus to pull on the circular muscles around the cervix, causing effacement (thinning) and dilation (opening) of the cervix. The contractions also pressure the baby to descend into the mother's pelvis, if it hasn't already. The entire process of labor and delivery usually takes between 2 and 36 hours, depending on the size of the baby, the baby's position in the uterus, the size of the mother's pelvis, the strength of the uterine contractions, the number of prior deliveries, and other factors. The length of labor is generally shorter for second and subsequent births.

The First Stage of Labor   The first stage of labor averages 13 hours for a first birth, although there is wide variation among women. It begins with cervical effacement and

TERMS

infant mortality   The death of a child at less than 1 year of age.

sudden infant death syndrome (SIDS)   The sudden death of an apparently healthy infant during sleep.

labor   The act or process of giving birth to a child, expelling it with the placenta from the mother's body by means of uterine contractions.

contraction   Shortening of the muscles in the uterine wall, which causes effacement and dilation of the cervix and assists in expelling the fetus.

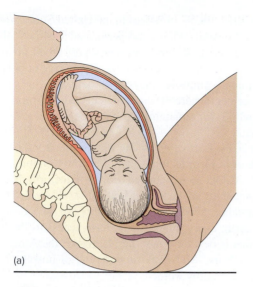

(a)

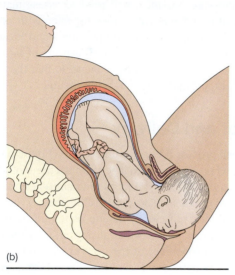

(b)

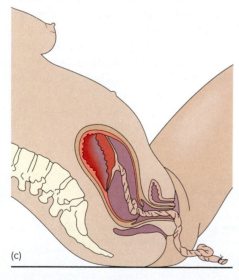

(c)

FIGURE 5.6 Birth: labor and delivery. (a) The first stage of labor; (b) the second stage of labor: delivery of the baby; (c) the third stage of labor: expulsion of the placenta.

dilation and continues until the cervix is completely dilated. Contractions usually last about 30 seconds and occur every 15–20 minutes at first. They occur more often later. The prepared mother relaxes as much as possible during these contractions to allow labor to proceed without being blocked by tension. Early in the first stage, a small amount of bleeding may occur as a plug of slightly bloody mucus that blocked the opening of the cervix during pregnancy is expelled. In some women, the amniotic sac ruptures and the fluid rushes out; this is sometimes referred to as "breaking the bag of water."

The last part of the first stage of labor, called **active labor,** is characterized by strong and frequent contractions, much more intense than in the early stages of labor. Contractions may last 60–90 seconds and occur every 1–3 minutes. During active labor the cervix opens completely, to a diameter of about 10 centimeters. When the head of the fetus is flexed forward, to present its smallest diameter, it measures 9–10 centimeters. Therefore, a completely dilated cervix should permit the passage of the fetal head.

The Second Stage of Labor

The second stage of labor is the "pushing phase." It begins with complete cervical dilation and ends with the delivery of the baby. With uterine contractions and maternal pushing, the baby descends through the bones of the pelvis, past the cervix, and into the vagina, which it stretches open. Some women find this the most difficult part of labor; others find that the contractions and bearing down bring a sense of relief. The baby's head and body turn to fit through the narrowest parts of the passageway, and the soft bones of the baby's skull move together and overlap as it is squeezed through the pelvis. When the top of the head appears at the vaginal opening, the baby is said to be *crowning*.

As the head of the baby emerges, the physician or midwife will check to ensure that the umbilical cord is not around the neck. With a few more contractions, the baby's shoulders and body emerge. As the baby is squeezed through the pelvis, cervix, and vagina, amniotic fluid in the lungs is forced out by the pressure on the baby's chest. Once this pressure is released as the baby emerges from the vagina, the chest expands and the lungs fill with air for the first time. The baby will appear wet and often is covered with a cheesy substance called *vernix*. The baby's head may be oddly shaped at first, due to the molding of the soft plates of bone during birth, but it usually takes on a more rounded appearance within 24 hours.

The Third Stage of Labor

In the third stage of labor, the uterus continues to contract until the placenta is expelled. This stage usually takes 5–30 minutes. The entire placenta must be expelled; if part remains in the uterus, it may cause bleeding and infection. Breastfeeding soon after delivery helps control uterine bleeding because it stimulates secretion of a hormone that makes the uterus contract.

active labor The last part of the first stage of labor, during which the cervix becomes fully dilated; characterized by intense and frequent contractions. **TERMS**

The baby's physical condition is assessed with the **Apgar score,** a formalized system for assessing the baby's physical condition and whether medical assistance is needed. Heart rate, respiration, color, reflexes, and muscle tone are rated individually with a score of 0–2, and a total score between 0 and 10 is given at 1 and 5 minutes after birth. A score of 7–10 at 5 minutes is considered normal. Most newborns are also tested for 29 specific disorders, some of which are life-threatening. The American Academy of Pediatrics endorses these tests, but they are not routinely performed in every state.

Pain Relief during Labor and Delivery

Women vary in how much pain they experience in childbirth. First babies are typically the most challenging to deliver because the birth canal has never stretched to this extent before. It is recommended that women and their partners learn about labor and what kinds of choices are available for pain relief. Childbirth preparation courses are a good place to start, and communicating with one's obstetrician or midwife is essential to assessing pain relief options. Pain can be modified by staying active in labor, laboring in water, and using breathing and relaxation techniques including hypnosis.

Medical pain relief can come in the form of intravenous narcotics, which are short-acting and can be used only in early labor. If a baby is born under the influence of narcotics, it can appear floppy and without vigor. The most commonly used medical intervention for pain relief is the *epidural injection.* This procedure involves placing a thin plastic catheter between the vertebrae in the lower back. Medication that reduces the transmission of pain signals to the brain is given through this catheter. Regional anesthetic drugs are given in low concentration to minimize weakening of the leg muscles so that the mother can push effectively during the birth. The advantage of the epidural is that the medication is used in low amounts in the confined space of the spinal column, protecting the fetus from the effect of the medication. The mother is awake and is an active participant in the birth.

Local anesthesia is available for repair of any tear or **episiotomy** (a surgical incision of the perineum to allow easier delivery of the baby) if the mother has not used an epidural for the labor.

Cesarean Delivery

In a **cesarean section,** the baby is removed through a surgical incision in the abdominal wall and uterus. Cesarean sections are necessary when a baby cannot be delivered vaginally—for example, if the baby's head is bigger than the mother's pelvis or if the baby is not head down at the time of labor. If the mother has a serious health condition such as high blood pressure, a cesarean may be safer for her than labor and a vaginal delivery. Cesareans are more common among women who are overweight or have diabetes. Other reasons for cesarean delivery include

abnormal or difficult labor, fetal distress, and the presence of a dangerous infection like herpes that can be passed to the baby during vaginal delivery.

Repeat cesarean deliveries are also very common. In 2014, 88.7% of American women who had had one child by cesarean had subsequent children delivered the same way. Although the risk of complications from a vaginal delivery after a previous cesarean delivery is low, there is a small (1%) risk of serious complications for the mother and baby if the previous uterine scar opens during labor (uterine rupture). For this reason, women and their physicians may choose to deliver by elective repeat cesarean.

Like any major surgery, cesarean section carries a longer recovery period and additional risks. Most cesarean deliveries are performed with regional anesthetic, which permits the mother to remain awake for the surgery with her partner present.

Ask Yourself

QUESTIONS FOR CRITICAL THINKING AND REFLECTION

If you are a woman, what are your views on labor and delivery options? If you have a child in the future, which facility, delivery, and pain management options do you think you would prefer? If you are a man, what are your views on participating in delivery? What steps do you think could be taken to help new mothers at home? In the workplace?

The Postpartum Period

The **postpartum period,** a stage of about three months following childbirth, is a time of critical family adjustments. Parenthood begins literally overnight, and the transition can cause considerable stress.

Breastfeeding

Lactation, the production of milk, begins about three days after childbirth. Prior to that time (sometimes as early as the second trimester), **colostrum** is

TERMS

Apgar score   A formalized system for assessing a newborn's need for medical assistance.

episiotomy   An incision made in the perineum to widen the vaginal opening to facilitate birth and prevent uncontrolled tearing during delivery.

cesarean section   A surgical incision through the abdominal wall and uterus, performed to deliver a fetus.

postpartum period   The period of about three months after delivering a baby.

lactation   The production of milk.

colostrum   A yellowish fluid secreted by the mammary glands around the time of childbirth until milk comes in, about the third day.

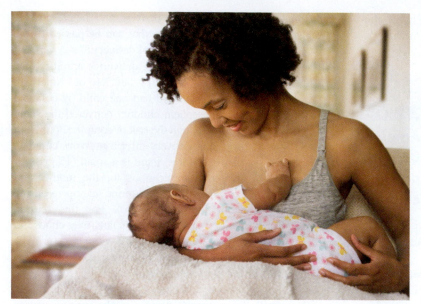

Breastfeeding can enhance the bond between mother and child. The American Academy of Pediatrics recommends breastfeeding exclusively for six months and then in combination with solid food until the baby is at least one year of age.

© KidStock/Getty Images

secreted by the nipples. Colostrum contains antibodies that help protect the newborn from infectious diseases; it is also high in protein.

The American Academy of Pediatrics recommends breastfeeding exclusively for six months, then in combination with solid food until the baby is one year of age, and then for as long after that as a mother and baby desire. Currently only 22.3% of U.S. mothers breastfeed exclusively for six months. Human milk is perfectly suited to the baby's nutritional needs and digestive capabilities, and it supplies the baby with antibodies. Breastfeeding decreases the incidence of infant infection and diarrhea and appears to decrease diabetes and childhood obesity.

Breastfeeding is beneficial to the mother as well. It stimulates contractions that help the uterus return to normal more rapidly, contributes to postpregnancy weight loss, and may reduce the risk of breast and ovarian cancers. Nursing also provides a sense of closeness and emotional well-being for mother and child. Less infection means more productive parents. Parents are able to miss less work. Avoiding formula is cost saving and good for the environment. For women who want to breastfeed but who have problems, help is available from support groups, books, or lactation consultants and health care providers.

However, bottlefeeding can also provide adequate nutrition, and it is easier to tell how much milk bottle-fed infant is taking in. Additionally, bottlefed infants tend to sleep longer. Both breastfeeding and bottlefeeding can be part of loving, secure parent-child relationships.

When a mother doesn't nurse, menstruation usually begins within about 10 weeks. Breastfeeding can prevent the return of menstruation for six months or longer because the hormone prolactin, which aids milk production, suppresses

hormones vital to the development of mature eggs. However, ovulation—and pregnancy—can occur before menstruation returns, so breastfeeding is not a reliable contraceptive method. If a woman wishes to avoid pregnancy, she should use a reliable method of birth control.

Postpartum Depression The physical stress of labor, blood loss, fatigue, decreased sleep, fluctuating postpartum hormone levels, and anxieties of becoming a new parent all contribute to emotional instability postpartum. About 50–80% of new mothers experience "baby blues," characterized by episodes of sadness, weeping, anxiety, headache, sleep disturbances, and irritability. A mother may feel lonely and anxious about caring for her infant.

About 9–16% of new mothers experience **postpartum depression.** Postpartum depression is characterized by a prolonged period of anxiety, guilt, fear, or self-blame; these feelings prevent the new mother from normal participation in everyday life or the normal care of her newborn. Those close to the affected woman may fear for the well-being of the mother or those in her care. Fortunately, postpartum depression can be prevented and treated effectively. Women with a history of depression or depression during pregnancy can benefit from early referral to an appropriate mental health care provider. Rest is a key component of recovery. The mother's support system should offer to take on important responsibilities to allow the mother to rest and recover, as well as encourage her to continue outside interests and share her concerns with a professional who can assess the need for therapy.

Some men also seem to get a form of postpartum depression, characterized by anxiety about their changing roles and feelings of inadequacy. Both mothers and fathers need time to adjust to their new roles as parents.

Attachment Another feature of the postpartum period is the development of attachment—the strong emotional tie that grows between the baby and the adult who cares for the baby. Parents can foster secure attachment relationships in the early weeks and months by responding sensitively to the baby's true needs. Parents who respond appropriately to the baby's signals of gazing, looking away, smiling, and crying establish feelings of trust in their child. They feed the baby when she's hungry, for example; respond when she cries; interact with her when she gazes, smiles, or babbles; and stop stimulating her when she frowns or looks away. A secure

postpartum depression An emotional low that may be experienced by the mother following childbirth.

TERMS

TIPS FOR TODAY AND THE FUTURE

A healthy sexual life is built on acceptance of yourself and good communication with your partners, as is recognizing that parenthood means making responsible choices and preparing for it long before pregnancy.

RIGHT NOW YOU CAN:

- Articulate to yourself exactly what your beliefs are about sexual relationships. Consider whether you are acting in accordance with your beliefs. Your beliefs may be different from those of your parents, family, and caregivers.
- If you're in a sexual relationship, consider the information you and your partner have shared about sex. Are you comfortable that you and your partner know enough about each other to have a safe, healthy sexual relationship?
- Take some time to think about whether you really *want* to have children. Cut through the cultural, societal, family, and personal expectations that may stand in the way of making the decision you really want to make.

IN THE FUTURE YOU CAN:

- If you're in a sexual relationship, or if you plan to begin one, open (or reopen) a dialogue about sex. Make time to talk at length about the responsibilities and consequences of a sexual relationship.
- If you want to be a parent someday, start looking at the many sources of information about pregnancy, childbirth, and parenting. This is a good idea for anyone—man or woman—who plans to have a family.

attachment relationship helps the child develop and function well socially, emotionally, and mentally.

For most people, the arrival of a child creates a deep sense of joy and accomplishment. However, adjusting to parenthood requires effort and energy. Talking with friends and relatives about their experiences during the first few weeks or months with a baby can help prepare new parents for the period when the baby's needs may require all the energy that both parents have to expend. But the pleasures of nurturing a new baby are substantial, and many parents look back on this time as one of the most significant and joyful of their lives.

SUMMARY

- The female external sex organs are referred to as the vulva, which includes the clitoris, the highly sensitive genital structure that plays an important role in sexual arousal and orgasm because of its high concentration of nerve endings. The vagina leads to the internal female sex organs, including the uterus, oviducts or fallopian tubes, and ovaries.

- The male external sex organs are the penis and the scrotum; the glans of the penis is an important site of sexual arousal because of the high concentration of nerve endings. Male internal sexual structures include the testes, epididymis, vasa deferentia, seminal vesicles, Cowper's gland, ejaculatory duct, and prostate gland.

- The menstrual cycle has four phases: menses, the estrogenic phase, ovulation, and the progestational phase.

- The ovaries gradually cease to function as women approach age 50 and enter menopause. The pattern of male sexual responses changes with age, and testosterone production gradually decreases.

- Sexual activity is based on stimulus and response. Stimulation may be physical or psychological. The sexual response cycle has four stages: excitement, plateau, orgasm, and resolution.

- Physical and psychological problems can interfere with sexual functioning. Treatment for sexual dysfunction first addresses any underlying medical conditions and then looks at psychosocial problems.

- In general, gender is distinct from sex in that the former refers to how people identify and feel about themselves, rather than the body parts and sexual organs they have.

- A person's sexual orientation can be heterosexual, homosexual, bisexual, asexual, or queer. Possible influences include genetics, hormonal factors, and early childhood experiences.

- Human sexual behaviors include celibacy, erotic fantasy, masturbation, touching, cunnilingus, fellatio, anal intercourse, and coitus. Responsible sexuality includes open, honest communication; consent to sexual activities; sexual privacy; contraception use; safe sex practices; sober sex; and the taking of responsibility for consequences.

- Fertilization is a complex process culminating when a sperm penetrates the membrane of the egg released from the woman's ovary.

- Early signs and symptoms of pregnancy include a missed menstrual period; slight bleeding; nausea; breast tenderness; increased urination; fatigue and emotional upset; and a softening of the uterus just above the cervix.

- During pregnancy, the uterus enlarges until it pushes up into the rib cage; the breasts enlarge and may secrete colostrum; the muscles and ligaments soften and stretch; and the circulatory system, lungs, and kidneys become more efficient.

- The fetal anatomy is almost completely formed in the first trimester and is refined in the second; during the third trimester, the fetus grows and gains most of its weight, storing nutrients in fatty tissues.

- Important elements of prenatal care include good nutrition; avoidance of drugs, alcohol, tobacco, infections, and other harmful environmental agents or conditions; and regular physical activity.

- Pregnancy usually proceeds without major complications. Problems that can occur include ectopic pregnancy, spontaneous abortion, preeclampsia, low birth weight, and preterm birth.

- The first stage of labor begins with contractions that exert pressure on the cervix, causing effacement and dilation. The second stage begins with complete cervical dilation and ends when the baby emerges. The third stage of labor is expulsion of the placenta.

• During the postpartum period, the mother's body begins to return to its prepregnancy state, and she may begin to breastfeed. Both mother and father must adjust to their new roles as parents as they develop a strong emotional bond with their baby.

FOR MORE INFORMATION

American Association of Sexuality Educators, Counselors, and Therapists (AASECT). Certifies sex educators, counselors, and therapists and provides listings of local therapists dealing with sexual problems.

http://www.aasect.org

American Congress of Obstetricians and Gynecologists (ACOG). Provides written materials relating to many aspects of preconception care, pregnancy, and childbirth.

http://www.acog.org

American Psychological Association: Answers to Your Questions about Transgender People, Gender Identity, and Gender Expression. Offers question-and-answer format sections on transgender and homosexuality.

http://www.apa.org/topics/sexuality/transgender.aspx

American Society for Reproductive Medicine. Provides up-to-date information about all aspects of infertility.

http://www.asrm.org

Centers for Disease Control and Prevention, National Center on Birth Defects and Developmental Disabilities. Provides information about a variety of topics related to birth defects, including fetal alcohol syndrome and the importance of folic acid.

http://www.cdc.gov/ncbddd

Children Now: Talking with Kids. Provides advice for parents about talking with children about difficult issues, including sex, relationships, and STIs.

https://www.childrennow.org/parenting-resources/

Eunice Kennedy Shriver *National Institute of Child Health and Human Development.* Provides information about reproductive and genetic problems; sponsors the "Safe to Sleep" campaign to fight SIDS.

http://www.nichd.nih.gov/sts

Health Resources and Services Administration (HRSA): Maternal and Child Health. Provides publications, videos, and other resources relating to maternal, infant, and family health.

http://www.mchb.hrsa.gov

The Kinsey Institute for Research in Sex, Gender, and Reproduction. One of the oldest and most respected institutions doing research on sexuality.

http://www.kinseyinstitute.org

Sexuality Information and Education Council of the United States (SIECUS). Provides information about many aspects of sexuality and has an extensive library and numerous publications.

http://www.siecus.org

See also the listings for Chapters 4, 6–8, and 18.

SELECTED BIBLIOGRAPHY

American Academy of Pediatrics, Task Force on Circumcision. 2012. Technical report: Male circumcision. *Pediatrics,* 130(3): e756–785.

American College Health Association. 2009. *American College Health Association—National College Health Assessment II: Reference Group Executive Summary Fall 2009.* Linthicum, MD: American College Health Association.

American Congress of Obstetricians and Gynecologists. 2007. Vaginal 'Rejuvenation' and Cosmetic Vaginal Procedures. Committee Opinion, Number 378 (affirmed 2014) (https://www.acog.org/-/media/Committee-Opinions/Committee-on-Gynecologic-Practice/co378.pdf?dmc=1&ts=20160130T1116423301).

American Pregnancy Association. 2015. *Depression During Pregnancy.* (http://americanpregnancy.org/pregnancy-health/depression-during-pregnancy/).

American Psychological Association. 2012. *Answers to Your Questions about Transgender People, Gender Identity, and Gender Expression* (http://www.apa.org/topics/sexuality/transgender.aspx).

American Psychological Association. 2012. *Answers to Your Questions for a Better Understanding of Sexual Orientation & Homosexuality* (http://www.apa.org/topics/sexuality/orientation.aspx).

American Psychological Association. 2016. *Answers to Your Questions About Individuals with Intersex Conditions* (http://www.apa.org/topics/lgbt/intersex.aspx).

Balter, M. 2015. Can epigenetics explain homosexuality puzzle? Science 350(6257): 148.

Basson, R. 2000. The female sexual response: A different model. *Journal of Sex & Marital Therapy* 26(1): 51–65.

Bogaert, A. F. 2006. Biological versus nonbiological older brothers and men's sexual orientation. *Proceedings of the National Academy of Sciences* 103(28): 10771–10774.

Bogle, K. 2008. *Hooking Up: Sex, Dating and Relationships on Campus.* New York: New York University Press.

Brewer, G., and C. Hendrie. 2011. Evidence to suggest that copulatory vocalizations in women are not a reflexive consequence of orgasm. *Archives of Sexual Behavior* 40(3): 559–564.

Burke, H., et al. 2012. Prenatal and passive smoke exposure and incidence of asthma and wheeze: Systematic review and meta-analysis. *Pediatrics* 129(4): 735–744.

Centers for Disease Control and Prevention. 2009. *Healthy Youth—Sexual Risk Behaviors* (http://www.cdc.gov/HealthyYouth/sexualbehaviors/index.htm).

Centers for Disease Control and Prevention. 2013. *Human Papillomavirus* (http://www.cdc.gov/hpv/index.html).

Centers for Disease Control and Prevention. 2013. *Prostate Cancer* (http://www.cdc.gov/cancer/prostate/index.htm).

Centers for Disease Control and Prevention. 2014. Youth Risk Behavior Surveillance System, United States, 2013. *MMWR Surveillance Summaries* 63(4) (http://www.cdc.gov/HealthyYouth/yrbs/index.htm).

Centers for Disease Control and Prevention. 2015. Fetal alcohol syndrome among children aged 7–9—Arizona, Colorado, and New York, 2010. *Morbidity and Mortality Weekly Report* 64(03): 54–57.

Centers for Disease Control and Prevention. 2015. *Sexually Transmitted Disease Surveillance 2014.* Atlanta, GA: U.S. Department of Health and Human Services.

Centers for Disease Control and Prevention. 2016. *Breastfeeding Report Card United States, 2016* (http://www.cdc.gov/breastfeeding/data/reportcard.htm).

Centers for Disease Control and Prevention. 2016. *ART Success Rates: Latest Data, 2014* (http://www.cdc.gov/art/artdata/index.html).

Centers for Disease Control and Prevention. 2016. STDs during Pregnancy—Fact Sheet (Detailed) (http://www.cdc.gov/std/pregnancy/stdfact-pregnancy-detailed.htm).

Centers for Disease Control and Prevention, American Society for Reproductive Medicine, and Society for Assisted Reproductive Technology. 2015. *2013 Assisted Reproductive Technology: Fertility Clinic Success Rates Report.* Atlanta, GA: U.S. Department of Health and Human

Services (ftp://ftp.cdc.gov/pub/Publications/art/ART-2013-Clinic-Report-Full.pdf).

Copen, C. E., A. Chandra, and I. Febo-Vazquez. 2016. Sexual behavior, sexual attraction, and sexual orientation among adults aged 18–44 in the United States: Data from the 2011–2013 National Survey of Family Growth. *National Health Statistics Report* No. 88. Hyattsville, MD: National Center for Health Statistics.

Crooks, R., and K. Baur. 2014. *Our Sexuality*. Belmont, CA: Wadsworth /Cengage Learning.

Dewitte, M., et al. 2015. Sex in its daily relational context. *Journal of Sexual Medicine* 12(12): 2436–2450.

Erickson-Schroth, L. ed. 2014. *Trans Bodies, Trans Selves*. Oxford, UK: Oxford University Press.

European Union. 2014. "Denmark: Combining Work and Family Life Successfully." European Platform for Investing in Children (http://europa .eu/epic/countries/denmark/index_en.htm).

Freeman, E. 2007. *Epidemiology and Etiology of Premenstrual Syndromes* (http://cme.medscape.com/viewarticle/553603).

Gades, N. M., et al. 2005. Association between smoking and erectile dysfunction: A population-based study. *American Journal of Epidemiology* 161(4): 346–351.

Garcia-Falgueras, A., and D. Swaab. 2010. Sexual hormones and the brain: An essential alliance for sexual identity and sexual orientation. *Pediatric Endocrinology* 17: 22–35.

Gilmore, A. K., and K. E. Bountress. 2016. Reducing drinking to cope among heavy episodic drinking college women: Secondary outcomes of a web-based combined alcohol use and sexual assault risk reduction intervention. *Addictive Behaviors* 61: 104–111.

Grant, Jamie M., et al. 2011. *Injustice at Every Turn: A Report on the National Transgender Survey*. Washington, DC: National Center for Transgender Equality and National Gay and Lesbian Task Force (http://www .thetaskforce.org/static_html/downloads/reports/reports/ntds_full.pdf).

HealthDay. 2016. U.S. health experts debate advice to women once Zika virus arrives (https://www.nlm.nih.gov/medlineplus/news/fullstory _158335.html).

Hock, R. R. 2012. *Human Sexuality*. Upper Saddle River, NJ: Pearson.

Institute of Medicine of the National Academies. 2011. *The Health of Lesbian, Gay, Bisexual, and Transgender People: Building a Foundation for Better Understanding*. Consensus Report, March 31. Washington, DC: Institute of Medicine of the National Academies (http://www.iom.edu/Reports/2011 /The-Health-of-Lesbian-Gay-Bisexual-and-Transgender-People.aspx).

Intersex Society of North America. n.d. *How Common Is Intersex?* (http:// www.isna.org/).

Iveniuk, J., C. O'Muircheartaigh, and K. A. Cagney. 2016. Religious influence on older Americans' sexual lives: A nationally representative profile. *Archives of Sexual Behavior* 45(1): 121–131.

Joannides, P. 2013. *Guide to Getting It On*. Waldport, OR: Goofy Foot Press.

Jordan-Young, R. M. 2010. *Brain storm: The Flaws in the Science of Sex Differences*. Cambridge, MA: Harvard University Press.

Kaplan, Helen. 1979. *Disorders of Sexual Desire (and Other New Concepts and Techniques in Sex Therapy)*. Bruner Meisel University.

Kaschak, E., and L. Tiefer, eds. 2001. *A New View of Women's Sexual Problems*. New York: Routledge.

Kelly, G. F. 2013. *Sexuality Today*, 11th ed. New York: McGraw-Hill.

Labuski, C. 2015. *It Hurts Down There: The Bodily Imaginaries of Female Genital Pain*. Albany: State University of New York Press.

Lindau, S. T., and N. Gavrilova. 2010. Sex, health, and years of sexually active life gained due to good health. *British Medical Journal* 340: c810.

May, P., et al. 2014. Prevalence and characteristics of fetal alcohol spectrum disorders. *Pediatrics* 134:855–866.

Mayo Clinic. 2014. *Premenstrual Syndrome* (http://www.mayoclinic.com /health/premenstrual-syndrome/DS00134/DSECTION=lifestyle-and-home-remedies).

Mayo Clinic. 2015. *Erectile Dysfunction* (http://www.mayoclinic.org /diseases-conditions/erectile-dysfunction/basics/definition/con-20034244).

McKee, R., & W. J. Taverner. 2013. *Taking Sides: Clashing Views on Controversial Issues in Human Sexuality,* 13th ed. New York: McGraw-Hill.

Meston, C., and D. Buss. 2009. *Why Women Have Sex: Understanding Sexual Motivation*. New York: Henry Holt.

National Center for Health Statistics. 2010. *Trends in Circumcision among Newborns* (http://www.cdc.gov/nchs/data/hestat/circumcisions/circumcisions .htm).

National Center for Health Statistics. 2015. Births: Final data for 2014. *National Vital Statistics Reports* 64(12).

National Center for Health Statistics. 2016. Births: Preliminary data for 2015. *National Vital Statistics Reports* 65(3): 1–15.

National Institutes of Health, National Cancer Institute. 2013. *Prostate Cancer* (http://www.cancer.gov/cancertopics/types/prostate).

National Library of Medicine. 2014. *MedlinePlus: Semen Analysis* (https://medlineplus.gov/ency/article/003627.htm).

National Women's Health Network. *Top Ten Things to Know about Addyi* (https://www.nwhn.org/wp-content/uploads/2015/10/NWHN_Addyi _Fact_Sheet_P2.pdf).

Ottaviani, G. 2014. *Crib Death—Sudden Infant Death Syndrome (SIDS): Sudden Infant and Perinatal Unexplained Death: The Pathologist's Viewpoint*. Berlin: Springer International

Pacik, P. T. 2009. Viewpoint: Botox treatment for vaginismus. *Plastic & Reconstructive Surgery* 124(6): 455e–456e.

Padilla, M. 2007. *Caribbean Pleasure Industry: Tourism, Sexuality, and AIDS in the Dominican Republic*. Chicago: University of Chicago Press.

Pandian, Z., A. Gibreel, and S. Bhattacharya. 2015. In vitro fertilization for unexplained infertility. *Cochrane Database Systemic Reviews* 19(11): CD003357.

Sample, I. 2011. Female orgasm captured in series of brain scans. *Guardian,* November 14, p. 9.

Savage, Dan. 2012. *It Gets Better*. New York: Penguin Books.

Slaughter, A.-M. 2015. *Unfinished Business: Women Men Work Family*. New York: Random House.

Snowden, J. M. 2015. Planned out-of-hospital birth and birth outcomes. *New England Journal of Medicine* 373(27): 2642–2653.

Sunderam, S., et al. 2015. Assisted reproductive technology surveillance—United States, 2013. *MMWR Surveillance Summaries* 64(SS11): 1–25.

U.S. Department of Health and Human Services. 2011. *Aging Male Syndrome* (http://womenshealth.gov/mens-health/teens-fathers-minorities -older-men/older-men.cfm#ams).

U.S. Department of Health and Human Services. n.d. *Surgeon General's Family Health History Initiative* (http://www.hhs.gov/familyhistory/, accessed 12/30/2015).

Wawer, M. J., et al. 2009. Circumcision in HIV-infected men and its effect on HIV transmission to female partners in Rakai, Uganda: A randomised controlled trial. *Lancet* 374(9685): 229–237.

WebMD. 2014. *Menopause and Hormone Replacement Therapy* (http://www. webmd.com/menopause/guide/menopause-hormone-therapy?page=2).

Wilcox, A. J., et al. 2000. The timing of the "fertile window" in the menstrual cycle: Day-specific estimates from a prospective study. *British Medical Journal* 321(7271): 1259–1262.

World Health Organization. 2010. *Female Genital Mutilation* (http://www .who.int/mediacentre/factsheets/fs241/en/).

World Health Organization. 2012. *Male Circumcision for HIV Prevention: Publications.* (http://www.who.int/hiv/pub/malecircumcision/en/).

Yarber, W. L., et al. 2012. *Human Sexuality: Diversity in Contemporary America,* 8th ed. New York: McGraw-Hill.

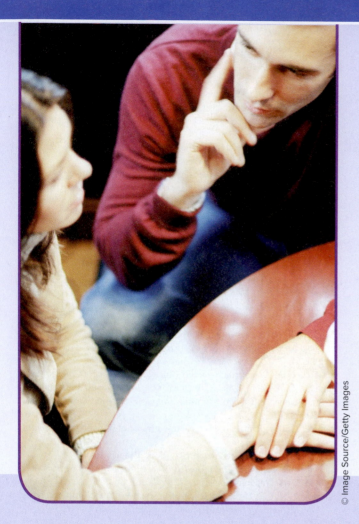

© Image Source/Getty Images

CHAPTER OBJECTIVES

- Explain how contraceptives work
- Explain the types of long-acting reversible contraceptives and how they work
- Explain the types of short-acting reversible contraceptives and how they work
- Explain approaches to emergency contraception
- Explain the types of permanent contraception
- Choose a contraceptive method that is right for you
- Summarize the history of abortion in the United States since the 19th century
- Discuss basic facts about abortion and the decision to have one
- Explain the methods of abortion
- Explain post-abortion care
- Describe the legal restrictions placed on abortion in the United States
- Explain the current debate over abortion

CHAPTER 6

Contraception and Abortion

For thousands of years, people have used **birth control** to manage **fertility** and prevent unwanted pregnancies. Records dating to the fourth century BCE describe foods, herbs, drugs, douches, and sponges used to prevent **conception**—the fusion of an ovum and a sperm that creates a fertilized egg, or *zygote*. Early attempts at **contraception** (the act of blocking conception through a device, substance, or method) followed the same principle as many modern birth control methods.

Today people can choose from many types of **contraceptives** to avoid unwanted pregnancies. *Modern* contraceptives—that is, female and male sterilization, oral hormonal pills, the intrauterine device (IUD), male and female condoms, injectables, implants, vaginal barrier methods, and emergency contraception—are much more predictable and effective than in the past. They are also more predictable and effective than *traditional* or *natural* methods of contraception, which include rhythm (periodic

abstinence); withdrawal; and the lactational amenorrhea method, based on the fact that breastmilk production causes lack of menstruation. Figure 6.1 provides data on the effectiveness of contraception in preventing unintended pregnancies. Of all unintended pregnancies, only 5% occurred in women who use

TERMS

birth control   The practice of managing fertility and preventing unwanted pregnancies.

fertility   The ability to reproduce.

conception   The fusion of ovum and sperm, resulting in a fertilized egg, or *zygote*.

contraception   The prevention of conception through the use of a device, substance, or method.

contraceptive   Any agent or method that can prevent conception.

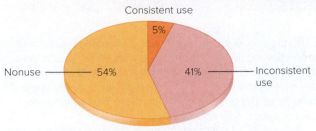

**Unintended Pregnancies
(3.1 Million)**

Consistent use 5%

Nonuse 54%

Inconsistent use 41%

By consistency of method use
during month of conception

FIGURE 6.1. **The number of unintended pregnancies in relation to contraception use.**

SOURCES: Curtin S. C., J. C. Abma, and K. Kost. 2015. 2010 Pregnancy rates among U.S. women (http://www.cdc.gov/nchs/data/hestat/pregnancy/2010 _pregnancy_rates.htm); Guttmacher Institute. March 2016. *Unintended Pregnancy in the United States* (https://www.guttmacher.org/fact-sheet /unintended-pregnancy-united-states).

contraception consistently. In addition to more efficacy, contraception is also now more available, at least to certain populations. With the implementation of the Affordable Care Act, privately insured women in the United States increasingly pay zero dollars for their birth control.

In addition to preventing pregnancy, some contraceptive products—the "barrier methods"—play an important role in protecting against **sexually transmitted infections (STIs).** (Chapter 13 provides a comprehensive overview of STIs, a term replacing *sexually transmitted diseases,* or *STDs.*) Informing yourself about the realities and risks and making responsible decisions about sexual and contraceptive behavior are crucial components of lifelong wellness.

HOW CONTRACEPTIVES WORK

Effective approaches to contraception include the following:

• **Barrier methods** work by physically blocking the sperm from reaching the egg. Condoms are the most popular method based on this principle.

• **Hormonal methods,** such as oral contraceptives (birth control pills), alter the biochemistry of the woman's body, preventing ovulation (the release of the egg) and producing changes that make it more difficult for the sperm to reach the egg if ovulation does occur.

• **Intrauterine device methods** prevent the sperm from reaching the egg through chemical or hormonal changes.

• **Natural methods** of contraception are based on the fact that the egg and the sperm have to be present at the same time for fertilization to occur; intercourse is avoided around the time of ovulation.

• **Surgical methods**—female and male sterilization— permanently prevent the union of sperm and eggs.

All contraceptive methods have advantages and disadvantages that make them appropriate for some people but not for others, and the best choice during one period of life may not be the best in another (see the box "Contraception Use and Pregnancy among College Students"). Factors that affect the choice of method include effectiveness, convenience, cost, reversibility, side effects and risks, and protection against STIs. This chapter helps you sort through these factors to decide which contraceptive method is best for you.

Contraceptive effectiveness is determined partly by the reliability of the method itself—the failure rate if it were always used exactly as directed ("perfect use"). Effectiveness is also determined by user characteristics, including fertility of the individual, frequency of intercourse, and how consistently and correctly the method is used. This "typical use" **contraceptive failure rate** is based on studies that directly measure the percentage of women experiencing an unintended pregnancy in the first year of contraceptive use. For example, the 9% failure rate of oral contraceptives means 9 out of 100 typical users will become pregnant in the first year. This failure rate is likely to be lower for women who are consistently careful in following instructions and higher for those who are frequently careless; the "perfect use" failure rate of oral contraceptives is 0.3%.

Another measure of effectiveness is the **continuation rate**—the percentage of people who continue to use the method after a specified period of time. This measure is important because many unintended pregnancies occur when a method is stopped and not immediately replaced with another. Thus a contraceptive with a high continuation rate would be more effective at preventing pregnancy than

sexually transmitted infection (STI) Any of several contagious infections contracted through intimate sexual contact. **TERMS**

barrier method A contraceptive that acts as a physical barrier, blocking sperm from uniting with an egg.

hormonal method A contraceptive that alters the biochemistry of a woman's body, preventing ovulation and making it more difficult for sperm to reach an egg if ovulation does occur.

intrauterine device method A form of contraception that prevents the sperm from reaching the egg through chemical or hormonal changes.

natural method An approach to contraception that does not use drugs or devices; requires avoiding intercourse during the period of the woman's menstrual cycle when an egg is most likely to be present at the site of conception and the risk of pregnancy is greatest.

surgical method Sterilization of a male or female to permanently prevent the transport of sperm or eggs to the site of conception.

contraceptive failure rate The percentage of women using a particular contraceptive method who experience an unintended pregnancy in the first year of use.

continuation rate The percentage of people who continue to use a particular contraceptive after a specified period of time.

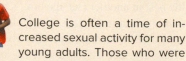

College is often a time of increased sexual activity for many young adults. Those who were sexually active in high school may have an increased number of partners or engage in riskier sexual behaviors once they enter college; those who abstained from intercourse during high school may begin to explore their sexuality once they enter this new environment. Surveys have shown that the majority of college students, up to 70%, engage in sexual activity, and some have more than one partner.

Concern about pregnancy is on the minds of students: 75% of students report that preventing unplanned pregnancy is very important to them. However, a large percentage of students report not using contraception during their most recent sexual activity. The study cited above found that only 56% of students used contraception during their most recent intercourse. Oral contraceptive pills were the most commonly used contraceptive, with about 60% of women using a contraceptive selecting this method; males who used a contraceptive at last intercourse reported having used the male condom approximately 66% of the time. Of note, the withdrawal method was used by 27% of respondents; this method does not protect against STIs and has a high failure rate.

Black and white college students differ somewhat in contraceptive use. Black students were more likely to have used a condom the last time they had vaginal intercourse, compared with white students (63% of blacks versus 58% of whites). White students were far more likely to use hormonal contraception than black students (66% versus 42%).

Although the oral contraceptive pill is a highly effective form of contraception when used as directed, and the male condom is effective at preventing the transmission of a wide variety of STIs, they must be used together to provide simultaneous protection against both pregnancy and STIs. This is particularly important for couples who are not in a long-term, mutually monogamous relationship. However, surveys show that college students use a male condom plus another form of contraception only about 45% of the time.

Around 2% of college women report having become pregnant in the prior year, many unintentionally. A disproportionate number of these pregnancies occur in students attending community colleges; a 2007 survey found that 5.3% of community college students reported a pregnancy during the year prior, whereas only 1.8% of students at four-year universities reported the same. Unintended pregnancies were nearly four times higher among black college students, compared with white students.

The consequences of pregnancy among college students can be significant. For example, studies have demonstrated that 60% of women who became pregnant while attending community college subsequently dropped out. Those who continue their education face added expenses and stress. Given the importance of education in achieving long-term career and financial goals, the implementation of effective contraception during the college years can have a significant impact on the lives of young women. Unfortunately, only 42% of students report that their college provided any information about pregnancy prevention.

SOURCES: National Campaign to Prevent Teen and Unplanned Pregnancy. 2015. *National College Health Assessment: Reference Group Executive Summary Spring 2011* (http://www.acha-ncha.org/docs/ACHA-NCHA-II_ReferenceGroup_ExecutiveSummary_Spring2011.pdf); National Center for Health Statistics. 2011. National Survey of Family Growth (http://www.cdc.gov/nchs/nsfg/).

---

one with a low continuation rate. A high continuation rate also indicates user satisfaction with a particular method.

Contraception is often divided into categories, or tiers, based on efficacy. Figure 6.2 offers a graphic depiction of these tiers along with the typical use effectiveness ratings and tips on how to improve efficacy.

LONG-ACTING REVERSIBLE CONTRACEPTION

Long-acting reversible contraception (LARC) consists of intrauterine devices (IUDs) and implants. These methods of contraception give very high satisfaction rates and have been shown to decrease instances of unintended pregnancy and abortion more than do other methods. According to the Institute of Medicine, "expanding access to LARC for all young women should be a national priority." The American College of Obstetricians and Gynecologists agrees that IUDs and implants should be encouraged for all appropriate candidates, including adolescents and women who have not yet given birth.

Intrauterine Devices (IUDs)

An **intrauterine device** (**IUD**) is a small plastic object placed in the uterus as a contraceptive. Three types of IUDs are now available in the United States: the Copper T-380A

> **TERMS**
>
> **long-acting reversible contraception (LARC)**   Intrauterine devices and implant methods of contraception, which last for several years, earn high satisfaction rates, and reduce rates of unintended pregnancy and abortion compared to other methods.
>
> **intrauterine device (IUD)**   A device inserted into the uterus as a contraceptive.

Effectiveness of Family Planning Methods

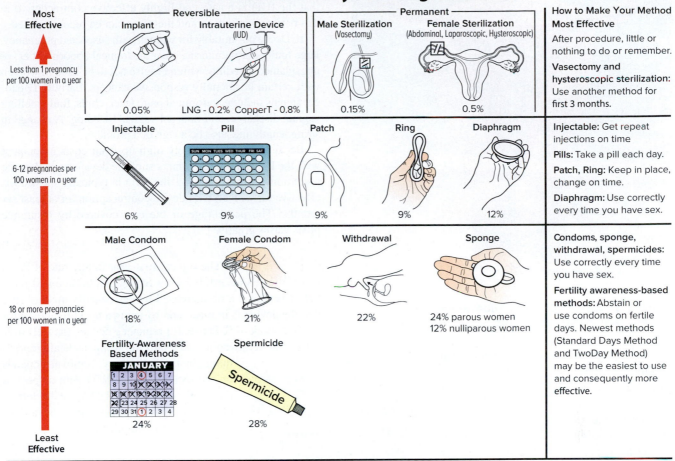

Most Effective	Reversible		Permanent		How to Make Your Method Most Effective

Reversible

Implant	Intrauterine Device (IUD)
0.05%	LNG - 0.2% CopperT - 0.8%

Permanent

Male Sterilization (Vasectomy)	Female Sterilization (Abdominal, Laparoscopic, Hysteroscopic)
0.15%	0.5%

Less than 1 pregnancy per 100 women in a year

How to Make Your Method Most Effective

After procedure, little or nothing to do or remember.

Vasectomy and hysteroscopic sterilization: Use another method for first 3 months.

Injectable	Pill	Patch	Ring	Diaphragm
6%	9%	9%	9%	12%

6-12 pregnancies per 100 women in a year

Injectable: Get repeat injections on time

Pills: Take a pill each day.

Patch, Ring: Keep in place, change on time.

Diaphragm: Use correctly every time you have sex.

Male Condom	Female Condom	Withdrawal	Sponge
18%	21%	22%	24% parous women 12% nulliparous women

Fertility-Awareness Based Methods	Spermicide
JANUARY — 24%	Spermicide — 28%

18 or more pregnancies per 100 women in a year

Condoms, sponge, withdrawal, spermicides: Use correctly every time you have sex.

Fertility awareness-based methods: Abstain or use condoms on fertile days. Newest methods (Standard Days Method and TwoDay Method) may be the easiest to use and consequently more effective.

Least Effective

CS 242797

CONDOMS SHOULD ALWAYS BE USED TO REDUCE THE RISK OF SEXUALLY TRANSMITTED INFECTIONS.

Other Methods of Contraception

Lactational Amenorrhea Method: LAM is a highly effective, temporary method of contraception.

Emergency Contraception: Emergency contraceptive pills or a copper IUD after unprotected intercourse substantially reduces risk of pregnancy.

Adapted from World Health Organization (WHO) Department of Reproductive Health and Research, Johns Hopkins Bloomberg School of Public Health/Center for Communication Programs (CCP). Knowledge for health project. Family planning: a global handbook for providers (2011 update). Baltimore, MD; Geneva, Switzerland: CCP and WHO; 2011; and Trussell J. Contraceptive failure in the United States. Contraception 2011;83:397–404.

U.S. Department of Health and Human Services
Centers for Disease Control and Prevention

FIGURE 6.2   Categorization of contraceptives based on efficacy. The percentages indicate the number out of every 100 women who experienced an unintended pregnancy within the first year of typical use of each contraceptive method.

SOURCE: Centers for Disease Control and Prevention. n.d. Effectiveness of family planning methods (http://www.cdc.gov/reproductivehealth/UnintendedPregnancy /PDF/Contraceptive_methods_508.pdf).

(also known as ParaGard), which provides protection for up to 12 years, and the Mirena and Skyla, both of which release small amounts of progestin (a synthetic progesterone) and remain effective for 5 and 3 years, respectively.

Current evidence suggests that ParaGard works primarily by preventing fertilization. This IUD contains copper, which is thought to cause biochemical changes in the uterus that affect the movement of sperm and eggs. ParaGard may also interfere with implantation of fertilized eggs. Like ParaGard, Mirena and Skyla also work primarily by preventing fertilization. As a result of the slow release of very small amounts of progestin, the cervical mucus thickens and stops fertilization.

An IUD must be inserted and removed by a trained professional. It can be inserted at any time during the menstrual cycle, as long as the woman is not pregnant. The device is threaded into a sterile inserter that is introduced through the cervix; a plunger pushes the IUD into the uterus. IUDs have two threads attached that protrude from the cervix into the vagina so that a woman can feel them to make sure the device is in place. These threads are trimmed so that only 1–1½ inches remain in the upper vagina (Figure 6.3).

Advantages   Intrauterine devices are highly reliable and are simple and convenient to use, requiring no attention. They do not require the woman to anticipate or interrupt sexual activity. IUDs have only local effects and tend to be very safe for all women, including those with complex medical problems. The long-term expense of using an IUD is also low. The main advantage is their low failure rate: Less than 1% of women using IUDs will get pregnant. In the absence of complications,

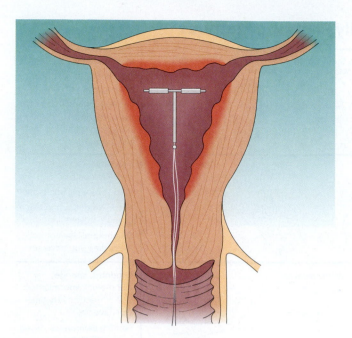

FIGURE 6.3 An IUD (Copper T-380A, or ParaGard) properly positioned in the uterus.

they are also fully reversible, meaning that fertility is restored as soon as the IUD is removed. Following IUD removal, the risk of ectopic pregnancy is decreased.

Mirena has the added advantage of greatly decreasing blood flow during menstruation and is often used as a treatment for excessive bleeding. In fact, after a year of using Mirena, menstrual bleeding is decreased by about 90%. Mirena generally reduces menstrual cramps and is often prescribed for that reason. The Mirena IUD has also been shown to prevent endometrial cancer (in the lining of the uterus) and even reverse the endometrial changes that precede endometrial cancer. ParaGard has been shown to decrease the risk of endometrial cancer, but the reasons for this are less clear.

Disadvantages   The IUD offers little to no protection against STIs. Most IUD side effects are limited to the genital tract. Side effects differ between the two types of IUD. Heavy menstrual flow and increased menstrual cramping sometimes occur with ParaGard, whereas Mirena causes a reduction in bleeding and cramping. Spontaneous expulsion of the IUD happens to 3% of women within the first year, most commonly during the first months after insertion. In rare cases, an IUD can puncture the uterine wall and migrate into the abdominal cavity.

A serious but rare complication of IUD use is pelvic inflammatory disease (PID). Most pelvic infections among IUD users occur shortly after insertion, are relatively mild, and can be treated successfully with antibiotics. For many years, IUD use was not recommended for women who had

never had a child. However, extensive research now reveals that the IUD is a safe and highly effective contraceptive in this patient population and therefore can be recommended.

IUDs are not suitable for women with suspected pregnancy, large tumors of the uterus, other anatomical abnormalities, or unexplained bleeding; Mirena is also not to be used in women with certain hormonally responsive cancers. Early IUD danger signals include abdominal pain, fever, chills, foul-smelling vaginal discharge, and unusual vaginal bleeding. A change in string length may also be a sign of a problem.

Because of the relatively high up-front costs associated with the IUDs, including the cost of the device as well as the practitioner's insertion fee, the IUD is typically most cost-effective for women who desire contraception for at least six months. The percentage of the cost covered by insurance plans varies greatly.

Effectiveness   The typical first-year failure rate of IUDs is 0.8% for ParaGard, 0.5% for Skyla, and 0.2% for Mirena. Effectiveness can be increased by periodically making sure that the device is in place and by using a backup method for the first week of IUD use. If pregnancy occurs, the IUD may need to be removed to safeguard the woman's health and to maintain the pregnancy; removal depends on the location of the IUD with respect to the pregnancy. If an IUD must be left in place during pregnancy, there is an increased risk of complications.

> **QUICK STATS**
>
> Use of long-acting reversible contraception (LARC) increased nearly fivefold in the past decade among women aged 15–44, from **1.5%** in 2002 to **7.2%** in 2011–2013.
>
> —Centers for Disease Control and Prevention, 2015

Contraceptive Implants

Contraceptive implants are placed under the skin of the upper arm and deliver a small but steady dose of progestin over a period of years. One such implant, called Nexplanon, is a single implant that is effective for three years and is considered to be one of the most effective forms of contraception (Figure 6.4). The progestins in implants have several contraceptive effects. They cause hormonal shifts that may inhibit ovulation and affect development of the uterine lining. The hormones also thicken the cervical mucus, inhibiting the movement of sperm. Contraceptive implants are best suited for women who wish to have continuous, highly effective, and long-term protection against pregnancy.

Advantages   Contraceptive implants are highly effective, with a failure rate of less than 1%. After insertion of the implants, no further action is required; contraceptive effects are reversed quickly upon removal. Because implants contain no estrogen, they carry a lower risk of certain side effects, such as blood clots (venous thromboembolism) and other cardiovascular complications. Menstrual bleeding tends to decrease but becomes irregular. Women who are breastfeeding can use Nexplanon.

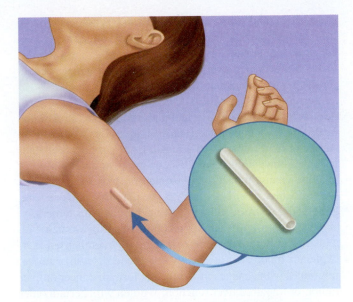

FIGURE 6.4 **Placement of contraceptive implant.** The Implanon/Nexplanon implant device has to be placed and removed by a trained medical professional.

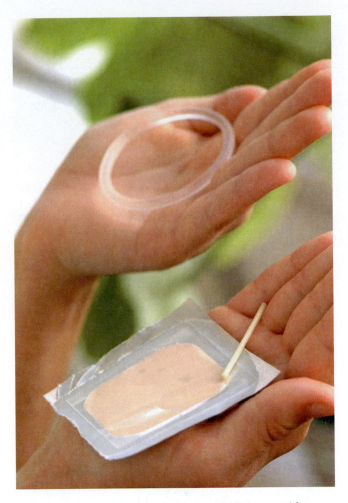

Reversible hormonal contraceptives are available in several forms. Shown here are the patch, the ring, and an implant.

© Phanie/Photo Researchers, Inc.

Disadvantages An implant provides little to no protection against STIs. Although the implants are barely visible, their presence may bother some women. Only specially trained practitioners can insert or remove the implants. The up-front costs associated with the implant, including the cost of the device as well as the practitioner's fees, can be significant; therefore, the device is cost-effective only for users desiring more than six months of contraception.

Common side effects of contraceptive implants are menstrual irregularities, including longer menstrual periods, spotting between periods, or having no bleeding at all. The menstrual cycle usually becomes more regular after one year of use. Less common side effects include headaches, weight gain, breast tenderness, nausea, acne, and mood swings.

Effectiveness The overall failure rate for Nexplanon is estimated at about 0.05%. It is one of the most effective methods of contraception and also one of the most discreet.

SHORT-ACTING REVERSIBLE CONTRACEPTION

A variety of hormonal and barrier methods fall into the group of short-acting reversible contraceptives. For these methods, the user must take action on a daily, weekly, or monthly basis, or at the time of intercourse. Such short-acting methods include, among others, oral contraceptives, skin patches, and vaginal rings.

Oral Contraceptives: The Pill

About a century ago, a researcher noted that ovulation does not occur during pregnancy. Further research revealed the hormonal mechanism: During pregnancy, the corpus luteum secretes progesterone and estrogen in amounts high enough to suppress ovulation. (See Chapter 5 for a complete discussion of the menstrual cycle.) **Oral contraceptives (OCs),** also known as *birth control pills* or "the pill," prevent ovulation by mimicking the hormonal activity of the corpus luteum. The active ingredients in OCs are estrogen and progestins, laboratory-made compounds that are closely related to progesterone. Today OCs are the most widely used form of contraception among unmarried women and are second only to sterilization among married women.

In addition to preventing ovulation, the birth control pill has other contraceptive effects. Its main mechanism of action is to inhibit the movement of sperm by thickening the cervical mucus. In the rare event that ovulation does occur, the pill alters the rate of ovum transport by means of its hormonal effects on the fallopian tubes, and it may prevent implantation by changing the lining of the uterus.

TERMS

oral contraceptive (OC) Hormone compounds (made of estrogen and progestins) in pill form that prevent conception by preventing ovulation; also called the *birth control pill* or "the pill."

Ask Yourself

QUESTIONS FOR CRITICAL THINKING AND REFLECTION

Prior to reading this section, how familiar were you with the variety of approaches to contraception? Did you know as much as you thought? Were you aware of the large number of contraceptive options that are currently available?

Advantages Oral contraceptives are fairly effective in preventing pregnancy. The majority of women who get pregnant while using the pill get pregnant because the pills were not taken as directed. The typical one-year failure rate is 9%. The pill is relatively simple to use and does not hinder sexual spontaneity. Most women also appreciate the predictable regularity of periods, as well as the reduction in cramps and blood loss. Women who have significant problems associated with menstruation may benefit from menstrual suppression with extended-cycle OCs. Finally, the pills are reversible and fertility returns shortly after stopping the pill.

Medical advantages include a decreased incidence of benign breast disease, acne, iron-deficiency anemia, ectopic pregnancy, colon and rectal cancer, endometrial cancer, and ovarian cancer. OC use reduces dysmenorrhea (painful periods), endometriosis, and polycystic ovary syndrome.

Disadvantages Although simple to ingest, remembering to take a pill every single day can be challenging. Furthermore, OCs do not protect against STIs. In some studies, OCs have been associated with increased risk of cervical chlamydia. If you are using the pill, you should also be using condoms regularly (an exception could be if you have a long-term, mutually monogamous relationship with an uninfected partner).

The majority of women do not experience any side effects associated with OC use. Among women who experience problems with OCs, the most common issue is bleeding during midcycle (called *breakthrough bleeding*), which is usually slight and tends to disappear after a few cycles. Symptoms of early pregnancy—such as morning nausea and swollen breasts—may appear during the first few months of OC use, although these side effects are uncommon with the low-dose pills in current widespread use. Other side effects can include depression, nervousness, changes in sex drive, dizziness, generalized headaches, migraine, and vaginal discharge.

Research shows that currently used low-dose OCs do not, on average, cause weight gain. Most women experience no change in their weight, while a small percentage lose weight, and about an equal percentage gain weight while taking OCs. The myth that OCs cause women to gain weight is actually dangerous because many unintended pregnancies have resulted when women avoided taking OCs due to unfounded fear of weight gain.

Another myth about OCs is that they can cause cancer. Actually, taking the pill greatly reduces a woman's risk for endometrial and ovarian cancers. OC use is associated with little, if any, increase in breast cancer and a slight increase in cervical cancer, but earlier detection and other variables (such as a woman's number of sexual partners) may account for much of this increase.

Serious OC side effects have been reported in a small number of women. These include blood clots, stroke, and heart attack, concentrated mostly in older women who smoke or have a history of circulatory disease. Recent studies have shown no increased risk of stroke or heart attack for healthy, young, nonsmoking women on lower-dosage pills. OC users may be slightly more prone to high blood pressure, gallbladder disease, and, very rarely, benign liver tumors.

Birth control pills are not recommended for women with a history of blood clots (or a close family member with unexplained blood clots at an early age), heart disease or stroke, migraines with changes in vision, any form of cancer or liver tumor, or impaired liver function. Women with certain other health conditions or behaviors, including migraines without changes in vision, high blood pressure, cigarette smoking, and sickle-cell disease, require close monitoring when taking the pill.

When deciding whether to use OCs, each woman needs to weigh the benefits against the risks. To make an informed decision, she should begin by getting advice from a health care professional. If you take the pill, you can take several steps to reduce the risks associated with OC use:

1. Request a low-dosage pill. (OCs recommended for most new users contain 20–35 micrograms of estrogen.)

2. Stop smoking.

3. Follow the directions carefully and consistently, making sure to take the pills at the same time every day.

4. Be alert to preliminary danger signals, which can be remembered by the word ACHES:

   Abdominal pain (severe)

   Chest pain (severe), cough, shortness of breath, or sharp pain on breathing in

   Headaches (severe), dizziness, weakness, or numbness, especially if one-sided

   Eye problems (vision loss or blurring) and/or speech problems

   Severe leg pain (calf or thigh)

5. Make sure your health practitioner knows your personal and family medical history to help determine whether OCs may be unsafe for you.

6. Have regular **Pap tests,** pelvic exams, and breast exams as recommended by your health practitioner.

Overall, OC risks are generally very small unless you are over 35, are a smoker, or have specific medical problems.

Pap test A scraping of cells from the cervix for examination under a microscope to detect cancer. **TERMS**

Table 6.1 — Risks of Contraception, Pregnancy, and Abortion

CONTRACEPTION	RISK OF DEATH
Oral contraceptives	
Nonsmoker	
Ages 15–34	1 in 1,667,000
Ages 35–44	1 in 33,300
Smoker	
Ages 15–34	1 in 57,800
Ages 35–44	1 in 5,200
IUDs	1 in 10,000,000
Barrier methods, spermicides	None
Fertility awareness–based methods	None
Tubal ligation	1 in 66,700
PREGNANCY	RISK OF DEATH
Pregnancy	1 in 6,900
ABORTION	RISK OF DEATH
Spontaneous abortion	1 in 142,900
Medical abortion	1 in 200,000
Surgical abortion	1 in 142,900

SOURCE: Hatcher, R. A., et al. *Contraceptive Technology*, 20th revised ed. 2011, Ardent Media.

For the vast majority of young women, the known, directly associated risk of death from taking birth control pills is much, much lower than the risk of death from pregnancy (Table 6.1).

Effectiveness   Oral contraceptive effectiveness varies substantially because it depends so much on individual factors. If taken as directed, the failure rate is as low as 0.3%. However, the typical user has a 9% failure rate. The continuation rate for OCs also varies; the average rate is 67% after one year. Besides forgetting to take the pill, another reason for OC failure is poor absorption of the drug due to vomiting or diarrhea, or to interactions with other medicines (including certain antibiotics, antiseizure medications, and the commonly used herb St. John's wort).

Contraceptive Skin Patch

The contraceptive skin patch, Ortho Evra, is a thin, 1¾-inch square patch that slowly releases an estrogen and a progestin into the bloodstream. The contraceptive patch prevents pregnancy in the same way as combination OCs, following a similar schedule. Each patch is worn continuously for one week and is replaced on the same day of the week for three consecutive weeks. The fourth week is patch-free, allowing a woman to have her menstrual period.

The patch can be worn on the upper outer arm, abdomen, buttocks, or upper torso (excluding the breasts); it is designed to stick to skin even during bathing or swimming. If a patch should fall off for more than a day, the U.S. Food and Drug Administration (FDA) advises starting a new four-week cycle of patches and using a backup method of contraception for the first week. Patches should be discarded according to the manufacturer's directions to avoid leakage of hormones into the environment.

Advantages   Because the patch provides the same combination of hormones as a combined birth control pill, the advantages are similar. The medical benefits of the patch include, but are not limited to, lighter, less painful menses; decreased risk of uterine and ovarian cancers; decreased anemia; and the ability to control your cycle. With both perfect and typical use, the patch is as effective as OCs in preventing pregnancy. Compliance seems to be higher with the patch than with OCs, probably because the patch requires weekly instead of daily action.

Disadvantages   Like other hormonal contraceptives, the patch doesn't protect against STIs. Patch users should also use condoms for STI protection unless they are in a long-term monogamous relationship with an uninfected partner. Minor side effects are similar to those of OCs, although breast discomfort may be more common in patch users. Some women also experience skin irritation around the patch. More serious complications are thought to be similar to those of OCs, including an increased risk of side effects among women who smoke. However, because Ortho Evra exposes users to higher doses of estrogen than most OCs, patch use may further increase the risk of blood clots. Recent studies show conflicting results regarding the risk of blood clots, but it is possible that the risk is slightly higher with the patch compared to low-dose OCs.

Effectiveness   With perfect use, the patch's failure rate is very low (0.3%) in the first year of use. The typical failure rate is approximately 9%, similar to that of the oral contraceptive pill. Failure rates have been shown to be higher in women weighing more than 198 pounds.

Vaginal Contraceptive Ring

The NuvaRing is a vaginal ring that is molded with a mixture of progestin and estrogen. The two-inch ring slowly releases hormones and maintains blood hormone levels comparable to those found with OC use. The ring prevents pregnancy in the same way as OCs. A woman inserts the ring anytime during the first five days of her menstrual cycle and leaves it in place for three weeks. During the fourth week, when the ring is removed, her next menstrual cycle occurs. A new ring is then inserted seven days later. Rings should be discarded according to the manufacturer's directions to avoid leakage of hormones into the environment. Backup contraception must be used for the first seven days of the first ring use or if the ring has been removed for more than three hours.

Advantages   The NuvaRing offers one month of protection with no daily or weekly action required. It does not require a fitting by a clinician, and exact placement in the vagina is not critical as it is with a diaphragm. Because the ring provides the same combination of hormones as a combined birth control pill, the advantages are similar. The medical benefits of the ring include, but are not limited to, lighter, less painful menses; decreased risk of uterine and ovarian cancer; decreased anemia; and the ability to control your cycle.

Disadvantages   The NuvaRing provides no protection against STIs. Side effects are roughly comparable to those seen with OC use, except for a lower incidence of nausea and vomiting. Other side effects may include vaginal discharge, vaginitis, and vaginal irritation. Medical risks also are similar to those found with OC use.

Effectiveness   As with the pill and patch, the perfect use failure rate is around 0.3%. The ring's typical use failure rate is similar to the pill's at 9%.

Injectable Contraceptives

Hormonal contraceptive injections were first developed in the 1960s. The first injectable contraceptive approved for use in the United States was Depo-Provera, which uses long-acting progestins. Injected into the arm or buttocks, Depo-Provera is usually given every 12 weeks, although it may provide effective contraception for a few weeks beyond that. The product prevents pregnancy by inhibiting ovulation.

Advantages   Injectable contraceptives are highly effective and require little action on the part of the user. Because the injections leave no trace and involve no ongoing supplies, injectable contraceptives allow women almost total privacy in their decision to use contraception. Depo-Provera has no estrogen-related side effects.

Disadvantages   Injectable contraceptives provide no protection against STIs. A woman must visit a health care facility every three months to receive the injections. The side effects of Depo-Provera are similar to those of implants: Menstrual irregularities are the most common, and after one year of using Depo-Provera many women have no menstrual bleeding at all. Weight gain is a common side effect. After discontinuing the use of Depo-Provera, women may experience temporary infertility for up to 12 months, making it less ideal for women who plan on conceiving in the near future.

Depo-Provera also has a unique risk: It can cause a reduction in bone density, especially in women who use it for an extended period. The rate of decline in bone density is most rapid in the first two years of use, but the good thing is that the bone density begins to increase shortly after discontinuation. Although decreased bone density is a risk factor for

osteoporosis (see Chapter 9) and fractures, no studies have shown that this decreased density actually leads to increased fractures. Nonetheless, women who use Depo-Provera are advised to do weight-bearing exercise and ensure an adequate intake of dietary calcium. Due to conflicting data, the FDA states that women should use Depo-Provera as a long-term contraceptive (longer than two years, for example) only if other methods are inadequate. However, multiple gynecologic associations believe that the benefits of this highly effective contraception outweigh the theoretical risks, and continuation should not be denied due to concerns regarding bone density.

Effectiveness   The perfect use failure rate is 0.2% for Depo-Provera. With typical use, the failure rate increases to 6% in the first year of use.

Male Condoms

The **male condom** is a thin sheath designed to cover the penis during sexual intercourse. Most brands available in the United States are made of latex, although condoms made of polyurethane and polyisoprene are also available. Condoms prevent sperm from entering the vagina and provide protection against most STIs. Condoms are the most widely used barrier method and the third most popular of all contraceptive methods used in the United States, after the pill and female sterilization.

Condom sales have increased dramatically in recent years, primarily because they are the only method of

male condom   A thin sheath that covers the penis during sexual intercourse; used for contraception and to prevent STI transmission.   **TERMS**

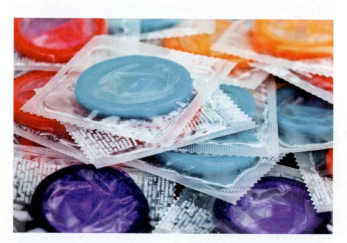

Condoms come in a variety of sizes, textures, and colors. Some brands have a reservoir tip designed to collect semen.
© Catherine Lane/Getty Images

contraception that provides substantial protection against HIV infection as well as some protection against other STIs. At least one-third of all male condoms are bought by women. This figure will probably increase as more women assume the right to insist on condom use. Many couples combine various contraceptives, using condoms for STI protection and another contraceptive method for greater protection against pregnancy.

The man or his partner must put the condom on the penis before it is inserted into the vagina because the small amounts of fluid that may be secreted unnoticed prior to **ejaculation** often contain sperm capable of causing pregnancy. The rolled-up condom is placed over the head of the erect penis and unrolled down to the base of the penis, leaving a half-inch space (without air) at the tip to collect semen (Figure 6.5). Some brands of condoms have a reservoir tip designed for this purpose. Uncircumcised men must first pull back the foreskin of the penis. Partners must be careful not to damage the condom with fingernails, rings, or other rough objects.

Many condoms are prelubricated with water-based or silicone-based lubricants. These lubricants make the condom more comfortable and less likely to break. Many people find that using extra, non-oil-based lubricant can be helpful. Prelubricated condoms are also available containing the **spermicide** nonoxynol-9, the same agent found in many of the contraceptive creams that women use. However, spermicidal condoms are no more effective than condoms without spermicide. They cost more and have a shorter shelf life than most other condoms. Further, condoms with nonoxynol-9 have been associated with urinary tract infections in women and, if they cause tissue irritation, an increased risk of HIV transmission. Planned Parenthood and many other public health agencies advise against the use of condoms lubricated with nonoxynol-9.

Water-based lubricants such as K-Y Brand Jelly or Astroglide can be used as needed. Any products that contain mineral or vegetable oil—including baby oil, many lotions, regular petroleum jelly, cooking oils (corn oil, shortening, butter, and so on), and some vaginal lubricants and antifungal or anti-itch creams—should not be used with latex condoms. Such products can cause latex to start disintegrating within 60 seconds, thus greatly increasing the chance of condom breakage. (Polyurethane is not affected by oil-based products.)

Advantages Condoms are easy to purchase and are available without prescription or medical supervision. In addition to being free of medical side effects (other than occasional allergic reactions), latex condoms help protect against STIs. A recent study determined that condoms may also protect women from human papillomavirus (HPV), which causes cervical cancer. Condoms made of polyurethane are appropriate for people who are allergic to latex. However, they are more likely to slip or break than latex condoms and therefore may give less protection against STIs and pregnancy. Polyisoprene condoms, marketed under the brand name SKYN, are safe for most people with latex allergies, stretchier, and less expensive than polyurethane condoms. Condoms made of lambskin are also available but permit the passage of HIV and other disease-causing organisms and are less effective for pregnancy prevention. Except for abstinence or intercourse within a monogamous relationship with an uninfected partner, the correct and consistent use of latex male condoms offers the most reliable available protection against the transmission of HIV.

Disadvantages The two most common complaints about condoms are that they diminish sensation and interfere with spontaneity. Although some people find these drawbacks serious, others consider them only minor distractions. Many couples learn to creatively integrate condom use into their sexual practices. Indeed, condom use can be a way to improve communication and share responsibility in a relationship.

Effectiveness During the first year of typical condom use among 100 users, approximately 18 pregnancies will occur. And even with perfect use, the first-year failure rate is

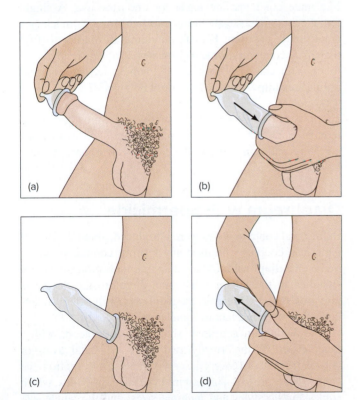

FIGURE 6.5 Use of the male condom. (a) Place the rolled-up condom over the head of the erect penis. Hold the top half-inch of the condom (with air squeezed out) to leave room for semen. (b) While holding the tip, unroll the condom onto the penis. Gently smooth out any air bubbles. (c) Unroll the condom down to the base of the penis. (d) To avoid spilling semen after ejaculation, hold the condom around the base of the penis as the penis is withdrawn. Remove the condom away from your partner, taking care not to spill any semen.

> **ejaculation**   An abrupt discharge of semen from the penis during sexual stimulation.
>
> **spermicide**   A chemical agent that kills sperm.
>
> TERMS

about 2%. At least some pregnancies happen because the condom is removed carelessly after ejaculation. Some may also occur because of breakage or slippage. Other contributing factors include poorly fitting condoms, insufficient lubrication (which increases the risk of breakage), excessively vigorous sex, and improper storage. (Because heat destroys rubber, latex condoms should not be stored for long periods in a wallet or a car's glove compartment.) To help ensure quality, condoms should not be used past their expiration date or more than five years past their date of manufacture (two years for those with spermicide).

If a condom breaks or is removed carelessly, a woman can reduce the risk of pregnancy somewhat by immediately taking an emergency contraceptive (discussed later in the chapter). By far the most common cause of pregnancy with condom users is "taking a chance"—that is, occasionally not using a condom at all—or waiting to use it until after preejaculatory fluid (which may contain some sperm) has already entered the vagina.

Female Condoms

The female condom is a clear, stretchy, disposable pouch with two rings that can be inserted into a woman's vagina. It was designed as an alternative to the male condom because the woman can control its use. It can be inserted up to eight hours before intercourse, so it need not interfere with the moment. It is about as effective in preventing pregnancy and the spread of STIs as the male condom.

The one-size-fits-all condom, called the FC2, consists of a soft, loose-fitting, nonlatex rubber sheath with two flexible rings. The ring at the closed end is inserted into the vagina and placed at the cervix much like a diaphragm. The ring at the open end remains outside the vagina. The female condom protects the inside of the vagina and part of the external genitalia.

The directions that accompany the FC2 should be followed closely. The manufacturer strongly recommends practicing inserting the female condom several times before actually using it for intercourse. Most women find that it is easy to use after they have practiced inserting the FC2 several times. The FC2 comes prelubricated with a silicone lubricant, but extra lubricant or a spermicide can be used if desired. As with male condoms, users need to take care not to tear the condom during insertion or removal. Following intercourse, the woman should remove the condom before standing up. By twisting and squeezing the outer ring, she can prevent the spilling of semen. A new condom should be used for each act of sexual intercourse. A female condom should not be used with a male condom because when the two are used together, tearing is more likely to occur.

Advantages   For many women, the greatest advantage of the female condom is the control it gives them over contraception and STI prevention. (Partner cooperation is still important, however.) Female condoms can be inserted up to

eight hours before sexual activity and are thus less disruptive than male condoms. Because the outer part of the condom covers the area around the vaginal opening as well as the base of the penis during intercourse, it offers potentially better protection against genital warts or herpes. The synthetic rubber pouch can be used by people who are allergic to latex. Because the material is thin and pliable, there is little loss of sensation. The FC2 is generously lubricated and the material conducts heat well, increasing comfort and natural feel during intercourse.

When used correctly, the female condom should theoretically provide protection against HIV transmission and STIs comparable to that of the latex male condom. However, in research involving typical users, the female condom was slightly less effective in preventing pregnancy and STIs. Effectiveness improves with careful practice and instruction.

Disadvantages   The female condom is unfamiliar to most people and requires practice to learn to use it effectively. The outer ring of the female condom, which hangs visibly outside the vagina, may be bothersome to some couples. During coitus, both partners must take care that the penis is inserted into the pouch, not outside it, and that the device does not slip inside the vagina. Female condoms, like male condoms, are made for one-time use. A single female condom costs about three to four times as much as a single male condom. Female condoms are harder to find than male condoms. Some pharmacies do not currently carry them. You can buy the FC2 at Planned Parenthood and online (see http://www.fc2.us.com/howtogetfc2.html).

Effectiveness   The typical first-year failure rate of the female condom is 21%. For women who follow instructions carefully and consistently, the failure rate is considerably lower—about 5%.

Diaphragm with Spermicide

Before oral contraceptives were introduced, about 25% of all American couples who used any form of contraception relied on the **diaphragm.** Many diaphragm users subsequently switched to the pill or IUDs, and therefore the device is rarely used now. However, the diaphragm still offers advantages that are important to some couples.

The diaphragm is a dome-shaped cup of silicone with a flexible rim. When correctly used with spermicidal cream or jelly, the diaphragm covers the cervix, blocking sperm from the uterus. There are two diaphragms available: The Milex, which comes in two styles and multiple sizes, and the single-size Caya, which became available in the United States in 2015.

> **diaphragm**   A contraceptive device consisting of a flexible, dome-shaped cup that covers the cervix and prevents sperm from entering the uterus.   **TERMS**

Diaphragms are available in the United States only by prescription. Because of individual anatomical differences among women, the round Milex diaphragm must be carefully fitted by a trained clinician to ensure both comfort and effectiveness. The fit should be checked with each routine annual medical examination, as well as after childbirth, abortion, abdominal or pelvic surgery, or a weight change of more than 10 pounds. Caya comes in only one size and does not require fitting; it is oval in shape and designed to fit most women. Caya is contoured for easier use and includes grip "dimples" on the sides to help with insertion and a small dome to aid in removal of the device.

A diaphragm should be used with spermicidal jelly or cream on the diaphragm before inserting it and checking its placement (Figure 6.6). If more than six hours elapse between the time of insertion and the time of intercourse, additional spermicide must be applied. The diaphragm must be left in place for at least six hours after the last act of coitus to give the spermicide enough time to kill all the sperm. With repeated intercourse, a condom should be used for additional protection.

To remove the diaphragm, the woman hooks the front rim (Milex) or small removal dome (Caya) down from the pubic bone with one finger and pulls it out. After each use, a diaphragm should be washed with mild soap and water, rinsed, patted dry, and examined for holes or cracks. Defects would most likely develop near the rim and can be spotted by looking at the diaphragm in front of a bright light. A diaphragm should be stored in its case.

Advantages   Diaphragm use is less intrusive than male condom use because a diaphragm can be inserted up to six hours before intercourse. Its use can be limited to times of sexual activity only, and it allows for immediate and total reversibility. The diaphragm is free of medical side effects (other than rare allergic reactions) and increased risk of urinary tract infection.

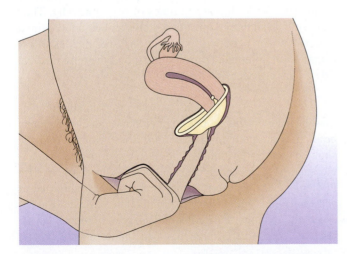

FIGURE 6.6   Positioning of the diaphragm. A diaphragm is positioned so that the cervix is completely covered and the front rim of the device is tucked behind the pubic bone. When correctly used with spermicidal jelly or cream, the diaphragm blocks sperm from reaching the uterus.

Disadvantages   Diaphragms must always be used with a spermicide, so a woman must keep both of these supplies with her whenever she anticipates sexual activity. Diaphragms require extra attention because they must be cleaned and stored with care to preserve their effectiveness. Some women cannot wear a diaphragm because of their vaginal or uterine anatomy. In other women, diaphragm use can cause bladder infections and may need to be discontinued if repeated infections occur.

Diaphragms have also been associated with a slightly increased risk of **toxic shock syndrome (TSS),** an occasionally fatal bacterial infection. To reduce the risk of TSS, a woman should wash her hands carefully with soap and water before inserting or removing the diaphragm, should not use the diaphragm during menstruation or when abnormal vaginal discharge is present, and should never leave the device in place for more than 24 hours.

Effectiveness   The diaphragm's effectiveness depends mainly on whether it is used properly. In actual practice, women rarely use it correctly every time they have intercourse and the typical failure rate is 12% during the first year of use. The main causes of failure are incorrect insertion, inconsistent use, and inaccurate fitting. If a diaphragm slips during intercourse, a woman should use emergency contraception.

Cervical Cap

The **cervical cap,** another barrier device, is a small flexible cup that fits snugly over the cervix and is held in place by suction. This cervical cap is a clear silicone cup with a brim around the dome to hold spermicide and trap sperm, and a removal strap over the dome. It comes in three sizes and must be fitted by a trained clinician. It is used like a diaphragm, with a small amount of spermicide placed in the cup and on the brim before insertion. The cervical cap is reusable but must be replaced annually.

Advantages   Advantages of the cervical cap are similar to those associated with diaphragm use. It is an alternative for women who cannot use a diaphragm because of anatomical reasons or recurrent urinary tract infections. The cap fits tightly, so it does not require backup condom use with repeated intercourse. It may be left in place for up to 48 hours.

Disadvantages   Along with most of the disadvantages associated with the diaphragm, difficulty with insertion and removal is more common for cervical cap users. Because there may be a slightly increased risk of TSS with prolonged use, the cap should not be left in place for more than 48 hours.

> **toxic shock syndrome (TSS)**   A bacterial **TERMS** disease usually associated with tampon use, and sometimes diaphragm use; symptoms include fever, rash, nausea, headache, dizziness, confusion, fainting, sore throat, cough, and abdominal pain.
>
> **cervical cap**   A small flexible cup that fits over the cervix; used with spermicide.

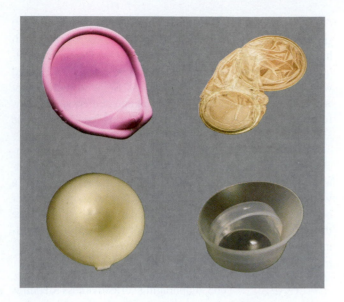

Many contraceptive methods work by blocking sperm from entering the cervix. While not as widely used as the hormonal methods, the barrier methods shown here—Caya diaphragm, cervical cap, female condom, and sponge—are important options for some couples.

© Phanie/Alamy; © McGraw-Hill Education/Christopher Kerrigan, photographer; © McGraw-Hill Education/Jill Braaten, photogapher

Effectiveness   Studies indicate that the average failure rate for the cervical cap is 16% for women who have never had a child and 32% for women who have had a child.

Contraceptive Sponge

The **contraceptive sponge** is a round, absorbent device about two inches in diameter with a polyester loop on one side (for removal) and a concave dimple on the other side, which helps it fit snugly over the cervix. The sponge is made of polyurethane and is presaturated with the same spermicide used in contraceptive creams and foams. The spermicide is activated when moistened with a small amount of water just before insertion. The sponge, which can be used only once, acts as a barrier and a spermicide and absorbs seminal fluid.

Advantages   The sponge offers advantages similar to those of the diaphragm and cervical cap. In addition, sponges can be obtained without a prescription or professional fitting, and they may be safely left in place for 24 hours without the addition of spermicide for repeated intercourse. Most women and men find the sponge to be comfortable and unobtrusive during sex.

Disadvantages   Reported disadvantages include difficulty with removal and an unpleasant odor if the sponge is left in place for more than 18 hours. Allergic reactions, such as irritation of the vagina, are more common with the sponge than with other spermicide products, probably because the overall dose of spermicide contained in each sponge is significantly higher than that used with other methods. (A sponge contains 1000 milligrams of spermicide compared with the 60–100 milligrams present in one application of other spermicidal products.) If irritation of the vaginal lining occurs, the risk of yeast infections and STIs (including HIV) may increase. The sponge is a single-use device and must be thrown away after each use. Additionally, the sponge cannot be used during menstruation.

Because the sponge has also been associated with toxic shock syndrome, the same precautions must be taken as those described for diaphragm use. A sponge user should be especially alert for symptoms of TSS when the sponge has been difficult to remove or was not removed intact.

Effectiveness   The typical effectiveness of the sponge is the same as that of the diaphragm (12% failure rate during the first year of use) for women who have never experienced childbirth. For women who have had a child, however, the failure rate rises to 24%.

Vaginal Spermicides

Spermicidal compounds developed for use with a diaphragm have been adapted for use without a diaphragm by combining them with a bulky base. Foams, creams, and jellies must be placed deep in the vagina near the cervical entrance and must be inserted no more than 60 minutes before intercourse. After an hour, their effectiveness is reduced drastically, and a new dose must be inserted. Another application is also required before each repeated act of coitus.

The spermicidal suppository is small and easily inserted like a tampon. The vaginal contraceptive film (VCF) is a paper-thin two-inch square of film that contains spermicide. It is folded over one or two fingers and placed high in the vagina, as close to the cervix as possible.

Advantages   The use of vaginal spermicides is relatively simple and can be limited to times of sexual activity. They are readily available in most drugstores and do not require a prescription or a pelvic examination. Spermicides allow complete and immediate reversibility, and the only medical side effects are occasional allergic reactions.

Disadvantages   When used alone, vaginal spermicides must be inserted shortly before intercourse, so their use may be seen as an annoying disruption. Some women find the slight increase in vaginal fluids after spermicide use unpleasant. Also, spermicides can alter the balance of bacteria in the vagina. Because this may increase the occurrence of yeast infections and urinary tract infections, women who are especially prone to these infections may want to avoid spermicides. Also, this contraception method does not protect

> **contraceptive sponge**   A contraceptive device about two inches in diameter that fits over the cervix and acts as a barrier and spermicide and absorbs seminal fluid.   **TERMS**

against STIs such as gonorrhea, chlamydia, or HIV. Overuse of spermicides can irritate vaginal tissues; if this occurs, the risk of HIV transmission may increase.

Effectiveness   Vaginal spermicides on their own are not very effective. The typical failure rate is about 28% during the first year of use. Spermicide is generally recommended only in combination with other barrier methods or as a backup to other contraceptives. Emergency contraceptives provide a better backup than spermicides, however.

Abstinence, Fertility Awareness, and Withdrawal

Millions of people worldwide do not use any of the contraceptive methods described earlier because of religious convictions, cultural prohibitions, poverty, or lack of information and supplies. If they use any method at all, they are likely to use one of the following relatively "natural" methods of attempting to prevent conception.

Abstinence   The decision not to engage in sexual intercourse for a chosen period of time, or **abstinence,** has been practiced throughout history for a variety of reasons. Until relatively recently, many people abstained because they had no other contraceptive measures. Concern about possible contraceptive side effects, STIs, and unwanted pregnancy may be factors. For others, the most important reason for choosing abstinence is a moral one, based on cultural or religious beliefs or strongly held personal values.

Fertility Awareness–Based Methods   Women who practice a **fertility awareness–based method** of contraception abstain from intercourse during the fertile phase of their menstrual cycle. Ordinarily only one egg is released by the ovaries each month, and it lives about 24 hours unless it is fertilized. Sperm deposited in the vagina may be capable of fertilizing an egg for up to six or seven days, so conception can theoretically occur only during six to eight days of any menstrual cycle. However, predicting which six to eight days is difficult. Recent studies show that even in women who have regular menstrual cycles, it is possible to become pregnant at any time during the menstrual cycle. It is even more difficult to predict the fertile time of the cycle in women who have irregular menses—a situation that is very common, especially in teenagers and women who are approaching menopause. Methods that attempt to predict the fertile times of a woman's cycle include calendar methods, temperature methods, and methods that rely on observation of the cyclical changes of the cervical mucus, as well as other characteristics of the cervix. Some women use a combination of methods to determine the time of ovulation.

Calendar methods are based on the idea that the average woman releases an egg 14–16 days before her period begins. To avoid pregnancy, she should abstain from intercourse for about eight days during her cycle, beginning several days before and during the time that ovulation is most likely to occur. However, in one recent study only about 10% of women with regular 28-day cycles actually ovulated 14 days before the next period. The situation is complicated further by the fact that many women have somewhat or very irregular cycles; calendar methods are extremely unreliable for these women.

Temperature methods are based on the knowledge that a woman's body temperature drops slightly just before ovulation and rises slightly after ovulation. A woman using the temperature method records her basal (resting) body temperature (BBT) every morning before getting out of bed and before eating or drinking anything. Once the temperature pattern is apparent (usually after about three months), the unsafe period for intercourse can be calculated as the interval from day 5 (day 1 is the first day of the period) until three days after the rise in BBT. To arrive at a shorter unsafe period, some women combine the calendar and temperature methods, calculating the first unsafe day from the shortest cycle of the calendar chart and the last unsafe day as the third day after a rise in BBT.

The *mucus method* (or Billings method) is based on changes in the cervical secretions throughout the menstrual cycle. During the estrogenic phase, cervical mucus increases and is clear and slippery. At the time of ovulation, some women can detect a slight change in the texture of the mucus and find that it is more likely to form an elastic thread when stretched between thumb and finger. After ovulation, these secretions become cloudy and sticky and decrease in quantity. Infertile, safe days are likely to occur during the relatively dry days just before and after menstruation. These additional clues have been found to be helpful by some couples who rely on fertility awareness–based methods. One problem that may interfere with this method is that vaginal infections, vaginal products, or medication can also alter the cervical mucus.

Any woman for whom pregnancy would be a serious problem should not rely on these methods alone because the failure rate is high—approximately 25% each year. Fertility awareness–based methods are not recommended for women who have very irregular cycles—about 15% of all menstruating women. Further, fertility awareness–based methods offer no protection against STIs. Some women use fertility awareness in combination with a barrier method to reduce their risk for unwanted pregnancy.

Withdrawal   In **withdrawal,** or *coitus interruptus,* the male removes his penis from the vagina just before he ejaculates. Withdrawal has a high failure rate because the male has to overcome a powerful biological urge. Further, because

---

> **TERMS**
>
> **abstinence**   Avoidance of sexual intercourse; a method of contraception.
>
> **fertility awareness–based method**   A method of preventing conception based on avoiding intercourse during the fertile phase of a woman's cycle.
>
> **withdrawal**   A method of contraception in which the man withdraws his penis from the vagina prior to ejaculation; also called *coitus interruptus.*

Table 6.2	Contraceptive Methods and STI Protection
METHOD	LEVEL OF PROTECTION
Hormonal methods	Do not protect against HIV or STIs in lower reproductive tract; may increase risk of cervical chlamydia; provide some protection against PID.
IUD	Does not protect against STIs.
Latex, polyisoprene, or polyurethane male condom	Best method for protection against STIs (if used correctly); does not protect against infections from lesions that are not covered by the condom. (Lambskin condoms do not protect against STIs.)
Female condom	Reduction of STI risk similar to that of male condom; may provide extra protection for external genitalia.
Diaphragm, sponge, or cervical cap	Provides some protection against cervical infections and PID. Diaphragms, sponges, and cervical caps should not be relied on for protection against HIV.
Spermicide	Modestly reduces the risk of some vaginal and cervical STIs; does not reduce the risk of HIV, chlamydia, or gonorrhea. If vaginal irritation occurs, infection risk may increase.
Fertility awareness–based methods	Do not protect against STIs.
Sterilization	Does not protect against STIs.
Abstinence	Complete protection against STIs (as long as all activities that involve the exchange of body fluids are avoided).

preejaculatory fluid may contain viable sperm, pregnancy can occur even if the man withdraws prior to ejaculation. Sexual pleasure is often affected because the man must remain in control and the sexual experience of both partners is interrupted. The failure rate for typical use is about 22% in the first year. Withdrawal does not protect against STIs.

Combining Methods

Couples can choose to combine the preceding methods in a variety of ways, both to add STI protection and to increase contraceptive effectiveness. For example, condoms are strongly recommended along with hormonal contraception whenever there is a risk of STIs (Table 6.2). For many couples, and especially for women, the added benefits far outweigh the extra effort and expense of using multiple methods.

EMERGENCY CONTRACEPTION

Emergency contraception (EC) refers to postcoital methods—those used after unprotected sexual intercourse. An emergency contraceptive may be appropriate if a regularly used method has failed (for example, if a condom breaks) or if unprotected sex has occurred. Sometimes called the "morning-after pill," emergency contraceptives are designed only for emergency use and should not be relied on as a regular birth control method; other methods of birth control are more effective.

When emergency contraceptives were first approved by the FDA, opponents feared that they might act as an **abortifacient**—preventing implantation of a fertilized egg, theoretically causing abortion. However, recent evidence indicates that emergency contraceptives do not interrupt an established pregnancy. Next-day or after-sex pills work primarily by inhibiting or delaying ovulation and by blocking the transport of sperm and eggs.

Plan B, Plan B One-Step, Next Choice One Dose, and Ella are now in common use and are more effective, with fewer side effects, than older methods of EC. Plan B One-Step, which replaced Plan B in 2009, contains a single progestin-only pill, whereas Next Choice One Dose has two pills that are taken 12 hours apart. The pills should be taken as soon as possible after inadequately protected sex. If taken within 24 hours after intercourse, emergency contraceptives may prevent as many as 75–95% of expected pregnancies. Overall they reduce pregnancy risk by about 89%. They are most effective if initiated in the first 12 hours, but they can be taken up to 120 hours (five days) after unprotected intercourse. Possible side effects include nausea, stomach pain, headache, dizziness, and breast tenderness. If a woman is already pregnant, these pills will not interfere with the pregnancy. Current emergency contraceptives are considered very safe.

Plan B One-Step is available over the counter (no prescription required) for everyone. Next Choice One Dose is available for persons 17 and older. To buy an emergency contraceptive, you need to ask for it at the pharmacy counter. It is recommended that you call ahead to make sure your pharmacy has EC on hand. The vast majority of pharmacies, especially the larger chains, currently carry emergency contraceptives.

Some clinicians advise women to keep a package of emergency contraceptives on hand in case their regular contraception method fails or they have unprotected intercourse. Research has found that ready access to emergency contraception improves the rate of use as well as decreasing the time to use. However, it does not lead to an increase in unprotected intercourse or STIs.

emergency contraception (EC) A birth control method used after unprotected sexual intercourse has occurred.

abortifacient An agent or substance that induces abortion.

TERMS

One reason women fail to take emergency contraceptives even when they have them may be that they underestimate their risk of pregnancy. Many women still believe that they can't get pregnant from a single act of intercourse. Expense is also an issue for some women. EC is covered by some health plans as well as by Medicaid in many states. However, many women must pay directly for EC, which costs about $50.

To find out more about emergency contraception and how to obtain it in your area, visit the Emergency Contraception website at http://ec.princeton.edu. Planned Parenthood is a good source of information, as are most pharmacies. Plan B One-Step has a website (http://www.planbonestep.com) that, as of this printing, contains a card you can print and hand to the pharmacist as an easy way to request EC. Next Choice One Dose, which is slightly less expensive than Plan B One-Step, also has a website (http://www.mynextchoice.com) where you can locate pharmacies in your area that carry the product. You can also call the Emergency Contraception Hotline (888-NOT-2-LATE) for more information about access.

Intrauterine devices can also be used for emergency contraception. If inserted within five days of unprotected intercourse, the Copper T ParaGard IUD (discussed earlier) is even more effective than pills for emergency contraception. It has the added benefit of providing up to 12 years of contraception.

PERMANENT CONTRACEPTION

Sterilization is permanent, and it is highly effective at preventing pregnancy. At present it is tied with the pill as the most commonly used contraceptive method in the United States and is by far the most common method used worldwide. It is especially popular among couples who have been married 10 or more years and have had all the children they intend to have. Sterilization does not protect against STIs.

An important consideration in choosing sterilization is that, in most cases, it cannot be reversed. Although the chances of restoring fertility are being increased by modern surgical techniques, such operations are costly, and pregnancy can never be guaranteed.

Many studies indicate that male sterilization is preferable to female sterilization for a variety of reasons. The overall cost of a female procedure is about four times that of a male procedure, the surgery itself is more complex, and women are much more likely than men to experience complications following the operation. Further, feelings of regret after sterilization seem to be more prevalent in women than in men. Before performing the procedure, most physicians require a thorough discussion with anyone considering sterilization.

Male Sterilization: Vasectomy

The procedure for male sterilization, **vasectomy,** involves severing the vasa deferentia, two tiny ducts that transport sperm from the testes to the seminal vesicles. After surgery, the testes continue to produce sperm, but the sperm are absorbed into the body. Because the testes contribute only about 10% of the total seminal fluid, the actual quantity of ejaculate is reduced only slightly. Hormone production from the testes continues with very little change, and secondary sex characteristics are not altered.

Vasectomy is ordinarily performed in a physician's office and takes about 30 minutes. A local anesthetic is injected into the skin of the scrotum. Small incisions are made at the upper end of the scrotum where it joins the body, and the vas deferens on each side is exposed, severed, and tied off or sealed by electrocautery. Some doctors seal each of the vasa with a plastic clamp, which is the size of a grain of rice. The incisions are then closed with sutures, and a small dressing is applied. Pain and swelling are usually slight and can be relieved with ice compresses and a scrotal support. Bleeding and infection occasionally develop but can be treated easily. After the procedure most men can return to work in two days.

Men can have sex after vasectomy as soon as they feel no discomfort, usually after about a week. Another method of contraception must be used for at least three months after vasectomy, however, because sperm produced before the operation may still be present in the semen.

Vasectomy is highly effective. In a small number of cases, a severed vas rejoins itself. The overall failure rate for vasectomy is 0.15%. About one-half of vasectomy reversals are successful, though this rate can vary significantly depending on the number of years since the initial surgery.

Female Sterilization

The most common method of female sterilization involves severing or blocking the oviducts, thereby preventing eggs from reaching the uterus, and sperm from entering the fallopian tubes. Ovulation and menstruation continue, but the unfertilized eggs are released into the abdominal cavity and absorbed. Hormone production by the ovaries and secondary sex characteristics are generally not affected.

TERMS

sterilization   Surgically altering the reproductive system to prevent pregnancy. Vasectomy is the procedure in males; tubal sterilization or hysterectomy is the procedure in females.

vasectomy   The surgical severing of the ducts that carry sperm to the ejaculatory duct.

Tubal sterilization (also called *tubal ligation*) is most commonly performed by a method called **laparoscopy**. A laparoscope, a camera containing a small light, is inserted through a small abdominal incision, and the surgeon looks through it to locate the fallopian tubes. Instruments are passed either through the laparoscope or through a second small incision, and the two fallopian tubes are sealed off with ties or staples or by electrocautery. General anesthesia is usually used. The operation takes about 30 minutes, and women can usually leave the hospital two to four hours after surgery. Tubal sterilization can also be performed shortly after a vaginal delivery through a small incision, or in the case of cesarean section during the same surgery.

Although tubal sterilization is riskier than vasectomy, with a rate of minor complications of about 6–11%, it is the more common procedure. Potential problems include bowel injury, wound infection, and bleeding. Serious complications are rare, and the death rate is low.

The failure rate for tubal sterilization is about 0.5%. When pregnancies occur, an increased percentage of them are ectopic (occurring outside the uterus). Ectopic pregnancy is dangerous and can even cause death, so any woman who suspects she might be pregnant after having tubal sterilization should seek medical help. Because successful reversal rates are low and the procedure is costly, female sterilization should be considered permanent.

A new form of incision-free female sterilization has also become available. This procedure can be performed with local anesthetic in a doctor's office and has a short recovery time. Called the Essure system, it consists of tiny springlike metallic implants that are inserted through the vagina and into the fallopian tubes, using a special catheter. Within three months, scar tissue forms over the implants, blocking the tubes.

Hysterectomy, removal of the uterus, is the preferred method of sterilization for only a small number of women, usually those with preexisting menstrual or other uterine problems.

WHICH CONTRACEPTIVE METHOD IS RIGHT FOR YOU?

The process of choosing and using a contraceptive method can be complex and varies from one couple to another (see the box "Barriers to Contraceptive Use"). Each person must consider many variables in deciding which method is most acceptable and appropriate for her or him. Key considerations include those listed here.

> **tubal sterilization**   Severing or blocking the oviducts to prevent eggs from reaching the uterus; also called *tubal ligation*.
>
> **laparoscopy**   Examining the internal organs by inserting a small camera through an abdominal incision.
>
> **hysterectomy**   Total or partial surgical removal of the uterus.
>
> **TERMS**

1. *The implications of an unplanned pregnancy and the efficacy of the method.* Many teens and young adults fail to consider how their lives would be affected by an unexpected pregnancy. People who choose to be sexually active but would be negatively affected by an unplanned pregnancy need to use an effective means of birth control and use it consistently.

2. *Health risks.* When considering any contraceptive method, determine whether it may pose a risk to your health. However, most women are candidates for most, if not all, methods of contraception. Remember that pregnancy carries significant health risks that are generally much greater than the risks of any method of contraception.

3. *STI risk.* STIs are another potential consequence of sex. In fact, several activities besides vaginal intercourse (such as oral and anal sex) can put you at risk for an STI. Condom use is of critical importance whenever any risk of STIs is present, even if you are using another contraceptive method to prevent pregnancy. This is especially true whenever you are not in an exclusive, long-term relationship.

4. *Convenience and comfort level.* The most convenient methods are the LARC methods (IUDs and implants) that do not require any work on the part of the user. Most women using hormonal methods also rank them high in convenience. If forgetting to take pills is a problem for you, a vaginal ring, contraceptive patch, implant, or injectable method may be a good alternative to the pill. For those who choose a barrier method, condoms are the most common. Some people think condom use disrupts spontaneity, but creative approaches to condom use can decrease these concerns. The diaphragm, cervical cap, contraceptive sponge, female condom, and spermicides can be inserted before intercourse begins, unlike condoms, which must be put on the erect penis.

5. *Type of relationship.* Barrier methods require more motivation and sense of responsibility from *each* partner than hormonal methods do. When the method depends on the cooperation of one's partner, assertiveness is necessary, no matter how difficult. This is especially true in new relationships, when condom use is most important.

6. *Ease and cost of obtaining and maintaining each method.* Investigate the costs of different methods. Under the Affordable Care Act, insurers (except for religious organizations) are required to cover the cost of contraception. On June 30, 2014, the Supreme Court ruled that closely held corporations with religious objections also may opt out of the contraception coverage. Remember that your student health clinic probably provides family planning services, and most communities have low-cost family planning clinics, such as Planned Parenthood.

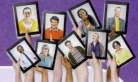

Even in ideal circumstances, raising children is challenging as well as exciting. The ideal situation is that a woman becomes pregnant only when she is ready to start a family. Why, then, when the stakes are so high, do so many unintended pregnancies occur? Well into the late 1960s birth control was barely adequate. But now, people have so many choices for effective contraception. Why doesn't everyone who wishes to prevent pregnancy use contraception consistently? Here are some of the reasons.

Long-acting reversible contraception (LARC) methods, such as implants and IUDs, are very effective, but some doctors have discouraged younger women from using them. Some reports indicate reasons that date back to 1980, when the most frequently used IUD, the Dalkon Shield, was recalled after it was linked to infertility and even death. Studies on current IUDs, however, have shown that they do not increase risk of death or infertility, and in fact, data suggest that Mirena (discussed earlier in the section on LARC) protects against STIs.

Economic and ethnic background as well as age are all factors that influence our behavior, and these factors often become difficult to disentangle. The cost for the medical exam, the IUD, the insertion of the IUD, and follow-up visits to a health care provider can range up to $1,000, depending on health insurance. This cost may deter some candidates. Studies show that ethnic and racial differences are significant in women under age 25 or who are unmarried: among sexually active single women aged 20–24, 4% of whites used no method of contraception, compared with 18% of blacks and 15% of Hispanics. In turn, the number of unintended pregnancies for black and Hispanic women is more than double that for white women, and the number of teen pregnancies is also much higher. In general, both LARC methods and sterilization are much more common among

older women, particularly those who are over 35 years of age or who have had children.

Cofounder of the Women of Color Sexual Health Network, Bianca Laureano, writes about other barriers young women may face when choosing a method of contraception. For example, they may be monitored by parents or guardians who do not believe in birth control. Laureano herself grew up in a Puerto Rican family who advised her that birth control kills Puerto Rican women.

Young women who are being closely monitored by anti-birth-control families must continue having a menstrual cycle, so they cannot use Depo-Provera, which, in some cases, causes menstrual bleeding to stop; they cannot wear a visible patch; and they cannot use a method that requires visits to a physician, especially if a parent or guardian attends their physical exams. In addition, some young people do not want a contraceptive method that requires them to remember to take a pill each day (oral birth control pills) or to touch their genitals (for example, the NuvaRing).

Although some health providers discourage LARC methods, many health advocates promote them among women seeking to avoid pregnancy. However, some observers are concerned that campaigns targeting "at-risk" women focus too much on minority, poor, and young women. In her book *Exposing Prejudice: Puerto Rican Experiences of Language, Race, and Class*, Bonnie Urciuoli gives a history of U.S. policies toward Puerto Rican immigrants, which included controlling their population through sterilization, enforced contraception, and migration. In *Killing the Black Body*, Dorothy Roberts describes the experiences of black women throughout U.S. history—from being forced to bear children during slavery to having their fertility controlled by modern-day welfare policies. Thus, one reason women of color may not use

LARC methods can be medical mistrust; another, as noted, may be having less access to these methods.

In general, contraception use has increased and teen pregnancies have decreased in recent decades. A study covering the years 2006 to 2010 found that about 89% of sexually active, single white teens aged 15–19 had used a form of contraception in the past three months. Among single, sexually active black teens of the same age, 81% had used contraception, as had 80% of Hispanic teens. Although the latter two groups are less likely to use the most effective forms of contraception, there is a movement toward LARC usage. A study comparing 2009 and 2012 found that women from all populations increasingly chose LARC methods but particularly Hispanic women, those with private insurance, those with fewer than two sexual partners in the previous year, and those who were *nulliparous* (had never given birth). Overall, then, a complex mix of factors relating to age, financial status, culture, history, and policy can create barriers to effective contraception.

SOURCES: England, P., et al. 2016. Why do young, unmarried women who do not want to get pregnant contracept inconsistently? Mixed-method evidence for the role of efficacy. *Socius: Sociological Research for a Dynamic World* 2. doi: 10.1177/2378023116629464; Kavanaugh, M. L., J. Jerman, and L. B. Finer. 2015. Changes in use of long-acting reversible contraceptive methods among U.S. women, 2009–2012. *Obstetrics & Gynecology* 126 (5): 917–927; Laureano, B. 2010. How accessible are IUDs? *Rewire*, April 19 (https://rewire.news /article/2010/04/19/accessible-iuds-0/); Melnick, M. 2010. The IUD makes a comeback. *Newsweek*, April 5 (http://www.newsweek.com /iud-makes-comeback-70545); Roberts, D. 1997. *Killing the Black Body: Race, Reproduction, and the Meaning of Liberty.* New York: Pantheon; Sweeney, M. M., and R. Kelly Raley. 2014. Race, ethnicity, and the changing context of childbearing in the United States. *Annual Review of Sociology* 40: 539–558; and Urciuoli, B. 1996. *Exposing Prejudice: Puerto Rican Experiences of Language, Race, and Class.* Boulder, CO: Westview.

7. *Religious or philosophical beliefs.* For some people, abstinence and/or fertility awareness–based methods may be the only permissible contraceptive methods.

8. *Potential noncontraceptive benefits.* Women with dysmenorrhea, irregular periods, acne, endometriosis, severe premenstrual syndrome (PMS), and other medical problems may benefit from using a particular method of contraception. Be sure to discuss these issues with your health care provider so that you can take advantage of the noncontraceptive benefits associated with many methods of birth control.

Whatever your needs, circumstances, or beliefs, *do* make a choice about contraception. Not choosing anything is the one method known *not* to work. Contraception is an area in which taking charge of your health has immediate and profound implications for your future.

ABORTION IN THE UNITED STATES SINCE THE 19TH CENTURY

While the methods have changed over time, the practice of abortion goes back thousands of years. Until the 19th century, abortion was largely a private affair in the United States: Women who conceived at times in their lives when having a child was unacceptable either ended the pregnancy themselves or sought help from others. Women turned to their midwives or purchased herbs or drugs from an apothecary or through the mail. Abortion services were also advertised in the newspapers, provided by individuals of varying medical competence. Without regulation or standards, in some circumstances having an abortion was dangerous and ineffective, resulting in physical harm to the woman or continuation of an undesired pregnancy.

The first anti-abortion campaign was launched in the mid-19th century; the result was that most abortion care provided at that time became criminalized. Physicians were at the forefront of this movement. They intended to raise the standard of abortion care, mandating that abortions should be provided only by physicians in a hospital setting for medical indications. For instance, a woman with a large family lacking the means to have another child did not qualify for an abortion unless it could be demonstrated that another pregnancy was life-threatening. Although improved safety was a goal, the techniques used by physicians in hospitals to terminate pregnancies were not necessarily safer than techniques used by nonphysicians in the community.

The new policies criminalizing much of abortion care greatly limited the supply of abortion services, but the demand did not change. During this time, there were few options to prevent pregnancy; methods of contraception were much less effective than the methods we have today, and women continued to have unintended pregnancies. Many women did not have an obvious medical indication to justify an abortion or could not pay for an abortion in the hospital. Consequently, thousands of women who sought to end their pregnancies had no choice but to seek illegal abortions.

In desperation, many found themselves using the services of unskilled individuals in unsanitary conditions, and suffered injury, subsequent infertility, or death.

By the mid-20th century, the medical profession started to recognize the harms of criminalizing abortion. Also during this time, women's status improved as they entered the labor force and demanded a say over reproductive decisions and access to safe abortion. Abortion was legalized in the United States in 1973 with the landmark Supreme Court decision in *Roe v. Wade,* determining that abortion is a fundamental right under the due process clause of the 14th Amendment.

Subsequently, legalization allowed significant improvements in abortion safety and technique. From a public health perspective, legalization of abortion ranks with the discovery of antibiotics in decreasing the overall death rate. New technologies expanded the provision of abortion in clinics rather than in hospitals exclusively, lowering cost and improving access for women nationwide. As a result, the abortion care we have today looks very different from pre-*Roe v. Wade*: The majority of women who obtain abortions do so in clinics specialized in abortion care. Abortions are rarely performed in the hospital as they once were, and it has become an extremely safe and effective process.

In terms of safety, the evolution of abortion care in the United States is overall a great success and has influenced abortion care worldwide; however, it is not without challenges. Using the legal system to restrict abortion has become an important strategy in state and national politics by groups opposed to abortion and has shifted the conversation away from the area of health and status of women in society. Over the past 40 years, some federal and many state laws have tested the limits of *Roe v. Wade* by making it more difficult for a woman to obtain an abortion, even if her decision to have one is not violated.

UNDERSTANDING ABORTION

The word **abortion** generally refers to a pregnancy ending. A **spontaneous abortion,** also called a miscarriage, is a pregnancy that ends on its own; it may be an emotionally trying event for some women and their families, and often experienced as a loss.

About 15% of pregnant women experience spontaneous abortions, which occur most frequently during the first trimester. Generally, chromosomal abnormalities lead to an abnormal pregnancy that is incompatible with life and that the body ultimately detects and ends. **Induced abortion,**

> **abortion** A pregnancy ending.
>
> **TERMS**
>
> **spontaneous abortion** Also known as *miscarriage* or *pregnancy loss;* a pregnancy that ends on its own.
>
> **induced abortion** An ongoing pregnancy that is ended deliberately; synonymous with pregnancy termination.

or pregnancy termination, is a pregnancy that is intentionally ended. The rest of this chapter focuses on induced abortion.

Abortion Statistics

The decision to have an abortion may be complex or emotional, and is usually in reaction to an unintended pregnancy. This is the reason for more than 95% of abortions. An **unintended pregnancy** includes pregnancies that are (1) *mistimed,* meaning that a woman or couple wanted to become pregnant but at a later date or (2) *unwanted,* meaning that a woman or couple had not wanted to become pregnant at that time at all. Mistimed pregnancies account for 65–75% of unintended pregnancies, a much larger percentage than unwanted pregnancies. More than half of women with unintended pregnancies continue their pregnancies and give birth. The remainder of women with unintended pregnancies have either an induced abortion or a miscarriage in relatively equal proportions.

About 1 million abortions are performed in the United States each year, making abortion the most common procedure that women of reproductive age undergo. In fact, one in four women has an abortion by age 30, making it very likely that each of us knows someone who has had one.

Researchers estimate that about 800,000 illegal abortions were performed annually in the years before *Roe v. Wade.* The number of legal abortions rose after 1973, reaching a peak in the early 1980s and then declining fairly steadily; the rate in 2011 was the lowest since 1973 (Figure 6.7). Stricter laws that limit access to abortion do not appear to be responsible for the drop, as the decrease has occurred across the nation and not just in states with the most significant restrictions. Pregnancy and birth rates have also declined, most likely due to increased access to and use of contraception to prevent unintended pregnancy. The timing of abortions has shifted to earlier in pregnancy, with over 90% taking place within the first 13 weeks (Figure 6.8).

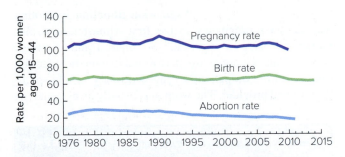

FIGURE 6.7 **Pregnancy (1976–2010), birth (1976–2014), and abortion rates (1976–2011).**

SOURCES: Curtin S. C., J. C. Abma, and K. Kost. 2015. 2010 Pregnancy rates among U.S. women (http://www.cdc.gov/nchs/data/hestat/pregnancy/2010 _pregnancy_rates.htm); Martin, J. A., et al. 2015. Births: Final data for 2013. *National Vital Statistics Reports* 64(1). Hyattsville, MD: National Center for Health Statistics; Jones, R. K., and J. Jerman. 2014. Abortion incidence and service availability in the United States, 2011. *Perspectives on Sexual and Reproductive Health*, 46(1): 3–14.

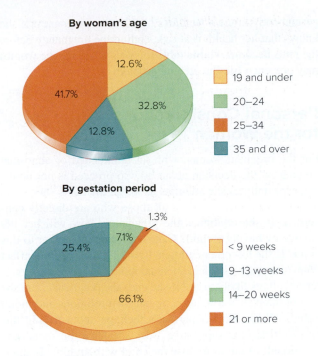

FIGURE 6.8 **Distribution of abortions by age and weeks of gestation: 2012.**

SOURCE: Centers for Disease Control and Prevention. 2015. Abortion surveillance—United States, 2012. *MMWR Surveillance Summaries* 64(SS10): 1-40.

Personal and Social Indicators Several personal and social indicators are commonly given as reasons for terminating a pregnancy. These reasons include lack of financial resources; interference with the woman's work, educational aspirations, or ability to care for dependents; reluctance to become a single mother; or problems in a relationship. Younger women who become pregnant often report that they are unprepared for the transition to motherhood, whereas older women regularly cite that a pregnancy would interfere with their responsibility to dependents.

Women who have abortions represent various ages, religions, races, and levels of education. Poverty has been identified as a key factor leading to an abortion. In 2008, 42% of women undergoing an abortion were poor by federal standards.

Fetal and Maternal Indicators Women or couples with a planned pregnancy may ultimately decide to end it if they learn that the fetus has a significant abnormality. Due to risks to their own health, pregnant women with serious medical conditions sometimes need to end their pregnancies. These conditions might include severe high blood pressure, a lung disease called pulmonary hypertension, severe kidney disease, advanced diabetes, and severe cardiac disease. Some conditions that already exist can worsen in pregnancy and

unintended pregnancy A mistimed (wrongly timed) or unwanted (not desired at all) pregnancy.

TERMS

permanently injure a woman's health after pregnancy. If she knows that her health is at risk, ending the pregnancy before the fetus becomes **viable** (able to survive outside the womb) may prevent a life-threatening problem.

Personal Considerations for the Woman

For the pregnant woman with an unintended or abnormal pregnancy, the decision about how to proceed is not political, especially as she attempts to weigh the many short- and long-term ramifications for all those who are directly concerned. If she continues the pregnancy, how will her life change by having a child? Can she become a mother to this child? If she has other children, how will another child affect them? How does she feel about adoption? What are her long-term feelings likely to be? If she ends the pregnancy, can she accept the decision in terms of her own religious and moral beliefs? What are her partner's feelings about having this child? If he is unsupportive, does she have the social and emotional resources to raise the child without him? If she is young, what will be the effects on her own growth? Will she be able to continue with her educational and personal goals? What about the ongoing financial responsibilities?

Personal Considerations for the Man

Men are often involved in the decision-making process with their partners, and they may experience a range of emotions similar to those felt by women. Men may also accompany their partners during the abortion process. Accompaniment may reflect an effort to share responsibility for the pregnancy as well as to provide emotional and practical support by providing transportation or helping to pay for the abortion. Supporting each other through the abortion process may strengthen their relationship. In some instances, men disagree with the woman's decision, and they may try to control the outcome of the pregnancy or may be abusive to their partners. Many abortion facilities are sensitive to creating a safe space for women in such situations.

METHODS OF ABORTION

The way a pregnancy is ended depends on how far along a woman is in her pregnancy. Ultrasound (a device that shows an image of the developing fetus) is the most accurate way to determine this. If an ultrasound is not available, the date of the woman's last period provides an estimate.

First-Trimester Abortion

As noted earlier, 90% of abortions in the United States take place in the first trimester. Women who are up to 2.5 months pregnant can choose between taking pills or having a procedure to end the pregnancy. Women who are 2.5–3.5 months pregnant undergo a procedure.

Medical Abortion **Medical abortion** entails taking two medications, mifepristone and misoprostol. Medical abortion is not the same as emergency contraception, also known as the "morning-after pill." Emergency contraception is designed to *prevent* pregnancy, whereas medical abortion *ends* an already existing pregnancy.

Women who have a medical abortion take mifepristone in a doctor's office and then go home. They take the second medication, misoprostol, on their own. This second medication causes period-like cramps and causes the pregnancy tissue to pass usually within 4 hours but up to 48 hours. The amount of bleeding is similar to that of a heavy period or miscarriage. Women return to see their provider 1–2 weeks later and have an ultrasound or a serum pregnancy test to confirm they are no longer pregnant. Medical abortion successfully ends pregnancies 95–97% of the time. If the woman continues to be pregnant, she may repeat the medications or undergo an aspiration procedure.

Aspiration Abortion **Aspiration abortion** is another way to end a pregnancy in the first trimester. It is also known as "suction abortion," or dilation and curettage (D&C). This is a procedure performed in a medical facility (usually in the outpatient setting and rarely in a hospital) by a trained provider. The woman is usually awake, and the

Ask Yourself

QUESTIONS FOR CRITICAL THINKING AND REFLECTION

Suppose one of your friends has an unplanned pregnancy and does not know what to do. How would you begin discussing how she feels and what options are available to her? What kind of support would you be willing to offer?

procedure is done through the vagina exclusively (no cut on the abdomen). The provider dilates the cervix (opening to the uterus) and inserts a slender tube (called a cannula or suction curette) into the uterus, which is attached to a vacuum device, and removes the pregnancy. The procedure may cause strong cramps and usually takes fewer than 10 minutes. Women undergoing the procedure receive a powerful oral or intravenous pain medication in addition to a numbing medication administered vaginally. The cramping subsides once the procedure is over. Women return home the same day—typically within 30 minutes to an hour after the pain medication has worn off.

Aspiration abortions are successful 98% of the time. Many women receive contraception such as an intrauterine device right after the abortion is completed, saving them an extra visit and protecting them from future pregnancy.

Medical vs. Aspiration Abortion in the First Trimester

Some women may have the option of selecting either medical or aspiration abortion to end a first-trimester pregnancy. A number of women feel that medical abortion allows them to take more control of the process and gives them more privacy than an aspiration abortion. Additionally, some women feel it is a more "natural" process because it mimics a miscarriage. It is also a noninvasive alternative to aspiration abortion because no instruments are introduced into the uterus. Most women who select a medical abortion are satisfied with this method.

A downside of medical abortion is that it takes longer to complete, typically at least 24 hours from the time the first pill is taken to the time the pregnancy passes, whereas an aspiration abortion takes about 10 minutes for the entire procedure. Side effects of one of the medications, misoprostol, include nausea, vomiting, diarrhea, fever, and abdominal pain for some women. Women undergoing a medical abortion are typically given additional medications to help with these symptoms. Medical abortion also generally requires more clinic visits, and there is a small risk of failure, which would then require another round of medications or an aspiration procedure. Vaginal bleeding is often more prolonged and in a few cases heavier than with aspiration abortion. The financial cost to the patient is generally about the same.

Second-Trimester Abortion

About 10% of abortions take place in the second trimester (greater than three months of pregnancy). Women who have an abortion at this stage in pregnancy may do so for a variety of reasons: They recognized they were pregnant later in the pregnancy; they had a difficult time finding a facility to have an abortion; they felt conflicted about ending the pregnancy and needed more time to decide; they discovered that the fetus had problems; or they became sick themselves, making it difficult or dangerous to continue the pregnancy. The approach to ending a second-trimester pregnancy depends on where the woman goes for care and how far along she is.

Some medical facilities offer termination of pregnancy by inducing labor with medications, a process called **induction abortion.** Other facilities offer surgery called **dilation and evacuation (D&E),** the most common method of second-trimester pregnancy termination in the United States. While similar to a first-trimester abortion, a D&E may take longer, and women typically receive stronger pain medications. Dilation and evacuation is typically done as outpatient surgery, but a woman may need to visit the health care provider or clinic the day before to take medications or begin the process of dilating the cervix. Under general or regional anesthesia, the fetus is surgically removed through the vagina, and suction is used to remove any remaining tissue; women can usually go home the same day. Soreness and cramping may occur for a day or two after the procedure, and some bleeding may last for 1–2 weeks. Second-trimester pregnancy termination is also very safe.

POSTABORTION CARE

Abortion is a safe procedure, usually performed at an outpatient clinic or doctor's office rather than a hospital, and women go home shortly after the visit. Abortion does not cause infertility, jeopardize a woman's ability to have children in the future, compromise her reproductive organs, or increase her chances of cancer in any way. Recovery is rapid, usually lasting just a few days.

Possible Physical Effects

The incidence of immediate problems following an abortion (infection, bleeding, trauma to the cervix or uterus, and incomplete abortion requiring repeat curettage) is rare. The potential for problems is reduced significantly by a woman's good health, early timing of the abortion, use of the suction method compared to an older technique using sharp curettage, performance by a well-trained clinician, and the availability and use of prompt follow-up care.

induction abortion A method to end a second-trimester pregnancy by administering medications to induce labor and delivery of a fetus. **TERMS**

dilation and evacuation (D&E) A vaginal procedure to end a second-trimester pregnancy that involves surgical removal of the pregnancy from the uterus.

Problems related to infection can be minimized through preabortion testing and treatment for gonorrhea, chlamydia, and other infections. Also, women are given antibiotics at the time of the procedure to decrease the likelihood of infection.

Possible Emotional Effects

Many women feel relief, guilt, regret, loss, or anger after an abortion. Some go through a period of sadness while making the decision to proceed with an abortion or shortly after it is performed. When a woman feels she was pressured into sexual intercourse or into the abortion, she may feel resentment. If she strongly believed abortion to be immoral, she may wonder if she is still a good person. Many of these feelings are strongest immediately after the abortion. Such feelings often pass rapidly. Others take time to resolve and fade only slowly. It is important for a woman to realize that a mixture of feelings is natural.

Researchers have found that women with resilient personalities (high self-esteem, perceived control over the situation, optimism) tend to view the unintended pregnancy in a more positive light and to adjust better than women with less resilient personalities (see Chapter 2 for more on resilience). Between 2008 and 2010, the Turnaway Study recruited women seeking abortions across the United States, some of whom succeeded in undergoing the procedure and others who were "turned away" because their pregnancies were too far along. Researchers found that a person's feelings toward an unintended pregnancy and feelings toward having an abortion are mixed—many women felt regret about an unwanted pregnancy and felt that the decision to have an abortion was the right decision for them.

Rates of mental health problems do not appear higher in those who had an abortion compared to those who gave birth or vice versa, suggesting that women are resilient despite their difficult circumstances. The most profound measurable effect observed in the group of women denied an abortion is that they were three times more likely to end up below the federal poverty line two years later compared to women who had abortions, though before the unintended pregnancy they had similar socioeconomic status. As many women predict when making a decision to have an abortion, having a child strains their resources to a significant degree.

LEGAL RESTRICTIONS ON ABORTION

In 1973 in the landmark case of *Roe v. Wade,* the U.S. Supreme Court made abortion legal in every state in the United States. To replace the restrictions most states still imposed at that time, the justices devised new standards to govern abortion decisions. They divided pregnancy into three parts, or *trimesters,* giving a woman less choice about abortion as her pregnancy advances toward full term. According to *Roe v. Wade,* in the first trimester, the abortion decision must be left to the judgment of the pregnant woman and her physician. During the second trimester, similar rights remain up to the point when the fetus becomes viable. Today most clinicians define this point as 24 weeks of gestation. When the fetus is considered viable, a state may regulate and even bar all abortions except those considered necessary to preserve the mother's life or health.

Three years after *Roe v. Wade,* Congress passed the Hyde Amendment, which prevents the use of federal funds (such as Medicaid) to pay for an abortion unless the pregnancy arises from incest or rape or if the woman's life is endangered. In practice, this amendment affects poor women (those who rely on Medicaid to pay for medical services). These women must pay out of pocket for abortion-related care, and if they are unable to pay or they take too long to raise funds, they may be compelled to continue their pregnancies. The Affordable Care Act (2010) explicitly permits states to dictate the circumstances under which abortions may be performed or insured. Currently 17 states provide nonfederal public money to assist some poor women seeking medically necessary abortions. Concerns have been raised that a two-tiered system has been created—one for women with means to pay for an abortion and another for those without.

Since 1973 many campaigns have been waged to overturn the *Roe v. Wade* decision, whereas other campaigns have tried to strengthen the rights provided by the decision. Although abortion remains legal throughout the United States, subsequent rulings by the Supreme Court, starting with *Planned Parenthood of Southeastern Pennsylvania v. Casey* (1992), have allowed states to regulate abortion throughout pregnancy as long as no "undue burden" is imposed on women seeking these services. The following are examples of restrictive laws that exist on the state level:

- *Physician and hospital requirements.* Thirty-eight states require an abortion to be performed by a licensed physician. Nineteen states require an abortion to be performed in a hospital after a specified point in the pregnancy, and 18 states require the involvement of a second physician after a specified point.

- *State-mandated counseling.* Seventeen states mandate that, before an abortion, women must be given counseling that includes information on at least one of the following: the purported link between abortion and breast cancer (5 states), the ability of a fetus to feel pain (12 states), or long-term mental health consequences for the woman (7 states).

- *Waiting periods.* Twenty-eight states require a woman seeking an abortion to wait a specified period of time, usually 24 hours, between the time she receives counseling and when the procedure is performed. Fourteen of these states have laws that effectively require the woman to make two separate trips to the clinic to obtain the procedure.

- *Parental involvement.* Thirty-eight states require some type of parental involvement in a minor's decision to have an abortion. Twenty-five states require one or both parents to consent to the procedure, whereas 13 require that one or both parents be notified and 5 states require both parental consent and notification.

THE PUBLIC DEBATE ABOUT ABORTION

Abortion is one of the most polarized and politicized issues of our times and has been since the 1960s. The American public has been willing to self-identify as "pro-life" or "pro-choice," though most hold middle-ground views and do not fall neatly into one of these two categories. A percentage of this middle-ground group instinctively feels that the fetus gains increasing human value as a pregnancy advances. In this view, first-trimester abortion is acceptable but later-term abortion should be performed only when the mother's health is in jeopardy.

Pro-life groups oppose abortion on the basis of their belief that life begins at conception. They believe that the fertilized egg must be afforded the same rights as a human being. This view holds that any woman who has sexual intercourse knows that pregnancy is a possibility; therefore, should she willingly have intercourse and get pregnant, she is morally obligated to carry the pregnancy through. For women who feel they are unable to raise a child, pro-life groups encourage adoption.

Pro-choice groups support the view that the decision to continue or end a pregnancy is a personal matter and that a woman should not be compelled to carry a pregnancy to term if she does not want to have a child. This view holds that distinctions

> **QUICK STATS**
>
> **More than one in three American women has an abortion before she turns 45.**
> —Guttmacher Institute, 2011

must be made between the stages of fetal development, that the fetus is part of the pregnant woman, and that she has priority over it. Members of this group argue that pregnancy can result from contraceptive failure or other factors out of a couple's control. (All contraceptive methods except abstinence have the potential for failure.) When pregnancy occurs, pro-choice supporters believe that the most moral decision possible must be determined according to each situation and that, in some cases, greater injustice could result if abortion were not an option.

Opinions about abortion have remained generally consistent over time. Although nearly half of Americans feel that abortion is morally wrong, an overwhelming majority supports legal availability of abortion services in some circumstances (see Figure 6.9). Most Americans oppose governmental regulation of women's reproductive decisions and also feel that paying for an abortion should be an individual's responsibility. Most do not support the use of public funds to help poor women obtain abortions; they also do not support inclusion of abortion benefits in a national basic health care plan.

Although the most vocal groups in the abortion debate tend to paint a black-or-white picture, most Americans view abortion as a complex issue and prefer to focus on preventive strategies. If the most common reason for abortion is unintended pregnancy, then more effort should be dedicated to sex education and promotion of consistent and effective contraception use. Also, more effort should be dedicated to creating a society with policies that make it easier to raise a child. Examples of such policies include parental leave, child care programs for working parents, and reduced costs for education and health care.

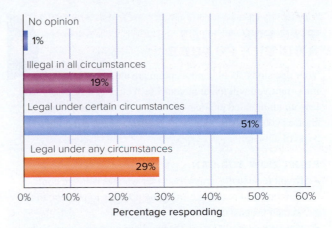

FIGURE 6.9 **Public opinion about abortion.**

SOURCE: Gallup Inc. 2016. *Public Opinion about Abortion* (http://www.gallup.com/poll/1576/abortion.aspx). Copyright 2016 Gallup Inc. All rights reserved. The content is used with permission; however, Gallup retains all rights to publication.

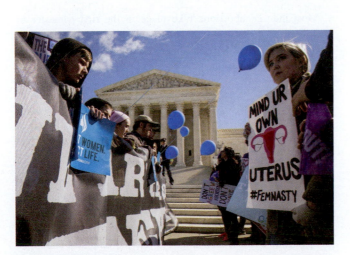

Pro-choice groups believe the decision to end or continue a pregnancy is a personal matter. Pro-life groups oppose abortion based on a belief that life begins at conception.

© Drew Angerer/Getty Images

TIPS FOR TODAY AND THE FUTURE

Your decisions about contraception are among the most important you will make in your life. You may never have to face an unintended pregnancy, but you should know what choices you would have as well as where you stand on the issue of abortion.

RIGHT NOW YOU CAN:

- If you're sexually active, consider whether you are confident that you're doing everything possible to prevent an unwanted pregnancy.
- If you're sexually active, discuss your contraceptive method with your partner. Make sure you are using the method that works best for you.
- Consider keeping an emergency contraceptive on hand in case of a slip-up.
- Consider your views on the morality of abortion, and whether it is acceptable under certain circumstances.

IN THE FUTURE YOU CAN:

- Talk to your physician about contraception and get his or her advice on choosing the best method.
- Occasionally discuss your contraceptive method with your partner to make sure it continues to meet your needs. A change in health status or lifestyle may make a different form of contraception preferable in the future.
- If you are sexually active or plan to become sexually active, talk to your partner about the possibility of pregnancy. How would you proceed? Do you share similar views and feelings, or do they differ? How would you resolve conflicts about this issue?

SUMMARY

- Barrier methods of contraception physically prevent sperm from reaching the egg; hormonal methods are designed to prevent ovulation, fertilization, and/or implantation; and surgical methods permanently block the movement of sperm or eggs to the site of conception.

- The choice of contraceptive method depends on effectiveness, convenience, cost, reversibility, side effects, risk factors, protection against STIs, and noncontraceptive benefits. Measures of effectiveness include failure rate and continuation rate.

- Hormonal methods may include a combination of estrogen and progestins, or progestins alone. Hormones may be delivered via pills, patch, vaginal ring, IUD, implants, or injections.

- Hormonal methods prevent ovulation, inhibit the movement of sperm, and affect the uterine lining so that implantation is prevented.

- IUDs can provide very effective long-term (3–12 years) contraception and are especially useful for women who want contraception for at least six months.

- Male condoms are simple to use, are immediately reversible, and provide STI protection; female condoms can be inserted hours before intercourse.

- The diaphragm, cervical cap, and contraceptive sponge cover the cervix and block sperm from entering; all need to be used with or contain spermicide.

- Vaginal spermicides come in the form of foams, creams, jellies, suppositories, and film.

- So-called natural methods include abstinence, withdrawal, and fertility awareness–based methods.

- Combining methods can increase contraceptive effectiveness and help protect against STIs. The most common combination is a hormonal method, such as the birth control pill, combined with condoms.

- The most commonly used emergency contraceptive, Plan B One-Step, is available without a prescription.

- Vasectomy—male sterilization—involves severing the vas deferens. Female sterilization involves severing or blocking the oviducts so that the egg cannot reach the uterus.

- Issues to be considered in choosing a contraceptive include the individual health risks of each method, the implications of an unplanned pregnancy, STI risk, convenience and comfort level, type of relationship, the cost and ease of obtaining and maintaining each method, and religious or philosophical beliefs.

- From the first anti-abortion campaigns of the mid-19th century, through the landmark *Roe v. Wade* Supreme Court decision of 1973, which legalized abortion in the United States, through the heated debate that continues today, abortion is a health issue that has also become politicized.

- In medical terms there are two distinct types of abortion: *spontaneous abortion* and *induced abortion*. A spontaneous abortion is a pregnancy that ends on its own and is referred to as *miscarriage* or *pregnancy loss*. Induced abortion is an ongoing pregnancy that is ended deliberately.

- Most induced abortions take place in the first trimester of pregnancy. Methods include taking medications or undergoing an aspiration procedure. Second-trimester abortions are less common than first-trimester abortions.

- Women's and men's emotional responses after an abortion include relief, happiness, regret, guilt, sadness, or anger; the strongest feelings usually occur immediately after the abortion. Research suggests that over 95% of women who have an abortion believe that it was the right decision for them.

- The controversy between pro-life and pro-choice viewpoints focuses on the issue of when life begins. Pro-life groups believe that a fertilized egg is a human life from the moment of conception and that a woman is obligated to carry a pregnancy to term. Pro-choice groups distinguish between stages of fetal development and argue that the fetus does not have an equal status to the pregnant woman and that the woman should make the final decision regarding her pregnancy. Most Americans are not completely pro-life or pro-choice but fall somewhere on the spectrum.

- Overall, public opinion in the United States supports legal abortion in at least some circumstances and opposes overturning *Roe v. Wade*.

FOR MORE INFORMATION

Association of Reproductive Health Professionals. Offers educational materials about family planning, contraception, and other reproductive health issues; the website includes an interactive questionnaire to help people choose contraceptive methods.

http://www.arhp.org

Bedsider.Org Provides information on all methods of contraception. Describes how to use a method, typical side effects, cost, and how to get the method.

https://bedsider.org/

Emergency Contraception Hotline. Provides information and referrals.

888-NOT-2-LATE

Emergency Contraception website. Provides extensive information about emergency contraception; sponsored by the Office of Population Research at Princeton University.

http://ec.princeton.edu

Guttmacher Institute. Provides reproductive health research, policy analysis, and public education.

http://www.guttmacher.org

It's Your Sex Life. Provides information about sexuality, relationships, contraceptives, and STDs; geared toward teenagers and young adults. Provided by the Kaiser Family Foundation and MTV.

http://www.itsyoursexlife.com

Kaiser Family Foundation: Women's Health Policy: Contraception. Provides information and reports focused on how policies affect reproductive health care and access to contraceptives.

http://kff.org/other/womens-health-policy-contraception/

Managing Contraception. Provides brief descriptions and tips for using many forms of contraception. Features a detailed survey to help with contraceptive choices.

http://www.managingcontraception.com

MedlinePlus: Abortion. Managed by the U.S. National Library of Medicine and the National Institutes of Health, this site provides a list of informational resources about various aspects of abortion.

http://www.nlm.nih.gov/medlineplus/abortion.html

National Abortion and Reproductive Rights Action League. Provides information about the politics of the pro-choice movement. Also provides information about the abortion laws and politics in each state.

http://www.prochoiceamerica.org

National Abortion Federation. Provides information and resources on medical and political issues relating to abortion; managed by health care providers.

http://www.prochoice.org

National Adoption Center. A national agency focused on finding adoptive homes for children with special needs or who are currently in foster care.

http://www.adopt.org

National Right to Life Committee. Provides information about pregnancy continuation and the politics of the pro-life movement.

http://www.nrlc.org

Planned Parenthood Federation of America. Provides information on family planning, contraception, and abortion and offers counseling services.

http://www.plannedparenthood.org

The following are some of the many organizations focusing on family planning and reproductive health issues worldwide:

International Planned Parenthood Federation

http://www.ippf.org

United Nations Population Fund

http://www.unfpa.org

SELECTED BIBLIOGRAPHY

Advancing New Standards in Reproductive Health. Turnaway Study (http://www.ansirh.org/research/turnaway.php).

Altshuler, A. L., et al. 2016. Male partners' involvement in abortion care: A mixed methods systematic review. *Perspectives on Sexual and Reproductive Health*. Forthcoming.

Altshuler, A., H. Gerns Storey, and S. Prager. 2015. Exploring abortion attitudes of US adolescents and young adults using social media. *Contraception* 91(3): 226–233.

American Congress of Obstetricians and Gynecologists. 2011. *Contraceptives* (http://www.acog.org/~/media/For%20Patients/faq021.pdf?dmc1&ts20120301T1336161249).

American College of Obstetricians and Gynecologists. 2015. Frequently Asked Questions: Induced Abortion. (http://www.acog.org/Patients/FAQs/Induced-Abortion).

Biggs, M., H. Gould, and D. Foster. 2013. Understanding why women seek abortions in the U.S. *BMC Women's Health* 13(1): 29.

Biggs, M., et al. 2014. Does abortion reduce self-esteem and life satisfaction? *Quality of Life Research* 23(9): 2505–2513.

Bitzer, J., and J. A. Simon. 2011. Current issues and available options in hormonal contraception. *Contraception* 84(4): 342–356.

Burke, A. E. 2011. The state of hormonal contraception today: Benefits and risks of hormonal contraceptives: Progestin-only contraceptives. *American Journal of Obstetrics and Gynecology* 205(4): S14–S17.

Cates, W., D. A. Grimes, and K. F. Schulz. 2004. The public health impact of legal abortion: 30 years later. *Perspectives on Sexual and Reproductive Health* 35(1): 25–28.

Centers for Disease Control and Prevention. 2012. Abortion surveillance—United States, 2008. *MMWR Surveillance Summaries* 60(SS15): 1–41.

Centers for Disease Control and Prevention. 2015. Abortion surveillance—United States, 2012. *MMWR Surveillance Summaries* 64(SS10): 1–40.

Centers for Disease Control and Prevention. 2015. Sexual activity, contraceptive use, a nd childbearing of teenagers aged 15–19 in the United States. *NCHS Data Brief,* No. 209.

Charles, V., et al. 2008. Abortion and long-term mental health outcomes: A systematic review of the evidence. *Contraception* 78(6): 436–450.

Cremer, M., and R. Masch. 2010. Emergency contraception: past, present and future. *Minerva Ginecologica* 62(4): 361–371.

Curtin S. C., J. C. Abma, and K. Kost. 2015. 2010 pregnancy rates among U.S. women (http://www.cdc.gov/nchs/data/hestat/pregnancy/2010_pregnancy_rates.htm).

Dehlendorf, C., et al. 2011. Race, ethnicity and differences in contraception among low-income women. *Perspectives on Sexual and Reproductive Health* 43(3): 181–187.

Fine, P., et al. 2010. Ulipristal acetate taken 48–120 hours after intercourse for emergency contraception. *Obstetrics and Gynecology* 115: 257–263.

Finer, L. B., and K. Kost. 2011. Unintended pregnancy rates at the state level. *Perspectives on Sexual and Reproductive Health* 43(2): 78–87.

Finer, L. B., and M. R. Zolna. 2011. Unintended pregnancy in the United States: Incidence and disparities, 2006. *Contraception* 84(5): 478–485.

Guttmacher Institute. 2012. *Facts on American Teens' Sexual and Reproductive Health* (http://www.guttmacher.org/pubs/FB-ATSRH.html).

Guttmacher Institute. 2012. *Update: U.S. Teenage Pregnancies, Births and Abortions: National and State Trends and Trends by Race and Ethnicity* (www.guttmacher.org/pubs/USTPtrends.pdf).

Guttmacher Institute. 2015. *Fact Sheet: Contraceptive Use in the United States* (http://www.guttmacher.org/pubs/fb_contr_use.html).

Guttmacher Institute. 2015. *Facts on Unintended Pregnancy in the United States* (http://www.guttmacher.org/pubs/FB-Unintended-Pregnancy-US.pdf).

Guttmacher Institute. 2016a. *Fact Sheet: Induced Abortion in the United States* (http://www.guttmacher.org/pubs/fb_induced_abortion.html).

Guttmacher Institute. 2016b. *State Funding of Abortion under Medicaid,* pp. 1–3 (http://www.guttmacher.org/statecenter/spibs/spib_SFAM.pdf).

Guttmacher Institute. 2016c. *State Policies in Brief: An Overview of Abortion Laws* (http://www.guttmacher.org/statecenter/spibs/spib_OAL.pdf).

Hatcher, R. A., et al. 2011. *Contraceptive Technology,* 20th ed. New York: Bridging the Gap Foundation.

Jick, S. S., et al. 2010. Postmarketing study of Ortho Evra and levonorgesterol oral contraceptives containing hormonal contraceptives with 30 mcg of ethinyl estradiol in relation to nonfatal venous thromboembolism. *Contraception* 81(1): 16–21.

Jones, R. K., and L. B. Finer. 2012. Who has second-trimester abortions in the United States? *Contraception* 85(6): 544–51.

Jones, R. K., and J. Jerman. 2014. Abortion incidence and service availability in the United States, 2011. *Perspectives on Sexual and Reproductive Health,* 46(1): 3–14.

Jones, R. K., and M. L. Kavanaugh. 2011. Changes in abortion rates between 2000 and 2008 and lifetime incidence of abortion. *Obstetrics and Gynecology* 117(6): 1358–1366.

Lopez, L. M., et al. 2011. Hormonal contraceptives for contraception in overweight or obese women. *Obstetrics and Gynecology* 116(5): 1206–1207.

Lopez, L. M., et al. 2011. Steroidal contraceptives: Effect on bone fractures in women. *Cochrane Database of Systematic Reviews,* 6 July (7): CD006033.

Lyus, R., et al. 2011. Use of the Mirena LNG-IUS and ParaGard CuT380A intrauterine devices in nulliparous women. *Contraception* 81(5): 367–371.

Mansour, D., et al. 2011. Fertility after discontinuation of contraception: A comprehensive review of the literature. *Contraception* 84(5): 465–477.

Meyer, J. L., et al. 2011. Advance provision of emergency contraception among adolescent and young adult women: A systematic review of the literature. *Journal of Pediatric and Adolescent Gynecology* 24(1): 2–9.

Mohamad, A. M., et al. 2011. Combined contraceptive ring versus combined oral contraceptive. *International Journal of Gynecology and Obstetrics* 114(2): 145–148.

Moore, A. M., L. Frohwirth, and N. Blades. 2011. What women want from abortion counseling in the United States: A qualitative study of abortion patients in 2008. *Social Work in Health Care* 50(6): 424–442.

National Center for Health Statistics. 2015. *National Survey of Family Growth: Emergency Contraception* (http://www.cdc.gov/nchs/nsfg/key_statistics/e.htm#emergency)

Ramasamy, R., and P. N. Schlegel. 2011. Vasectomy and vasectomy reversal: An update. *Indian Journal of Urology* 27(1): 92–97 (http://www.ncbi.nlm.nih.gov/pmc/articles/PMC3114592/).

Raymond, E. G., and D. A. Grimes. 2012. The comparative safety of legal induced abortion and childbirth in the United States. *Obstetrics and Gynecology* 119(2.1): 215–219.

Richardson, A. R., and F. N. Maltz. 2012. Ulipristal acetate: Review of the efficacy and safety of a newly approved agent for emergency contraception. *Clinical Therapeutics* 34(1): 24–36.

Rocca, C., et al. 2015. Decision rightness and emotional responses to abortion in the United States: A longitudinal study. *PLoS ONE* 10(7): e0128832.

Sedgh, G., S. Singh, and R. Hussain. 2014. Intended and unintended pregnancies worldwide in 2012 and recent trends. *Studies in Family Planning* 45(3): 301–314.

Sedgh, G., et al. 2015. Adolescent pregnancy, birth, and abortion rates across countries: Levels and recent trends. *Journal of Adolescent Health.* 56(2): 223–230.

Shellenberg, K. M., and A. O. Tsui. 2012. Correlates of perceived and internalized stigma among abortion patients in the USA: An exploration by race and Hispanic ethnicity. *International Journal of Gynecology & Obstetrics* 118(Suppl. 2):S152–S159.

Sonfield A., et al. 2015. The impact of the federal contraceptive coverage guarantee on out-of-pocket payments for contraceptives: 2014 update. *Contraception* 91: 44–48.

United Nations, Department of Economic and Social Affairs, Population Division. 2015. *Trends in Contraceptive Use Worldwide 2015* (http://www.un.org/en/development/desa/population/publications/pdf/family/trendsContraceptiveUse2015Report.pdf).

Upadhyay, U. D., et al. 2014. Denial of abortion because of provider gestational age limits in the United States. *American Journal of Public Health* 104(9): 1687–1694.

Ventura, S. J., et al. 2014. Estimated pregnancy rates and rates of pregnancy outcomes for the United States, 1990–2008. *National Vital Statistics Report* 60(7): 1–22.

Winner, B., et al. 2012. Effectiveness of long-acting reversible contraception. *New England Journal of Medicine* 366(21) 1998–2007.

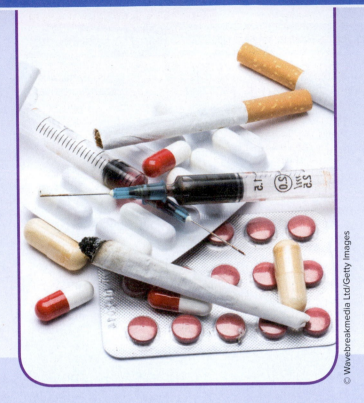
© Wavebreakmedia Ltd/Getty Images

CHAPTER 7

Drug Use and Addiction

The use of **drugs** for both medical and social purposes is widespread in the United States (Table 7.1). Many Americans believe that every problem has or should have a chemical solution. For fatigue, many turn to caffeine; for insomnia, sleeping pills; for anxiety or boredom, prescription medication, alcohol, or other recreational drugs. Advertisements, social pressures, and the human desire for quick solutions to difficult problems all contribute to the prevailing attitude that drugs can ease all pain. But benefits often come with the risk of harmful consequences, and drug use can—and in many cases does—pose serious or even life-threatening risks.

This chapter introduces the concepts of addiction and misuse, and then focuses on the major classes of misused drugs, their effects, their potential for addiction and impairment, and other issues related to their use. Alcohol and nicotine—two of the most widely used and most problematic psychoactive drugs—are discussed in Chapter 8.

ADDICTION

The most serious drug-related risks are addiction and impairment of daily activities. The drugs most often associated with addiction and impairment are **psychoactive drugs**—those that alter a person's experiences or consciousness. In the short term, psychoactive drugs can cause **intoxication,** a state in which, sometimes, unpredictable physical and emotional changes occur. A person who is intoxicated may experience potentially serious changes in physical functioning. His or her emotions and judgment may be affected in ways that lead to uncharacteristic and unsafe behavior. Recurrent drug use can have profound physical, emotional, and social effects.

Although addiction is most often associated with drug use, many experts now extend the concept of addiction to

> **TERMS**
>
> **drug**   Any chemical other than food intended to affect the structure or function of the body.
>
> **psychoactive drug**   A drug that can alter a person's consciousness or experience.
>
> **intoxication**   The state of being mentally affected by a chemical (literally, a state of being poisoned).

| Table 7.1 | Nonmedical Drug Use among Americans, 2015 (percent using in past month) |

	YOUNG ADULTS AGE 18–25	YOUTHS AGE 12–17	ALL AMERICANS AGE 12 AND OVER
ILLICIT DRUGS	22.3	8.8	10.1
Marijuana* and hashish	19.8	7.0	8.4
Cocaine	1.7	0.2	0.7
Heroin	0.3	0.0	0.1
Hallucinogens	1.8	0.5	0.5
Ecstasy	0.9	0.1	0.2
Inhalants	0.4	0.7	0.2
Methamphetamine	0.4	0.1	0.3
NONMEDICAL USE OF PSYCHOTHERAPEUTICS	5.1	2.0	2.4
Pain relievers	2.4	1.1	1.4
Tranquilizers	1.7	0.7	0.7
Stimulants	2.2	0.5	0.6
Sedatives	0.2	0.1	0.2
TOBACCO (ALL FORMS)	33.0	6.0	23.9
Cigarettes	26.7	4.2	19.4
Smokeless tobacco	5.4	1.5	3.4
Cigars	8.9	2.1	4.7
ALCOHOL	58.3	9.6	51.7
Binge alcohol use	39.0	5.8	24.9
Heavy alcohol use	10.9	0.9	6.5

*See the section titled "Marijuana and Other Cannabis Products" for information about the legal status of marijuana.

SOURCE: SAMHSA Center for Behavioral Health Statistics and Quality 2016: *Results from the 2015 National Survey on Drug Use and Health*. Retrieved from http://www.samhsa.gov/data/sites/default/files/NSDUH-DetTabs-2015/NSDUH-DetTabs-2015/NSDUH-DetTabs-2015.htm

other behaviors. **Addictive behaviors** are habits that have gotten out of control, with resulting negative effects on a person's health. The most characteristic feature of addiction is a loss of control caused by a disruption in the brain's system that regulates motivation and reward. It manifests as an unrelenting pursuit of a physical or psychological reward and/or relief through substance use or behaviors, such as gambling, despite unwanted consequences. Addiction involves craving and the inability to recognize significant risk or other problems with behaviors, interpersonal relationships, and emotional response. Like other chronic diseases, addiction often involves cycles of relapse and remission. Without treatment, addiction is progressive and can result in disabling or deadly health consequences.

addictive behavior Compulsive behavior that is both rewarding and reinforcing and is often pursued to the marginalization or exclusion of other activities and responsibilities.

addiction A chronic disease that disrupts the brain's system of motivation and reward, characterized by a compulsive desire and increasing need for a substance or behavior, and by harm to the individual and/or society.

tolerance Lower sensitivity to a drug or substance so that a given dose no longer exerts the usual effect and larger doses are needed.

TERMS

What Is Addiction?

Today scientists view **addiction** as a chronic disease that involves disruption of the brain's systems related to reward, motivation, and memory. Dysfunction in these systems leads to biological, psychological, and social effects associated with pathologically pursuing pleasure or relief by substance use and other behaviors. The American Psychiatric Association (APA) defines addiction as a "complex condition, a chronic brain disease that causes compulsive substance use despite harmful consequences." In addition to disorders related to drugs, the APA also includes a new category of behavioral addictions such as gambling disorder and Internet gaming disorder in the *Diagnostic and Statistical Manual of Mental Disorders (DSM-5)*, the standard classification system used by mental health professionals.

Although experts now agree that addiction is more fully defined by behavioral characteristics, they also agree that changes in the brain underlie addiction. One such change is **tolerance,** in which the body adapts to a drug so that the initial dose no longer produces the original emotional or psychological effects. This process means the user has to take larger and larger doses of a drug to achieve the same high. The concept of addiction as a disease process, one based in identifiable changes to brain cells and brain chemistry rather than a moral failing, has led to many advances in the understanding and treatment of drug addiction.

As noted, many researchers now view activities like gambling, eating, exercising, and sex as potential behavioral addictions, and some scientists assert that these activities release brain chemicals that cause a pleasurable rush in much the same way that psychoactive drugs do. The brain's own chemicals thus become the "drug" that can cause addiction. These theorists suggest that all addictions—whether to drugs or to pleasurable activities—have a common mechanism in the brain. In this view, addiction is partly the result of our own natural wiring.

The view that addiction is based in our brain chemistry does *not* imply that people are not responsible for their addictive behavior. Many experts believe it is inaccurate and counterproductive to think of all bad habits and excessive behaviors as diseases. All addictions involve an initial voluntary step, and other factors such as lifestyle, personality traits, and environmental factors play key roles in the development of addiction.

Diagnosing Substance Misuse and Addiction

In general terms, **substance misuse** is use of a substance that is not consistent with medical or legal guidelines. Misuse is a broad concept and can include use of illegal drugs, prescription drugs in greater-than-prescribed amounts, another person's prescription drug, or a legal substance like alcohol in an unsafe manner. Some researchers distinguish between misuse and abuse on the basis of an individual's intent. For example, taking double a prescribed dose of sleeping medication because the first dose didn't seem to help would be an example of drug *misuse*. The situation in which a person takes multiple painkillers in an effort to get high would be considered drug *abuse*. However, either scenario could be dangerous, and any drug misuse carries the risk of negative effects. You do not have to be addicted to a drug or even misuse it more than once to suffer serious consequences.

In the *DSM-5*, the APA provides criteria for diagnosing problems associated with regular drug use. Classifying a person as having a substance use disorder is not as simple as applying a label; instead, an individual is classified based on symptoms ranging from mild (an average college binge drinker) to severe (a person who is out of control).

The latest version of the *DSM* dropped the past distinction between *dependence* and *abuse* in diagnosing drug-related disorders; however, both terms are still used in other contexts. Note that physical dependence, in a narrow sense, can be a normal bodily response to use of a substance. For example, regular coffee drinkers may experience caffeine withdrawal symptoms if they reduce their intake; however, that does not mean they have a substance use disorder. In the context of addiction and substance use disorders, the National Institute on Drug Abuse specifies that **dependence** may involve this type of physical dependence but must also meet other criteria, such as compulsive use.

Addiction is a psychological or physical dependence on a substance or behavior that has undesirable, negative consequences. According to the APA, people with addiction are focused on a particular drug or behavior to the point that it takes over their lives; they use the substance or engage in the behavior compulsively despite knowing it will cause problems. We refer to the *DSM-5* definition of **substance use disorders** in this chapter but also recognize the terms *dependence, abuse,* and *addiction,* which are commonly used in mental health literature. The term *abuse,* however, is slowly falling out of favor and being replaced with such terms as *misuse, disorder,* and *dependence.*

The 11 *DSM-5* criteria for a substance use disorder are listed below; they are grouped in four categories. The severity of the disorder is determined by the number of criteria a person meets:

- 2–3 criteria indicate a mild disorder.
- 4–5 criteria point to a moderate disorder.
- 6 or more criteria are evidence of a severe disorder.

Impaired Control

1. *Taking the substance in larger amounts or over a longer period than was originally intended.*
2. *Expressing a persistent desire to cut down on or regulate substance use, but being unable to do so.*
3. *Spending a great deal of time getting the substance, using the substance, or recovering from its effects.*
4. *Craving or experiencing an intense desire or urge to use the substance.*

Social Problems

5. *Failing to fulfill major obligations at work, school, or home.*
6. *Continuing to use the substance despite having persistent or recurrent social or interpersonal problems caused or worsened by the effects of its use.*
7. *Giving up or reducing important social, school, work, or recreational activities because of substance use.*

TERMS

substance misuse or abuse The use of any substance in a manner inconsistent with legal or medical guidelines; may be associated with adverse social, psychological, or medical consequences; the use may be intermittent and with or without tolerance and physical dependence.

dependence Frequent or consistent use of a drug or behavior that makes it difficult for the person to get along without it; the result of physiological and/or psychological adaptation that occurs in response to the substance or behavior; typically associated with tolerance and withdrawal but can also be based solely on behavioral factors such as compulsive use.

substance use disorder A cluster of symptoms involving cognitive, bodily, and social impairment related to the continued use of a substance; a single disorder measured on a continuum from mild to severe.

Risky Use

8. *Using the substance in situations in which it is physically hazardous to do so.*

9. *Continuing to use the substance despite the knowledge of having persistent or recurrent physical or psychological problems caused or worsened by substance use.*

Drug Effects

10. *Developing tolerance to the substance.* When a person requires increased amounts of a substance to achieve the desired effect or notices a markedly diminished effect with continued use of the same amount, he or she has developed tolerance to the substance.

11. *Experiencing withdrawal.* In someone who has maintained prolonged, heavy use of a substance, a drop in its concentration within the body can result in unpleasant physical and cognitive **withdrawal** symptoms. Withdrawal symptoms are different for different drugs. For example, nausea, vomiting, and tremors are common withdrawal symptoms in people dependent on alcohol, opioids, or sedatives.

The Development of Addiction

An addiction often starts when a person does something to bring pleasure or avoid pain. The activity may be drinking a beer, using the Internet, playing the lottery, or shopping. If it works, the person is likely to repeat it. Reinforcement leads to an increasing dependence on the behavior. Tolerance—caused by physical changes to brain cells and reward pathways in the brain—develops, and the person needs more of the substance or behavior to feel the expected effect. Eventually the behavior becomes a central focus of the person's life, and other areas such as school performance or relationships deteriorate. The behavior no longer brings pleasure, but repeating it is necessary to avoid withdrawal.

Although many common behaviors are potentially addictive, most people who engage in them do not develop problems. The reason lies in the combination of factors involved in the development of addiction, including personality, lifestyle, heredity, the social and physical environment, and the nature of the substance or behavior in question.

Examples of Addictive Behaviors

As noted, behaviors that are not related to drugs can become addictive for some people. Such behaviors can include eating, gambling, and playing Internet games. Any substance or activity that becomes the focus of a person's life at the expense of other needs and interests can be damaging to health. Like addiction to drugs, behavioral or nondrug addiction involves symptoms such as craving, loss of control over the behavior, tolerance, withdrawal, and a repeating pattern of recovery and relapse. These symptoms support the theory that nondrug addictions promote changes in the brain regions and systems associated with misuse of and addiction to alcohol, nicotine, or other drugs.

Compulsive Gambling Compulsive gamblers cannot control the urge to gamble, even in the face of ruin. The consequences of compulsive gambling are not just financial; the suicide rate of compulsive gamblers is 20 times higher than that of the general population. About 1% of adult Americans are compulsive (pathological) gamblers, and another 2% are "problem gamblers." Some 42% of college students gamble at least once in a year, and about 3% gamble at least once a week. Sixty-five percent of pathological gamblers commit crimes to support their gambling habit.

The APA recognizes gambling disorder as a behavioral addiction associated with at least four of 10 characteristic behaviors, including preoccupation with gambling, unsuccessful

> ### QUICK STATS
> **48** states and the District of Columbia allow some form of legalized gambling. (No form of gambling is legal in Hawaii or Utah.)
> —National Council on Problem Gambling, 2016

When taken to an extreme, even healthy activities such as exercise can become addictive.

© Dirima/Getty Images

> **withdrawal** Physical and psychological symptoms that follow the interrupted use of a drug on which a user is physically dependent; symptoms may be mild or life threatening. **TERMS**

efforts to quit, using gambling to escape problems, and lying to family members to conceal the extent of gambling. These characteristics have much in common with the behavioral dysfunctions used to describe addiction. Many compulsive gamblers also have drug and alcohol misuse problems.

Internet Gaming Disorder   Recognized as a potentially addictive behavior by the APA but indicated for further study is Internet gaming. Similar to other addictions, Internet gaming disorder can be classified as mild, moderate, or severe based on the impact on a person's life. Characteristic behaviors include preoccupation with Internet games, loss of interest in other activities, using gaming to relieve anxiety or guilt, and risking opportunities or relationships due to time spent gaming. The disorder is separate from gambling disorder and different from general use of social media or the Internet.

Compulsive Exercising   When taken to a compulsive level, even healthy activity can turn into harmful addictions. For example, compulsive exercising is now recognized as a serious departure from normal behavior. Compulsive exercising is often accompanied by more severe psychiatric disorders such as anorexia nervosa and bulimia (see Chapter 11). Traits often associated with compulsive exercising include an excessive preoccupation and dissatisfaction with body image, use of laxatives or vomiting to lose weight, and development of other obsessive-compulsive symptoms.

Work Addiction   People who are excessively preoccupied with work are often called *workaholics*. Work addiction, however, is based on a set of specific symptoms, including an intense work schedule, the inability to limit your own work schedule, the inability to relax, even when away from work, and failed attempts at curtailing the intensity of work (in some cases).

A person with a work addiction is likely to neglect other aspects of life. For example, she or he may exercise less, spend less time with family and friends, and avoid social activities.

Work addiction typically coincides with a well-known risk factor for cardiovascular disease—the Type A personality (see Chapter 12). Traits associated with Type A personality include competitiveness, ambition, drive, time urgency, restlessness, hyper-alertness, and hostility.

Sex Addiction   More controversial is the notion of addiction to sex. Behaviors associated with sex addiction include an extreme preoccupation with sex, a compulsion to have sex repeatedly in a given period of time, a great deal of time and energy spent looking for partners or having sex, sex used as a means of relieving painful feelings, and the experience of negative emotional, personal, and professional consequences as a result of sexual activities. Even therapists who challenge the concept of sex addiction recognize that some people become overly preoccupied with sex, cannot seem to control their sex drive, and act in potentially harmful ways in order to stay satisfied.

Compulsive Buying or Shopping   A compulsive buyer repeatedly gives in to the impulse to buy more than he or she needs or can afford. Compulsive spenders usually buy luxury items rather than daily necessities, even though they are usually distressed by their behavior and its social, personal, and financial consequences. Some experts link compulsive shopping with neglect or abuse during childhood; it also seems to be associated with eating disorders, depression, and bipolar disorder.

Internet Addiction   In the years since the Internet became widely available, millions of Americans have become compulsive Internet users—as many as one out of eight people; among college students, approximately one out of seven fit this description. To spend more time online, Internet addicts skip other important activities. Compulsive Internet users often spend their work time online, a fact that has led many employers to adopt strict Internet usage policies. Despite negative financial, social, or academic consequences, compulsive Internet users don't feel able to stop. As with other addictive behaviors, Internet addiction may result when people use their behavior to alleviate stress or avoid painful emotions.

WHY PEOPLE USE AND MISUSE DRUGS

Using drugs to alter consciousness is an ancient and universal pursuit. People have used alcohol for celebration and intoxication for thousands of years. People in all parts of the world have exploited the psychoactive properties of plants, such as the coca plant in South America and the opium poppy in the Far East. But many drugs have addictive properties and change the chemistry of the brain; their use can open the door to the problems of misuse and dependence.

The Allure of Drugs

Young people may be drawn to drugs by the allure of the exciting and illegal. They may be curious, rebellious, or vulnerable to peer pressure. Young people may want to imitate adult models in their lives or in the movies. Most people who take illicit drugs do so experimentally, typically trying a drug one or more times but not continuing. The main factors in the initial choice of a drug are whether it is available and whether peers are using it.

Although some people use drugs because they have a desire to alter their mood or are seeking a spiritual experience, others are motivated by a desire to escape boredom, anxiety, depression, feelings of worthlessness, or other distressing symptoms. They use drugs to cope with the difficulties they experience in life. For people living in poverty, many of these reasons for using drugs are magnified. They may be dealing with dangerous environments, unstable family situations, severe financial stress, and lack of access to mental health services. Further, the buying and selling of drugs provide access to an unofficial alternative economy that may seem like an opportunity for success.

How do some people use psychoactive drugs without becoming addicted? The answer seems to be a combination of

Ask Yourself

QUESTIONS FOR CRITICAL THINKING AND REFLECTION

Have you ever repeatedly or compulsively engaged in a behavior that had negative consequences? What was the behavior, and why did you continue? Did you ever worry that you were losing control? Were you able to bring the behavior under control?

Table 7.2	Psychoactive Drugs and Their Potential for Substance Use Disorder and Addiction

Very high	Heroin
High	Nicotine, morphine
Moderate/high	Cocaine, pentobarbital
Moderate	Alcohol, ephedra, Rohypnol
Moderate/low	Caffeine, marijuana, MDMA (methylenedioxymethamphetamine), nitrous oxide
Low/very low	Ketamine, LSD (lysergic acid diethylamide), mescaline, psilocybin

SOURCE: Adapted from Gable, R. S. 2006. Acute toxicity of drugs versus regulatory status. In J. M. Fish (Ed.), *Drugs and Society: U.S. Public Policy*, pp. 149-162. Lanham, MD: Rowman & Littlefield.

physical, psychological, and social factors. Research indicates that some people may be born with a brain chemistry or metabolism that makes them more vulnerable to addiction. Other research suggests that people who were exposed to drugs in the womb may have an increased risk of abusing drugs themselves later in life.

Research shows that about one-third of people with psychological disorders also have a substance use disorder; about one-third of those have a second mental disorder. Diagnosing psychological problems among people with substance use disorders can be difficult because drug intoxication and withdrawal can mimic the symptoms of a mental illness.

Social factors can influence drug dependence. These include factors discussed earlier—growing up with a family member who uses drugs, belonging to a peer group that emphasizes or encourages drug use, and living in poverty. Because they have easy access to drugs, health care professionals are also at a higher risk.

Risk Factors for Drug Misuse and Addiction

The causes and course of an addiction are varied, but people with addictions (commonly referred to as *addicts*) share some characteristics. As mentioned, many use a substance or activity as a substitute for healthier coping strategies. People vary in their ability to manage their lives, and those who have trouble dealing with stress and painful emotions may be susceptible to addiction.

Some people may have a genetic predisposition to addiction to a particular substance based on a variation in brain chemistry. People with addictive disorders usually have a distinct preference for a particular addictive behavior. They also often have problems with impulse control and self-regulation and tend to be risk takers.

Nevertheless, drug misuse and addiction occur at all income and education levels, among all ethnic groups, and across all age groups (see the box "Drug Use among College Students"). Society is concerned with the casual or recreational use of illegal drugs because it is not possible to know when it will lead to addiction. Some casual users develop substance-related problems; others do not. Some drugs are more likely than others to lead to addiction (Table 7.2), but even some heroin or cocaine users do not meet the APA's criteria for substance use disorder.

QUICK STATS

27.1 million Americans age 12 and over used an illicit drug in the past 30 days; this averages to about 1 in 10 Americans.

—Substance Abuse and Mental Health Services Administration, 2016

Factors Associated with Trying Drugs It isn't possible to accurately predict who will misuse drugs or become addicted, but young people at a high risk of *trying* drugs—the first step toward misuse—tend to share the following characteristics:

• *Male.* Males are more likely than females to use almost all types of illicit drugs. National overdose deaths from prescription drugs, cocaine, and heroin are consistently higher in males than females. However, females are just as likely as males to eventually become addicted.

• *Troubled childhood.* Teens are more likely to try drugs if they have had behavioral issues in childhood, have suffered sexual or physical abuse, used tobacco at a young age, or suffer from certain mental or emotional problems.

• *Thrill-seeker.* Impulsivity and a sense of invincibility is a factor in drug experimentation.

• *Dysfunctional family.* A chaotic home life with poor supervision, constant tension or arguments, or parental abuse increases the risk of teen drug use. Having parents who misuse drugs or alcohol increases the risk for teen drug and alcohol use.

• *Peer group that accepts drug use.* Young people who are uninterested in school, have problems at school, have difficulty fitting in, or view illicit substances with an accepting attitude are more likely to try drugs.

• *Poor.* Young people who live in disadvantaged areas are more likely to be around drugs at a young age.

• *Girl dating an older boy.* Adolescent girls who date boys two or more years older than themselves are more likely to use drugs.

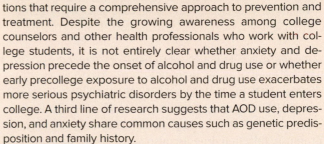

Drug use in college has long been recognized as a significant health problem that affects many students. According to the most recent survey data from the NSDUH, 22.3% of young adults aged 18–25 reported using an illicit drug in the past 30 days, with marijuana the most commonly used drug (refer to Table 7.1). Other surveys show that recreational drug use is fairly common among college students. According to the 2015 American College Health Association–National College Health Assessment, 15.0% of college students reported using marijuana at least once in the past 30 days. Nearly 6% of student reported nonmedical use of prescription stimulants within the past year.

Drug use on college campuses has been examined extensively, and many experts believe that no single factor can explain the widespread impact of this phenomenon. Family history, peer pressure, depression, anxiety, low self-esteem, and the dynamics of college life (for example, the drive to compete and a distorted perception of drug use among peers) have been suggested as potential explanations for college-age drug use.

Excessive alcohol use often accompanies illicit drug use and the risk of combining drugs and alcohol increases with the number of drinks a young adult consumes during a single session. In 2015, among the 17.3 million heavy drinkers age 12 and over, 32.5 percent were also current illicit drug users. Persons who were not current alcohol users were less likely to have used illicit drugs in the past month.

The term *AOD* (alcohol and other drug) has been coined to refer to this type of substance use among college students.

Further, AOD use and depression and/or anxiety are generally recognized as coexisting conditions that require a comprehensive approach to prevention and treatment. Despite the growing awareness among college counselors and other health professionals who work with college students, it is not entirely clear whether anxiety and depression precede the onset of alcohol and drug use or whether early precollege exposure to alcohol and drug use exacerbates more serious psychiatric disorders by the time a student enters college. A third line of research suggests that AOD use, depression, and anxiety share common causes such as genetic predisposition and family history.

However, one aspect of drug use among college students remains clear: AOD use has dramatic consequences for the educational, family, and community lives of students. Poor academic performance has been linked with AOD use. Further, driving while intoxicated remains one of the most dangerous outcomes associated with AOD use affecting families and communities.

Several AOD prevention programs are now under way at college campuses. Several federal laws have been enacted to provide resources and a legislative framework for addressing AOD use at schools. The 1989 Drug-Free Schools and Communities Act and the 1998 Higher Education Amendments are examples of concerted federal legislative efforts to encourage the development of educational policies for preventing alcohol and other drug use and providing assistance to college students at risk for these harmful behaviors.

Factors Associated with Not Using Drugs As a group, nonusers also share some characteristics. Not surprisingly, people who perceive drug use as risky and who disapprove of it are less likely to use drugs than those who believe otherwise. Drug use is also less common among people who have positive self-esteem and self-concept and who are assertive, independent thinkers who are not controlled by peer pressure. Self-control, social competence, optimism, academic achievement, and religiosity (religious beliefs and attendance of religious services) are also linked to lower rates of drug use.

Home environments are also influential: Coming from a strong family, one that has a clear policy on drug use, is another characteristic of people who don't use drugs. Young people who communicate openly with and feel supported by their parents are also less likely to use drugs.

RISKS ASSOCIATED WITH DRUG MISUSE

Addiction is not the only serious potential consequence of drug misuse. In 2011 nearly 2.5 million emergency department visits were related to drug misuse or abuse. The following are serious concerns as well:

- *Intoxication.* People who are under the influence of drugs—intoxicated—may act in uncharacteristic and unsafe ways because their physical and mental functioning are impaired. They are more likely to be injured from a variety of causes, to have unsafe sex, and to be involved in incidents of aggression and violence.

- *Unexpected side effects.* Psychoactive drugs have many physical and psychological effects beyond the alteration of consciousness. These effects range from nausea and constipation to paranoia, depression, and heart failure. Some drugs also carry the risk of fatal overdose.

- *Unknown drug constituents.* There is no quality control in the illegal drug market, so the composition, dosage, and toxicity of street drugs are highly variable. Studies indicate that half of all street drugs don't contain their promised primary ingredient. In some cases, a drug may be present in unsafe dosages or mixed with other drugs to boost its effects. Makers of street drugs aren't held to any safety standards, so illicit drugs can be contaminated or even poisonous.

- *Infection and injection drug use.* Many injection drug users (IDUs) share or reuse needles, syringes, and other injection supplies, which can easily become contaminated

Ask Yourself

QUESTIONS FOR CRITICAL THINKING AND REFLECTION

Have you ever tried a psychoactive drug for fun? What were your reasons for trying it? Whom were you with, and what were the circumstances? What was your experience? What would you tell someone who was thinking about trying a drug?

with the user's blood. Small amounts of blood can carry enough human immunodeficiency virus (HIV) and hepatitis C virus (HCV) to be infectious. In 2014, 5% of new diagnoses of HIV infection in men were due to injection drug use and another 3% to male-to-male sexual contact and injection drug use. Injection drug use also accounts for nearly half of new HCV infections.

The surest way to prevent diseases related to injection drug use is to never inject drugs. Syringe exchange programs (SEPs)—where IDUs can trade a used syringe for a new one—have been advocated to help slow the spread of HIV and reduce the rates and cost of other health problems associated with injection drug use. Getting people off drugs is clearly the best solution, but there are far more IDUs than treatment facilities can currently handle.

• *Legal consequences.* Many psychoactive drugs are illegal, so possessing them can result in large fines and imprisonment. According to the Federal Bureau of Investigation (FBI), the highest arrest counts for all types of crimes were for drug use violations (estimated at 1.6 million out of 11.2 million total arrests in 2014).

HOW DRUGS AFFECT THE BODY

The drugs discussed in this chapter have complex and variable effects, many of which can be traced to changes in brain chemistry. However, the same drug may affect different people differently or the same person in different ways under different circumstances. Beyond a fairly predictable general change in brain chemistry, the effects of a drug may vary depending on drug factors, user factors, and social factors.

Changes in Brain Chemistry

Once a psychoactive drug reaches the brain, it acts on one or more **neurotransmitters,** either increasing or decreasing their concentration and actions. Cocaine, for example, affects dopamine, a neurotransmitter thought to play a key role in the process of reinforcement—the brain's way of telling itself, "That's good; do the same thing again." When a

QUICK STATS

68.2% of new HCV infections in 2014 occurred among people who used injection drugs two weeks to six months before they noticed symptoms.

—Centers for Disease Control and Prevention, 2016

neurotransmitter is released by one neuron, it travels across a gap, called a synapse, to signal another neuron.

The duration of a drug's effect depends on many factors and may range from 5 minutes (crack cocaine) to 12 or more hours (LSD). As drugs circulate through the body, they are metabolized by the liver and eventually excreted by the kidneys in urine. Small amounts may also be eliminated in other ways, including in sweat, in breast milk, and via the lungs.

Drug-Related Factors

When different drugs or dosages produce different effects, the differences are usually caused by one or more of five different drug factors:

1. The **pharmacological properties** of a drug are its effects on a person's body chemistry, behavior, and psychology. Pharmacological properties also include the amount of a drug required to exert various effects, the time course of the effects, and other characteristics such as a drug's chemical composition.

2. The **dose-response function** is the relationship between the amount of drug taken and the type and intensity of its effects. Many psychological effects of drugs reach a plateau in the dose-response function, so that increasing the dose does not increase the effect any further. With LSD, for example, the maximum changes in perception occur at a certain dose, and no further changes in perception take place if higher doses are taken. However, all drugs have more than one effect, and the dose-response functions usually are different for different effects. This means that increasing the dose of any drug may begin to result in additional effects, which are likely to be more unpleasant or dangerous at high doses.

3. The **time-action function** is the relationship between the time elapsed since a drug was taken and the intensity of its effect. A drug's effects are greatest when its concentrations in body tissues are changing fastest, especially if they are increasing.

TERMS

neurotransmitter A brain chemical that transmits nerve impulses.

pharmacological properties The overall effects of a drug on a person's behavior, psychology, and chemistry.

dose-response function The relationship between the amount of a drug taken and the intensity and type of the resulting effect.

time-action function The relationship between the time elapsed since a drug was taken and the intensity of its effect.

4. The person's *drug use history* may influence the effects of a drug. A given amount of alcohol, for example, will affect a habitual drinker less than an occasional drinker. Tolerance to some drugs builds rapidly. To experience the same effect, a user has to abstain from the drug for a period of time before that dosage will again exert its original effects.

5. The *method of drug use* directly affects the strength of the response. Methods of use include ingestion, inhalation, injection, and absorption through the skin or tissue linings. Drugs are usually injected in one of three ways: intravenously (IV, or mainlining), intramuscularly (IM), or subcutaneously (SC, or skin popping).

Physical Factors

Certain physical characteristics help determine how a person will respond to a drug. Body mass is one variable: The effects of a certain dose of a drug on a 150-pound person will be greater than its effect on a 200-pound person. Other variables include general health and genetic factors. For example, some people have an inherited ability to rapidly metabolize a cough suppressant called dextromethorphan, which also has psychoactive properties. These people must take a higher-than-normal dose to get a given cough suppressant effect.

If a person's biochemical state is already altered by another drug, this too can make a difference. Some drugs intensify the effects of other drugs, as is the case with alcohol and sedatives. Some drugs block the effects of other drugs, such as when a tranquilizer is used to relieve anxiety caused by cocaine. Interactions between drugs, including many prescription and over-the-counter (OTC) medications, can be unpredictable and dangerous.

One physical condition that requires special precautions is pregnancy. It can be risky for a woman to use any drugs at all during pregnancy, including alcohol and common OTC products like cough medicine. The risks are greatest during the first trimester, when the fetus's body is forming rapidly and even small biochemical alterations in the mother can have a devastating effect on fetal development (see Chapter 5). Even later, the fetus is more susceptible than the mother to the adverse effects of any drugs she takes. The fetus may even become physically dependent on a drug being taken by the mother and suffer withdrawal symptoms after birth.

high The subjectively pleasing effects of a drug, usually felt quite soon after the drug is taken.

placebo effect A response to an inert or innocuous substance given in place of an active drug.

TERMS

Psychological Factors

Sometimes a person's response to a drug is strongly influenced by the user's expectations about how he or she will react (the psychological *set*). With large doses, the drug's chemical properties seem to have the strongest effect on the user's response. But with small doses, psychological (and social) factors are often more important. When people want to believe that a given drug will affect them a certain way, they are likely to experience those effects regardless of the drug's pharmacological properties. In one study, regular users of marijuana reported a moderate level of intoxication (**high**) after using a cigarette that smelled and tasted like marijuana but contained no THC, the active ingredient in marijuana. This is an example of the **placebo effect**—when a person receives an inert substance yet responds as if it were an active drug. In other studies, subjects who smoked low doses of real marijuana that they believed to be a placebo experienced no effects from the drug. Clearly the user's expectations had a greater effect than the drug itself.

Social Factors

The *setting* is the physical and social environment surrounding the drug use. If a person uses marijuana at home with trusted friends and pleasant music, the effects are likely to be different from the effects if the same dose is taken in an austere experimental laboratory with an impassive research technician. Similarly, a dose of alcohol that produces mild euphoria and stimulation at a noisy, active cocktail party might induce sleepiness and slight depression when taken at home while alone.

GROUPS OF PSYCHOACTIVE DRUGS

The following sections and Figure 7.1 introduce six representative groups of psychoactive drugs: opioids, central nervous system (CNS) depressants, central nervous system stimulants, marijuana and other cannabis products, hallucinogens, and inhalants. Some of these drugs are classified according to how they affect the body. Others—the opioids and the cannabis products—are classified according to their chemical makeup.

Category	Representative drugs	Street names	Appearance	Methods of use	Short-term effects
Opioids 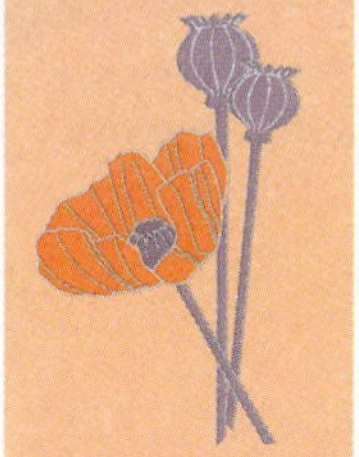	Heroin	Dope, H, junk, brown sugar, smack	White/dark brown powder; dark tar or coal-like substance	Injected, smoked, snorted	Relief of anxiety and pain; euphoria; lethargy, apathy, drowsiness, confusion, inability to concentrate; nausea, constipation, respiratory depression
	Opium	Big O, black stuff, hop	Dark brown or black chunks	Swallowed, smoked	
	Morphine	M, Miss Emma, monkey, white stuff	White crystals, liquid solution	Injected, swallowed, smoked	
	Oxycodone, codeine, hydrocodone	Oxy, O.C., killer, Captain Cody, schoolboy, vike	Tablets, powder made from crushing tablets	Swallowed, injected, snorted	
Central nervous system depressants 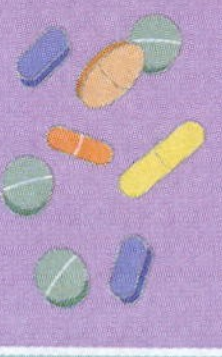	Barbiturates	Barbs, reds, red birds, yellows, yellow jackets	Colored capsules	Swallowed, injected	Reduced anxiety, mood changes, lowered inhibitions, impaired muscle coordination, reduced pulse rate, drowsiness, loss of consciousness, respiratory depression
	Benzodiazepines (e.g., Valium, Xanax, Rohypnol)	Candy, downers, tranks, roofies, forget-me pill	Tablets	Swallowed, injected	
	Methaqualone	Ludes, quad, quay	Tablets	Injected, swallowed	
	Gamma hydroxy butyrate (GHB)	G, Georgia home boy, grievous bodily harm	Clear liquid, white powder	Swallowed	
Central nervous system stimulants 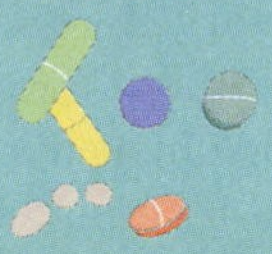	Amphetamine, methamphetamine	Bennies, speed, black beauties, uppers, chalk, crank, crystal, ice, meth	Tablets, capsules, white powder, clear crystals	Injected, swallowed, smoked, snorted	Increased and irregular heart rate, blood pressure, metabolism; increased mental alertness and energy; nervousness, insomnia, impulsive behavior; reduced appetite
	Cocaine, crack cocaine	Blow, C, candy, coke, flake, rock, toot, snow	White powder, beige pellets or rocks	Injected, smoked, snorted	
	Ritalin	JIF, MPH, R-ball, Skippy	Tablets	Injected, swallowed, snorted	
	Synthetic cathinones ("bath salts")	Bliss, Blue Silk, Flakka, Ivory Wave, Meow Meow, Vanilla Sky, White Lightning	Fine white, off-white, or slightly yellow-colored powder or crystals; can be tablets or capsules	Swallowed, smoked, vaporized, sniffed, snorted, and injected	Increased blood pressure, rapid heart beat, panic attacks in some people
Marijuana and other cannabis products 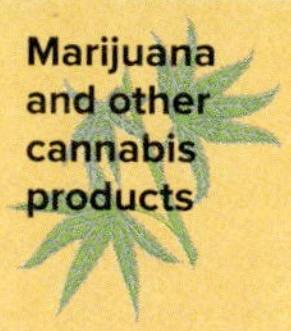	Marijuana	Dope, grass, joints, Mary Jane, reefer, skunk, weed, pot	Dried leaves and stems	Smoked, swallowed	Euphoria, slowed thinking and reaction time, confusion, anxiety, impaired balance and coordination, increased heart rate
	Hashish	Hash, hemp, boom, gangster	Dark, resin-like compound formed into rocks or blocks	Smoked, swallowed	
	K-2, Spice	Black Mamba, Bliss, Bombay Blue, Fake Weed, Genie, Spice, Zohai	Dried leaves	Smoked, teas	Increased blood pressure and heart beat, paranoia, panic attacks
Hallucinogens 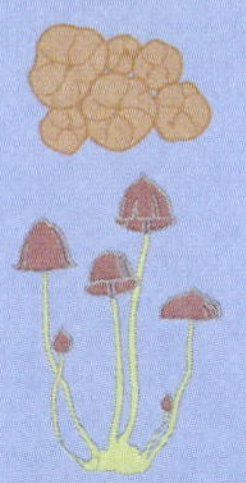	LSD	Acid, boomers, blotter, yellow sunshines	Blotter paper, liquid, gelatin tabs, pills	Swallowed, absorbed through mouth tissues	Altered states of perception and feeling; nausea; increased heart rate, blood pressure; delirium; impaired motor function; numbness, weakness
	Mescaline (peyote)	Buttons, cactus, mesc	Brown buttons, liquid	Swallowed, smoked	
	Psilocybin	Shrooms, magic mushrooms	Dried mushrooms	Swallowed	
	Ketamine	K, special K, cat valium, vitamin K	Clear liquid, white or beige powder	Injected, snorted, smoked	
	PCP	Angel dust, hog, love boat, peace pill	White to brown powder, tablets	Injected, swallowed, smoked, snorted	
	MDMA (ecstasy)	X, peace, clarity, Adam, Molly	Tablets	Swallowed	
Inhalants 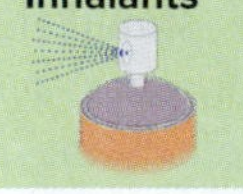	Solvents, aerosols, nitrites, anesthetics	Laughing gas, poppers, snappers, whippets	Household products, sprays, glues, paint thinner, petroleum products	Inhaled through nose or mouth	Stimulation, loss of inhibition, slurred speech, loss of motor coordination, loss of consciousness

FIGURE 7.1 Commonly misused drugs and their effects.

SOURCES: The Partnership for a Drug-Free America. 2016. *Drug Guide* (http://www.drugfree.org/drug-guide/); National Institute on Drug Abuse. 2016. *Commonly Abused Drugs Chart* (https://www.drugabuse.gov/drugs-abuse/commonly-abused-drugs-charts)

Opioids

Opioids are natural or synthetic (laboratory-made) drugs that relieve pain, cause drowsiness, and induce **euphoria.** Natural opioid-like hormones released by the brain, called endorphins, can inhibit pain and induce euphoria. Opium, morphine, heroin, methadone, codeine, hydrocodone, oxycodone, meperidine, and fentanyl are opioids. When taken at prescribed doses, opioids have beneficial medical uses, including pain relief and cough suppression. Opioids tend to reduce anxiety and produce lethargy, apathy, and an inability to concentrate.

Although the euphoria associated with opioids is an important factor in their misuse, many people experience a feeling of uneasiness when they first use these drugs. Even so, the misuse of opioids often results in addiction. Tolerance can develop rapidly and be pronounced. Withdrawal symptoms include cramps, chills, sweating, nausea, tremors, irritability, and feelings of panic.

According to the Substance Abuse and Mental Health Services Administration (SAMHSA), heroin use has been rising since 2007, increasing from 373,000 yearly users to 828,000 users in 2015. Heroin overdose deaths have also spiked alarmingly, increasing from 3,036 deaths in 2010 to 10,574 deaths in 2014. The potentially high but variable purity of street heroin poses a risk of unintentional overdose (see Figure 7.2). Symptoms of overdose include respiratory depression, coma, and constriction of the pupils; death can result.

When taken as prescribed in tablet form, these drugs treat moderate to severe chronic pain and do not typically lead to misuse. However, as is the case with other opioids, use of prescription painkillers can lead to misuse and addiction. When taken in large doses or combined with other drugs, oxycodone and hydrocodone can cause fatal

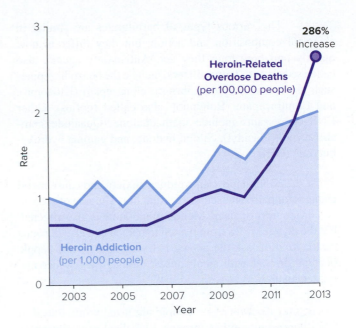

FIGURE 7.2 **Heroin addictions and deaths, 2002-2013.**

SOURCE: Centers for Disease Control and Prevention. 2015. *Today's Heroin Epidemic Infographics* (http://www.cdc.gov/vitalsigns/heroin/infographic.html).

> ### QUICK STATS
>
> **In 2014, deaths from opioid overdose surpassed car crashes as the leading cause of injury-related death in the United States.**
>
> —Centers for Disease Control and Prevention, 2016

respiratory depression. Some people who become addicted to prescription opioid painkillers may eventually turn to heroin because heroin is far cheaper than prescription opioids.

Recent surveys have found that people who are addicted to opioid painkillers are 40 times more likely to also be addicted to heroin; 45% of heroin users are also addicted to prescription painkillers. In 2014, pharmacies in the United States dispensed 245 million prescriptions for opioid painkillers, enough for every American adult to have a bottle of pills. In 2016, the Centers for Disease Control and Prevention announced a new effort to reduce the number of inappropriate prescriptions written for opioid painkillers.

Central Nervous System Depressants

Central nervous system **depressants,** also known as **sedative-hypnotics,** depress the **central nervous system (CNS).** The result can range from mild **sedation** to death.

Prescription painkillers such as oxycodone and hydrocodone are opioids that can have serious consequences such as fatal respiratory depression. The recreational use of these drugs is reported in about 2% of the population aged 12 and over.

© Education Images/Universal Images Group/Getty Images

> ### TERMS
>
> **opioid** Any of several natural or synthetic drugs that relieve pain and cause drowsiness and/or euphoria; examples are opium, morphine, and heroin; also called a *narcotic*.
>
> **euphoria** An exaggerated feeling of well-being.
>
> **depressant, sedative-hypnotic** A drug that decreases nervous or muscular activity, causing drowsiness or sleep.
>
> **central nervous system (CNS)** The brain and spinal cord.
>
> **sedation** The induction of a calm, relaxed, often sleepy state.

Types The various types of barbiturates are similar in chemical composition and action, but they differ in how quickly and how long they act. Antianxiety agents, also called sedatives or **tranquilizers,** include the benzodiazepines such as Xanax, Valium, Librium, clonazepam (Klonopin), and flunitrazepam (Rohypnol, also called roofies). Other CNS depressants include methaqualone (Quaalude), ethchlorvynol (Placidyl), chloral hydrate, and gamma hydroxybutyrate (GHB).

Effects CNS depressants reduce anxiety and cause mood changes, impaired muscular coordination, slurring of speech, and drowsiness or sleep. Mental functioning is also affected, but the degree varies from person to person and also depends on the kind of task the person is trying to do. Most people become drowsy with small doses, although a few become more active.

From Use to Misuse People are usually introduced to CNS depressants either through a medical prescription or through drug-using peers. The use of Rohypnol and GHB (discussed in greater detail later in this chapter) is often associated with dance clubs and raves. The misuse of CNS depressants by a medical patient may begin with repeated use for insomnia and progress to dependence through increasingly larger doses at night, coupled with doses during stressful times of the day.

Most CNS depressants, including alcohol, can lead to addiction. Tolerance, sometimes for up to 15 times the usual dose, can develop with repeated use. Tranquilizers can produce physical dependence even at ordinary prescribed doses. Withdrawal symptoms can be more severe than those accompanying opioid addiction and are similar to the DTs of alcoholism (see Chapter 8). They may begin as anxiety, shaking, and weakness but may turn into convulsions and possibly cardiovascular collapse and death.

While intoxicated, people on depressants cannot function well. They are often confused and may be obstinate, irritable, or abusive. Long-term use of depressants like alcohol can lead to serious physical effects, including brain damage, with impaired ability to reason and make judgments.

Overdosing with CNS Depressants Too much depression of the central nervous system slows respiration and may stop it entirely. CNS depressants are particularly dangerous in combination with another depressant, such as alcohol. People who combine depressants with alcohol account for thousands of emergency department visits and hundreds of overdose deaths each year.

Club Drugs Some people refer to club drugs as soft drugs because they see them as recreational—for the casual weekend user—rather than as addictive. But club drugs have many potential negative effects and are particularly potent and unpredictable when mixed with alcohol. Substitute drugs are often sold in place of club drugs, putting users at risk for taking dangerous combinations of unknown drugs.

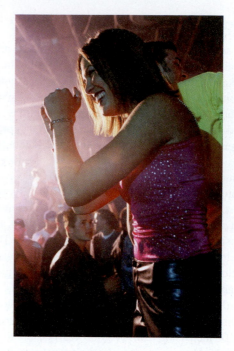

Club drugs such as Rohypnol are referred to as "date rape drugs" because they can be added surreptitiously to drinks.
© Rubberball/Getty Images

Rohypnol (flunitrazepam) is a sedative that is 10 times more potent than Valium. Its effects, which are magnified by alcohol, include reduced blood pressure, dizziness, confusion, gastrointestinal disturbances, and loss of consciousness. Users of Rohypnol may develop physical and psychological dependence on the drug. Rohypnol has never been approved for medical use by the U.S. Food and Drug Administration (FDA); along with some other club drugs, it is used as a "date rape drug." Because they can be added to beverages surreptitiously, these drugs may be unknowingly consumed by intended rape victims. In addition to depressant effects, some drugs also cause *anterograde amnesia*—the loss of memory of things occurring while under the influence of the drug. Rohypnol can be fatal if combined with alcohol.

GHB (gamma hydroxybutyrate) can be produced in clear liquid, white powder, tablet, and capsule form. GHB is a CNS depressant that in large doses or when taken in combination with alcohol or other depressants can cause sedation, loss of consciousness, respiratory arrest, and death. GHB may cause prolonged and potentially life-threatening withdrawal symptoms. GHB is often produced clandestinely,

TERMS

tranquilizer A central nervous system (CNS) depressant that reduces tension and anxiety.

Rohypnol (flunitrazepam) A sedative that is 10 times more potent than Valium; used as a "date rape drug."

GHB (gamma hydroxybutyrate) A central nervous system depressant that can be produced in clear liquid, white powder, tablet, and capsule form.

resulting in widely varying degrees of purity; it has been responsible for many poisonings and deaths.

Central Nervous System Stimulants

Central nervous system **stimulants** speed up the activity of the nervous or muscular system. Under their influence, the heart rate accelerates, blood pressure rises, blood vessels constrict, the pupils and bronchial tubes dilate, and gastric and adrenal secretions increase. There is greater muscular tension and sometimes an increase in motor activity. Small doses usually make people feel more awake and alert, and less fatigued and bored. The most common CNS stimulants are cocaine, amphetamines, nicotine (see Chapter 8), ephedrine, and caffeine.

Cocaine   Usually derived from the leaves of coca shrubs that grow high in the Andes in South America, cocaine is a potent CNS stimulant. Cocaine is usually snorted and absorbed through the nasal mucosa or injected intravenously, providing rapid increases of the drug's concentration in the blood and therefore fast, intense effects. Another method of use involves processing cocaine with baking soda and water, yielding the ready-to-smoke form of cocaine known as crack. Crack is typically available as small beads or pellets smokable in glass pipes.

EFFECTS   The effects of cocaine are usually intense but short-lived. The euphoria lasts from 5 to 20 minutes and ends abruptly, to be replaced by irritability, anxiety, or slight depression. When cocaine is absorbed via the lungs by either smoking or inhalation, it reaches the brain in about 10 seconds, and the effects are particularly intense. This is part of the appeal of smoking crack. The effects from IV injections occur almost as quickly—in about 20 seconds. Since the mucous membranes in the nose briefly slow absorption, the onset of effects from snorting takes 2–3 minutes. Heavy users may inject cocaine intravenously every 10–20 minutes to maintain the effects.

The larger the cocaine dose and the more rapidly it is absorbed into the bloodstream, the greater the immediate—and sometimes lethal—effects. Sudden death from cocaine is most commonly the result of excessive CNS stimulation that causes convulsions and respiratory collapse, irregular heartbeat, extremely high blood pressure, blood clots, and possibly heart attack or stroke. Although rare, fatalities can occur in healthy young people; among people aged 18–59, cocaine users are seven times more likely than nonusers to have a heart attack. Chronic cocaine use produces inflammation of the nasal mucosa, which can lead to persistent bleeding and ulceration of the septum

> **stimulant**   A drug that increases nervous or muscular activity.
>
> **state dependence**   A situation in which information learned in a drug-induced state is difficult to recall when the effect of the drug wears off.
>
> **TERMS**

between the nostrils. The use of cocaine may also cause paranoia and aggressiveness. When steady cocaine users stop taking the drug, they experience a sudden "crash" characterized by depression, agitation, and fatigue, followed by a period of withdrawal.

COCAINE USE DURING PREGNANCY   Cocaine rapidly passes from the mother's bloodstream into the placenta and can have serious effects on the fetus. A woman who uses cocaine during pregnancy is at higher risk for miscarriage, premature labor, and stillbirth. She is more likely to deliver a low-birth-weight baby who has a small head circumference. Her infant may be at increased risk for defects of the genitourinary tract, cardiovascular system, central nervous system, and extremities. It is difficult to pinpoint the effects of cocaine because many women who use cocaine also use tobacco and alcohol.

Infants whose mothers use cocaine may also be born intoxicated. Cocaine also passes into breast milk and can intoxicate a breastfeeding infant.

Amphetamines   Amphetamines (uppers) are a group of synthetic chemicals that are potent CNS stimulants. Some common drugs in this family are amphetamine (Benzedrine), dextroamphetamine (Dexedrine), and methamphetamine (Methedrine). Crystal methamphetamine (also called ice) is a smokable, high-potency form of methamphetamine, or meth.

EFFECTS   Small doses of amphetamines usually make people feel more alert. Amphetamines generally increase motor activity but do not measurably alter a normal, rested person's ability to perform tasks calling for challenging motor skills or complex thinking. When amphetamines improve performance, it is primarily by counteracting fatigue and boredom. In small doses, amphetamines increase heart rate and blood pressure and change sleep patterns.

Amphetamines are sometimes used to curb appetite, but after a few weeks the user develops tolerance and higher doses are necessary. When people stop taking the drug, their appetite usually returns, and they gain back the weight they lost.

MISUSE AND ADDICTION   Much amphetamine misuse begins as an attempt to cope with a temporary situation. A student cramming for an exam or an exhausted long-haul truck driver can go a little longer by taking amphetamines, but the results can be disastrous. The likelihood of making bad judgments increases significantly. The stimulating effects may also wear off suddenly, and the user may precipitously feel exhausted or fall asleep ("crash").

Another problem is **state dependence,** the phenomenon whereby information learned in a certain drug-induced state is difficult to recall when the drug wears off. Performance may deteriorate when students use drugs to study and then take tests in their normal, nondrug state. (Users of antihistamines may also experience state dependence.) Repeated use of amphetamines, even in moderate doses, often leads to tolerance and the need for increasingly larger doses. The result can be severe disturbances in behavior, including a

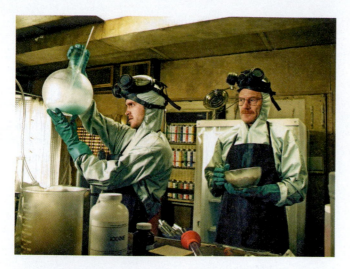

Crystal meth is often manufactured in small, home "laboratories," like the one featured in the RV in the popular television series *Breaking Bad*.

© A.F. Archive/Alamy

temporary state of paranoid **psychosis,** with delusions of persecution and episodes of unprovoked violence.

Methamphetamine is more addictive than other forms of amphetamine. It also is more dangerous because it is more toxic and its effects last longer. In the short term, meth can cause rapid breathing, increased body temperature, insomnia, tremors, anxiety, and convulsions. Meth use has been linked to high-risk sexual behavior and increased rates of sexually transmitted infections, including HIV infection. In the long term, the effects of meth can include weight loss, severe acne, hallucinations, paranoia, violence, and psychosis. Meth use may cause extensive tooth decay and tooth loss, a condition referred to as "meth mouth," but this may be due to poor hygiene associated with chronic meth use and severe drug dependence in general. Meth takes a toll on the user's heart and can cause heart attack and stroke. Methamphetamine users have signs of brain damage similar to those seen in Parkinson's disease patients. These symptoms can persist even after drug use ceases, causing impaired memory and motor coordination problems. Withdrawal from meth causes symptoms that may include muscle aches and tremors, profound fatigue, deep depression, despair, and apathy. Addiction to methamphetamine is associated with pronounced psychological cravings and obsessive drug-seeking behavior.

Women who use amphetamines during pregnancy risk premature birth, stillbirth, low birth weight, and early infant death. Babies born to amphetamine-using mothers have a higher incidence of cleft palate, cleft lip, and deformed limbs. They may also experience symptoms of withdrawal.

psychosis A severe mental disorder characterized by a distortion of reality; symptoms might include delusions or hallucinations.

TERMS

Ritalin A stimulant with amphetamine-like effects, Ritalin (methylphenidate) is used to treat attention-deficit/hyperactivity disorder (ADHD). When methylphenidate is injected or snorted, dependence and tolerance can result rapidly.

Caffeine Caffeine is a very popular psychoactive drug and also one of the most ancient. It is found in coffee, tea, cocoa, soft drinks, headache remedies, and OTC preparations like NoDoz. (Table 7.3 lists typical levels of caffeine in several popular beverages.) In ordinary doses, caffeine produces greater alertness and a sense of well-being.

Table 7.3	Caffeine Content of Popular Beverages	
COFFEE	SERVING SIZE (OZ.)	TYPICAL CAFFEINE LEVEL (MG)*
Regular coffee, brewed	8	95
Regular coffee, instant	8	93
Espresso	1	64
Decaffeinated coffee, brewed	8	5
Decaffeinated coffee, instant	8	2
TEA		
Regular tea, brewed	8	47
Decaffeinated tea, brewed	8	2
Green tea, brewed	8	Varies
SODA		
Code Red Mountain Dew	12	54
Mello Yello	12	53
Diet Coke	12	47
Dr. Pepper, Diet Dr. Pepper	12	41
Sunkist Orange Soda	12	41
Pepsi	12	38
Coca-Cola Classic, Diet Pepsi	12	35
ENERGY DRINKS		
No Name	8.4	280
SoBe No Fear	16	174
Monster Energy, Rockstar	16	160
SoBe Adrenaline Rush	16	152
Full Throttle, Full Throttle Fury	16	144
AMP Energy Drink	16	143
Red Bull	8.3	76
Vault	8	47

*Caffeine levels vary greatly by brand of product, manner of preparation, and amount consumed. The amounts shown here are averages based on tests conducted by a variety of organizations. The FDA limits the amount of caffeine in cola and pepper soft drinks to 71 milligrams per 12-ounce serving. To find the exact amount of caffeine in any product, check that product's label.

SOURCES: Center for Science in the Public Interest. 2007. *Caffeine Content of Food & Drugs* (http://www.cspinet.org/new/cafchart.htm); Mayo Clinic. 2008. *Caffeine Content in Tea, Soda, and More* (http://www.mayoclinic.com /health/caffeine/AN01211); U.S. Department of Agriculture, Agricultural Research Service. 2009. *USDA National Nutrient Database for Standard Reference, Release 22* (http://www.ars.usda.gov/ba/bhnrc/ndl).

It also decreases feelings of fatigue or boredom, so using caffeine may enable a person to keep at physically tiring or repetitive tasks longer. Such use is usually followed, however, by a sudden letdown. Caffeine does not noticeably influence a person's ability to perform complex mental tasks unless fatigue, boredom, or other factors have already affected normal performance.

Caffeine mildly stimulates the heart and respiratory system, increases muscular tremor, and enhances gastric secretion. Higher doses may cause nervousness, anxiety, irritability, headache, disturbed sleep, and gastric irritation or peptic ulcers. In people with high blood pressure, caffeine can cause blood pressure to rise even further above normal; in people with type 2 diabetes, caffeine may cause glucose and insulin levels to rise after meals.

Drinks containing caffeine are rarely harmful for most people, but some tolerance develops, and withdrawal symptoms of irritability, headaches, and even mild depression occur. People can usually avoid problems by simply decreasing their daily intake of caffeine.

ENERGY "SHOTS" The popularity of small (1.5- to 3-ounce) energy drinks has increased dramatically in recent years. Because these products are sold as dietary supplements rather than food, their caffeine content is not regulated by the FDA. Each two-ounce "shot" typically contains the same amount of caffeine (roughly 100 mg) as a regular-size cup of coffee.

Marijuana and Other Cannabis Products

With approximately 22.2 million current users, marijuana is the most widely used illegal drug in the United States. This status may be changing as more states—25 and the District of Columbia (DC) at the time of writing—legalize medical marijuana as well as regulate recreational usage. THC (tetrahydrocannabinol) is the main active ingredient in marijuana. Marijuana plants that grow wild often have less than 1% THC in their leaves. When selected strains are cultivated by separation of male and female plants (*sinsemilla*), the bud leaves from the flowering tops may contain 7–8% THC. Hashish, a potent preparation made from the thick resin that exudes from the marijuana leaves, may contain up to 14% THC.

These various preparations have all been known and used for centuries, so the frequently heard claim that today's marijuana is more potent than the marijuana of the 1970s is not strictly true. However, because a greater proportion of the marijuana sold today is the higher-potency (and more expensive) sinsemilla, the average potency of street marijuana has increased.

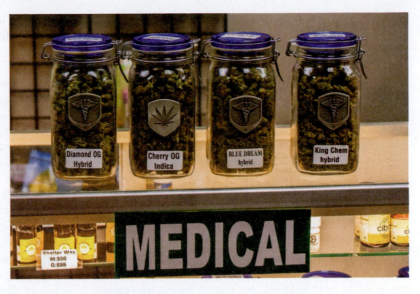

Some states permit the sale of both medical and recreational marijuana. The regulations typically differ for the two types of sales: In Colorado, for example, medical marijuana is taxed at a lower rate and is less expensive than recreational marijuana.
© Blaine Harrington III/Getty Images

Short-Term Effects and Uses As is true with most psychoactive drugs, the effects of a low dose of marijuana are strongly influenced both by the user's expectations and by past experiences. At low doses, marijuana users typically experience euphoria, a heightening of subjective sensory experiences, a slowing down of the perception of passing time, and a relaxed attitude. These pleasant effects are the reason this drug is so widely used. With moderate doses, marijuana's effects become stronger, and the user can also expect to have impaired memory function, disturbed thought patterns, lapses of attention, and feelings of **depersonalization,** in which the mind seems to be separated from the body.

Very high doses produce feelings of depersonalization, marked sensory distortion, and changes in body image (such as a feeling that the body is very light). Inexperienced users sometimes think these sensations mean they are going crazy and become anxious or even panicky.

Physiologically, marijuana increases heart rate and dilates certain blood vessels in the eyes, which creates the characteristic bloodshot eyes. The user may also feel less inclined toward physical exertion and may feel particularly hungry or thirsty. Because THC affects parts of the brain controlling balance, coordination, and reaction time, marijuana use impairs driving performance. The combination of alcohol and marijuana significantly impairs driving performance and increases crash risk.

Colorado, Washington, Alaska, Oregon, and the District of Columbia permit the recreational use of marijuana.

> **depersonalization** A state in which a person loses the sense of his or her reality or perceives his or her body as unreal. **TERMS**

The Supreme Court has held that state laws permitting medical marijuana use cannot supersede federal law. Thus, anyone using marijuana can still be prosecuted under federal drug laws, although the Obama administration indicated that it would not pursue such prosecutions.

Research shows benefits for using cannabis to treat muscle spasms in multiple sclerosis and cancer-related pain that is not otherwise relieved by opioid medications. Many cancer patients and people with AIDS use marijuana because they find it effective in relieving nausea and restoring appetite.

Long-Term Effects

The most probable long-term effect of smoking marijuana is respiratory damage, including impaired lung function and chronic bronchial irritation. Although no evidence links marijuana use to lung cancer, it may cause changes in lung tissue that promote cancer growth. Marijuana users may be at increased risk for emphysema and cancer of the head and neck, and among people with chronic conditions like cancer and AIDS, marijuana use is associated with increased risk of fatal lung infections. (These are key reasons why the Institute of Medicine has recommended the development of alternative methods of delivering the potentially beneficial compounds in marijuana.) Heavy users may experience learning problems, as well as subtle impairments of attention and memory that may or may not be reversible following long-term abstinence. Long-term use may also affect sperm productivity and quality.

Studies show that marijuana use during pregnancy may affect neural development. Children exposed to cannabis in-utero showed cognitive deficits, suggesting that maternal use of marijuana has interfered with the proper development of the brain. Babies born to mothers who used marijuana during pregnancy also had increased startles and tremors as well as difficulty adjusting to light. Their sleep patterns were altered, and they showed increased irritability. As children developed into adolescents, memory, impulsivity, and attention problems emerged. Moreover, THC rapidly enters breast milk and may impair an infant's early motor development.

Hallucinogens

As shown in Figure 7.1, **hallucinogens** are a group of drugs whose predominant pharmacological effect is to alter the user's perceptions, feelings, and thoughts.

LSD

LSD (lysergic acid diethylamide) is one of the most powerful psychoactive drugs. Tiny doses will produce noticeable effects in most people, such as an altered sense of time, visual disturbances, an improved sense of hearing, mood changes, and distortions in how people perceive their bodies. Dilation of the pupils and slight dizziness, weakness, and nausea may also occur. With larger doses, users may experience a phenomenon known as **synesthesia**: feelings of depersonalization and other alterations in the perceived relationship between the self and external reality.

A severe panic reaction, which can be terrifying in the extreme, can result from taking any dose of LSD. Even after the drug's chemical effects have worn off, spontaneous **flashbacks** and other psychological disturbances can occur.

MDMA

MDMA (methylenedioxymethamphetamine), and variants called ecstasy (MDMA with a stimulant such as caffeine added) and molly (a powder said to be "purer" than ecstasy), may be classified as a hallucinogen or a stimulant, having both hallucinogenic and amphetamine-like properties. Tolerance to MDMA develops quickly, leading users to take the drug more frequently, use higher doses, or combine MDMA with other drugs to enhance the drug's effects, and high doses can cause anxiety, delusions, and paranoia. Users may experience euphoria, increased energy, and a heightened sense of belonging. Using MDMA can produce dangerously high body temperature and potentially fatal dehydration; several cases have been reported of low total body salt concentrations (hyponatremia). Some users experience confusion, depression, anxiety, paranoia, muscle tension, involuntary teeth clenching, blurred vision, nausea, and seizures. Even low doses can affect concentration, judgment, and driving ability.

Other Hallucinogens

Most other hallucinogens have the same general effects as LSD, but there are some variations. For example, a DMT (dimethyltryptamine) or ketamine high does not last as long as an LSD high; an STP (4-methyl-2,5-dimethoxyamphetamine) high lasts longer.

PCP (phencyclidine) reduces and distorts sensory input, especially proprioception—the sensation of body position and movement—and creates a state of sensory deprivation. PCP was initially used as an anesthetic but was unsatisfactory because it caused agitation, confusion, and delirium (loss of contact with reality). Because it can be easily made, PCP is often available illegally and is sometimes used as an inexpensive replacement for other psychoactive drugs.

Mescaline, derived from the peyote cactus, is the ceremonial drug of the Native American Church. It causes effects similar to LSD, including altered perception and feeling; increased body temperature, heart rate, and blood pressure; weakness and trembling; and sleeplessness. Mescaline is expensive, so most street mescaline is diluted LSD or a mixture of other drugs. Hallucinogenic effects can be obtained from certain mushrooms (*Psilocybe mexicana*, or "magic mushrooms"), certain morning glory seeds, nutmeg, jimsonweed, and other botanical products; but unpleasant side effects, such as dizziness, have limited the popularity of these products.

> **TERMS**
>
> **hallucinogen**   Any of several drugs that alter perception, feelings, or thoughts; examples are LSD, mescaline, and PCP.
>
> **synesthesia**   A condition in which a stimulus evokes not only the sensation appropriate to it but also another sensation of a different character, such as when a color evokes a specific smell.
>
> **flashback**   A perceptual distortion or bizarre thought that recurs after the chemical effects of a drug have worn off.

Inhalants

Inhaling certain chemicals can produce effects ranging from heightened pleasure to delirium and death. Inhalants fall into several major groups: (1) volatile solvents, which are found in products such as paint thinner, glue, and gasoline; (2) aerosols, which are sprays that contain propellants and solvents; (3) nitrites, such as butyl nitrite and amyl nitrite; and (4) anesthetics, which include nitrous oxide (laughing gas).

Inhalant use tends to be highest among younger adolescents and declines with age. Inhalant use is difficult to control because inhalants are easy to obtain. They are present in a variety of seemingly harmless products, from dessert-topping sprays to underarm deodorants, that are both inexpensive and legal. Using the drugs also requires no illegal or suspicious paraphernalia. Inhalant users get high by sniffing, snorting, "bagging" (inhaling fumes from a plastic bag), or "huffing" (placing an inhalant-soaked rag in the mouth).

Although different in makeup, nearly all inhalants produce effects similar to those of anesthetics, which slow down body functions. Low doses may cause users to feel slightly stimulated; at higher doses, users may feel less inhibited and less in control. Sniffing high concentrations of the chemicals in solvents or aerosol sprays can cause a loss of consciousness, heart failure, and death. High concentrations of any inhalant can also cause death from suffocation by displacing oxygen in the lungs and central nervous system. Deliberately inhaling from a bag or in a closed area greatly increases the chances of suffocation. Other possible effects of the excessive or long-term use of inhalants include damage to the nervous system; hearing loss; increased risk of cancer; and damage to the liver, kidneys, and bone marrow.

Prescription Drug Misuse

The National Institute on Drug Abuse describes prescription drug abuse as the use of a medication without a prescription, in a way other than as prescribed, or for the experience or feelings elicited. Over the past decade, misuse of prescription drugs has increased and national surveys now show that prescription medications—such as those used to treat pain, ADHD, and anxiety—are being abused at a rate second only to marijuana and alcohol among Americans age 12 and over. More people died from drug overdoses in the United States in 2014 than in any previous year on record, outnumbering motor vehicle crashes one and a half times.

Among high school seniors, abuse of Adderall—the prescription form of amphetamine used to treat ADHD—has become a significant problem. In 2015, 7.5% of seniors reported nonmedical use of Adderall within the past year, up from 5.4% in 2009. More than one in five seniors (21.5%) have used at least one prescription medication without a doctor's orders at least once; 15.0% report use within the previous year. A study of college students

found that almost two-thirds (61.8%) were offered prescription stimulants for nonmedical use by their senior year and 31.0% used them. Studying was the predominant motive, and the most common source was a friend with a prescription.

Synthetic Recreational Drugs

In recent years, herbal or synthetic recreational drugs have become increasingly available. These "designer drugs" are intended to have pharmacological effects similar to those of illicit drugs but to be chemically distinct from them and therefore either legal or impossible to detect in drug screening. The drugs fall into two main groups. One group is marketed as synthetic marijuana and sold as "herbal incense," or "herbal highs," with names such as Spice, K2, Genie, and Mr. Nice Guy. The other group is marketed as stimulants with properties like those of cocaine or amphetamine and sold as "bath salts" with names such as Zoom, Ivory Wave, and White Rush.

Spice and other synthetic mimics of THC are distributed in the form of dried leaves or powder. They are typically smoked, using a pipe or by rolling in a cigarette paper, but can also be ingested as an infusion such as tea, or inhaled. The active ingredients in Spice and similar products are synthetic cannabinoids that act on brain cells to produce effects similar to those of THC, such as physical relaxation, changes in perception, elevated mood, and mild euphoria. Synthetic marijuana went through a period of initial popularity among teens and young adults. In 2011, 11.4% of high school seniors reported having used synthetic marijuana at least once during the year, according to the Monitoring the Future survey conducted by the University of Michigan. Usage dropped sharply beginning in 2013, and had declined to 5.2% by 2015; still, that represented use by 1 in 20 twelfth graders. A similar pattern was seen among full-time college students, with usage reported at 8.5% in 2011, declining to 1.5% in 2015.

Spice and similar products have not been included in any wide-scale animal or human studies, and little information is available in international medical databases. The blends of ingredients vary widely, but these products typically contain more than a dozen different plant-derived compounds, which give rise to a variety of drug combinations. Calls to poison control centers for exposure to synthetic marijuana doubled between 2010 and 2011, with patients describing symptoms that include rapid heart rate, vomiting, agitation, confusion, and hallucinations. In March 2011, the U.S. Drug Enforcement Administration (DEA) banned five synthetic cannabinoids used in Spice and similar products.

"Bath salts," marketed as cocaine or methamphetamine substitutes, are widely available on the Internet. They contain synthetic cathinones such as mephedrone, methylone, or methylenedioxypyrovalerone (MDPV). Emergency department admissions have increased for bath salts, with MDPV the most common synthetic cathinone found in blood and urine of patients. Similar in effect to MDMA (ecstasy), these cathinones are synthetic versions of the active ingredient found in the stimulant khat, a chewable leaf that is widely used in countries of the Middle East and Africa. The products are sold in small packets of salt-like crystals with warnings like "novelty only" and "not for human consumption." Bath salts can be ingested by smoking, eating, or injecting or by crushing them and snorting the powder. The speed of onset is up to 15 minutes depending on how the drug is ingested, and the effects may last as long as six hours. The effects of bath salts can be severe and include combative violent behavior, extreme agitation, confusion, hallucinations, hypertension, chest pain, and suicidal thoughts. In 2010, poison control centers in the United States received 304 calls about reactions to bath salts; the number rose to 6,138 calls in 2011. In September 2011, the DEA banned three of the drugs found in bath salts; possession or sale of the chemicals or products that contain them is now illegal.

PREVENTING DRUG-RELATED PROBLEMS

Although the use of some drugs, both legal and illegal, has declined dramatically since the 1970s, the use of others has held steady or increased. Mounting public concern has led to great debate and a wide range of opinions about what should be done. Efforts to address the problem include workplace drug testing, tougher law enforcement and prosecution, and treatment and education. With drugs entering the country on a massive scale from South America, Southeast Asia, and elsewhere, and being distributed through tightly controlled drug-smuggling organizations and street gangs, the success of any program is uncertain.

Drugs, Society, and Families

According to the U.S. Department of Justice, the National Drug Intelligence Center, and the National Institute on Drug Abuse, the cost to society of illicit drug use alone is $193 billion annually. That figure is higher than the cost of many major health problems, including diabetes, obesity, and smoking. But the costs are more than just financial—they are also paid in human pain and suffering.

The criminal justice system is inundated with people accused of crimes related to drug possession, sale, or use.

The FBI reports that roughly 1.5 million arrests are made annually for drug violations. In 2013, the most recent year for which data are available, about 16% of state prison inmates (208,000) were serving time for drug offenses. In 2015, almost half of federal inmates (86,080) were in prison because of drug offenses. The Bureau of Justice Statistics reports that about half of all state and federal prisoners—roughly 850,000 men and women—meet diagnostic criteria for drug abuse or addiction. Many assaults and murders are committed when people try to acquire or protect drug territories, settle disputes about drugs, or steal from dealers. Violence and gun use are common in neighborhoods where drug trafficking is prevalent. Addicts commit more robberies and burglaries than criminals not on drugs. People under the influence of drugs, especially alcohol, are more likely to commit violent crimes like rape and murder than are people who do not use drugs.

To what extent is drug misuse also a health care issue for society? In the United States, illegal drug use leads to more than 800,000 emergency department admissions and nearly 20,000 deaths annually. It is in the best interest of society to treat drug addiction in those who want help, but there is not nearly enough space in treatment facilities to help the millions of Americans who need immediate treatment.

Drug use takes a toll on individuals and families. Children born to women who use drugs such as alcohol, tobacco, or cocaine may have long-term health problems. Drug misuse in families can become a vicious cycle. Children who observe the adults around them using drugs assume it is acceptable. Abuse, neglect, lack of opportunity, and unemployment become contributing factors to drug use, perpetuating the cycle. Research also reveals some correlations between drug use and particular population groups (see box "Drug Use and Race/Ethnicity").

Legalizing Drugs

Pointing out that many of the social problems associated with drugs are related to prohibition (which failed for alcohol from 1920-1933) rather than to the effects of the drugs themselves, some people have argued for various forms of drug legalization or decriminalization. Proposals range from making drugs such as marijuana and heroin available by prescription to allowing licensed dealers to sell some of these drugs to adults. Proponents argue that legalizing some currently illicit drugs—but putting controls on them similar to those used for alcohol, tobacco, and prescription drugs—could eliminate many problems. Some states have adopted policies that decriminalize possession of small amounts of marijuana—that is, possession for recreational use either is legal or is treated as a misdemeanor crime without significant penalty. Opponents of drug legalization argue that allowing easier access to drugs would expose many more people to possible addiction. Drugs would be cheaper and easier to obtain, and drug use would be more socially acceptable. Legalizing drugs could cause an increase in drug use among children and teenagers. Opponents point out that

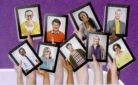

DIVERSITY MATTERS
Drug Use and Race/Ethnicity

Surveys of the U.S. population find a variety of trends in drug use and misuse among racial and ethnic groups (see the accompanying table). In addition to these general trends, there are also trends relating to specific drugs.

According to the Monitoring the Future survey, African American high school students have for many years had significantly lower rates of illicit drug use compared to white students. The gap has narrowed in recent years, however, due to increased rates of marijuana use among black students and a leveling off of marijuana use among whites. African American high school students at all grade levels report higher usage of bath salts and lower usage of hallucinogens than other groups. Among twelfth graders in 2015, heroin use was higher among black students (1.0%) than among whites (0.4%) and Hispanics (0.5%).

A similar rise in marijuana use has been seen among Hispanic students in recent years, with Hispanics reporting the highest levels of past-year marijuana use among students at grades 8, 10, and 12. Among twelfth graders, Hispanic students report the highest past-year use of synthetic marijuana,

Past-Month Illicit Drug Use among People Age 12 and Over by Race/Ethnicity, 2015

Race/Ethnicity	Percentage
Not Hispanic or Latino	
White	10.2
Black or African American	12.5
American Indian or Alaska Native	14.2
Native Hawaiian or Other Pacific Islander	9.8
Asian	4.0
Two or more races	17.2
Hispanic or Latino	9.2

cocaine, and inhalants. Overall, Hispanic students report the highest levels of illicit drug use in eighth grade, with the gap among groups narrowing by twelfth grade; the higher dropout rates among Hispanic students compared to whites and African Americans may contribute to this pattern.

White twelfth graders report the highest nonmedical use of several prescription drugs, including Oxycontin and Vicodin. In 2015, nonmedical use of Adderall among twelfth graders was reported by 8.4% of white students, 5.9% of black students, and 4.4% of Hispanic students. Alcohol use was also

highest among white students: the 30-day prevalence of alcohol use reported in 2015 among twelfth graders was 24.0% among blacks, 36.3% among Hispanics, and 40.9% among whites.

SOURCES: Johnston, L. D., et al. 2016. *Monitoring the Future National Survey Results on Drug Use, 1975–2015: Overview, Key Findings on Adolescent Drug Use.* Ann Arbor: Institute for Social Research, The University of Michigan; SAMHSA Center for Behavioral Health Statistics and Quality. 2016. *Results from the 2015 National Survey on Drug Use and Health* (http://www.samhsa.gov/data/sites/default/files/NSDUH-DetTabs-2015/NSDUH-DetTabs-2015/NSDUH-DetTabs-2015.htm).

---

alcohol and tobacco—drugs that already are legal—are major causes of disease and death in our society.

Drug Testing

According to data from recent surveys, the majority of substance users hold full-time jobs. Drug use in the workplace not only creates health problems for individual users but also has a negative effect on productivity and on safety of coworkers.

Statistics from the federal government show that 8.4% of full-time workers were illicit drug users in 2007, the most recent year for which data are available. In absolute numbers, approximately 13.1 million illicit drug users and 13.0 million heavy alcohol users were full-time workers in 2007. Illicit drug use is highest among workers in the food industry and construction sectors, while heavy alcohol use is greatest

> **QUICK STATS**
>
> In 2015, **3.7 million** people age 12 and over (1.4% of the population) received treatment for a problem related to the use of alcohol or illicit drugs.
>
> —Substance Abuse and Mental Health Services Administration, 2016

among construction, mining, and repair workers. The economic burden of lost productivity resulting from premature death, illness, and disability is estimated to run as high as $114 billion for drug misuse and $179 billion for heavy alcohol use.

The extent of the drug problem has given rise to the development of workplace policies to help workers regain their health and well-being. Workplace policies developed to address the problem often include drug testing and referral services. Despite controversial aspects of drug testing in the workplace, a growing number of U.S. workers recognize the need for such screening.

Most drug testing involves a urine test. Testing for alcohol may involve a blood or breath test. The accuracy of these tests has improved in recent years, so there are fewer opportunities for people to cheat or for the tests to yield inaccurate results. If a person tests positive for drugs, the employer may provide drug counseling or treatment, suspend the employee until he or she tests negative, or fire the individual.

Treating Drug Addiction

Under the Affordable Care Act, all insurance sold on health insurance exchanges or provided by Medicaid to certain newly eligible adults must include services for treatment of substance use disorders such as alcohol or drug addiction. Treatment for addiction often is characterized by discrete and repeated episodes of short-term abstinence and relapse. Regardless of the therapeutic approach, many individuals undergoing treatment often return to drug or alcohol use. Relapse, which commonly occurs within one year after treatment, can result in worsening of the original substance use problem.

Preventing relapse and maintaining long-term cessation of drug use is an exceedingly complex medical goal. Medical interventions based on pharmaceutical aids to enhance the individual's long-term commitment to change and stay drug-free remain challenging. Relapse prevention research includes expanding the repertoire of behavioral skills individuals need to decrease the risk of recidivism.

Medication-Assisted Treatment   Medications are increasingly being used in addiction treatment to reduce the craving for the abused drug or to block or oppose its effects. Perhaps the best-known medication for drug use is methadone, a synthetic drug used as a substitute for heroin. Methadone prevents withdrawal reactions and reduces the craving for heroin. Its use enables heroin-addicted people to function normally in social and vocational activities, although they remain dependent on methadone. The drug buprenorphine in combination with naloxone, approved for treatment of opioid addiction, reduces cravings and relapse.

Medication therapy can appear more efficacious and efficient and is therefore popular among patients and health care providers. However, the relapse rate remains high. Combining drug therapy with psychological and social services improves success rates, underscoring the importance of psychological factors in drug dependence.

Treatment Centers   Treatment centers offer a variety of short-term and long-term services, including hospitalization, detoxification, counseling, and other mental health services. The therapeutic community is a specific type of center, a residential program run in a completely drug-free atmosphere. Administered by ex-addicts, these programs use confrontation, strict discipline, and unrelenting peer pressure to attempt to resocialize the addicted individual with a different set of values. Halfway houses, which are transitional settings between a 24-hour-a-day program and independent living, are an important phase of treatment for some people.

Groups and Peer Counseling   Groups such as Alcoholics Anonymous (AA) and Narcotics Anonymous (NA)

have helped many people. People receiving treatment in drug substitution programs or substance use treatment centers are often urged or required to join a mutual-help group as part of their recovery. Many of these groups follow a 12-step program. Group members' first step is to acknowledge that they have a problem over which they have no control. Peer support is a critical ingredient of these programs, and members usually meet at least once a week. As part of a 12-step program, each member is paired with a sponsor to call on for advice and guidance in working through the 12 steps and getting support if the temptation to relapse becomes overwhelming. With such support, thousands of substance-dependent people have been able to recover, remain abstinent, and reclaim their lives. Chapters of AA and NA meet on some college campuses; community-based chapters are listed in the phone book, in local newspapers, and online. Other organizations provide an alternative to the 12 steps such as LifeRing Secular Recovery, Rational Recovery, SMART Recovery, Women for Sobriety, and Refuge Recovery.

Many colleges also have peer counseling programs, in which students are trained to help other students who have drug problems. A peer counselor's role may be as limited as referring a student to a professional with expertise in substance dependence for an evaluation or as involved as helping arrange a leave of absence from school for participation in a drug treatment program (see the box "If Someone You Know Has a Drug Problem . . .").

Harm Reduction Strategies   Because many attempts at treatment are at first unsuccessful, some experts advocate the use of harm reduction strategies. The goal of harm reduction is to minimize the negative effects of drug use and misuse: A common example is the use of designated drivers to reduce alcohol-related motor vehicle crashes. Drug substitution programs such as methadone maintenance are another well-known form of harm reduction; although participants remain drug dependent, the negative consequences of their drug use are reduced. Additional examples of harm reduction strategies include the following:

- Syringe exchange programs, designed to reduce transmission of HIV and hepatitis C
- Safe injection facilities or sites where heroin users can go to inject heroin under medical supervision
- Provision of easy-to-use forms of naloxone, a drug that rapidly reverses opioid overdose, to family members and caregivers of heroin users; in 2014, the FDA approved a hand-held naloxone autoinjector
- Free testing of street drugs for purity and potency to help users avoid unintentional toxicity or overdose

Codependency   Many treatment programs also offer counseling for those who are close to drug abusers. Drug misuse takes a toll on friends and family members, and counseling can help people work through painful feelings of guilt and

Changes in behavior and mood in someone you know may signal a growing dependence on drugs. Signs that a person's life is beginning to focus on drugs include the following:

- Sudden withdrawal or emotional distance
- Rebellious or unusually irritable behavior
- A loss of interest in usual activities or hobbies
- A decline in school performance
- A sudden change in the chosen group of friends
- Changes in sleeping or eating habits
- Frequent borrowing of money or stealing
- Secretive behavior about personal possessions, such as a backpack or the contents of a drawer
- Deterioration of physical appearance

If you believe a family member or friend has a drug problem, locate information about drug treatment resources available on campus or in your community. Communicate your concern, provide him or her with information about treatment options, and offer your support during treatment. If the person continues to deny having a problem, talk with an experienced counselor about setting up an intervention—a formal, structured confrontation designed to end denial by having family, friends, and other caring people present their concerns to the drug user. Participants in an intervention would indicate the ways in which the individual is hurting others as well as himself or herself. If your friend or family member agrees to treatment, encourage him or her to attend a support group such as Narcotics Anonymous or Alcoholics Anonymous.

And finally, examine your relationship with the abuser for signs of codependency. If necessary, get help for yourself; friends and family of drug users can often benefit from counseling.

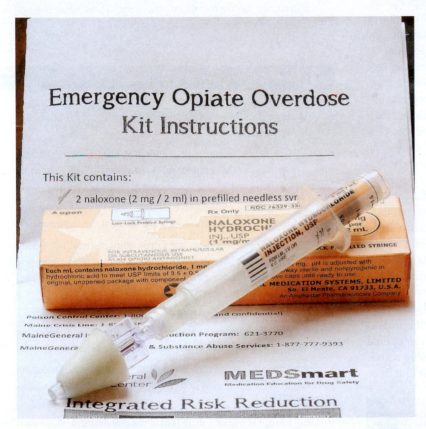

A naloxone kit is an example of a harm reduction strategy for people at risk of an opioid overdose.

© Portland Press Herald/Joe Phelan/Getty Images

approval, and security are contingent on their taking care of the abuser. People can become codependent naturally because they want to help when someone they love becomes dependent on a drug. They may assume that their good intentions will persuade the drug user to stop.

Codependent people often engage in behaviors that remove or soften the effects of drug use on the user—so-called *enabling* behaviors. The habit of enabling can inhibit a drug abuser's recovery because the person never has to experience the consequences of his or her behavior. Often the enabler is dependent, too—on the patterns of interaction in the relationship. People who need to take care of others often marry people who need to be taken care of. Children in these families often develop the same behavior pattern as one of their parents—either becoming helpless or becoming a caregiver. For this reason, many treatment programs involve the whole family.

Have you ever been an enabler in a relationship? You may have if you've ever done any of the following:

- Given someone countless chances to stop abusing drugs
- Made excuses or lied for someone to his or her friends, teachers, or employer

powerlessness. **Codependency,** in which a person close to the drug abuser is controlled by the abuser's behavior, sometimes develops. Codependent people may come to believe that love,

- Joined someone in drug use and blamed others for your behavior
- Lent money to someone to continue drug use
- Stayed up late waiting for or gone out searching for someone who uses drugs
- Felt embarrassed or angry about the actions of someone who uses drugs
- Ignored the drug use because the person got defensive when you brought it up
- Avoided confronting a friend or relative who was obviously intoxicated or high on a drug

If you come from a codependent family or see yourself developing codependency relationships or engaging in enabling behaviors, consider acting now to make changes in your patterns of interaction. Remember, you cannot cause or cure drug addiction in another person.

Preventing Drug Misuse

Obviously the best solution to drug misuse is prevention. Government attempts at controlling the drug problem have historically focused on stopping the production, importation, and distribution of illegal drugs. A national drug policy announced in 2010, however, redirects federal funding and efforts into stopping the demand for drugs. Developing persuasive antidrug educational programs may offer the best hope for solving the drug problem in the future. Indirect approaches to prevention involve building young people's self-esteem, improving their academic skills, and increasing their recreational opportunities. Direct approaches involve providing information about the adverse effects of drugs and teaching tactics that help students resist peer pressure to use drugs in various situations. Developing strategies for resisting peer pressure is one of the more effective techniques.

Prevention efforts need to focus on the different motivations individuals have for using and misusing specific drugs at different ages. For example, grade-school children seem receptive to programs that involve their parents or well-known adults such as professional athletes. Adolescents in junior or senior high school are often more responsive to peer counselors. Many young adults tend to be influenced by efforts that focus on health education. For all ages, it is important to provide nondrug alternatives—such as recreational facilities, counseling, greater opportunities for leisure activities, and places to socialize—that speak to the individual's or

group's specific reasons for using drugs. Reminding young people that most people, no matter what age, are *not* users of illegal drugs, do *not* smoke cigarettes, and do not get drunk frequently is a critical part of preventing substance misuse.

TIPS FOR TODAY AND THE FUTURE

RIGHT NOW YOU CAN:
- Look for ways to cut back on caffeine if you are a regular user.
- Consider whether you or someone you know might benefit from drug counseling. Find out what types of services are available on campus or in your area.

IN THE FUTURE YOU CAN:
- Think about the drug-related attitudes of people you know. For example, talk to two older adults and two fellow students about their attitudes toward legalizing marijuana. What are the differences in their opinions, and how do they account for them?
- Analyze media portrayals of drug use. As you watch television shows and movies, note the way they depict drug use among people of different ages and backgrounds. How realistic are the portrayals, in your view? Think about the influence they have on you and your peers.

SUMMARY

- Addiction is a bio-psycho-social-spiritual process that is a chronic medical condition.

- Addictive behaviors are self-reinforcing. Addicts experience a strong compulsion for the behavior and a loss of control over it; an escalating pattern of misuse with serious negative consequences may result.

- Drug misuse is a maladaptive pattern of drug use that persists despite adverse social, psychological, or medical consequences.

- Drug addiction involves taking a drug compulsively, neglecting constructive activities because of it, and continuing to use it despite the adverse effects resulting from its use. Tolerance and withdrawal symptoms are often present.

- The sources or causes of addiction include heredity, personality, lifestyle, and environmental factors. People may use an addictive behavior as a means of alleviating stress or painful emotions.

- Some common behaviors are potentially addictive, including gambling, shopping, sexual activity, Internet use, eating, exercising, and working.

- Drug misuse is use of a drug that is not consistent with medical or legal guidelines.

- Criteria for a substance use disorder are grouped in four categories: impaired control, social problems, risky use, and drug effects.

- Reasons for using drugs include the lure of the illicit, curiosity, rebellion, peer pressure, and the desire to alter your mood or escape boredom, anxiety, depression, or other psychological problems.

Ask Yourself

QUESTIONS FOR CRITICAL THINKING AND REFLECTION

Do you know someone who may have a drug problem? What steps, if any, have you taken to help that person? If you were using drugs and felt that things had gone out of control, what would you want your friends to do for you?

- Risks associated with drug misuse include intoxication, unexpected side effects, the ingestion of unknown drug constituents, injection-related infections, and legal consequences.

- Psychoactive drugs affect the mind and body by altering brain chemistry. The effect of a drug depends on its properties and on how it's used (drug factors), the physical and psychological characteristics of the user (user factors), and the physical and social environment surrounding the drug use (social factors).

- Opioids relieve pain, cause drowsiness, and induce euphoria; they reduce anxiety and produce lethargy, apathy, and an inability to concentrate.

- CNS depressants slow down the overall activity of the central nervous system; they reduce anxiety and cause mood changes, impaired muscular coordination, slurring of speech, and drowsiness or sleep.

- CNS stimulants speed up the activity of the central nervous system, causing acceleration of the heart rate, a rise in blood pressure, dilation of the pupils and bronchial tubes, and an increase in gastric and adrenal secretions.

- Marijuana usually causes euphoria and a relaxed attitude at low doses; very high doses produce feelings of depersonalization and sensory distortion. Use during pregnancy may impair fetal growth.

- Hallucinogens alter perception, feelings, and thoughts and may cause an altered sense of time, visual disturbances, and mood changes.

- Inhalants are present in a variety of everyday products; they can cause delirium. Their use can lead to loss of consciousness, heart failure, suffocation, and death.

- Economic and social costs of drug misuse include the financial costs of law enforcement, treatment, and health care and the social costs of crime, violence, and family problems. Drug testing and drug legalization have been proposed to address some of the problems related to drug use.

- Approaches to treatment include medication, treatment centers, self-help groups, and peer counseling; many programs also offer counseling to family members.

FOR MORE INFORMATION

American Society of Addiction Medicine: Patient Resources. Provides information about treatment and support groups.
http://www.asam.org/quality-practice/patient-guidelines-resources

Do It Now Foundation. Provides youth-oriented information about drugs.
http://www.doitnow.org

Drug Enforcement Administration (DEA): Drug Facts Sheets. Provides basic facts about major drugs of abuse.
https://www.dea.gov/druginfo/factsheets.shtml

Go Ask Alice. A health question-and-answer resource produced by Columbia University; see "Alcohol & Other Drugs" in the Health Answers section.
http://goaskalice.columbia.edu

National Center on Addiction and Substance Abuse. Provides information on addiction, including prevention and treatment.
http://www.centeronaddiction.org

National Council on Problem Gambling. Provides information and help for people with gambling problems and their families.
http://www.ncpgambling.org

National Drug Information, Treatment, and Referral Hotlines (SAMHSA: see below)
800-662-HELP
800-729-6686 (Spanish)
800-487-4889 (TDD for hearing impaired)

National Institute on Drug Abuse (NIDA). Develops and supports research on drug addiction prevention; provides background information on drugs of abuse.
http://www.drugabuse.gov

Net Addiction: FAQs. Provides background information on Internet Addiction Disorder.
http://netaddiction.com

Partnership for Drug-Free Kids: Drug Guide. A comprehensive source of information on specific drugs.
http://www.drugfree.org/drug-guide

Substance Abuse and Mental Health Services Administration (SAMHSA). Provides statistics, information, and other resources related to substance abuse prevention and treatment.
http://www.samhsa.gov

The following additional organizations/websites provide support services:

Alcoholics Anonymous (AA)
http://www.aa.org/

Cocaine Anonymous (CA)
https://ca.org

Debtors Anonymous (DA)
http://debtorsanonymous.org

Gamblers Anonymous (GA)
http://www.gamblersanonymous.org/ga/

LifeRing® Secular Recovery
http://lifering.org/

Marijuana Anonymous (MA)
http://www.marijuana-anonymous.org

Narcotics Anonymous (NA)
http://www.na.org

Overeaters Anonymous (OA)
https://oa.org

Refuge Recovery
http://www.refugerecovery.org

Sex Addicts Anonymous (SAA)
https://saa-recovery.org

SMART® Recovery
http://www.smartrecovery.org

Women For Sobriety
http://www.womenforsobriety.org

SELECTED BIBLIOGRAPHY

American College Health Association. 2014. *American College Health Association-National College Health Assessment II: Reference Group Executive Summary Spring 2014.* Hanover, MD: American College Health Association.

American Psychiatric Association. 2013. *Diagnostic and Statistical Manual of Mental Disorders,* 5th ed. Washington, DC: American Psychiatric Publishing

American Psychiatric Association. 2015. *What Is Addiction?* (https://www.psychiatry.org/patients-families/addiction/what-is-addiction).

Centers for Disease Control and Prevention. 2015. *HIV Surveillance Report, 2014;* vol. 26. http://www.cdc.gov/hiv/library/reports/surveillance.

Centers for Disease Control and Prevention. 2015. *Today's Heroin Epidemic* (http://www.cdc.gov/vitalsigns/heroin/index.html).

Centers for Disease Control and Prevention. 2016. Increases in drug and opioid overdose deaths—United States, 2000-2014. *MMWR* 64(50): 1378-1382.

Centers for Disease Control and Prevention. 2016. *Surveillance for Viral Hepatitis–United States, 2014* (http://www.cdc.gov/hepatitis/statistics/2014surveillance/commentary.htm).

Drug Enforcement Administration, U.S. Department of Justice. 2011. *Drugs of Abuse: A DEA Resource Guide, 2011 Edition* (http://www.justice.gov/dea/pubs/drugs_of_abuse.pdf).

Garnier-Dykstra, L. M., et al. 2012. Nonmedical use of prescription stimulants during college: Four-year trends in exposure opportunity, use, motives, and sources. *Journal of American College Health* 60(3): 226–234.

Johnston, L. D., et al. 2016. *Monitoring the Future National Survey Results on Drug Use, 1975–2015.* Vol. 2: *College Students and Adults Ages 19–55.* Ann Arbor: Institute for Social Research, University of Michigan.

National Council on Problem Gambling. 2016. *What Is Problem Gambling?* (http://www.ncpgambling.org/help-treatment/faq/).

National Institute on Drug Abuse. 2014. *The Science of Drug Abuse and Addiction: The Basics* (https://www.drugabuse.gov/publications/media-guide/science-drug-abuse-addiction-basics).

Office of National Drug Control Policy. 2015. *National Drug Control Strategy* (https://www.whitehouse.gov/ondcp/national-drug-control-strategy).

Rudd, R. A., et al. 2016. Increases in drug and opioid overdose deaths—United States, 2000–2014. *MMWR* 64(50): 1378-1382.

SAMHSA Center for Behavioral Health Statistics and Quality. 2016. *Results from the 2015 National Survey on Drug Use and Health* (http://www.samhsa.gov/data/sites/default/files/NSDUH-DetTabs-2015/NSDUH-DetTabs-2015/NSDUH-DetTabs-2015.htm).

Swan, S. C., et al. 2016. Just a dare or unaware? Outcomes and motives of drugging ("drink spiking") among students at three college campuses. *Psychology of Violence,* 23 May (advance online publication).

U.S. Department of Justice, Federal Bureau of Investigation. 2014. *Crime in the United States: 2014* (https://www.fbi.gov/about-us/cjis/ucr/crime-in-the-u.s/2014/crime-in-the-u.s.-2014/persons-arrested/main).

U.S. Food and Drug Administration. 2014. FDA approves new hand-held auto-injector to reverse opioid overdose (http://www.fda.gov/NewsEvents/Newsroom/PressAnnouncements/ucm391465.htm).

U.S. Food and Drug Administration. 2015. Combating misuse and abuse of prescription drugs: Q&A with Michael Klein, Ph.D. (http://www.fda.gov/ForConsumers/ConsumerUpdates/ucm220112.htm).

Volkow, N. D., and A. T. McLellan. 2016. Opioid abuse in chronic pain—misconceptions and mitigation strategies. *New England Journal of Medicine* 374: 1253-1263.

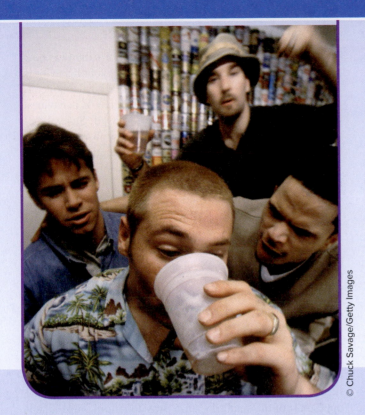
© Chuck Savage/Getty Images

CHAPTER 8

Alcohol and Tobacco

CHAPTER OBJECTIVES

- Understand how alcoholic beverages affect your body
- Describe the immediate and long-term effects of drinking alcohol
- Understand what constitutes excessive use of alcohol
- Explain the demographic patterns related to tobacco use
- List the reasons why people use tobacco
- Explain the health hazards associated with tobacco use
- Discuss the effects of smoking on nonsmokers
- List social and legislative actions that can be taken to combat smoking
- Explain strategies that help people stop using tobacco

Despite numerous prohibitions against it throughout history, alcohol has remained the most popular psychoactive drug in the Western world. Alcohol plays contradictory roles in human behavior. Used in moderation, alcohol can enhance social occasions by loosening inhibitions and creating pleasant feelings of relaxation. But alcohol can also be unhealthful. Like other drugs, alcohol produces physiological effects that can impair functioning in the short term while causing devastating damage in the long term. For some people, alcohol use can fuel an addiction, leading to a lifetime of recovery or, for a few, to debilitation and death.

This chapter discusses the complexities of alcohol and tobacco use and provides information that will help you make choices that are right for you. See Chapter 7 for a discussion of the terms *abuse, use,* and *misuse.* Here they are used somewhat interchangeably.

alcohol The intoxicating ingredient in fermented or distilled beverages; a colorless, pungent liquid.
TERMS

ALCOHOLIC BEVERAGES AND THEIR EFFECTS ON THE BODY

If you are ever around people who are drinking, you probably notice that alcohol affects different people in different ways. One person may seem to get drunk after just a drink or two, while another appears to tolerate a great deal of alcohol without becoming intoxicated. These differences make alcohol's effects on the body seem mysterious and help explain why many misconceptions have evolved about alcohol use. The following sections examine how alcohol works in the body.

Common Alcoholic Beverages

Technically speaking, there are many kinds of **alcohol,** and each is an organic compound. In this book, however, the term *alcohol* refers only to ethyl alcohol (or ethanol). Several kinds of alcohol are chemically similar to ethyl alcohol, such as methanol (wood alcohol) and isopropyl alcohol (rubbing alcohol), but they are highly toxic; if consumed, these forms of alcohol can cause serious illness, blindness, and even death.

There are several basic types of alcoholic beverages. Ethanol is the psychoactive ingredient in each of them:

• Beer is a mild intoxicant brewed from a mixture of grains. By volume, beer usually contains 3–6% alcohol.

• Ales and malt liquors, which also have grain bases and are similar to beer in their processing, typically contain 6–8% alcohol by volume.

• Wines are made by fermenting the juices of grapes or other fruits. During *fermentation*, sugars from the fruit react with yeast to create ethanol and other by-products. In table wines, the concentration of alcohol is about 9–14%. A more potent type of wine, *fortified wine*, is called this because extra alcohol is added during its production. Fortified wines—such as sherry, port, and Madeira—contain about 20% alcohol.

• Hard liquor—such as gin, whiskey, rum, tequila, vodka, and liqueur—is made by *distilling* brewed or fermented grains or other plant products. Hard liquors usually contain 35–50% alcohol but can be much stronger.

The concentration of alcohol in a beverage is indicated by its **proof value,** which amounts to two times the percentage concentration. For example, if a beverage is 100 proof, it contains 50% alcohol by volume. Two ounces of 100-proof whiskey contain one ounce of pure alcohol. The proof value of hard liquor can usually be found on the bottle's label.

"Standard Drinks" versus Actual Servings When discussing alcohol consumption, the term **one drink** or (*a standard drink*) refers to the amount of a beverage that typically contains about 0.6 ounce of alcohol. A 12-ounce bottle of beer, a 5-ounce glass of wine, and a 1.5 ounce shot of hard liquor are all considered one drink.

A typical serving of most alcoholic beverages is larger (sometimes significantly larger) than a single standard drink. This is particularly true of mixed drinks, which often include more than one type of hard liquor.

Caloric Content Alcohol provides 7 calories per gram, and the alcohol in one drink (14–17 grams) supplies about 100–120 calories. Most alcoholic beverages also contain some carbohydrate; for example, one beer provides about 150 total calories. The "light" in light beer refers to calories; a light beer typically has close to the same alcohol content as a regular beer and about 100 calories. A 5-ounce glass of red wine has 100 calories; white wine has 96. A 3-ounce margarita supplies 157 calories, a 6-ounce cosmopolitan has 143 calories, and a 6-ounce rum and Coke contains about 180 calories.

> **proof value**   Two times the percentage of alcohol, by volume, in an alcoholic beverage; a "100-proof" beverage is 50% alcohol by volume.
>
> **one drink**   The amount of a beverage that typically contains about 0.6 ounce of alcohol; also called a *standard drink*.
>
> **TERMS**

Absorption

The rate at which your body absorbs alcohol will affect how quickly you feel drunk and also how quickly your behavior is impaired. In fact, the speed at which your blood alcohol concentration rises has been linked to the degree of behavioral impairment, more than the concentration itself. Several factors determine the rate of absorption: how fast you drink, how fast your stomach empties its contents, and how much and what type of food and other drugs are in your system. Food in the stomach slows the rate of absorption.

The kind of alcohol (volume, concentration, and nature) also affects absorption. For example, the carbonation in a beverage like champagne increases the rate of alcohol absorption, as do artificial sweeteners (commonly used in drink mixers). You may be surprised to know that drinking highly concentrated alcoholic beverages such as hard liquor slows absorption. And a biological influence on rate of absorption is the gender and ethnic group to which you belong, a topic discussed later in the chapter.

How does absorption occur? When a person ingests alcohol, a small amount diffuses into the lining of the mouth. From the stomach, about 20% goes directly into the bloodstream, and about 75% of the alcohol is absorbed through the upper part of the small intestine. Any remaining alcohol enters the bloodstream farther along the gastrointestinal (GI) tract. Once in the bloodstream, alcohol produces sensations of intoxication.

Metabolism and Excretion

Once alcohol has been absorbed, it metabolizes, meaning that it transforms into usable substances and waste. The usable parts are transformed into energy and fat reserves in the following way.

The circulatory system quickly transports alcohol throughout the body. Because alcohol easily moves through most biological membranes, it is rapidly distributed throughout most body tissues. Although a small amount of alcohol is metabolized in the stomach, most metabolization occurs in the liver. The alcohol is converted first to acetaldehyde, then to acetate through the help of several enzymes. Individuals vary slightly in the enzymes they have inherited and so can display different reactions to alcohol. (See the box "Metabolizing Alcohol: Our Bodies Work Differently.")

About 2–10% of ingested alcohol is not metabolized in the liver or other tissues but is excreted unchanged by the lungs, kidneys, and sweat glands. Excreted alcohol causes the telltale smell on a drinker's breath and is the basis of breath and urine analyses for alcohol levels.

Alcohol readily enters the human brain, affecting neurotransmitters—the chemicals that carry messages between brain cells. These changes are temporary, creating many of the immediate effects of drinking alcohol. With chronic heavy use, however, alcohol's disruptive effects can become permanent, resulting in loss of brain function and changes in brain structure.

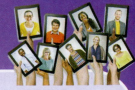
Do you and your friends react differently to alcohol? If so, your reactions may be affected by genetic differences in alcohol metabolism. **Metabolism** refers to the chemical transformation of alcohol and other substances in your body into energy and waste. Alcohol is metabolized mainly in the liver, where an enzyme, alcohol dehydrogenase, converts the alcohol into a toxic substance called acetaldehyde. Acetaldehyde causes many of alcohol's noxious effects. Ideally it is quickly broken down to a less active by-product, acetate, by another enzyme, acetaldehyde dehydrogenase (ALDH). Acetate can then separate into water and carbon dioxide and easily be eliminated. But people vary in the length of time it takes to break down the toxins in alcohol and in how efficiently they can process them. Some differences in metabolism are associated with ethnicity.

Some people, primarily those of Asian descent, inherit ineffective or inactive variations of that latter enzyme, acetaldehyde dehydrogenase. Others, including some people of African and Jewish descent, have forms of alcohol dehydrogenase that metabolize alcohol to acetaldehyde very quickly. Either way, toxic acetaldehyde builds up when these people drink alcohol. They experience a reaction called *flushing syndrome*. Their skin feels hot, their heart and respiration rates increase, and they may get a headache, vomit, or break out in hives. The severity of their reactions is affected by the inherited form of their alcohol-metabolizing enzymes. Drinking makes some people so uncomfortable that they are unlikely to develop alcohol addiction.

The body's response to acetaldehyde is the basis for treating alcohol misuse with the drug disulfiram (Antabuse), which inhibits the action of acetaldehyde dehydrogenase. When a person taking disulfiram ingests alcohol, acetaldehyde levels increase rapidly, and he or she develops an intense flushing reaction along with weakness, nausea, vomiting, and other disagreeable symptoms.

How people behave in relation to alcohol is influenced in complex ways by a wide range of factors, including liver size, body mass, and social and cultural influences. But individual choices and behavior are also strongly influenced by specific genetic characteristics.

Alcohol Intake and Blood Alcohol Concentration

Blood alcohol concentration (BAC) is the ratio of alcohol in a person's blood by weight, expressed as the percentage of alcohol measured in a deciliter of blood. BAC is affected by the amount of alcohol consumed in a given amount of time and by individual factors:

- *Body weight.* In most cases, a smaller person develops a higher BAC than a larger person after drinking the same amount of alcohol (Figure 8.1). A smaller person has less overall body tissue into which alcohol can be distributed.

- *Percentage of body fat.* A person with a higher percentage of body fat will usually develop a higher BAC than a more muscular person of the same weight. Alcohol does not concentrate as much in fatty tissue as in muscle and most other tissues, in part because fat has fewer blood vessels.

- *Sex.* Women metabolize less alcohol in the stomach than men do because the stomach enzyme that breaks down alcohol before it enters the bloodstream is four times more active in men than in women, thus releasing more unmetabolized alcohol into the bloodstream in women. Hormonal fluctuations may also affect the rate of alcohol metabolism, making a woman more susceptible to high BACs at certain times during her menstrual cycle.

> **QUICK STATS**
>
> In the United States, about **90,000** deaths are related to excessive alcohol use each year.
>
> —Centers for Disease Control and Prevention, 2015a

BAC also depends on the balance between the rate of alcohol absorption and the rate of alcohol metabolism. A man who weighs 150 pounds and has normal liver function metabolizes about 0.3 ounce of alcohol per hour, the equivalent of about half a 12-ounce bottle of beer or half a 5-ounce glass of wine.

The rate of alcohol metabolism varies among individuals and is determined largely by genetic factors and drinking behavior. Chronic drinking activates enzymes that metabolize alcohol in the liver, so people who drink frequently metabolize alcohol at a more rapid rate than nondrinkers. Although the rate of alcohol absorption can be slowed by factors like food, the metabolic rate *cannot* be influenced by exercise, breathing deeply, eating, drinking coffee, or taking other drugs. Whether a person is asleep or awake, the rate of alcohol metabolism is the same.

> **TERMS**
>
> **metabolism** The chemical transformation of food and other substances in the body into energy and wastes, first through breaking apart the components and then using them in other forms.
>
> **blood alcohol concentration (BAC)** The amount of alcohol in the blood expressed as the percentage of alcohol in a deciliter of blood; used as a measure of intoxication.

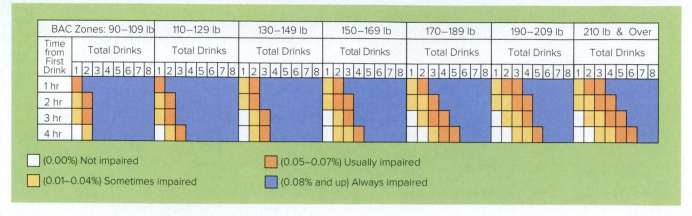

BAC Zones:	90–109 lb	110–129 lb	130–149 lb	150–169 lb	170–189 lb	190–209 lb	210 lb & Over
Time from First Drink	Total Drinks	Total Drinks	Total Drinks	Total Drinks	Total Drinks	Total Drinks	Total Drinks
	1 2 3 4 5 6 7 8	1 2 3 4 5 6 7 8	1 2 3 4 5 6 7 8	1 2 3 4 5 6 7 8	1 2 3 4 5 6 7 8	1 2 3 4 5 6 7 8	1 2 3 4 5 6 7 8
1 hr							
2 hr							
3 hr							
4 hr							

☐ (0.00%) Not impaired   ☐ (0.05–0.07%) Usually impaired
☐ (0.01–0.04%) Sometimes impaired   ☐ (0.08% and up) Always impaired

FIGURE 8.1 **Approximate blood alcohol concentration (BAC) and body weight.** This chart illustrates the BAC an average person of a given weight would reach after drinking the specified number of drinks in the time shown. The federal legal limit for BAC for drivers is 0.08%; for drivers under 21 years of age, many states have zero-tolerance laws that set BAC limits of 0.01% or 0.02%.

If a person absorbs slightly less alcohol each hour than he or she can metabolize in an hour, the BAC remains low. People can drink large amounts of alcohol this way over a long period of time without becoming noticeably intoxicated. Even so, they run the risk of long-term health problems (described later in the chapter). If a person drinks alcohol more quickly than it can be metabolized, the BAC will increase steadily, and he or she will become more and more intoxicated (see Figure 8.2).

ALCOHOL'S IMMEDIATE AND LONG-TERM EFFECTS

The effects of alcohol consumption on health depend on the individual, the circumstances, and the amount of alcohol consumed.

Immediate Effects

Blood alcohol concentration is a primary factor determining the effects of alcohol. At low concentrations, alcohol tends to make people feel relaxed and jovial, but at higher concentrations, people are more likely to feel angry, sedated, or sleepy. In general, alcohol slows reactions, impairs coordination and judgment, and eventually, sedates to inactivity. The senses become less acute.

Low Concentrations of Alcohol The effects of alcohol can first be felt at a BAC of 0.03–0.05%. These effects may include lightheadedness, relaxation, and a release of inhibitions. Most drinkers experience mild euphoria and become more sociable. When people drink in social settings, alcohol often seems to act as a stimulant, enhancing conviviality or assertiveness. This apparent stimulation occurs because alcohol depresses inhibitory centers in the brain.

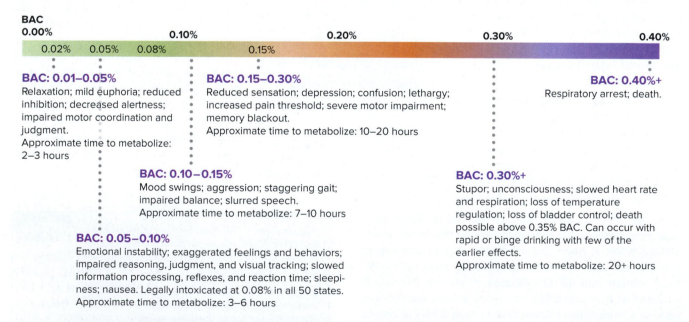

BAC: 0.01–0.05%
Relaxation; mild euphoria; reduced inhibition; decreased alertness; impaired motor coordination and judgment.
Approximate time to metabolize: 2–3 hours

BAC: 0.05–0.10%
Emotional instability; exaggerated feelings and behaviors; impaired reasoning, judgment, and visual tracking; slowed information processing, reflexes, and reaction time; sleepiness; nausea. Legally intoxicated at 0.08% in all 50 states.
Approximate time to metabolize: 3–6 hours

BAC: 0.10–0.15%
Mood swings; aggression; staggering gait; impaired balance; slurred speech.
Approximate time to metabolize: 7–10 hours

BAC: 0.15–0.30%
Reduced sensation; depression; confusion; lethargy; increased pain threshold; severe motor impairment; memory blackout.
Approximate time to metabolize: 10–20 hours

BAC: 0.30%+
Stupor; unconsciousness; slowed heart rate and respiration; loss of temperature regulation; loss of bladder control; death possible above 0.35% BAC. Can occur with rapid or binge drinking with few of the earlier effects.
Approximate time to metabolize: 20+ hours

BAC: 0.40%+
Respiratory arrest; death.

FIGURE 8.2 **Effects of blood alcohol concentration (BAC) at each stage of intoxication.**

Remember: Being very drunk is potentially life-threatening. Helping a drunken friend could save a life.

• Be firm but calm. Don't engage the person in an argument or discuss her drinking behavior while she is intoxicated.

• Get the person out of harm's way. Don't let her drive, wander outside, or drink any more alcohol. Reduce stimuli and create a safe, quiet place.

• If possible without distressing the person, try to find out what and how much she drank, and when as well as what other drugs or medications she took, how much, and when.

• If the person is unconscious, don't assume she is just "sleeping it off." Place her on her side with her knees up. This position helps prevent choking if she vomits.

• Monitor airway, breathing, and circulation (check pulse).

• Stay with the person. You need to be ready to help if she vomits or stops breathing.

• Don't try to give the person anything to eat or drink, including coffee or other drugs. Don't give cold showers or try to make her walk around. None of these things help anyone to sober up, and they can be dangerous.

Call 911 immediately in any of the following instances:

• You can't wake the person even with shouting or shaking.

• The person is taking fewer than eight breaths per minute, or her breathing seems shallow or irregular.

• You think the person took other drugs with alcohol.

• The person has had an injury, especially a blow to the head.

• The person drank a large amount of alcohol in a short period of time and then became unconscious. Death caused by alcohol poisoning most often occurs when the blood alcohol level rises very quickly due to rapid ingestion of alcohol.

If you aren't sure what to do, call 911. You may save a life.

Higher Concentrations of Alcohol At higher concentrations, the pleasant effects tend to be replaced by more negative ones: interference with motor coordination, verbal performance, and intellectual functions. The drinker often becomes irritable and may be easily angered or given to crying. When the BAC reaches 0.1%, most sensory and motor functioning is reduced, and many people become sleepy. Vision, smell, taste, and hearing become less acute. At 0.2%, most drinkers are completely unable to function, either physically or psychologically, because of the pronounced depression of the central nervous system, muscles, and other body systems. Coma usually occurs at a BAC of 0.35%, and any higher level can be fatal.

Alcohol Hangover The symptoms include headache, shakiness, nausea, diarrhea, fatigue, and impaired mental functioning. A hangover is probably caused by a combination of the toxic products of alcohol breakdown, dehydration, and hormonal effects. During a hangover, heart rate and blood pressure increase, making some individuals more vulnerable to heart attacks. Electroencephalography (brain wave measurement) shows diffuse slowing of brain waves for up to 16 hours after BAC drops to 0.0%. Studies of pilots, drivers, and skiers all indicate that coordination and cognition are impaired in a person with a hangover, increasing the risk of injury.

Alcohol Poisoning Drinking large amounts of alcohol in a short time can rapidly raise the BAC into the lethal range. Alcohol, either alone or in combination with other drugs, is responsible for more toxic overdose deaths than any other drug. Death from alcohol poisoning may be caused either by central nervous system and respiratory depression or by inhaling fluid or vomit into the lungs. The amount of alcohol that renders a person unconscious is dangerously close to a fatal dose. Although passing out may prevent someone from drinking more, BAC can keep rising during unconsciousness because the body continues to absorb ingested alcohol into the bloodstream. Special care should be taken to ensure the safety of anyone who has been drinking heavily, especially if he or she passes out (see the box "Dealing with an Alcohol Emergency").

Using Alcohol with Other Drugs Alcohol-drug combinations are a leading cause of drug-related deaths. Using alcohol while taking a medication that depresses the CNS increases the effects of both drugs, potentially leading to coma, respiratory depression, and death. Such drugs include barbiturates, Valium-like drugs, narcotics such as codeine, and over-the-counter antihistamines such as Benadryl. For people who consume three or more drinks per day, use of over-the-counter pain relievers like aspirin, ibuprofen, or

Ask Yourself
QUESTIONS FOR CRITICAL THINKING AND REFLECTION
Have you ever had a hangover or watched someone else suffer through one? Did the experience affect your attitude about drinking? In what way?

Alcoholic Energy Drinks: The Dangers of Being "Drunk and Wide Awake"

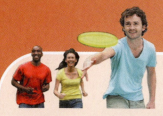

A striking problem of caffeinated alcoholic beverages (CABs) is that the consumer *perceives* himself or herself to be more alert than he or she actually is. Whereas combining energy drinks with alcohol increases alcohol absorption, caffeine does nothing to speed metabolism of the alcohol by the liver. A 2014 study of 744 college students over 56 days showed that for those who mixed energy drinks with alcohol, the number of drinks they consumed increased, as did the amount of time they spent drinking and, thus, the negative experiences associated with drinking alcohol. These negative consequences include hangover and "getting into trouble." The perception that energy drinks offset the effects of alcohol and that their consumers are not as impaired as when drinking alcohol alone leads to an increased risk for injury, aggression, and impaired decision making.

Since Red Bull was introduced to the U.S. market in 1997, and dozens of other energy drink brands followed, consumption of these drinks has become increasingly popular. The caffeine content may be five times greater than that in a typical cup of coffee. Energy drink marketing targets primarily adolescents and young adults. In surveys, 30–50% of young people and 40–60% of college students report consuming energy drinks in the past month.

According to researchers from SAMHSA, 1 in 10 emergency department visits related to the highly caffeinated drinks were reported in 2011. These were patients age 12 and over, and nearly half the emergencies occurred after the beverages were mixed with alcohol or other drugs.

Mixing alcohol with energy drinks is fairly common. In one study, 34% of college students had done so in the past year. Among energy drink consumers, 54% reported mixing in alcohol.

A growing body of evidence highlights the risks associated with the use of CABs. For example, studies cited by the Centers for Disease Control and Prevention (CDC) have reported the following:

- Being in a "drunk/awake" state can lead to risky behaviors such as drunk driving, unplanned sex or sexual assault, and aggression.

- CAB drinkers are three times as likely as non-CAB drinkers to binge-drink.

- CAB drinkers are about twice as likely as non-CAB drinkers to report being taken advantage of sexually, taking advantage of someone sexually, or riding with a driver who was under the influence of alcohol.

- Emerging evidence indicates that CAB use, especially by adolescents, may lead to an increased risk of alcohol or drug dependence later in life.

In 2009, the U.S. Food and Drug Administration (FDA) launched an investigation into the safety, and even the legality, of commercial CABs. It sent letters to nearly 30 CAB manufacturers, asking them to prove that their products met "generally regarded as safe" criteria. Manufacturers that could not provide sufficient evidence of their products' safety risked having them removed from the marketplace. In 2010, the FDA reported that CABs are a public health concern and that adding caffeine to malt alcoholic beverages is an "unsafe food additive" in violation of the Federal Food, Drug, and Cosmetic Act.

Effectively, the FDA banned the sale of premixed drinks. Still, a general lack of regulation of energy drinks has led to vigorous marketing campaigns by CAB manufacturers, making unsubstantiated claims about the performance-enhancing properties of their product. It is important that individual consumers personally investigate what they are consuming.

SOURCES: Polak, K., et al. 2016. Energy drink use is associated with alcohol and substance use in eight, tenth, and twelfth graders. *Preventive Medicine Reports* 4: 381–384. Patrick, M. E., and J. L. Maggs. 2014. Energy drinks and alcohol: Links to alcohol behaviors and consequences across 56 days. *Journal of Adolescent Health* 54(4): 454–459; Substance Abuse and Mental Health Services Administration. 2014. *The DAWN Report: 1 in 10 Energy Drink-Related Emergency Department Visits Results in Hospitalization.* Rockville, MD: Substance Abuse and Mental Health Services Administration (http://www.samhsa.gov/data/sites/default/files/spot124-energy-drinks-2014.pdf).

acetaminophen increases the risk of stomach bleeding and liver damage. Some antacids, antibiotics, and diabetes medications can also interact dangerously with alcohol.

Many illegal drugs are especially dangerous when combined with alcohol. Life-threatening overdoses occur at much lower doses when heroin and other narcotics are combined with alcohol. When cocaine and alcohol are used together, they form a toxic substance in the liver called cocaethylene, which can produce effects that neither drug alone does.

A recent trend among young drinkers involves mixing alcoholic beverages with caffeinated ones, especially highly caffeinated energy drinks (see the box "Alcoholic Energy Drinks: The Dangers of Being 'Drunk and Wide Awake'").

Alcohol-Related Injuries and Violence   The combination of impaired judgment, weakened sensory perception, reduced inhibitions, impaired motor coordination, and increased aggressiveness and hostility that characterizes alcohol intoxication can be dangerous. Through homicide, suicide, automobile crashes, and other traumatic incidents, alcohol use is linked to about 90,000 deaths each year in the United States. The majority of people who attempt suicide have been drinking. Among successful suicides, alcohol use is common as well; an analysis of studies involving over 420,000 participants reveals that alcohol use disorder is an important predictor of suicide. Alcohol use more than triples the risk of fatal injuries during leisure activities such as swimming and boating. More than 50% of fatal falls and serious burns happen to people who have been drinking.

Alcohol and Aggression Eighty percent of arrests happen for drug- and alcohol-related offenses (domestic violence, driving under the influence of alcohol, public drunkenness, and property and drug offenses). Alcohol use contributes to 40% of all murders, assaults, and rapes. It is frequently found in the bloodstream of victims as well as perpetrators. Some people become violent under alcohol's influence, and alcohol is an important component of gang life, maintaining the solidarity of the group, and contributing to gang violence.

Alcohol misuse can wreak havoc on home life. Marital discord and domestic violence often exist in the presence of excessive alcohol consumption. Heavy drinking by parents is associated with abuse of their children, typically emotional or psychological abuse.

Alcohol and Sexual Decision Making Alcohol seriously impairs a person's ability to make wise decisions about sex. A recent survey of college students revealed that frequent binge drinkers were five times more likely to engage in unplanned sexual activity and five-and-a-half times more likely to have unprotected sex than non–binge drinkers. **Binge drinking** is a pattern of rapid, periodic drinking that brings a person's blood alcohol concentration up to 0.08% or higher, typically with five or more drinks for men, or four drinks for women, typically within about two hours. The difference between *bingeing* and *heavy drinking*, according to the Substance Abuse and Mental Health Services Administration (SAMHSA) is that heavy drinking involves bingeing on five or more days in the past month.

Heavy drinkers are also more likely to have multiple sex partners and to engage in other forms of high-risk sexual behavior. Rates of sexually transmitted infections (including HIV) and unwanted pregnancy are higher among people who drink heavily than among people who drink moderately or not at all.

Drinking and Driving

In 2014, 9,967 Americans were killed in accidents involving alcohol-impaired drivers—close to one-third of all traffic fatalities for the year. The National Highway Transportation Safety Administration (NHTSA) estimates that someone is killed in an alcohol-related crash every 53 minutes.

QUICK STATS

In 2015, **13.8%** of drivers aged 18–25 years reported driving under the influence of alcohol at least once in the past year, down from **19.9%** in 2000.

—Substance Abuse and Mental Health Services Administration, 2016

The NHTSA further reports that, of all drivers involved in fatal crashes, those aged 21–24 had the highest percentage of BACs of 0.08% or higher.

People who drink are unable to drive safely because their judgment is impaired, their reaction time is slower, and their coordination is reduced. Some driving skills are affected at BACs of 0.02% and lower.

The *dose-response function* (see Chapter 7) is the relationship between the amount of alcohol or drug consumed and the type and intensity of the resulting effect. Higher doses of alcohol are associated with a much greater probability of automobile crashes (Figure 8.3). A person driving with a BAC of 0.14% is over 40 times more likely to be involved in a crash than someone with no alcohol in his or her blood.

In addition to an increased risk of injury and death, driving while intoxicated can have serious legal consequences. Drunk driving is against the law. The legal limit for BAC is 0.08% in all states, the District of Columbia, and Puerto Rico. Stiff penalties for drunk driving include fines, loss of license, confiscation of vehicle, and jail time. Under current zero-tolerance laws in many states, drivers under age 21 who have consumed *any* alcohol may have their licenses suspended. If you are out of your home and drinking, find alternative transportation or appoint a *designated driver* who doesn't drink and can provide safe transportation home.

It's more difficult to protect yourself against someone else who drinks and drives. Learn to be alert to the erratic driving that signals an impaired driver. Warning signs include wide, abrupt, and illegal turns; straddling the center line or lane

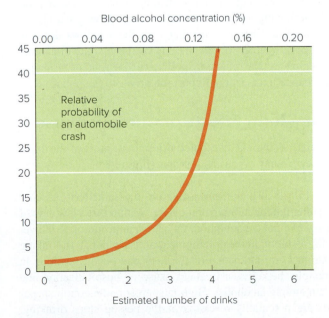

FIGURE 8.3 **The dose-response relationship between BAC and automobile crashes.**

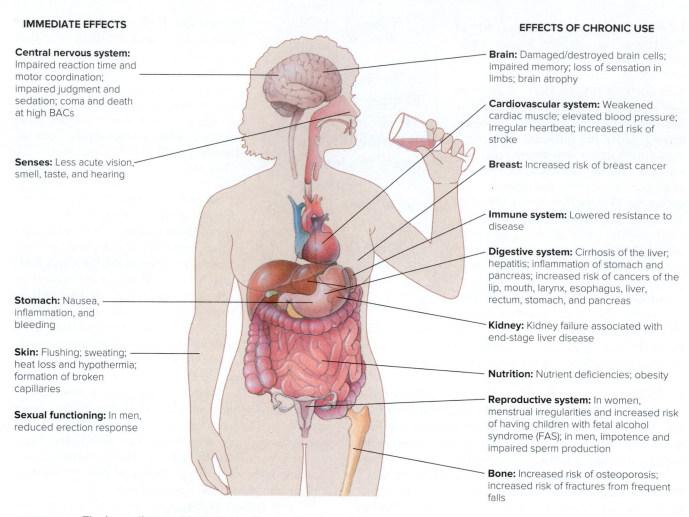

IMMEDIATE EFFECTS

Central nervous system: Impaired reaction time and motor coordination; impaired judgment and sedation; coma and death at high BACs

Senses: Less acute vision, smell, taste, and hearing

Stomach: Nausea, inflammation, and bleeding

Skin: Flushing; sweating; heat loss and hypothermia; formation of broken capillaries

Sexual functioning: In men, reduced erection response

EFFECTS OF CHRONIC USE

Brain: Damaged/destroyed brain cells; impaired memory; loss of sensation in limbs; brain atrophy

Cardiovascular system: Weakened cardiac muscle; elevated blood pressure; irregular heartbeat; increased risk of stroke

Breast: Increased risk of breast cancer

Immune system: Lowered resistance to disease

Digestive system: Cirrhosis of the liver; hepatitis; inflammation of stomach and pancreas; increased risk of cancers of the lip, mouth, larynx, esophagus, liver, rectum, stomach, and pancreas

Kidney: Kidney failure associated with end-stage liver disease

Nutrition: Nutrient deficiencies; obesity

Reproductive system: In women, menstrual irregularities and increased risk of having children with fetal alcohol syndrome (FAS); in men, impotence and impaired sperm production

Bone: Increased risk of osteoporosis; increased risk of fractures from frequent falls

FIGURE 8.4   The immediate and long-term effects of alcohol misuse.

marker; driving against traffic; driving on the shoulder; weaving, swerving, or nearly striking objects or other vehicles; following too closely; erratic speed; driving with headlights off at night; and driving with the windows down in very cold weather. If you see any of these signs in another driver, avoid that vehicle by pulling off the road or turning at the nearest intersection. Report the driver to the police.

Long-Term Effects of Chronic Abuse

Because alcohol is distributed throughout most of the body, it affects many organs and tissues (Figure 8.4).

The Digestive System   Even in the short term, alcohol can alter the functioning of the liver. Within just a few days of heavy alcohol consumption, fat begins to accumulate in liver cells, resulting in the development of "fatty liver." If drinking continues, inflammation of the liver can occur, resulting in alcoholic hepatitis, a frequent cause of hospitalization and death among alcoholics. Both fatty liver and alcoholic hepatitis are potentially reversible if the person stops drinking. With continued alcohol use, however, liver cells are progressively damaged and then destroyed. The destroyed cells are

replaced by fibrous scar tissue, a condition known as **cirrhosis.** People with cirrhosis who continue to drink have only a 50% chance of surviving five or more years.

Alcohol can inflame the pancreas, causing nausea, vomiting, abnormal digestion, and severe pain. Acute alcoholic pancreatitis generally occurs in binge drinkers. Unlike cirrhosis, which usually occurs after years of heavy alcohol use, pancreatitis can occur after one or two severe binge-drinking episodes. Acute pancreatitis is often fatal; in survivors it can become a chronic condition.

The Cardiovascular System   The effects of alcohol on the cardiovascular system depend on the amount of alcohol consumed. Moderate doses of alcohol—one drink or less a day for women and one to two drinks a day for men—may reduce the risk of heart disease and heart attack in some people. (The possible health benefits of alcohol are discussed later in this chapter.)

> **cirrhosis**   A disease in which the liver is severely damaged by alcohol, other toxins, or infection.   **TERMS**

However, higher doses of alcohol harm the cardiovascular system. In some people, more than two drinks a day will elevate blood pressure, making stroke and heart attack more likely. Some alcoholics show a weakening of the heart muscle, a condition known as **cardiac myopathy.** Binge drinking can cause "holiday heart," characterized by serious abnormal heart rhythms, which usually appear within 24 hours of a binge episode.

Cancer In 2000, the U.S. Department of Health and Human Services added alcoholic beverages to its list of known human carcinogens. Chronic alcohol consumption is a clear risk factor for cancers of the mouth, throat, larynx, and esophagus. (These cancers are also associated with use of tobacco, with which alcohol frequently acts as a cocarcinogen.) Five or six daily drinks, especially combined with smoking, increases the risk of these cancers by a factor of 50 or more. Heavy drinking also puts users at risk for colorectal cancer and the most common form of liver cancer; and continued heavy drinking in people with hepatitis accelerates progression to this cancer.

Studies have also found that light to moderate drinking can increase your risk. A 2015 study suggests that consuming even one drink per day increases the risk of breast cancer. In all alcohol-related cancers, however, genetics and other biological factors play important roles and help explain why some chronic alcohol abusers do not get cancer.

Brain Damage Brain damage due to chronic alcohol abuse is also tempered by a person's physiology and genetics. Imaging studies document that many alcoholics experience brain shrinkage with loss of both gray and white matter, reduced blood flow, and slowed metabolic rates in some brain regions. To some extent, brain shrinkage can be reversed over time with abstinence. About half of the alcoholics in the United States have cognitive impairments, ranging from mild to severe. These include memory loss, dementia, and compromised problem-solving and reasoning abilities. Malnutrition, particularly thiamine deficiency, contributes to severe brain damage.

Mortality Excessive alcohol consumption is a factor in several leading causes of death for Americans. Average life expectancy among people with alcohol use disorder is about 15 years less than among people who do not have the disorder. About half the deaths caused by alcohol are due to chronic conditions such as cirrhosis and cancer; the other half are due to acute conditions or events such as car crashes, falls, and suicide.

Alcohol Use during Pregnancy

During pregnancy, alcohol and its metabolic product acetaldehyde readily cross the placenta, harming the developing fetus. Damage to the fetus depends on the amount of alcohol consumed and the stage of the pregnancy. Early in pregnancy, heavy drinking can cause spontaneous abortion or miscarriage. Alcohol in early pregnancy, during critical fetal development periods, can also cause a collection of birth defects known as *fetal alcohol syndrome (FAS)*, which was discussed in Chapter 5.

Because rapid brain development continues throughout pregnancy, the fetal brain stays vulnerable to alcohol use until birth. Although effects of drinking later in pregnancy do not typically cause the characteristic physical deformities of FAS, getting drunk just once during the final three months of pregnancy can damage a fetal brain.

FAS is a permanent, incurable condition that causes lifelong disability. CDC studies identify the number of FAS cases as ranging from two to nine infants for every 10,000 live births in the United States. About three times as many babies are born with **alcohol-related neurodevelopmental disorder (ARND).** Children with ARND appear physically normal but often have significant learning and behavioral disorders. As adults, they are more likely to develop substance use disorders and to have criminal records. ARND must be treated as early as possible to avoid long-term physiological as well as social consequences. Treatments include medical care, medication, behavior and education therapy, parent training, and other approaches such as biofeedback, yoga, and art therapy. The whole range of FAS and ARND is commonly called *fetal alcohol spectrum disorder (FASD)*.

No one is sure exactly how much alcohol causes FASD. Like other untoward effects of alcohol, genetics and individual differences in metabolism, along with environmental factors such as diet, are thought to affect vulnerability. But a 2015 report from the American Academy of Pediatrics stresses that no amount of alcohol at any point during pregnancy is considered safe.

Women who are trying to conceive, or who are sexually active without using effective contraception, should abstain from alcohol to avoid inadvertently harming their fetus in the first few days or weeks of pregnancy, before they know they're expecting. Binge drinking among women of childbearing age is a particular concern. And because any alcohol consumed by a nursing mother quickly enters her milk, many physicians advise nursing mothers to abstain from drinking alcohol.

> **QUICK STATS**
>
> About **10%** of pregnant women drink alcohol, and **3%** are binge drinkers.
>
> —Centers for Disease Control and Prevention, 2015b

> **TERMS**
>
> **cardiac myopathy** Weakening of the heart muscle through disease.
>
> **alcohol-related neurodevelopmental disorder (ARND)** Cognitive and behavioral problems seen in people whose mothers drank alcohol during pregnancy.

Ask Yourself

QUESTIONS FOR CRITICAL THINKING AND REFLECTION

Have you ever witnessed or been involved in an alcohol emergency? Did you think the situation was urgent at the time? What were the circumstances surrounding the event? How did the people involved deal with it?

Possible Health Benefits of Alcohol?

Researchers are changing their tune on the effects of moderate drinking. Previous studies showed that light to moderate drinking may improve heart health by raising blood levels of HDL (the beneficial form of cholesterol), by thinning the blood, and by reducing inflammation and the risk of dangerous blood clots, all of which can contribute to the risk of a heart attack.

Newer studies, however, cast doubt on such benefits. A recent study published in the *British Medical Journal* suggests that, if anyone benefits, it is women age 65 and over, and that even this finding may be explained by a selection bias (the results come from a survey). But even older women may do well to minimize their drinking behavior: The American Heart Association reports on new research among the elderly showing that women who drank moderately had small reductions in heart function.

There is no evidence that drinking in one's twenties and thirties has any health benefits. Although some studies have shown lower death rates for moderate or light drinkers, and fewer heart attacks and strokes, these studies fail to identify alcohol as the cause.

EXCESSIVE USE OF ALCOHOL

As discussed in Chapter 7, the *DSM-5* is refocusing general understanding of excessive alcohol use. It diagnoses behavior based on a continuum of mild, moderate, and severe. Rather than using the terms *alcoholic* or *non-alcoholic,* the *DSM-5* prefers **alcohol use disorder.** If a person meets two of the following criteria, she or he has an alcohol use disorder; two to three symptoms indicates a mild disorder, four to five a moderate disorder, and six or more a severe disorder.

To determine a person's place on the disorder spectrum, you could ask these questions:

1. Do you often consume alcohol in large amounts over a long period?
2. Do you find that your efforts to control your alcohol use are unsuccessful?
3. Do you spend excessive time using alcohol or recovering from its effects?
4. Do you have a strong desire or craving to use alcohol?
5. Does your persistent alcohol use cause a failure to fulfill obligations at work, school, or home?
6. Do you continue using alcohol despite recurrent social or interpersonal problems caused by its effects?
7. Have you reduced important social or recreational activities because of your alcohol use?
8. Do you persist in using alcohol in situations that are physically risky?
9. Do you continue using alcohol despite knowing that it can cause or worsen a recurrent physical or psychological problem?
10. Do you have a need for increased amounts of alcohol to achieve a desired effect (increased tolerance)?
11. Do you experience symptoms of withdrawal, such as sweating, increased pulse rate, hand tremor, insomnia, nausea, and anxiety?

Alcohol Use Disorder: From Mild to Severe

Severe *alcohol use disorder,* or **alcoholism,** involves more extensive problems with alcohol use, usually involving physical tolerance and withdrawal. Alcoholism is discussed in greater detail later in the chapter.

How can you tell if you or someone you know has serious problems with alcohol? Look for the following warning signs:

- Drinking alone or secretively
- Using alcohol deliberately and repeatedly to perform or get through difficult situations
- Using alcohol as a way to "self-medicate" in order to dull strong emotions or negative feelings
- Feeling uncomfortable on certain occasions when alcohol is not available
- Escalating alcohol consumption beyond an already established drinking pattern
- Consuming alcohol heavily in risky situations, such as before driving
- Getting drunk regularly or more frequently than in the past
- Drinking in the morning

Binge Drinking

In 2015, 26.9% of Americans age 18 and over reported that they engaged in binge drinking in the past month; 7.0% reported that they engaged in heavy drinking in the past month.

> **alcohol use disorder** Abuse of alcohol that leads to clinically significant impairment.
>
> **alcoholism** A pathological use of alcohol or impairment in functioning due to alcohol; characterized by tolerance to alcohol and withdrawal symptoms.
>
> **TERMS**

Among Americans under age 21, most drinking occurs in the form of bingeing, and over 90% of the alcohol they drink is consumed while binge drinking. Over half the alcohol consumed by all adults in the United States is downed during binge drinking.

Binge drinking caused more than half of the 90,000 deaths and three-fourths of the estimated economic cost of excessive drinking—$249 billion—in 2010 (the latest available data). Students also often mention that they pay in other, nonmonetary ways when they binge drink (see the box "Peer Pressure and College Binge Drinking"). Frequent binge drinkers are three to seven times more likely than non–binge drinkers to engage in unplanned or unprotected sex, drive after drinking, get hurt or injured, fall behind in school work, or argue with friends.

Alcoholism

As mentioned earlier, alcoholism is usually characterized by tolerance to alcohol and withdrawal symptoms. Everyone who drinks—even if not suffering from an alcohol use disorder—develops tolerance after repeated alcohol use.

Patterns and Prevalence   Alcoholism occurs among people of all racial and ethnic groups and at all socioeconomic levels. There are different patterns of excessive alcohol use, including these four common ones:

1. Regular daily intake of large amounts
2. Regular heavy drinking limited to weekends
3. Long periods of sobriety interspersed with binges of daily heavy drinking lasting for weeks or months
4. Heavy drinking limited to periods of stress

Once established, alcoholism often exhibits a pattern of exacerbations and remissions. The person may stop drinking and abstain from alcohol for days or months after a frightening problem develops. Alcoholism is not hopeless, however. Many alcoholics achieve permanent abstinence.

Health Effects   As described in Chapter 7, *tolerance* means that a drinker needs more alcohol to achieve intoxication or the desired effect, that the effects of continued use of the same amount of alcohol are diminished, or that the drinker can function adequately at doses or a BAC that would produce significant impairment in a casual user. Heavy users of alcohol may need to consume about 50% more than they originally needed in order to experience the same degree of intoxication.

Withdrawal symptoms include trembling hands (shakes or jitters), a rapid pulse and accelerated breathing rate, insomnia, nightmares, anxiety, and GI upset. More severe withdrawal symptoms occur in about 5% of alcoholics. These include seizures (sometimes called "rum fits"), confusion,

and **hallucinations** such as seeing visions or hearing voices. Still less common is **delirium tremens (the DTs)**, a medical emergency characterized by severe disorientation, confusion, epileptic-like seizures, and vivid hallucinations, often of vermin and small animals. The mortality rate from the DTs can be as high as 15%.

Alcoholics face all the physical health risks associated with intoxication and chronic drinking described earlier in the chapter. Some damage is compounded by nutritional deficiencies that often accompany alcoholism. A mental problem associated with alcohol use is profound memory gaps (commonly known as blackouts).

Social and Psychological Effects   Alcohol use causes more serious social and psychological problems than all other forms of drug abuse combined. For every person who is an alcoholic, another three or four people are directly affected.

People suffering from an alcohol use disorder frequently have mental disorders. They are much more likely to have clinical depression, panic disorder, schizophrenia, borderline personality disorder, or antisocial personality disorder. People with anxiety or panic attacks may try to use alcohol to lessen their anxiety, even though alcohol often makes these disorders worse. Alcohol use disorder often co-occurs with other substance abuse problems as well.

Causes of Alcoholism   The precise causes of alcoholism are unknown, but many factors are probably involved. Some studies suggest that as much as 50–60% of a person's risk for alcoholism is determined by genetic factors. Not all children of alcoholics become alcoholic, however, and it is clear that other factors are involved. A person's risk of developing alcoholism may be increased by having certain personality disorders, having grown up in a violent or otherwise troubled household, and imitating the alcohol abuse of peers and other role models. People who begin drinking excessively in their teens are especially prone to binge drinking and alcoholism later in life.

Treatment   Some alcoholics recover without professional help. How often this occurs is unknown, but it is estimated that as many as one-third stop drinking on their own or reduce their drinking enough to eliminate problems. Most alcoholics, however, require a treatment program of some kind in order to stop drinking. Many different kinds of programs exist.

> **TERMS**
>
> **hallucination**   A false perception that does not correspond to external reality, such as seeing visions or hearing voices that are not there.
>
> **delirium tremens (the DTs)**   A state of confusion brought on by the reduction of alcohol intake in an alcohol-dependent person; other symptoms are sweating, trembling, anxiety, hallucinations, and seizures.

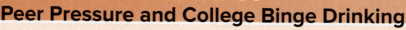

WELLNESS ON CAMPUS
Peer Pressure and College Binge Drinking

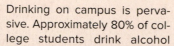

Drinking on campus is pervasive. Approximately 80% of college students drink alcohol and, of those, about half report having binged on alcohol. Every year, more than 1,800 college students aged 18–24 die from alcohol-related injuries. Another 600,000 sustain unintentional alcohol-related injuries; 700,000 are assaulted by other students who have been drinking; and close to 100,000 are victims of alcohol-related date rape or sexual assault.

These statistics have shocked many students, administrators, and parents into demanding changes in college attitudes and policies regarding alcohol. In response, the National Institute on Alcohol Abuse and Alcoholism (NIAAA) created task forces that bring together research and calls for action. Its reports focus on three levels of action:

1. Ultimately *each student* is accountable and must take responsibility for his or her own behavior. Programs that encourage and support development of healthy attitudes toward alcohol are needed. These programs should target students at increased risk of developing alcohol problems: first-year students, Greek organization members, and athletes. Treatment should be readily available for problem drinkers.

2. The *student body as a whole* must work to discourage alcohol abuse. These efforts include promoting alcohol-free activities, reducing availability of alcohol, and avoiding social and commercial promotion of alcohol on campus. The environment should be designed to accept students who choose to abstain and disapprove of students who drink to excess. Fraternities, sororities, eating clubs, and other campus organizations should be held accountable for inappropriate alcohol use, especially involving underage students, that takes place on their premises.

3. *Colleges and surrounding communities* must cooperate to discourage excessive drinking. College administrators, law enforcement, bar and liquor store owners, residents who live near campus, and the court system must all do their part to reduce the availability of cheap alcohol and to enforce existing laws. Those who enable students to drink irresponsibly must be held accountable.

Peer Pressure

The pressure to think and act along certain peer-prescribed guidelines plays a major role in drinking motivations. Late adolescence and early adulthood are times of life in which we are particularly susceptible to frequent alcohol abuse, risky behavior, and peer pressure. A 2014 study of young adult men examined direct versus indirect peer pressure. The researchers found that indirect pressure, as in the ideas contributing to our beliefs about alcohol, had more influence than direct pressure, such as offers or dares to drink at parties. The most common motivations of the young adult men were to get high and to forget their worries, rather than to fit in socially or make their social gatherings more fun. Thus, the authors of the study recommend targeting motives over peer pressure as a way to change behaviors.

A vehicle for peer-pressuring young people in particular is the display of drinking and smoking on social media. A study of high school social media users emphasizes that exposure—at any time of day, in any setting, alone or with others—to a friend's risky displays contributed to their drinking and smoking. Parents and teachers could consider teaching adolescents about the effects of posting online about risky behaviors.

No single treatment works for everyone, so a person may have to try different programs before finding the right one.

One of the oldest and best-known recovery programs is Alcoholics Anonymous (AA). In many communities, AA consists of self-help groups that meet several times each week and follow a 12-step program. Important steps for people in these programs include recognizing that they are "powerless over alcohol" and must seek help from a "higher power" to regain control of their lives. By verbalizing these steps, the alcoholic directly addresses the denial that is often prominent in alcoholism and other addictions. Many AA members have a sponsor of their choosing who is available by phone 24 hours a day for individual support and crisis intervention.

Other recovery approaches are available. Some, like Rational Recovery and Women for Sobriety, deliberately avoid any emphasis on higher spiritual powers. A more controversial approach to problem drinking is offered by the group Moderation Management, which encourages people to manage their drinking behavior by limiting intake or abstaining.

Al-Anon and Alateen are companion programs to AA for families and friends of alcoholics. In Al-Anon, spouses and others explore how they enable the alcoholic to drink by denying, rationalizing, or covering up his or her drinking and how they can change this codependent behavior.

Inpatient hospital rehabilitation is useful for some alcoholics, especially if they have serious medical or mental problems or if life stressors threaten to overwhelm them. There are also several medical treatments for alcoholism.

• *Disulfiram* (*Antabuse*) inhibits the metabolic breakdown of acetaldehyde and causes patients to flush and feel ill when they drink, theoretically inhibiting impulse drinking. However, disulfiram is potentially dangerous if the user continues to drink.

• *Naltrexone* (ReVia, Depade) binds to a brain pleasure center that reduces the craving for alcohol and decreases its pleasant, reinforcing effects. When taken correctly, naltrexone usually does not make the user feel ill.

Ten Ways to Decline a Drink

1. No thanks.
2. My religious beliefs or health condition prohibit me from drinking.
3. I have offered to be the designated driver.
4. I am an athlete or musician who cannot compromise my general performance.
5. I must do something tomorrow, and I won't be able to do it if I drink tonight (could be babysitting, taking a test, visiting a relative, attending a concert).
6. I'm dancing (or DJing).
7. I already have a drink (whether alcoholic or not can be hard to tell).
8. I'm cutting calories.
9. I don't like the taste of alcohol.
10. The last time I drank I became violent.

What Schools Are Doing

Some schools have attempted to shift classes to Fridays and even Saturdays after they found that binge drinking increases when students don't have Friday classes. Increasingly, incoming students are required to take a three-hour online class about alcohol. And some campuses apply stricter punishment for underage drinking and public drunkenness, with the likelihood of suspension for repeat offenders.

Many colleges ban ads for alcoholic drinks in college newspapers and during broadcasts of college athletic events. Flyers, posters, and other promotions for cheap drinks, such as two-for-one specials, happy hours, all you can drink, and

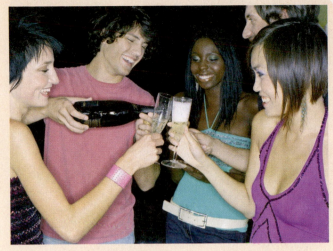
© Paul Bradbury/Getty Images

ladies' night, are banned on many campuses. In these college communities, bars and restaurants that cater to students are discouraged from offering patrons cheap alcohol.

SOURCES: Huang, G. C., et al. 2014. Peer influences: The impact of online and offline friendship networks on adolescent smoking and alcohol use. *Journal of Adolescent Health* 54(5): 508–514; National Institute on Alcohol Abuse and Alcoholism. 2015. *College Drinking* (http://www.niaaa.nih.gov/alcohol-health/special-populations-co-occurring-disorders/college-drinking); National Institute on Drug Abuse. 2015. *6 Tactful Tips for Resisting Peer Pressure to Use Drugs and Alcohol* (https://teens.drugabuse.gov/blog/post/6-tactful-tips-resisting-peer-pressure-to-use-drugs-and-alcohol); Studer, J., et al. 2014. Peer pressure and alcohol use in young men: A mediation analysis of drinking motives. *International Journal of Drug Policy* 25(4): 700–708.

• *Injectable naltrexone* (Vivitrol) acts the same as oral naltrexone, but it is a single monthly shot administered by a health professional. Compliance with a monthly regimen may be better for some alcoholics.

• *Acamprosate* (Campral) helps people maintain abstinence after they have stopped drinking. It is unclear how acamprosate works, but it appears to act on brain pathways related to alcohol abuse.

Alcohol treatment programs are successful in achieving an extended period of sobriety for about half of those who participate. Success rates of conventional treatment programs are about the same for men and women and for people from different racial and ethnic groups. AA remains the mainstay of treatment for most people and is often a component of even the most expensive treatment programs.

Gender and Ethnic Differences

Alcohol abusers come from all socioeconomic levels and cultural groups, but notable differences appear in drinking patterns between men and women and among different racial and ethnic groups (Table 8.1).

Men Men are more likely than women to drink alcohol, to misuse alcohol, and to develop an alcohol use disorder. Among white American men, excessive drinking often begins in the teens or twenties and progresses gradually through the thirties until the man is clearly identifiable as an alcoholic by the time he is in his late thirties or early forties. Other men may remain controlled drinkers until later in life, sometimes becoming alcoholic in association with retirement, the loss of friends and loved ones, boredom, illness, or psychological disorders.

Table 8.1 — Alcohol Use and Binge Alcohol Use by Sex and Race/Ethnicity in 2015, Age 12 and Over

	PAST MONTH PREVALENCE (PERCENTAGE OF TOTAL POPULATION)	
	ALCOHOL USE	BINGE ALCOHOL USE
Gender		
Male	56.2	29.6
Female	47.4	20.5
Race and Ethnicity		
Not Hispanic or Latino		
White	57.0	26.0
Black or African American	43.8	23.4
American Indian and Alaska Native	37.9	24.1
Native Hawaiian/Pacific Islander	33.8	17.8
Asian American	39.7	14.0
Two or more races	42.8	22.9
Hispanic or Latino	42.4	25.7
Total Population	**51.7**	**24.9**

SOURCE: Substance Abuse and Mental Health Services Administration Center for Behavioral Health Statistics and Quality. 2016. *Results from the 2015 National Survey on Drug Use and Health* (http://www.samhsa.gov/data/sites/default/files/NSDUH-DetTabs-2015/NSDUH-DetTabs-2015/NSDUH-DetTabs-2015.htm).

Women Women tend to become alcoholic at later ages and with fewer years of heavy drinking. It is not unusual for women in their forties or fifties to succumb to alcoholism after years of controlled drinking.

Women alcoholics develop cirrhosis and other medical complications more often and after a shorter period of heavier drinking than men, and have higher death rates—including deaths from cirrhosis—than male alcoholics. Some alcohol-related health problems are unique to women, including increased risk of breast cancer, menstrual disorders, infertility, and bearing children with FAS. Women are more vulnerable to the anticlotting effects of alcohol, which can raise the risk of bleeding strokes. Female alcoholics are less likely to seek early treatment for drinking problems, possibly because of the social stigma attached to problem drinking.

African Americans As a group, African Americans use less alcohol than the average for American adults, but they face disproportionately high levels of alcohol-related birth defects, cirrhosis, cancer, hypertension, and other medical problems. In addition, African Americans are more likely than members of other racial or ethnic groups to be victims of alcohol-related homicides, criminal assaults, and injuries. African American women are more likely to abstain from alcohol use than white women, but among black women who drink there is a higher percentage of heavy drinkers.

AA groups of predominantly African Americans are effective, perhaps because essential elements of AA—sharing common experiences, mutual acceptance of one another as human beings, and trusting a higher power—are already a part of African American culture.

Latinos Drinking patterns among Latinos vary significantly, depending on their specific cultural background and level of acculturation. Drunk driving and cirrhosis are the most common causes of alcohol-related death and injury among Hispanic men. Hispanic women are more likely to abstain from alcohol than white or black women, but those who drink are at special risk for problems. Treating the entire family as a unit is an important part of treatment because family pride, solidarity, and support are important aspects of Latino culture.

Asian Americans As a group, Asian Americans have lower-than-average rates of alcohol abuse. However, acculturation may somewhat weaken the generally strong Asian taboos and community sanctions against alcohol use. Asian American men consume much more alcohol than do Asian American women (60% versus 39%). For many Asian Americans, though, the genetically based physiological aversion to alcohol remains a deterrent to abuse. Ethnic agencies, health care professionals, and ministers seem to be the most effective sources of treatment for members of this group, when needed. That alcohol may interact with hepatitis B virus is of special concern because Asian Americans have a higher prevalence of this hepatitis infection.

American Indians and Alaska Natives As a group, American Indians and Alaska Natives have a relatively low rate of drinking overall (more abstainers) and a rate of binge drinking that is similar to the overall population rate. However, alcohol use disorder is significantly more prevalent among Native Americans compared to other groups, as is the death rate from alcohol-related causes such as motor vehicle crashes. Socioeconomic disadvantage can be a barrier to adequate health care. Treatment may be more effective if it reflects tribal values.

Helping Someone with an Alcohol Problem

Helping a friend or relative with an alcohol problem requires skill and tact. Start by making sure you are not enabling someone to continue excessive use of alcohol. Enabling

QUICK STATS

On an average day, **1.2 million** out of **9 million** full-time college students and **240,000** out of **2 million** part-time college students drink alcohol.

—Substance Abuse and Mental Health Services Administration, 2016

The responsible use of alcohol includes understanding your own attitudes and behaviors, managing your behavior, and encouraging responsible behavior in others.

Examine Your Attitudes and Behavior

• Consider your feelings about alcohol and drinking. Do you care if alcohol is available at social activities? How do you feel about people who don't drink?

• Consider where your attitudes toward drinking and alcohol come from. How was alcohol used in your family when you were growing up? How is it used—or how do you think it is used—on your campus? How is it portrayed in ads? In other words, what influences might be shaping your alcohol use?

• Consider your own drinking behavior. If you drink, what are your reasons? Is your drinking moderate and responsible? Or do you drink too much and experience negative consequences?

Drink Moderately and Responsibly

• Drink slowly and space your drinks. Sip your drinks and alternate them with nonalcoholic choices. Don't drink alcoholic beverages to quench your thirst. Avoid drinks made with carbonated mixers. Watch your drinks being poured or mixed so that you can be sure of what you're drinking.

• Eat before and while drinking. Don't drink on an empty stomach. Food in your stomach will slow the rate at which alcohol is absorbed and thus often lower the peak BAC.

• Know your limits and your drinks. Learn how different BACs affect you and how to keep your BAC under control.

• Be aware of the setting. In dangerous situations, such as driving, abstinence is the only appropriate choice.

• Use designated drivers. Arrange carpools to and from parties or events where alcohol will be served. Rotate the responsibility for acting as a designated driver.

• Learn to enjoy activities without alcohol. If you can't have fun without drinking, you may have a problem with alcohol.

Encourage Responsible Drinking in Others

• Encourage responsible attitudes. Learn to express disapproval about someone who has drunk too much. Don't treat the choice to abstain as strange. The majority of American adults drink moderately or not at all.

• Be a responsible host. Serve only enough alcohol for each guest to have a moderate number of drinks, and offer nonalcoholic choices. Always serve food along with alcohol. Stop serving alcohol an hour or more before people will leave. Insist that a guest who drank too much take a taxi or rideshare, ride with someone else, or stay overnight rather than drive.

• Hold drinkers fully responsible for their behavior. Pardoning unacceptable behavior fosters the attitude that the behavior is due to the drug rather than the person.

• Take community action. Find out about prevention programs on your campus or in your community. Consider joining an action group such as Students Against Destructive Decisions (SADD).

---

takes many forms, such as making excuses for the alcohol abuser—for example, saying "he has the flu" when it is really a hangover.

Another important step is open, honest labeling—"I think you have a problem with alcohol." Such explicit statements usually elicit emotional rebuttals and may endanger a relationship. However, you are not helping your friends by allowing them to deny their problems with alcohol or other drugs. Taking action shows that you care.

Even when problems are acknowledged, there is usually reluctance to get help. You can't cure a friend's drinking problem, but you can guide him or her to appropriate help. Your best role might be to obtain information about the available resources and persistently encourage their use.

See the box "Drinking Behavior and Responsibility" for additional strategies for cultivating a responsible relationship with alcohol.

WHO USES TOBACCO?

Rates of smoking vary based on gender, age, race and ethnicity, and education level (Figure 8.5). According to the CDC National Health Interview Survey, 16.8% of Americans age 18 and over were cigarette smokers in 2014. About 18.8% of men and 14.8% of women reported that they currently smoked cigarettes. Adults with a twelfth-grade education or less were much more likely to smoke cigarettes than were those with a college degree. The number of people in the

Ask Yourself
QUESTIONS FOR CRITICAL THINKING AND REFLECTION

Do you know anyone with a serious alcohol problem? From what you have read in this chapter, would you say that this person abuses alcohol or is dependent on it? What effects, if any, has this person's problem had on your life? Have you thought about getting support or help?

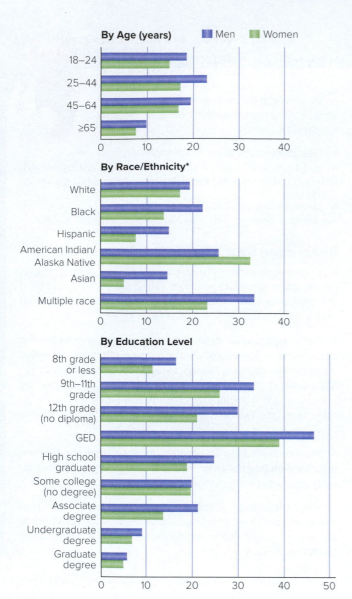

By Age (years) ■ Men ■ Women

By Race/Ethnicity*

By Education Level

FIGURE 8.5 Who smokes cigarettes? Overall 16.8% of American adults currently smoke cigarettes—18.8% of men and 14.8% of women. However, smoking rates vary significantly by age, race/ethnicity, and education level.

*Unless noted, all racial/ethnic groups are non-Hispanic; Hispanics can be of any race.

SOURCE: Centers for Disease Control and Prevention. 2015. Current cigarette smoking among adults—United States, 2005–2014. *Morbidity and Mortality Weekly Report* 64(44): 1233–1240.

United States who smoke (every day or some days) has been decreasing overall, however, with about a 20% decline since 2005. The largest decrease has been in adults aged 18–24, with a 31.6% decrease from 2005 to 2014.

WHY PEOPLE USE TOBACCO

Although people start smoking for a variety of reasons, they usually become long-term smokers after becoming addicted to nicotine—the key psychoactive ingredient in tobacco smoke.

Ask Yourself

QUESTIONS FOR CRITICAL THINKING AND REFLECTION
Do any of your friends or family members smoke or use smokeless tobacco? What effect has it had on their health and relationships? Have you ever discussed their tobacco use with them? Why or why not?

Nicotine Addiction

The primary reason why people continue to use **tobacco** is that they have become addicted to a powerful **psychoactive drug: nicotine.** Although the tobacco industry long maintained that nicotine had not been proved to be addictive, scientific evidence overwhelmingly shows that it is highly addictive. In fact, many researchers consider nicotine to be the most physically addictive of all the psychoactive drugs, including cocaine and heroin.

Some neurological studies indicate that nicotine acts on the brain in much the same way as cocaine and heroin. Nicotine reaches the brain via the bloodstream seconds after it is inhaled or, in the case of spit tobacco, absorbed through membranes of the mouth or nose. It triggers the release of powerful chemical messengers in the brain, including epinephrine, norepinephrine, and dopamine. But unlike street drugs, most of which are used to achieve a high, nicotine's primary attraction seems to lie in its ability to modulate everyday emotions.

At low doses, nicotine acts as a stimulant, increasing heart rate and blood pressure. In adults, nicotine can enhance alertness, concentration, information processing, memory, and learning. The opposite effect, however, occurs in teens who smoke; they show impairment in memory and other cognitive functions.

In some circumstances, nicotine acts as a mild sedative. Most commonly, nicotine relieves symptoms such as anxiety, irritability, and mild depression in tobacco users who are experiencing withdrawal. Some studies have shown that high doses of nicotine and rapid smoking cause increases in levels of glucocorticoids and endorphins, hormones that moderate moods and reduce stress. Tobacco users are able to fine-tune nicotine's effects and regulate their moods by increasing or decreasing their intake of the drug. Studies have shown that smokers experience milder mood variation than nonsmokers while performing long, boring tasks or while watching emotional movies, for example.

All tobacco products contain nicotine, and using any of them can lead to addiction. Nicotine addiction fulfills the

TERMS

tobacco The leaves of cultivated tobacco plants prepared for smoking, chewing, or use as snuff.

psychoactive drug A chemical substance that affects brain function and changes perception, mood, or consciousness.

nicotine A toxic, addictive substance found in tobacco and responsible for many of the effects of tobacco.

criteria for substance misuse described in Chapter 7, including loss of control, tolerance, and withdrawal.

Loss of Control   About 69% of smokers say they want to quit completely, but only about 43% of smokers try to quit each year. Regular tobacco users live according to a rigid cycle of need and gratification. On average, they can go no more than 40 minutes between doses of nicotine; otherwise, they begin feeling edgy and irritable and have trouble concentrating. Tobacco users may plan their daily schedule around opportunities to satisfy their nicotine cravings; this loss of control and personal freedom can affect all the dimensions of wellness.

Tolerance and Withdrawal   Tobacco users build up **tolerance** to nicotine—a condition in which higher doses of nicotine are required to produce the same initial effect. Whereas one cigarette may make a beginning smoker nauseated and dizzy, a long-term smoker may have to chain-smoke a pack or more to experience the same effects. For most regular tobacco users, sudden abstinence from nicotine produces predictable **withdrawal** symptoms. These symptoms, which come on several hours after the last dose of nicotine, can include severe cravings, insomnia, confusion, tremors, difficulty concentrating, fatigue, muscle pains, headache, nausea, irritability, anger, and depression. Although most of these symptoms of physical dependence pass in two or three days, the craving associated with addiction persists. Even years after quitting, many ex-smokers report intermittent, intense urges to smoke.

Social and Psychological Factors

Why do tobacco users have such a hard time quitting even when they want to? Social and psychological forces combine with physiological addiction to maintain the tobacco habit. Many people, for example, have established habits of smoking while doing something else—while talking, working, drinking, and so on. The spit tobacco habit is also associated with certain situations—studying, drinking coffee, or playing sports. These associations can make it more difficult for users to break their habits because the activities they associate with tobacco use continue to trigger urges. Such activities are called **secondary reinforcers;** they act together with physiological addiction to keep the user dependent on tobacco.

Genetic Factors

Genetics play an important role in some aspects of tobacco use. Specific genes may affect how nicotine is metabolized in the body, increasing or decreasing an individual's risk for

addiction. Inherited factors may be more important than social and environmental factors in smoking initiation and in the development of nicotine dependence.

Why Start in the First Place?

In the United States, the legal age to purchase cigarettes is 18 in most states, and 21 in California and Hawaii (as of 2016). Despite this, nearly 90% of all adult smokers report that they started smoking before age 18. The average age for starting smokers and smokeless tobacco users is around 15. The earlier people begin smoking, the more likely they are to become heavy smokers—and to die of tobacco-related disease.

Young people start using tobacco for a variety of reasons. Many young, white, male athletes, for example, begin using spit tobacco to emulate professional athletes. Young women commonly take up smoking because they think it will help them lose weight or stay thin. Most often, however, young people start smoking simply because their peers are already doing it; smoking gives them a way to fit in with a crowd or to look cool.

Rationalizing the Dangers   Making the decision to smoke requires minimizing or denying both the health risks and the tremendous pain, disability, emotional trauma, family stress, and financial expense involved in tobacco-related diseases such as cancer and emphysema. A sense of invincibility, characteristic of many adolescents and young adults, also contributes to the decision to use tobacco.

Many teenagers believe they can stop smoking when they want. In fact, adolescents are more vulnerable to nicotine than are older tobacco users. Compared with older smokers, adolescents become heavy smokers and develop dependence after fewer cigarettes. Nicotine addiction can start within a few days of smoking and after just a few cigarettes. Over half of teenagers who try cigarettes progress to daily use, and about half of those who ever smoke daily progress to nicotine dependence. One National Institute of Drug Abuse (NIDA) survey revealed that about 75% of smoking teens state they wish they had never started.

HEALTH HAZARDS

Tobacco adversely affects nearly every part of the body, including the brain, stomach, mouth, and reproductive organs.

Tobacco Smoke: A Toxic Mix

Tobacco smoke contains thousands of chemical substances, several hundred of which are known to be harmful to humans, including acetone (found in nail polish remover), ammonia, hexamine (lighter fluid), and toluene (industrial solvent). Smoke from a typical unfiltered cigarette contains about 5 billion particles per cubic millimeter—50,000 times as many as are found in an equal volume of smoggy urban air. These particles, when condensed, form a brown, sticky mass called **cigarette tar.**

Carcinogens and Poisons   At least 69 chemicals in tobacco smoke are linked to the development of cancer. Some, such as benzo(a)pyrene and urethane, are **carcinogens**—that is, they directly cause cancer. Other chemicals, such as formaldehyde, are **cocarcinogens;** they do not themselves cause cancer but combine with other chemicals to stimulate the growth of certain cancers, at least in laboratory animals. Other substances in tobacco cause health problems because they damage the lining of the respiratory tract or decrease the lungs' ability to fight off infection.

Cigarette smoke contains carbon monoxide, the deadly gas in automobile exhaust, in concentrations 400 times greater than is considered safe in industrial workplaces. Not surprisingly, smokers often complain of breathlessness when they exert themselves. Carbon monoxide displaces oxygen in red blood cells, depleting the body's supply of oxygen needed for extra work. Carbon monoxide also impairs visual acuity, especially at night.

Additives   Tobacco manufacturers use additives to manipulate the taste and effect of cigarettes and other tobacco products. Additives account for roughly 10%, by weight, of a cigarette, and include sugars and other flavoring agents, humectants (compounds that keep tobacco from drying

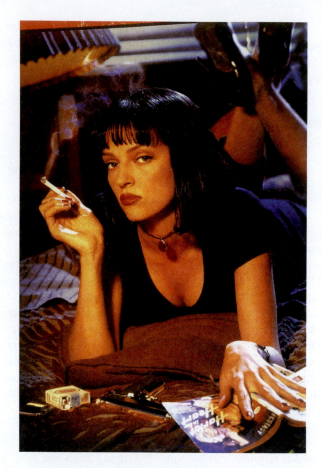

Although not its primary intent, this shot of Uma Thurman smoking, in the film *Pulp Fiction,* works as a successful advertisement for the tobacco industry.
© Ullstein Bild/Pressefoto Kindermann/Getty Images

Emulating Smoking in the Media
Media portrayals of smoking are a key influence on young people. In fact, studies by the National Cancer Institute have concluded that a direct causal relationship exists between media portrayals of smoking and smoking initiation. And a study conducted by researchers at the Dartmouth Medical School found that more than 50% of young people surveyed began smoking after watching repeated favorable portrayals of smoking in movies.

In general, the fictional portrayal of smoking in films and television does not reflect actual U.S. patterns of tobacco use. The prevalence of smoking among lead characters is three to four times that among comparable Americans. Films typically show smokers as white, male, well educated, successful, and attractive. In reality, smokers tend to be poor and to have less education (see Figure 8.5). Public campaigns to reduce images of smoking in movies have succeeded somewhat; smoking is shown less often in films and television shows now than even just a few years ago. Still, antismoking advocates say that films are still a critical and highly successful form of advertising for the tobacco industry.

QUICK STATS

More than 264 billion cigarettes were sold in the United States in 2015.
—The Maxwell Report: Year End & Fourth Quarter 2015 Cigarette Industry

TERMS

cigarette tar   A brown, sticky mass created when the chemical particles in tobacco smoke condense.

carcinogen   Any substance that causes cancer.

cocarcinogen   A substance that works with a carcinogen to cause cancer.

out), and chemicals that enhance the addicting properties of nicotine. Some additives and their uses are described below:

- *Sugars (such as licorice, cocoa, honey).* These mask the bitter taste of tobacco, allowing for deeper inhalation. Burning sugar produces acetaldehyde, which is an addictive carcinogen.

- *Other flavorings.* Theobromine and glycyrrhizin are flavorings that also act as bronchodilators, opening the lungs' airways and making it easier for nicotine to get into the bloodstream.

- *Ammonia.* The main purpose of this additive is to boost nicotine delivery. Ammonia reduces the acidity of tobacco smoke and releases nicotine in the form of a base (alkaline) rather than a salt, which would bind to other acid components of smoke. As a free base, nicotine is more readily absorbed into the blood.

- *Potassium citrate, aluminum, and clay.* These additives make **sidestream smoke** (the uninhaled smoke from a burning cigarette) less obvious and objectionable. They are added to cigarette wrappers to convert particulate ash into an invisible gas with less irritating odor than would be given off by a conventional paper wrapper. Additives such as these are intended to reduce social pressures from nonsmokers.

Nearly 600 chemicals, approved as safe when used as food additives, are used in manufacturing cigarettes.

"Reduced Harm" Cigarettes   Some smokers prefer low-tar, low-nicotine, or filtered cigarettes because they believe them to be less dangerous alternatives. The tobacco industry has long promoted such products as "reduced harm" cigarettes, meaning they are supposedly less damaging to their users' health. But there is no such thing as a safe cigarette, and smoking behavior is a more important factor in tar and nicotine intake than the type of cigarette smoked. Smokers who switch to a low-nicotine brand often compensate by smoking more cigarettes, inhaling more deeply, taking larger or more frequent puffs, or blocking ventilation holes with lips or fingers to offset the effects of filters.

In 2010, federal regulations prohibited cigarette manufacturers from labeling their products with descriptors such as "light," "mild," or "low"—terms that have effectively convinced many consumers that such cigarettes are safer alternatives to higher-tar cigarettes.

Ask Yourself

QUESTIONS FOR CRITICAL THINKING AND REFLECTION

What has influenced your decision to smoke, not to smoke, or to quit smoking? Have you ever felt that images or messages in the media were encouraging you to use tobacco? How do you react to such messages?

Menthol Cigarettes   About 70% of African American smokers smoke these cigarettes, as compared to 30% of European American smokers. Studies have found that African Americans absorb more nicotine than other groups and metabolize it more slowly; they also have lower rates of successful quitting. The anesthetizing effect of menthol, which may allow smokers to inhale more deeply and hold smoke in their lungs for a longer period, may be partly responsible for these differences.

The Immediate Effects of Smoking

The beginning smoker often has symptoms of mild nicotine poisoning, including the following: dizziness; faintness; rapid pulse; cold, clammy skin; nausea; vomiting; diarrhea.

The effects of nicotine on smokers vary, largely depending on the size of the nicotine dose and how much tolerance the smoker has built up through previous smoking. Nicotine can either excite or tranquilize the nervous system, depending on dosage, and it has many other immediate effects (see Figure 8.6). It stimulates the part of the brain called the **cerebral cortex.** It also stimulates the adrenal glands to release adrenaline. Nicotine inhibits the formation of urine; constricts the blood vessels, especially in the skin; accelerates the heart rate; and elevates blood pressure. Smoking depresses hunger sensations and dulls the taste buds.

The Long-Term Effects of Smoking

Smoking is linked to many deadly and disabling diseases (again, refer to Figure 8.6). Research indicates that the total amount of tobacco smoke inhaled is a key factor contributing to disease. People who smoke more cigarettes per day, inhale deeply, puff frequently, smoke cigarettes down to the butts, or begin smoking at early ages run a greater risk of disease than do those who smoke more moderately or who do not smoke at all.

Cardiovascular Disease   Although lung cancer tends to receive the most publicity, one form of cardiovascular disease, **coronary heart disease (CHD),** is actually the most widespread single cause of death for cigarette smokers. CHD often results when the arteries that supply the heart muscle with blood develop **atherosclerosis.** In

TERMS

sidestream smoke   The uninhaled smoke from a burning cigarette.

cerebral cortex   The outer region of the brain, which controls complex behavior and mental activity.

coronary heart disease (CHD)   Cardiovascular disease caused by hardening of the arteries that supply oxygen to the heart muscle; also called *coronary artery disease.*

atherosclerosis   Cardiovascular disease caused by the deposit of fatty substances (called *plaque*) in the walls of the arteries.

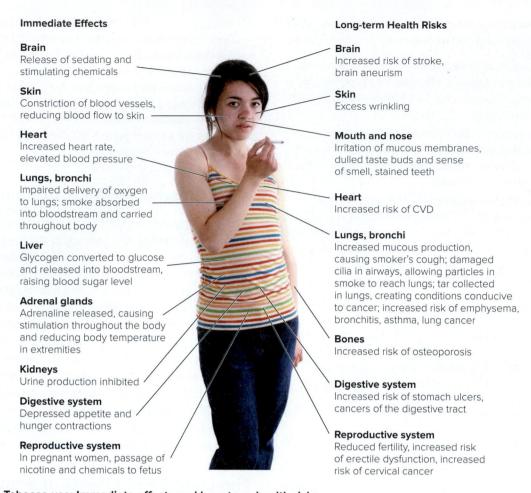

Immediate Effects

Brain
Release of sedating and
stimulating chemicals

Skin
Constriction of blood vessels,
reducing blood flow to skin

Heart
Increased heart rate,
elevated blood pressure

Lungs, bronchi
Impaired delivery of oxygen
to lungs; smoke absorbed
into bloodstream and carried
throughout body

Liver
Glycogen converted to glucose
and released into bloodstream,
raising blood sugar level

Adrenal glands
Adrenaline released, causing
stimulation throughout the body
and reducing body temperature
in extremities

Kidneys
Urine production inhibited

Digestive system
Depressed appetite and
hunger contractions

Reproductive system
In pregnant women, passage of
nicotine and chemicals to fetus

Long-term Health Risks

Brain
Increased risk of stroke,
brain aneurism

Skin
Excess wrinkling

Mouth and nose
Irritation of mucous membranes,
dulled taste buds and sense
of smell, stained teeth

Heart
Increased risk of CVD

Lungs, bronchi
Increased mucous production,
causing smoker's cough; damaged
cilia in airways, allowing particles in
smoke to reach lungs; tar collected
in lungs, creating conditions conducive
to cancer; increased risk of emphysema,
bronchitis, asthma, lung cancer

Bones
Increased risk of osteoporosis

Digestive system
Increased risk of stomach ulcers,
cancers of the digestive tract

Reproductive system
Reduced fertility, increased risk
of erectile dysfunction, increased
risk of cervical cancer

FIGURE 8.6 Tobacco use: Immediate effects and long-term health risks.

© Tim Large–Youth Social Issues/Alamy

atherosclerosis, fatty deposits called **plaques** form on the inner walls of arteries, causing them to narrow and stiffen. Smoking and exposure to environmental tobacco smoke (ETS) permanently accelerate the rate of plaque accumulation in the coronary arteries—50% for smokers, 25% for ex-smokers, and 20% for people regularly exposed to ETS. The crushing chest pain of **angina pectoris,** a primary symptom of CHD, results when the heart muscle, or *myocardium,* does not get enough oxygen. Sometimes a plaque forms at a narrow point in a main coronary artery. If the plaque completely blocks the flow of blood to a portion of the heart, that portion may die. This type of heart attack is called a **myocardial infarction.**

CHD can also interfere with the heart's electrical activity, resulting in disturbances of the normal heartbeat rhythm.

Smokers have a death rate from CHD that is 70% higher than that of nonsmokers. The risks of CHD decrease rapidly when a person stops smoking. This is particularly true for younger smokers, whose coronary arteries have not yet been damaged extensively. Cigarette smoking has been linked to other cardiovascular diseases, including the following:

• *Stroke.* A sudden interference with the circulation of blood in a part of the brain, resulting in the destruction of brain cells.

• *Aortic aneurysm.* A bulge in the aorta caused by a weakening in its walls.

• *Pulmonary heart disease.* A disorder of the right side of the heart, caused by changes in the blood vessels of the lungs.

Lung Cancer and Other Cancers   Cigarette smoking is the primary cause of lung cancer. Those who smoke two or more packs of cigarettes a day have lung cancer death rates 12–25 times greater than those of nonsmokers. The dramatic rise in lung cancer rates among women in the past 40 years clearly parallels the increase in smoking in this

TERMS

plaque   A deposit on the inner wall of blood vessels; blood can coagulate around plaque and form a clot.

angina pectoris   Chest pain due to coronary heart disease.

myocardial infarction   A heart attack caused by the complete blockage of a main coronary artery.

group; lung cancer now exceeds breast cancer as the leading cause of cancer deaths among women. The risk of developing lung cancer increases with the number of cigarettes smoked each day and the number of years of smoking. Evidence suggests that after 1 year without smoking, the risk of lung cancer decreases substantially. After 10 years, the risk of lung cancer among ex-smokers is 50% lower than for those who continue to smoke.

Research has also linked smoking to cancers of the trachea, mouth, pharynx, esophagus, larynx, pancreas, bladder, kidney, breast, cervix, stomach, liver, colon, and skin.

Chronic Obstructive Pulmonary Disease The stresses placed on the lungs by smoking can permanently damage lung function and lead to *chronic obstructive pulmonary disease (COPD),* also known as chronic obstructive lung disease or chronic lower respiratory disease. COPD is a disorder that consists of several diseases, including emphysema and chronic bronchitis. It is caused by the overtaxing of smokers' lungs, which need to work harder in response to the constant exposure to chemicals and irritants. COPD was the third leading cause of death in the United States in 2013 (the most recent year for which complete data are available).

Smoking is the primary cause of **emphysema,** a disabling condition in which the air sacs in the walls of the lungs lose their elasticity and are gradually destroyed. The lungs' ability to take in oxygen and expel carbon dioxide is impaired. A person with emphysema is often breathless, gasps for air, and has the feeling of drowning. The heart must pump harder and may become enlarged. People with emphysema often die from a damaged heart. There is no known way to reverse this disease.

Persistent, recurrent inflammation of the bronchial tubes characterizes **chronic bronchitis.** When the cell lining of the bronchial tubes is irritated, it secretes excess mucus. Bronchial congestion is followed by a chronic cough, which makes breathing more and more difficult. If smokers have chronic bronchitis, they face a greater risk of lung cancer, no matter how old they are or how many cigarettes they smoke.

Even when the smoker shows no signs of lung impairment or disease, cigarette smoking damages the respiratory system. Normally the cells lining the bronchial tubes secrete *mucus,* a sticky fluid that collects particles of soot, dust, and other substances in inhaled air. Mucus is cleared out of the lungs into the throat by the continuous motion of *cilia,* which are hairlike structures that protrude from the inner surface of the bronchial tubes. If the cilia are destroyed or impaired, or if inhaled air contains more pollutants than the system can remove, the protection provided by cilia is lost.

Cigarette smoke first slows and then stops the action of the cilia. Eventually it destroys them, leaving delicate membranes exposed to injury from substances inhaled in cigarette smoke or from the polluted air in which the person lives or works. Special cells called *macrophages* (a type of white blood cell) also work to remove foreign particles from the respiratory tract by engulfing them. Smoking appears to make macrophages work less efficiently. This interference with the functioning of the respiratory system often leads rapidly to the conditions known as *smoker's throat* and *smoker's cough,* as well as to shortness of breath. Even smokers of high school age show impaired respiratory function compared with nonsmokers of the same age. Other respiratory effects of smoking include a worsening of allergy and asthma symptoms and an increase in the smoker's susceptibility to colds.

Additional Health, Cosmetic, and Economic Concerns

People who smoke are more likely to develop peptic ulcers and are more likely to die from them (especially stomach ulcers) because smoking impairs the body's healing ability. Smoking also increases the risk of gastroesophageal reflux, which causes heartburn and can, if severe, raise the risk of esophageal cancer. Smoking affects blood flow in the veins and arteries of the penis and is an independent risk factor for erectile dysfunction (impotence). Smoking is linked to reduced fertility in both men and women. Smokers are at increased risk for tooth decay and gum and periodontal diseases, with symptoms appearing by the mid-twenties. Smoking dulls the senses of taste and smell. Over time it increases the risk of hearing loss and of macular degeneration and cataracts (both are serious eye conditions that can result in partial or total blindness). Smokers have higher rates of motor vehicle crashes, fire-related injuries, and back pain. Smoking can cause premature skin wrinkling, premature baldness, stained teeth, discolored fingers, and a persistent tobacco odor in clothes and hair. In September 2015, the average per-pack price of cigarettes was $5.51, although the price in most states is from $6 to $8. A pack-a-day habit could cost more than $2000 per year for cigarettes alone, or over $20,000 after 10 years. In addition, smoking contributes to osteoporosis, increases the risk of complications from diabetes, and accelerates the course of multiple

emphysema A disease characterized by a loss of lung tissue elasticity and destruction of the air sacs, impairing the lungs' ability to take in oxygen and expel carbon dioxide.

chronic bronchitis Recurrent, persistent inflammation of the bronchial tubes.

TERMS

sclerosis. Further research may link tobacco use to other disorders.

Cumulative Effects The cumulative effects of tobacco use fall into two general categories. The first category is reduced life expectancy. A male who takes up smoking before age 15 and continues to smoke is only half as likely to live to age 75 as a male who never smokes. Females who have similar smoking habits also have a reduced life expectancy.

The second category involves quality of life. A national health survey begun in 1964 shows that smokers spend one-third more time away from their jobs because of illness than nonsmokers.

Both male and female smokers have a greater rate of acute and chronic disease than people who have never smoked. Smokers become disabled at younger ages than nonsmokers and have more years of unhealthy life as well as shorter life spans.

Gender Differences in Health Hazards Although overall risks of tobacco-related illness are similar for women and men, sex appears to make a difference in some diseases. Women, for example, are more at risk for smoking-related blood clots and strokes than are men, and the risk is even greater for women using oral contraceptives. Among men and women with the same smoking history, the odds for developing three major types of cancer, including lung cancer, are 1.2–1.7 times higher in women than in men.

Women who smoke also have risks associated with reproduction and the reproductive organs. Smoking is associated with greater menstrual bleeding, greater duration of painful menstrual cramps, and more variability in menstrual cycle length. Smokers have a more difficult time becoming pregnant, and they reach menopause on average a year or two earlier than nonsmokers. When women smokers become pregnant, they face increased chances of miscarriage or placental disorders that lead to bleeding and premature delivery; rates of ectopic pregnancy, preeclampsia, and stillbirth are also higher among women who smoke. In addition, smoking is a risk factor for cervical cancer.

Risks Associated with Other Forms of Tobacco Use

Many smokers have switched from cigarettes to other forms of tobacco, such as spit (smokeless) tobacco, cigars, pipes, clove cigarettes, bidis, hookahs, and e-cigarettes. These alternatives, however, can be just as harmful as cigarettes.

Spit (Smokeless) Tobacco More than 8.2 million adults and about 7.7% of all high school students are current spit tobacco users, with a higher prevalence of current smokeless tobacco use among male (12.8%) than female

(2.5%) students. About 80% of users start by the ninth grade.

Spit tobacco comes in two major forms: snuff and chewing tobacco (chew). In snuff, the tobacco leaf is processed into a coarse, moist powder and mixed with flavorings. Snuff is usually sold in small tins. Users place a wad of tobacco in their mouths and then chew or suck it to release the nicotine. All types of smokeless tobacco cause an increase in saliva production, and the resulting tobacco juice is spit out or swallowed.

The nicotine in spit tobacco—along with flavorings and additives—is absorbed through the gums and lining of the mouth. Holding an average-size dip in the mouth for 30 minutes delivers about the same amount of nicotine as two or three cigarettes. Because of its nicotine content, spit tobacco is highly addictive. Some users keep it in their mouths even while sleeping.

Although not as dangerous as smoking cigarettes, the use of spit tobacco carries many health risks. Gums and lips become dried and irritated and may bleed. White or red patches may appear inside the mouth; this condition, known as *leukoplakia,* can lead to oral cancer. About 25% of regular spit tobacco users have *gingivitis* (inflammation) and recession of the gums and bone loss around the teeth, especially where the tobacco is typically placed. The senses of taste and smell are usually dulled.

One of the most serious effects of spit tobacco is an increased risk of oral cancer—cancers of the lip, tongue, cheek, throat, gums, roof and floor of the mouth, and larynx. Spit tobacco contains at least 28 chemicals known to cause cancer, and long-term snuff use may increase the risk of oral cancer by as much as 50 times. Surgery to treat oral cancer is often disfiguring and may involve removing parts of the face, tongue, cheek, or lip.

Cigars and Pipes Cigar smoking increased steadily since the early 1990s but then dropped somewhat in 2014. Cigars are most popular among white males aged 18–44 with higher-than-average income and education, but women are also smoking cigars in record numbers. In government surveys, 13% of American high school students reported having smoked at least one cigar in the previous month. Fewer than 1% of Americans, mostly males who also smoke cigarettes, are pipe smokers.

Because cigar and pipe smoke is more alkaline than cigarette smoke, users of cigars and pipes do not need to inhale in order to ingest nicotine; instead they absorb nicotine through the gums and lining of the mouth. Cigars contain more tobacco than cigarettes and so contain more nicotine and produce more tar when smoked. Large cigars may contain as much tobacco as a whole pack of cigarettes and may take one or two hours to smoke.

The health risks of cigars depend on the number of cigars smoked and whether the smoker inhales. Because most cigar and pipe users do not inhale, they have a lower risk of cancer and cardiovascular and respiratory diseases than cigarette smokers. However, their risks are substantially higher than those of nonsmokers. For example, compared to nonsmokers, people who smoke one or two cigars per day without inhaling have six times the risk of cancer of the larynx. The risks are much higher for cigar smokers who inhale: They have 27 times the risk of oral cancer and 53 times the risk of cancer of the larynx compared to nonsmokers, and their risk of heart and lung diseases approaches that of cigarette smokers. Smoking a cigar immediately impairs the ability of blood vessels to dilate, reducing the amount of oxygen delivered to tissues, including the heart muscle, especially during stress. Pipe and cigar smoking are also risk factors for pancreatic cancer, which is almost always fatal.

Nicotine addiction is another concern. The recent rise in cigar use among teens has raised concerns because nicotine addiction almost always develops in the teen or young adult years. More research is needed to determine if cigar use by teens will develop into nicotine addiction and frequent use of either cigarettes or spit tobacco.

Clove Cigarettes and Bidis

Clove cigarettes, also called *kreteks* or *chicartas,* are made of tobacco mixed with chopped cloves; they are imported primarily from Indonesia and Pakistan. Clove cigarettes contain almost twice as much tar, nicotine, and carbon monoxide as conventional cigarettes and so present all the same health hazards. Some chemical constituents of cloves may also be dangerous. A number of serious respiratory injuries and deaths have resulted from the use of clove cigarettes.

Bidis, or "beadies," are small cigarettes imported from India that contain species of tobacco different from those used by U.S. cigarette manufacturers. The tobacco in bidis is hand-rolled in Indian ebony leaves (tendu) and then often flavored; clove, mint, chocolate, and fruit varieties are available. Bidis contain up to four times more nicotine than U.S. cigarettes and twice as much tar.

Hookah

Hookahs—sometimes called water pipes or *shisha*—are pipes used for smoking specially flavored tobacco (e.g., apple, mint, cherry). The hookah has four main parts: the head, body, hose, and water urn. As the smoke is inhaled through the mouthpiece attached to the hose that passes through the water urn, the water cools the smoke and emits it as vapor.

Hookah use originated in ancient Persia and India, but it has gained popularity around the globe in recent years. In 2006, an estimated 300 hookah bars operated in the United States; since then the number has grown and continues to grow.

> **hookah** A pipe used for smoking specially flavored tobacco (e.g., apple, mint, cherry); sometimes called a water pipe or *shisha*.
>
> **TERMS**

Although high school and middle school students' use of cigarettes, cigars, smokeless tobacco, pipe tobacco, and bidis declined significantly during 2011–2015, their use of e-cigarettes and hookahs increased dramatically. A drop in hookah use among high school students was observed during 2014–2015, but not among middle school students. About 30% of college students have smoked hookah tobacco at least once.

Hookah smoking carries many of the same health risks as cigarette smoking; it is therefore *not* a safe alternative. In fact, due to the mode of smoking (inhalation), hookah smokers may absorb higher concentrations of the toxins commonly found in cigarette smoke. One hour of hookah smoking involves 200 puffs, whereas an average cigarette involves 20 puffs. The volume of smoke inhaled during a typical hookah session is about 90,000 milliliters (ml), compared with 500–600 ml inhaled when smoking a cigarette.

E-Cigarettes

The electronic cigarette, also known as an *e-cigarette* or *e-cig,* is a battery-powered device that resembles a real cigarette. Instead of containing tobacco, the device uses a changeable filter that contains one or more chemicals, such as nicotine, flavorings, and other compounds. The user "smokes" an e-cig by sucking the filtered end; the device's battery heats the chemicals to create an inhalable vapor. During use (vaping), the device's tip even glows like the burning end of a real cigarette. Although electronic cigarettes have been advertised as a way to help smokers quit smoking—in a 2014 survey, the CDC reported that individuals trying to quit likely chose e-cigarettes over tobacco cigarettes—no evidence submitted to the FDA supports this claim.

Electronic cigarettes get hot enough to produce carcinogens and other toxic chemicals like formaldehyde, also found in traditional cigarettes, or diethylene glycol, which is a toxic chemical in antifreeze. Moreover, a recent study found that

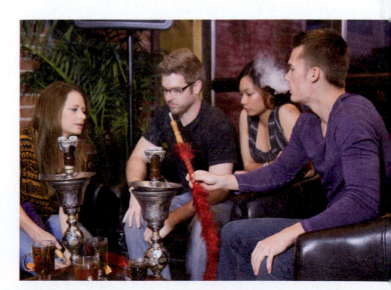

Although cigarette smoking has decreased among high school and college students, hookah smoking has increased.

© Inkk Studios/Getty Images

even nicotine-free e-cigarette solutions and vapor caused disruptions and damage to lung cells in humans and mice. The authors of this study postulated that this was due to chemicals they detected in the e-cigarette solution and vapor, including acrolein, propylene glycol, and glycerol.

E-cigarettes also produce nanoparticles, which have been linked to inflammation leading to asthma, stroke, and heart disease. One study found that vaping may make antibiotic-resistant bacteria even harder to kill. In another recent study, e-cigarette flavoring chemicals were linked to an irreversible respiratory disease called bronchiolitis obliterans, or "popcorn lung," in which the airways become inflamed and scarred, resulting in a permanent cough and shortness of breath.

Between 2011 and 2015, the rate of e-cigarette use among high school students increased more dramatically than it did for any other tobacco product. During 2015, e-cigarettes were the most popular tobacco product among both middle school (5.3%) and high school (16.0%) students. Although e-cigarettes were not previously regulated under the FDA, a new ruling in May 2016 extended the FDA's authority over all forms of tobacco products. These new rules ban the sale of e-cigarettes to minors and require identification for purchase.

Marketers of e-cigarettes have claimed that the devices deliver only nicotine, making them a safe cigarette that does not cause cancer and can serve as an alternative to other nicotine replacement products such as gum and patches. According to the FDA, however, not all e-cigarettes contain nicotine. Further, the FDA has warned that some varieties of e-cigarettes are flavored, apparently to make them appeal to teenagers and other first-time smokers. The products do not carry the same types of warnings required on tobacco products. Eight senators have called on the FDA to focus on the harmful vapors that e-cigarettes produce as well as the ingredients they contain. New York City, Chicago, and Los Angeles have recently banned e-cigarettes from some private and public places.

Ask Yourself

QUESTIONS FOR CRITICAL THINKING AND REFLECTION

Do you know anyone who has suffered from an illness related to tobacco use? If so, what problems did that person face? What was the outcome? Did the experience have any effect on your views about using tobacco?

THE EFFECTS OF SMOKING ON THE NONSMOKER

Tobacco users aren't the only ones who suffer ill effects. Tens of thousands of nonsmokers die each year because of exposure to secondhand smoke. Further, the medical and societal costs of tobacco use are enormous.

Environmental Tobacco Smoke

The U.S. Environmental Protection Agency (EPA) has designated **environmental tobacco smoke (ETS)**—more commonly called *secondhand smoke*—a Class A carcinogen. The HHS National Toxicology Program classifies ETS as a "known human carcinogen." The Surgeon General has concluded that for some people there is no safe level of exposure to ETS; even brief exposure can cause serious harm.

Environmental tobacco smoke consists of mainstream smoke and sidestream smoke. Smoke exhaled by smokers is referred to as **mainstream smoke.** Sidestream smoke enters the atmosphere from the burning end of a cigarette, cigar, or pipe. Nearly 85% of the smoke in a room where someone is smoking comes from sidestream smoke. Sidestream smoke is unfiltered (it is not filtered through either a cigarette filter or a smoker's lungs) and has twice as much tar and nicotine, three times as much benzo(a)pyrene, almost three times as much carbon monoxide, and three times as much ammonia as mainstream smoke.

In rooms where people are smoking, levels of carbon monoxide can exceed those permitted by Federal Air Quality Standards for outside air. In a typical home with the windows closed, it takes about six hours for 95% of the airborne cigarette smoke particles to clear. The carcinogens in the secondhand smoke from a single cigar exceed those of three cigarettes, and cigar smoke contains up to 30 times more carbon monoxide.

ETS Effects Nonsmokers subjected to ETS frequently develop coughs, headaches, nasal discomfort, and eye irritation. Other symptoms range from breathlessness to sinus problems. People with allergies tend to suffer the most.

ETS causes an estimated 7300 lung cancer deaths and 34,000 deaths from heart disease each year in people who do not smoke. Exposure to ETS is also associated with a 20% increase in the progression of atherosclerosis. ETS aggravates asthma and increases the risk for breast and cervical cancers.

Scientists have been able to measure changes that contribute to lung tissue damage and potential tumor promotion in the bloodstreams of healthy young test subjects who spend just three hours in a smoke-filled room. After just 30 minutes of exposure to ETS, the function in the coronary arteries of healthy nonsmokers is reduced to the same level as that of smokers.

> **environmental tobacco smoke (ETS)** **TERMS**
> Smoke that enters the atmosphere from the burning end of a cigarette, cigar, or pipe, as well as smoke that is exhaled by smokers; also called *secondhand smoke*.
>
> **mainstream smoke** Smoke that is inhaled by a smoker and then exhaled into the atmosphere.

Infants, Children, and ETS Infants and children are perhaps the group most vulnerable to the harmful effects of ETS. Recent studies have shown that infants exposed to smoke from more than 21 cigarettes a day are more than *23 times* more likely to die of sudden infant death syndrome (SIDS) than are babies not exposed to ETS. Chemicals in tobacco smoke also show up in breast milk, and breastfeeding may pass more chemicals to the infant of a smoking mother than the infant receives through direct exposure to ETS.

ETS triggers bronchitis, pneumonia, and other respiratory infections in infants and toddlers up to age 18 months, resulting in as many as 15,000 hospitalizations each year.

Older children suffer, too. ETS is a risk factor for asthma and aggravates symptoms in children who already have asthma. ETS is also linked to reduced lung function and fluid buildup in the middle ear, a contributing factor in middle-ear infections, a leading reason for childhood surgery. Children and teens exposed to ETS score lower on tests of reading and reasoning. Later in life, people exposed to ETS as children are at increased risk for lung cancer, emphysema, and chronic bronchitis.

Smoking and Pregnancy

Smoking almost doubles a pregnant woman's chance of having a miscarriage, and it significantly increases her risk of ectopic pregnancy. Maternal smoking causes hundreds of infant deaths in the United States each year, primarily due to premature delivery and smoking-related problems with the placenta. Maternal smoking is a major factor in low birth weight, which puts newborns at high risk for infections and other serious problems. If a nonsmoking mother is regularly exposed to ETS, her infant is also at greater risk for low birth weight.

Babies born to mothers who smoke more than two packs a day perform poorly on developmental tests in the first hours after birth, compared to babies of nonsmoking mothers. Later in life, obesity, hyperactivity, short attention span, and lower scores on spelling and reading tests all occur more frequently in children whose mothers smoked during pregnancy than in those born to nonsmoking mothers. Prenatal tobacco exposure has also been associated with behavioral problems in children.

Ask Yourself

QUESTIONS FOR CRITICAL THINKING AND REFLECTION

What antismoking ordinances are in effect in your community? Does your school prohibit smoking on campus? Do you think these rules have been effective in reducing smoking or exposure to ETS? Do you support such regulations? Why or why not?

WHAT CAN BE DONE TO COMBAT SMOKING?

There are many ways to act against this public health threat.

Action at Many Levels

Thousands of local ordinances across the nation now restrict or ban smoking in restaurants, stores, workplaces, and even public outdoor areas. An assessment made in 2010 found that nearly 80% of Americans live in municipalities that restrict or ban smoking in public buildings, workplaces, restaurants, and bars. Hundreds of colleges and universities now have totally smoke-free campuses or prohibit smoking in residential buildings. As local nonsmoking laws proliferate, evidence mounts that environmental restrictions are effective in encouraging smokers to quit.

At the state level, many tough anti-tobacco laws have been passed. As of 2015, comprehensive smoke-free air laws were in effect in 28 states, the District of Columbia, and Puerto Rico. California has one of the most aggressive—and successful—tobacco control programs, combining taxes on cigarettes, graphic advertisements, and bans on smoking in bars and restaurants.

Regulation of Tobacco

Until 2009, the U.S. FDA did not have the power to regulate tobacco products. That changed when Congress passed the

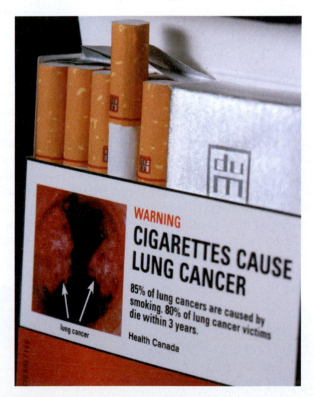

Canada's graphic cigarette labels have greatly helped reduce smoking rates.

© Bloomberg/Norm Betts/Getty Images

Family Smoking Prevention and Tobacco Control Act, which gives the agency the power to dictate how much nicotine is included in tobacco products. Under this law the FDA can eliminate or control levels of the thousands of chemical additives used to make tobacco more appealing and addictive. In addition, the legislation strengthens health warnings and places even greater limits on tobacco advertising, both of which have had a significant impact on smoking prevalence. For instance, larger graphic warnings in Canada have been attributed to an estimated 12–20% reduction in smoking rates between 2000 and 2009. Similar reductions in smoking rates could emerge in the United States once graphic warning labels like those in Canada are implemented.

The World Health Organization has taken the lead in international anti-tobacco efforts by sponsoring the Framework Convention on Tobacco Control. Another international activity is the annual commemoration of World No Tobacco Day (May 31), on which smokers are encouraged to stop smoking for one day.

Such efforts at the local, state, national, and international levels represent progress, but health activists warn that tobacco industry influence remains strong. The tobacco industry contributes heavily to sympathetic legislative officeholders and candidates. The tobacco industry has also focused increasing attention on the developing world, exporting its products to countries with few or no consumer protection laws in place.

QUICK STATS

In many states the price of a pack of cigarettes can exceed **$6.00**. But each pack of cigarettes creates **$35** dollars of health-related costs for the smoker.
—American Cancer Society, 2015

Individual Action

Nonsmokers have the right not only to breathe clean air but also to take action to help solve one of society's most serious public health threats. Here are just some of the many actions you can take. When a smoker violates a no-smoking designation, complain. If your favorite restaurant or shop doesn't have a nonsmoking policy, ask the manager to adopt one. If you see children buying tobacco, report this illegal activity to the facility manager or the police. Learn more about addiction and tobacco cessation so that you can better support the tobacco users you know. Vote for candidates who support anti-tobacco measures; contact local, state, and national representatives to express your views.

Ask Yourself

QUESTIONS FOR CRITICAL THINKING AND REFLECTION

What are your views on the government's role in regulating tobacco products? Is current regulation enough, or should the government go further in controlling the production and marketing of these products? What events or experiences have shaped your views on this issue?

HOW A TOBACCO USER CAN QUIT

Giving up tobacco is a long-term, intricate process. Research shows that tobacco users move through predictable stages—from being uninterested in stopping, to thinking about change, to making a serious effort to stop, to finally maintaining abstinence. But most attempt to quit several times before they finally succeed. Relapse is a normal part of the process.

Benefits of Quitting

Giving up tobacco provides immediate health benefits to men and women of all ages (Table 8.2). The younger people are when they stop smoking, the more pronounced the health improvements. And these improvements gradually but invariably increase as the period of nonsmoking lengthens. It's never too late to quit, though. According to a Surgeon General's report, people who quit smoking, regardless of age, live longer than people who continue to smoke.

Options for Quitting

Most tobacco users—69% in a recent survey—want to quit, and half of those who want to quit will make an attempt this year. What are their options? No single method works for everyone, but each does work for some people some of the time.

Behavior Change   Choosing to quit requires developing a strategy for success. Some people quit cold turkey, whereas others taper off slowly. Over-the-counter and prescription products help many people. Support from others and regular exercise are behavioral factors that have been shown to increase the chances that a smoker will stop smoking permanently. Support can come from friends and family and/or formal group programs sponsored by organizations such as the American Cancer Society and the American Lung Association, or by a college health center or community hospital. Programs that combine group support with nicotine replacement therapy have rates of continued abstention as high as 35% after one year.

Most smokers in the process of quitting experience both physical and psychological effects of nicotine withdrawal, and exercise can help with both. For many smokers, tobacco use is associated with certain times and places—following a meal, for example. Resolving to walk after dinner instead of lighting up provides a distraction from cravings and eliminates the cues that trigger a desire to smoke. In addition, many people worry about weight gain associated with quitting. Although most ex-smokers do gain a few pounds, at least temporarily, incorporating exercise into a new tobacco-free routine lays the foundation for healthy weight management. The health risks of adding a few pounds are minimal compared to the risks of continued smoking.

Table 8.2 — Benefits of Quitting Smoking

Within 20 minutes of your last cigarette:
- Blood pressure drops to normal
- Pulse rate drops to normal
- Temperature of hands and feet increases to normal
- You stop polluting the air

8 hours:
- Carbon monoxide level in blood drops to normal
- Oxygen level in blood increases to normal

24 hours:
- Chance of heart attack decreases

48 hours:
- Nerve endings start regrowing
- Ability to smell and taste is enhanced

2–3 months:
- Circulation improves
- Walking becomes easier
- Lung function increases up to 30%

1–9 months:
- Coughing, sinus congestion, fatigue, and shortness of breath all decrease

1 year:
- Heart disease death rate is half that of a smoker

5 years:
- Stroke risk drops nearly to the risk for nonsmokers

10 years:
- Lung cancer death rate drops to 50% of that of continuing smokers
- Incidence of other cancers (mouth, throat, larynx, esophagus, bladder, kidney, and pancreas) decreases
- Risk of ulcer decreases

15 years:
- Risk of lung cancer is about 25% of that of continuing smokers
- Risks of heart disease and death are close to those of nonsmokers

SOURCES: BeTobaccoFree.gov. n.d. *Get on a Path to a Healthier You (Quitting)* (http://betobaccofree.hhs.gov/gallery/quit.html); U.S. National Library of Medicine. 2013. *Benefits of Quitting Tobacco* (https://www.nlm.nih.gov/medlineplus/ency/article/007532.htm).

Free telephone quitlines are emerging as a popular and effective way to get help to stop smoking. Quitlines are staffed by trained counselors who help each caller plan a personal quitting strategy, usually including a combination of nicotine replacement therapy, changes in daily habits, and emotional support.

HHS has a national toll-free number, 1-800-QUITNOW (1-800-784-8669), to serve as a single access point for smokers seeking information and assistance in quitting. As with any significant change in health-related behavior, giving up tobacco requires planning, sustained effort, and support. It is an ongoing process, not a one-time event. The "Kicking the Tobacco Habit" box at the end of the chapter describes the steps that successful quitters follow.

Smoking Cessation Products Each year millions of Americans visit their doctors in the hope of finding a drug that can help them stop smoking. Although pharmacological options are limited, the few available drugs have proved successful.

CHANTIX (VARINICLINE) The newest smoking cessation drug, marketed under the name Chantix, works in two ways: It reduces nicotine cravings, easing the withdrawal process, and it blocks the pleasant effects of nicotine. The drug acts on neurotransmitter receptors in the brain.

Unlike most smoking cessation products currently on the market, Chantix is not a nicotine replacement. For this reason, smokers may be advised to continue smoking for the first few days of treatment to avoid withdrawal and to allow the drug to build up in their bodies. The approved course of treatment is 12 weeks, but the duration and recommended dosage depend on several factors, including the smoker's general health and the length and severity of his or her nicotine addiction.

Side effects reported with Chantix include nausea, headaches, vomiting, sleep disruptions, and changes in taste perception. People with kidney problems or who take certain medications should not take Chantix, and it is not recommended for women who are pregnant or nursing. Further, the FDA has been investigating reports of the drug causing adverse reactions, such as behavioral changes, agitation, depression, suicidal thoughts, and attempted suicide. Anyone taking Chantix should immediately notify his or her doctor of any sudden change in mood or behavior.

ZYBAN (BUPROPION) Bupropion is an antidepressant (prescribed under the name Wellbutrin) as well as a smoking cessation aid (prescribed under the name Zyban). As a smoking cessation aid, bupropion eases the symptoms of nicotine withdrawal and reduces the urge to smoke. Like Chantix, it acts on neurotransmitter receptors in the brain.

Bupropion users have reported an array of side effects, but they are rare. Side effects may be reduced by changing the dosage, taking the medicine at a different time of day, or taking it with or without food. Bupropion is not recommended for people with specific physical conditions or who take certain drugs. Zyban and Wellbutrin should not be taken together.

NICOTINE REPLACEMENT PRODUCTS The most widely used smoking cessation products replace the nicotine that the user would normally get from tobacco. The user continues to get nicotine, so withdrawal symptoms and cravings are reduced. Although still harmful, nicotine replacement products provide a cleaner form of nicotine without

> **QUICK STATS**
> **77% of American college students report that they have never smoked a cigarette.**
> —American College Health Association, 2016

the thousands of poisons and tars produced by burning tobacco. Less of the product is used over time as the need for nicotine decreases.

Nicotine replacement products come in several forms, including patches, gum, lozenges, nasal sprays, and inhalers. They are available in a variety of strengths and can be worked into many different smoking cessation strategies. Most are available without a prescription.

The nicotine patch is popular because it can be applied and forgotten until it needs to be removed or changed, usually every 16 or 24 hours. Placed on the upper arm or torso, it releases a steady stream of nicotine, which is absorbed through the skin. The main side effects are skin irritation and redness. Nicotine gum and nicotine lozenges have the advantage of allowing the smoker to use them whenever he or she craves nicotine. Side effects of nicotine gum include mouth sores and headaches; nicotine lozenges can cause nausea and heartburn. Nicotine nasal sprays and inhalers are available only by prescription.

Although all these products have proved to be effective in helping users stop smoking, experts recommend them only as one part of a complete smoking cessation program. Such a program should include regular professional counseling and physician monitoring.

TIPS FOR TODAY AND THE FUTURE

The responsible use of alcohol means drinking in moderation or not at all. The best approach to tobacco use is never to start.

RIGHT NOW YOU CAN:

- Consider whether there is a history of alcohol abuse or dependence in your family.
- Think about your current drinking habits. For example, count the number of parties you attended in the past month and how many drinks you had at each one.
- If you smoke, throw the pack and lighter away.
- If you use tobacco, go outside for a short walk or a stretch to limber up. Breathe deeply. Tell a friend you've just decided to quit.

IN THE FUTURE YOU CAN:

- Think about the next party you plan to attend. Decide how much you will drink at the party, and how you will get home afterward.
- Watch your friends' behavior at events where drinking is involved. Do any of them show signs of a drinking problem? If so, consider what you can do to help.
- Resolve to quit smoking. Research your options for quitting and choose the one you think will work best for you.
- Recruit a friend or family member to help you quit smoking. Arrange to talk to this person whenever you feel the urge to smoke.

SUMMARY

- Although alcohol has long been a part of human celebrations, it is a psychoactive drug capable of causing addiction.

- After being absorbed into the bloodstream in the stomach and small intestine, alcohol is transported throughout the body. The liver metabolizes alcohol as blood circulates through it.

- If people drink more alcohol each hour than the body can metabolize, blood alcohol concentration (BAC) increases. The rate of alcohol metabolism depends on a variety of individual factors.

- Alcohol is a CNS depressant. At low doses, it tends to make people feel relaxed.

- At higher doses, alcohol interferes with motor and mental functioning; at very high doses, alcohol poisoning, coma, and death can occur. Effects may be increased if alcohol is combined with other drugs.

- Alcohol use increases the risk of injury and violence; drinking before driving is particularly dangerous, even at low doses.

- Chronic alcohol use has negative effects on the digestive and cardiovascular systems and increases cancer risk and overall mortality.

- Pregnant women who drink risk giving birth to children with a cluster of birth defects known as fetal alcohol syndrome (FAS). Even occasional drinking during pregnancy can cause brain injury in the fetus.

- Alcohol misuse involves drinking in dangerous situations or drinking to a degree that causes academic, professional, interpersonal, or legal difficulties.

- Alcoholism is characterized by more extensive problems with alcohol, usually involving tolerance and withdrawal.

- Binge drinking is a common form of alcohol abuse that has negative effects on both drinkers and nondrinkers. For numerous reasons, college students may be especially prone to binge drinking.

- Physical consequences of alcoholism include the direct effects of tolerance and withdrawal, as well as all the problems associated with chronic drinking. Psychological problems associated with alcoholism include memory loss and additional mental disorders such as depression.

- Alcoholism treatment approaches include mutual support groups like AA, job- and school-based programs, inpatient hospital programs, and pharmacological treatments.

- Helping someone who abuses alcohol means avoiding being an enabler, and obtaining information about available resources and persistently encouraging their use.

- Smoking is the largest preventable cause of premature disease and death in the United States. Nevertheless, millions of Americans use tobacco.

- Regular tobacco use causes physical dependence on nicotine, characterized by loss of control, tolerance, and withdrawal. Habits can become associated with tobacco use and trigger the urge for a cigarette.

- People who begin smoking are usually imitating others or responding to seductive advertising. Smoking is associated with low education level and the use of other drugs.

- Tobacco smoke is made up of thousands of chemicals, including some that are carcinogenic or toxic or that damage the respiratory system.

- Nicotine acts on the nervous system as a stimulant or a depressant. It can cause blood pressure and heart rate to increase, straining the heart.

- Cardiovascular disease is the most widespread cause of death for cigarette smokers. Cigarette smoking is the primary cause of lung cancer and is linked to many other cancers and respiratory diseases.

- Cigarette smoking is linked to ulcers, impotence, reproductive health problems, dental diseases, and other conditions. Tobacco use leads to lower life expectancy and to a diminished quality of life.

- The use of spit tobacco leads to nicotine addiction and is linked to a variety of cancers of the head and neck.

- Cigars, pipes, clove cigarettes, bidis, hookahs, and e-cigarettes are not safe alternatives to cigarettes. Using them results in lung, lip, larynx, and pancreatic cancers, COPD, and emphysema, among other conditions.

- Environmental tobacco smoke (ETS) contains high concentrations of toxic chemicals and can cause headaches, eye and nasal irritation, and sinus problems. Long-term exposure to ETS causes cancer and heart disease.

- Infants and young children take in more pollutants than adults do; children whose parents smoke are especially susceptible to respiratory diseases.

- Smoking during pregnancy increases the risk of miscarriage, stillbirth, congenital abnormalities, premature birth, and low birth weight. SIDS, behavior problems, and long-term impairments in development are also risks to infants and children of mothers who smoke during pregnancy.

- Individuals and groups have many options for acting against tobacco use. Nonsmokers can use social pressure and legislative channels to assert their rights to breathe clean air.

- Giving up smoking is a difficult and long-term process. Although most ex-smokers quit on their own, some smokers benefit from stop-smoking programs, over-the-counter and prescription medications, and support groups.

FOR MORE INFORMATION

Action on Smoking and Health (ASH). Provides statistics, news briefs, and other information.

http://ash.org

Al-Anon Family Group Headquarters. Provides information and referrals to local Al-Anon and Alateen groups. The website includes a self-quiz to determine if you are affected by someone's drinking.

http://www.al-anon.alateen.org

Alcoholics Anonymous (AA) World Services. Provides general information about AA, literature about alcoholism, and information about AA meetings and related 12-step organizations.

http://www.aa.org

AlcoholScreening.Org. Provides information about alcohol and health, referrals for treatment and support groups, and a drinking self-assessment.

http://www.alcoholscreening.org

Alcohol Treatment Referral Hotline. Provides referrals to local intervention and treatment providers.

800-ALCOHOL

American Cancer Society (ACS). Provides information about the dangers of tobacco, as well as tools for prevention and cessation for both smokers and users of spit tobacco; sponsors the annual Great American Smokeout.

http://www.cancer.org

American Lung Association. Provides information about lung diseases, tobacco control, and environmental health.

http://www.lungusa.org

Bacchus Network. An association of college- and university-based peer education programs that focus on prevention of alcohol abuse and promotion of campus health safety.

https://www.naspa.org/constituent-groups/groups/bacchus-initiatives

The College Alcohol Study. Harvard School of Public Health. Provides information about and results from the recent studies of binge drinking on college campuses.

http://www.hsph.harvard.edu/news/magazine/winter09binging-problems/

CDC's Tobacco Information and Prevention Source (TIPS). Provides research results, educational materials, and tips on how to quit smoking; website includes special sections for kids and teens.

http://www.cdc.gov/tobacco

College Drinking: Changing the Culture. Created by the National Institute on Alcohol Abuse and Alcoholism (NIAAA), this site gives comprehensive research-based information on issues related to alcohol abuse and binge drinking among college students.

http://www.collegedrinkingprevention.gov

Environmental Protection Agency Indoor Air Quality/ETS. Provides information and links about secondhand smoke.

https://www.epa.gov/indoor-air-quality-iaq/secondhand-tobacco-smoke-and-smoke-free-homes

Mothers Against Drunk Driving (MADD). Supports efforts to develop solutions to the problems of drunk driving and underage drinking and provides news, information, and brochures about many topics, including a guide for giving a safe party.

http://www.madd.org

National Association for Children of Alcoholics (NACoA). Provides information and support for children of alcoholics.

888-554-COAS

http://www.nacoa.org

National Council on Alcoholism and Drug Dependence (NCADD). Provides information and counseling referrals.

212-269-7797

800-NCA-CALL (24-hour Hope Line)

http://www.ncadd.org

National Institute on Alcohol Abuse and Alcoholism (NIAAA). Provides booklets and other publications on a variety of alcohol-related topics, including fetal alcohol syndrome, alcoholism treatment, and alcohol use and minorities.

http://www.niaaa.nih.gov

Nicotine Anonymous. A 12-step program for tobacco users.

http://www.nicotine-anonymous.org

Smokefree.gov. Provides step-by-step strategies for quitting as well as expert support via telephone or instant messaging.

http://www.smokefree.gov

Substance Abuse and Mental Health Services Administration. Provides statistics and information about alcohol abuse, including resources for people who want to help friends and family members overcome alcohol abuse problems.

http://www.samhsa.gov

See also the listings for Chapter 7.

World Health Organization Tobacco Free Initiative. Promotes the goal of a tobacco-free world.

http://www.who.int/tobacco/en

World No Tobacco Day (WNTD). Provides information about the annual worldwide event to encourage people to quit smoking; includes general information about tobacco use and testimonials of ex-smokers.

http://www.who.int/campaigns/no-tobacco-day/2016/en/

See also the listings for Chapters 7 and 12.

SELECTED BIBLIOGRAPHY

Allen, J. G., et al. 2016. Flavoring chemicals in e-cigarettes: Diacetyl, 2, 3-pentanedione, and acetoin in a sample of 51 products, including fruit-, candy-, and cocktail-flavored e-cigarettes. *Environmental Health Perspectives* 124(6) (http://ehp.niehs.nih.gov/15-10185/).

American Cancer Society. 2016. *Cancer Facts and Figures, 2016.* Atlanta, GA: American Cancer Society.

American College Health Association. 2016. *American College Health Association–National College Health Assessment IIc: Reference Group Executive Summary Fall 2015.* Hanover, MD: American College Health Association.

American Heart Association. 2015. The downside to alcohol: Moderate drinking in later years may damage heart. *Heart Insight* (http://heartinsight .heart.org/Fall-2015/The-Downside-to-Alcohol/).

American Lung Association. 2016. *State of Tobacco Control 2016* (http:// www.lung.org/our-initiatives/tobacco/reports-resources/sotc/at-a -glance/).

American Psychiatric Association. 2013. *Diagnostic and Statistical Manual of Mental Disorders,* 5th ed. *(DSM-5).* Washington, DC: American Psychiatric Publishing.

Campaign for Tobacco-Free Kids. 2016. *State Cigarette Excise Tax Rates and Rankings.* Washington, DC: Campaign for Tobacco-Free Kids.

Campaign for Tobacco-Free Kids. 2016. Tobacco Company Political Action Committee (PAC) Contributions to Federal Candidates (https://www .tobaccofreekids.org/what_we_do/federal_issues/campaign_contributions).

Cao, Y., et al. 2015. Light to moderate intake of alcohol, drinking patterns, and risk of cancer: Results from two prospective US cohort studies. *British Medical Journal* 351: h4238.

Centers for Disease Control and Prevention. 2010. Vital signs: Nonsmokers' exposure to secondhand smoke—United States, 1999–2009. *MMWR* 59(35): 1141–1146.

Centers for Disease Control and Prevention. 2011. Quitting smoking among adults—United States, 2001–2010. *MMWR* 60(44).

Centers for Disease Control and Prevention. 2012. Vital signs: Current cigarette smoking among adults—United States, 2011. *MMWR* 61(44): 889–894.

Centers for Disease Control and Prevention. 2014. *Smoking and Tobacco Use Fact Sheet: Tobacco-Related Mortality* (http://www.cdc.gov /tobacco/data_statistics/fact_sheets/health_effects/tobacco_related _mortality).

Centers for Disease Control and Prevention. 2015. Current cigarette smoking among adults—United States, 2005–2014. *MMWR* 64(44): 1233–1240.

Centers for Disease Control and Prevention. 2015a. *Alcohol and Public Health: Fact Sheets—Binge Drinking* (http://www.cdc.gov/alcohol/fact -sheets/binge-drinking.htm).

Centers for Disease Control and Prevention. 2015b. Alcohol use and binge drinking among women of childbearing age—United States, 2011– 2013. *MMWR* 64(37): 1042–1046.

Centers for Disease Control and Prevention. 2016. Tobacco use among middle and high school students—United States, 2011-2015. *MMWR* 65(14): 361–367.

Centers for Disease Control and Prevention. 2016. State Tobacco Activities Tracking and Evaluation (STATE) System (http://www.cdc.gov /STATESystem).

College Drinking Prevention. 2013. *A Snapshot of Annual High-Risk College Drinking Consequences* (http://www.collegedrinkingprevention .gov/StatsSummaries/snapshot.aspx).

Cunningham, J. K., T. A. Solomon, and M. L. Muramoto. 2016. Alcohol use among Native Americans compared to whites: Examining the veracity of the 'Native American elevated alcohol consumption' belief. *Drug and Alcohol Dependence* 160: 65–75.

Darvishi, N., et al. 2015. Alcohol-related risk of suicidal ideation, suicide attempt, and completed suicide: A meta-analysis. *PLOS ONE* e0126870.

Daube, M. 2015. Alcohol's evaporating health benefits. *British Medical Journal* 350: h407.

Division of Reproductive Health, National Center for Chronic Disease Prevention and Health Promotion. 2013. *Tobacco Use and Pregnancy* (http://www.cdc.gov/reproductivehealth/TobaccoUsePregnancy/index .htm).

Federal Trade Commission. 2016. *Federal Trade Commission Cigarette Report for 2013.* Washington, DC: Federal Trade Commission.

Huang, J., F. J. Chalupka, and G. T. Fong. 2013. Cigarette graphic warning labels and smoking prevalence in Canada: A critical examination and reformulation of the FDA regulatory impact analysis. *Tobacco Control.* DOI: 10.1136/tobaccocontrol-2013-051170.

Jha, P., et al. 2013. 21st century hazards of smoking and benefits of cessation in the United States. *New England Journal of Medicine* 368: 341–350.

Johnston, L. D., et al. 2016. *Monitoring the Future National Results on Adolescent Drug Use 1975–2015: Overview of Key Findings.* Ann Arbor: Institute for Social Research, University of Michigan.

Kane, J. C., et al. 2016. Differences in alcohol use patterns between adolescent Asian American ethnic groups: Representative estimates from the National Survey on Drug Use and Health 2002-2013. *Addictive Behaviors* 64: 154–158.

Klarich, D. S., Brasser, S. M., and M. Y. Hong. 2015. Moderate alcohol consumption and colorectal cancer risk. *Alcoholism: Clinical and Experimental Research* 398(8): 1280–1291.

Lipari, R. N., and B. Jean-Francois. 2016. *A Day in the Life of College Students Aged 18 to 22: Substance Use Facts.* Rockville, MD: Center for Behavioral Health Statistics and Quality, Substance Abuse and Mental Health Services Administration.

Mallett, K. A., et al. 2013. An update of research examining college student alcohol-related consequences: New perspectives and implications for interventions. *Alcoholism: Clinical and Experimental Research* 37(5): 709–716.

Maxwell J. C. 2016. *The Maxwell Report: Year End & Fourth Quarter 2015 Cigarette Industry.* Richmond, VA: John C. Maxwell, Jr.

National Council on Alcoholism and Drug Dependence. 2015. *Alcohol, Drugs and Crime* (https://ncadd.org/about-addiction/alcohol-drugs -and-crime).

National Highway Traffic Safety Administration. 2015. *Traffic Safety Facts 2014: Alcohol-Impaired Driving*. Washington, DC: National Highway Traffic Safety Administration, DOT HS. 812–231.

Sacks, J., et al. 2015. 2010 national and state costs of excessive alcohol consumption. *American Journal of Preventive Medicine* 49(5): e73–e79.

SAMHSA Center for Behavioral Health Statistics and Quality. 2016. *Results from the 2015 National Survey on Drug Use and Health* (http://www.samhsa.gov/data/sites/default/files/NSDUH-DetTabs-2015/NSDUH-DetTabs-2015/NSDUH-DetTabs-2015.htm).

Schweitzer, K. S., et al. 2015. Endothelial disruptive pro-inflammatory effects of nicotine and e-cigarette vapor exposures. *American Journal of Physiology-Lung Cellular and Molecular Physiology*. DOI: 10.1152/ajplung.00411.2014.

Substance Abuse and Mental Health Services Administration. 2012. *Nearly Half of College Student Treatment Admissions Were for Primary Alcohol Abuse* (http://www.samhsa.gov/data/spotlight/Spotlight054College2012.pdf).

Substance Abuse and Mental Health Services Administration. 2015. *Behavioral Health Trends in the United States: Results from the 2014 National Survey on Drug Use and Health* (HHS Publication No. SMA 15-4927, NSDUH Series H-41). Rockville, MD: Substance Abuse and Mental Health Services Administration.

Substance Abuse and Mental Health Services Administration Center for Behavioral Health Statistics and Quality. 2016. *Results from the 2015 National Survey on Drug Use and Health* (http://www.samhsa.gov/data/sites/default/files/NSDUH-DetTabs-2015/NSDUH-DetTabs-2015/NSDUH-DetTabs-2015.htm).

Svanberg, J., et al., eds. 2014. *Alcohol and the Adult Brain*. London: Taylor and Francis.

Torre, L. A., et al. 2016. Cancer statistics for Asian Americans, Native Hawaiians, and Pacific Islanders, 2016: Converging incidence in males and females. *CA: A Cancer Journal for Clinicians* 66(3): 182–202.

U.S. Department of Health and Human Services. 2007. *The Surgeon General's Call to Action to Prevent and Reduce Underage Drinking*. Washington, DC: Department of Health and Human Services, Office of the Surgeon General.

U.S. Department of Justice, Federal Bureau of Investigation. 2013. *Crime in the United States: 2012* (http://http://www.fbi.gov/about-us/cjis/ucr/crime-in-the-u.s/2012/crime-in-the-u.s.-2012/tables/29tabledatadecpdf).

U.S. Department of Health and Human Services. 2014. *The Health Consequences of Smoking—50 Years of Progress: A Report of the Surgeon General*. Atlanta, GA: HHS, Centers for Disease Control and Prevention, National Center for Chronic Disease Prevention and Health Promotion, Office on Smoking and Health.

U.S. Surgeon General. 2006. *The Health Consequences of Involuntary Exposure to Tobacco Smoke* (http://www.surgeongeneral.gov/library/secondhandsmoke/report/).

Vander Ven, T. 2011. *Getting Wasted: Why College Students Drink Too Much and Party So Hard*. New York: NYU Press.

Williams, J. F., and V. C. Smith, the Committee on Substance Abuse. 2015. Fetal alcohol spectrum disorders. *American Academy of Pediatrics* 136(5): e1395–e1406.

Zhang, J., et al. 2014. Comparison of clinical features between non-smokers with COPD and smokers with COPD: A retrospective observational study. *International Journal of Chronic Obstructive Pulmonary Disease* 9: 57–63.

BEHAVIOR CHANGE STRATEGY
Kicking the Tobacco Habit

Congratulations! You've decided to quit smoking. You likely already know that your first day without cigarettes may be difficult. Here are six steps you can take to handle your "quit day" and be confident about being able to stay quit.

1. Make a Quit Plan

Having a quit plan helps you stay focused, confident, and motivated to quit. No single approach to quitting works for everyone. If you don't know what quit method might be right for you, visit the Quit Smoking Methods Explorer (http://smokefree.gov/explore-quit-methods) to learn more. As part of your plan, identify your reasons for quitting: for example, to be healthier, save money, smell better, relieve the worrying of your loved ones.

2. Set a Quit Date

Choose a date within the next two weeks. This will give you enough time to prepare:

- Start to get rid of smoking reminders—e.g., wash your clothes, clean your car, get rid of matches and ashtrays.
- Identify your smoking triggers. Triggers are the people, places, things, and situations that set off your urge to smoke. Some are emotional, such as feeling stressed or down; others are habitual, such as talking on the phone or drinking alcohol; still others are social, such as going to a bar or a party. Being aware of your triggers

will help you avoid them or think of strategies for defusing them.

- Consider how you will fight the inevitable cravings—for example, think of ways to keep your hands and mouth busy; find new ways to relieve stress or improve your mood.

3. Stay Busy on Your Quit Day

Being busy will help you keep your mind off smoking and distract you from cravings. Try some of these activities:

- Go out for walks. Notice details about your neighborhood.
- Chew gum or hard candy.
- Keep your hands busy with a pen or toothpick.
- Drink lots of water.
- Relax with deep breathing.
- Go to a movie.
- Spend time with nonsmoking friends and family.
- Go to dinner at your favorite smoke-free restaurant.

4. Avoid Smoking Triggers

On your quit day, try to avoid all your triggers.

- Throw away all your cigarettes, lighters, and ash trays if you haven't already.
- Avoid caffeine, which can make you feel jittery. Try drinking water instead.

- Spend time with nonsmokers.
- Go to places where smoking isn't allowed.
- Get plenty of rest and eat healthy foods. Being tired can trigger you to smoke.
- Change your routine to avoid the things you associate with smoking.

5. Stay Positive

Quitting smoking is difficult. It happens one minute... one hour... one day at a time. Try not to think of quitting as forever. Pay attention to *today,* and the time will add up. Your quit day might not be perfect; what matters is that you don't smoke—not even one puff. Reward yourself for being smoke-free for 24 hours. You deserve it.

6. Ask for Help

You don't need to rely on willpower alone to be smoke-free. Tell your family and friends when your quit day is. Ask them for support on quit day and in the first few days and weeks after. Let them know exactly how they can support you. Don't assume they'll know. Be honest about your needs. If using nicotine replacement therapy is part of your plan, be sure to start using it first thing in the morning. Finally, Smokefree.gov has many tools to help you, including a text message program, apps to help you track cravings and monitor your progress, online chats with a cessation counselor, and a Facebook page.

SOURCES: Smokefree.gov. n.d. *Build Your Quit Plan* (http://smokefree.gov/build-your-quit-plan); Smokefree.gov. n.d. *Quit Day: 5 Steps* (http://smokefree.gov /steps-on-quit-day).

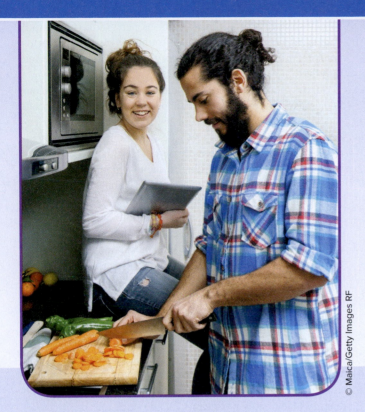

© Maica/Getty Images RF

CHAPTER 9

CHAPTER

CHAPTER OBJECTIVES

- List the components of a healthy diet
- Explain how to make informed choices about foods
- Put together a personal nutrition plan

Nutrition Basics

Choosing foods that provide the nutrients you need while limiting the substances linked to disease should be an important part of your daily life. Your dietary needs change as you go through different life stages, guided by your current energy needs, daily nutrient requirements, locally available foods, foods you choose to eat, and your health condition. When you are actively involved in sports, for example, your energy needs will be higher than when you are inactive, even if your age and body size remain the same. Similarly, energy needs for lactating mothers are higher than those for nonlactating mothers with similar body size and physical activity levels.

This chapter examines the role of personal dietary choices and the basic principles of **nutrition.** It introduces the six classes of essential nutrients and explains their roles in health and disease. It also provides guidelines for designing a healthy diet plan.

COMPONENTS OF A HEALTHY DIET

If you're like most people, you think about your diet in terms of the foods you like to eat. More important for your health, though, are the nutrients contained in those foods. Your body requires proteins, fats, carbohydrates, vitamins, minerals, and water—about 45 **essential nutrients.** In this context, the word *essential* means that you must get these substances from food because your body is unable to manufacture them or make an adequate amount to meet your physiological needs. The body needs some essential nutrients in relatively large amounts; these **macronutrients** include protein, fat, carbohydrate, and water. **Micronutrients,** such as vitamins and minerals, are required in much smaller amounts.

TERMS

nutrition   The science of food and dietary supplements, and how the body uses them in health and disease.

essential nutrients   Dietary components the body must get from foods or supplements because it cannot manufacture them to meet its needs.

macronutrient   An important nutrient required by the body in relatively large amounts.

micronutrient   An important nutrient required by the body in minute amounts.

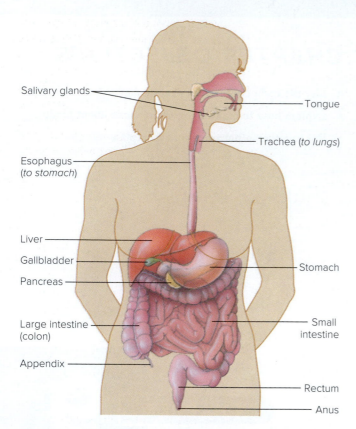

FIGURE 9.1 **The digestive system.** Food is partially broken down by being chewed and mixed with saliva in the mouth. After traveling to the stomach via the esophagus, food is broken down further by stomach acids and other secretions. As food moves through the digestive tract, it is mixed by muscular contractions to facilitate further digestion and absorption. Most absorption of nutrients occurs via the lining of the small intestine. The large intestine reabsorbs excess water; the remaining solid wastes are collected in the rectum and excreted through the anus.

Most nutrients become available to the body through the process of **digestion,** in which the foods we eat are broken down into compounds the gastrointestinal tract can absorb and that the body processes further and uses for normal body functions (Figure 9.1). An adequate diet must provide enough essential nutrients and energy to support and regulate various vital body functions.

The amount of energy in foods is expressed as **kilocalories (kcal)**. One kilocalorie represents the amount of heat required to raise the temperature of 1 liter of water by 1°C. An average person needs about 2000 kilocalories per day to meet his or her energy needs. Although technically inaccurate, people usually refer to kilocalories as *calories*; you'll also find the word *calorie* used on food labels. What's the difference between "energy" and "calorie?" **Energy** is the capacity to do work. Calories are used to measure energy. The energy in food is chemical energy, which the body converts to mechanical, electrical, or heat energy.

Of the six broad classes of essential nutrients, fat supplies the most energy per gram (9 calories) followed by protein and carbohydrate, which each supply 4 calories per gram. Alcohol, though not an essential component of the diet, also

supplies energy, providing 7 calories per gram. (One gram equals a little less than 0.04 ounce.) Certain calories consumed in excess of your energy needs may be converted into fat that is then stored in the body.

Just meeting energy needs is not enough. As noted earlier, our bodies also need an adequate amount of the essential nutrients to function properly. Many Americans consume sufficient or excess calories but not enough of all essential nutrients. Nearly all foods contain combinations of nutrients, although foods are sometimes classified according to their predominant nutrient; for example, spaghetti and other pasta are carbohydrates.

For many people, nutrient density is an important concept related to food energy. Nutrient-dense foods are those that are high in essential nutrients but relatively low in calories. You can think of your daily calorie intake as a budget: You need to spend your calories wisely on nutrient-dense foods to obtain all essential nutrients while staying within your budget.

Proteins—The Basis of Body Structure

Proteins form important parts of the body's main structural components: muscles and bones. Proteins also form important parts of blood, enzymes, some hormones, and cell membranes. When consumed, proteins also provide energy (4 calories per gram) for the body.

Amino Acids   The building blocks of proteins are called **amino acids.** Twenty common amino acids are found in food proteins. Nine of these amino acids are essential (sometimes called indispensable). As long as foods supply certain nutrients, the body can produce the other 11 amino acids.

Complete and Incomplete Proteins   Individual protein sources are considered *complete* if they supply all the essential amino acids in adequate amounts and *incomplete* if they do not. Meat, fish, poultry, eggs, milk, cheese, and soy provide complete proteins. Incomplete proteins, which come from other plant sources such as nuts and legumes (dried beans and peas), are good sources of most essential amino acids but are usually low in one or more.

TERMS

digestion   The process of breaking down foods into compounds the gastrointestinal tract can absorb and the body can use.

kilocalorie   A measure of energy content in food; 1 kilocalorie represents the amount of heat needed to raise the temperature of 1 liter of water 1°C; commonly referred to as a *calorie*.

energy   The capacity to do work, measured by calories. We get energy from certain nutrients in food.

protein   An essential nutrient that forms important parts of the body's main structures (muscles and bones) as well as blood, enzymes, hormones, and cell membranes; also provides energy.

amino acid   One of the building blocks of proteins; 20 common amino acids are found in foods.

Certain combinations of vegetable proteins, such as grains and legumes, or wheat and peanuts in a peanut butter sandwich, for example, allow each vegetable protein to make up for the amino acids missing in the other protein. The combination yields a complete protein. Many traditional food pairings, such as beans and rice or corn and beans, have emerged as dietary staples because they are complementary proteins.

Recommended Protein Intake   The Food and Nutrition Board of the Institute of Medicine has established goals to help ensure adequate intake of protein as well as the other macronutrients (Table 9.1). For protein, adequate daily intake for adults is 0.8 gram per kilogram (0.36 gram per pound) of body weight. So, if you weigh 140 pounds, you should consume at least 50 grams of protein per day, and if you weigh 180 pounds, then 65 grams of protein per day represents adequate intake.

Most Americans meet or exceed the protein intake needed for adequate nutrition. If you consume substantially more protein than your body needs, the extra energy from protein is synthesized into fat for storage or burned for energy requirements, depending on your overall energy intake.

Consuming some protein above the amount needed for adequate nutrition is not harmful; suggested daily intake limits have been set as a proportion of overall calories rather than as specific amounts. The Food and Nutrition Board recommendations for how much protein (and other energy-supplying nutrients) to consume as a percentage of total daily energy intake are called Acceptable Macronutrient Distribution Ranges (AMDRs); the AMDRs aim to ensure adequate intake of essential nutrients and also reduce the risk of chronic diseases. The AMDR for protein for adults age 19 years and over is 10–35% of total daily calorie intake (see Table 9.1): For someone consuming a 2000-calorie diet, this percentage range corresponds to a suggested daily intake of between 50 and 175 grams per day. Healthy protein-rich food choices are described in detail later in the chapter.

Fats—Essential in Small Amounts

At 9 calories per gram, fats, also known as *lipids,* are the most concentrated source of energy. The fats stored in your body represent usable energy, help insulate your body, and support and cushion your organs. Fats in the diet help your body to absorb fat-soluble vitamins, and they add important flavor and texture to foods. Fats are the major fuel for the body during rest and light activity. Two fats, linoleic acid and alpha-linolenic acid, are essential fatty acids and necessary components of the diet. They are used to make compounds that are key regulators of body functions such as the maintenance of blood pressure and the progress of a healthy pregnancy.

Types and Sources of Fats   Called *triglycerides,* most of the fats in foods are fairly similar in composition, generally including a molecule of glycerol (an alcohol) with three fatty acid chains attached to it. Animal fat, for example, is made primarily of triglycerides.

Within a triglyceride, differences in the fatty acid structure result in different types of fats. Depending on this structure, a fat may be saturated or unsaturated, monounsaturated or polyunsaturated, depending on how many double bonds exist in the structure of the fatty acid chains. The essential fatty acids linoleic acid and alpha-linolenic acid are both polyunsaturated (they have two or more double bonds). Different types of fatty acids have different characteristics and therefore varied effects on health, as discussed in the box "Fats and Health."

Food fats are usually composed of both saturated and unsaturated fatty acids. The dominant type of fatty acid determines the fat's characteristics. Food fats containing large amounts of saturated fatty acids or trans fatty acids are usually solid at room temperature; they are generally found naturally in animal products or in products containing hydrogenated oils.

Table 9.1	Goals for Protein, Fat, and Carbohydrate Intake		
	DAILY ADEQUATE INTAKE DISTRIBUTION (GRAMS)*		ACCEPTABLE MACRONUTRIENT DISTRIBUTION RANGE (PERCENTAGE OF TOTAL DAILY CALORIES)
	MEN	WOMEN	
Protein**	56	46	10–35
Fat (total)			20–35
Linoleic acid	17	12	
Alpha-linolenic acid	1.6	1.1	
Carbohydrate	130	130	45–65

*To meet daily energy needs, you must consume more than the minimally adequate amounts of the energy-providing nutrients listed here, which alone supply only 800-900 calories. Use the AMDRs to set overall daily goals.

**Protein-intake goals can be calculated more specifically by multiplying your body weight in pounds by 0.36.

NOTE: Individuals can allocate total daily energy intake among the three classes of macronutrients to suit individual preferences. To translate percentage goals into daily-intake goals expressed in calories and grams, multiply the appropriate percentages by your total daily energy intake and then divide the results by the corresponding calories per gram. For example, a fat limit of 35% applied to a 2200-calorie diet would be calculated as follows: 0.35 × 2200 = 770 calories of total fat; 770 ÷ 9 calories per gram = 86 grams of total fat.

SOURCE: Recommendations from Food and Nutrition Board, Institute of Medicine. 2005. *Dietary Reference Intakes for Energy, Carbohydrate, Fiber, Fat, Fatty Acids, Cholesterol, Protein, and Amino Acids.* Washington, DC: National Academies Press.

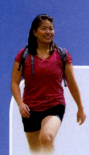

TAKE CHARGE
Fats and Health

Scientists are still unraveling the complex effects that individual types of fats, total fat intake, and overall dietary patterns have on health and the risk for specific diseases.

Artificial Trans Fats: Heading for the Exit

Most health experts and public health recommendations agree on the dangers of artificial trans fats because of their double-negative effect on heart health—raising LDL and lowering HDL. Consuming trans fats appears to increase the risk of both cardiovascular disease and type 2 diabetes. As awareness of these health risks grew, cities and states banned the use of trans fats in restaurants and foods prepared for retail sales, and food manufacturers reduced the amount of trans fats in processed foods. According to the U.S. Food and Drug Administration (FDA), trans fat consumption declined by almost 80% between 2003 and 2012.

In 2015, the FDA removed partially hydrogenated oils (the primary source of artificial trans fats) from the category of food additives "generally regarded as safe" for use in human foods. The FDA gave food companies until June 2018 to remove them from products. This change will substantially lower trans fat consumption in the United States and is expected to reduce the incidence of coronary heart disease and prevent thousands of fatal heart attacks each year.

Until trans fats are eliminated from processed foods, consumers can check for them by examining the ingredient list of a food for "partially hydrogenated oil" or "vegetable shortening." In addition, if a food contains 0.5 g or more of trans fats, the amount will be listed on the Nutrition Facts label.

Saturated Fats: Mixed Evidence?

Many studies have examined the effects of dietary-fat intake on blood cholesterol levels and the risk of heart disease. Long-standing advice has been to limit saturated fat; however, a 2014 analysis published in *Annals of Internal Medicine* challenged the widely accepted saturated-fat hypothesis that butter and other sources of saturated fat cause coronary heart disease. Researchers analyzed multiple studies, consisting of more than 600,000 participants. They concluded that "current evidence does not clearly support cardiovascular guidelines that encourage high consumption of polyunsaturated fatty acids and low consumption of total saturated fats." Other scientists challenged the methods and findings of the study, and the recommendations from the American Heart Association and American College of Cardiology strongly advise lowering saturated-fat intake for reducing cardiovascular risk, especially for those people with risk factors for heart disease.

Research on the health effects of saturated fats is ongoing. For example, do saturated fats in beef, butter, milk, and chocolate all have the same effect on heart disease risk? And what are the health effects of shifts in the intake of particular fats within the overall context of the diet? Also, dietary fat—and the foods that contain it—affect health in other ways besides heart disease risk. Diets high in saturated-fat-rich fatty red meats are associated with an increased risk of certain forms of cancer, especially colon cancer.

A Focus on Total or Type?

Both the latest federal dietary guidelines and changes coming to food labels reflect a greater emphasis on the types of fats consumed rather than the total. Overall fat intake is important, especially if the fats are in foods with few other nutrients. Experts generally agree that limiting saturated and trans fats is a more important goal than cutting total fats. On average, Americans' intake of total fats is within the AMDR, but saturated-fat intake is over the recommended levels.

What does this mean for you? Although more research is needed on the precise effects of different types and amounts of fat on overall health, evidence suggests that most people benefit from keeping their saturated-fat consumption within recommended intake levels and avoiding all trans fats. But dietary patterns are more important for health than is a focus on a single nutrient. The fats in your diet are found in foods that contain other nutrients, and the foods you consume are in the pattern of your overall diet. Increased body weight, aging, and gender are more important for predicting negative health events than is eating one kind of dietary fat rather than another.

The U.S. Department of Agriculture recommends that Americans limit their intake of saturated fat to less than 10% of total calories per day—but that they do so in the context of an overall healthy dietary pattern. Replace excess saturated fats with healthier fat options (unsaturated fats) and not with refined carbohydrates and sugar. Don't replace one less-than-healthy choice with another. Healthy dietary patterns are described in detail later in the chapter.

SOURCES: U.S. Department of Health and Human Services and U.S. Department of Agriculture. 2015. *2015–2020 Dietary Guidelines for Americans,* 8th ed. (http://health.gov/dietaryguidelines/2015/guidelines); U.S. Food and Drug Administration. 2015. *The FDA Takes Steps to Remove Artificial Trans Fats in Processed Foods* (http://www.fda.gov/NewsEvents/Newsroom/PressAnnouncements/ucm451237.htm); Chowdhury, R., et al. 2014. Association of dietary, circulating, and supplement fatty acids with coronary risk: A systematic review and meta-analysis. *Annals of Internal Medicine* 160(6): 398–406.

The leading sources of saturated fat in the American diet are red meats (hamburger, steak, roasts), whole milk, cheese, hot dogs, and lunchmeats. Palm and coconut oils, also known as "tropical oils," although derived from plants, are also highly saturated and are solid or semisolid at room temperature. Most monounsaturated and polyunsaturated fatty acids in foods usually come from plant sources and are liquid at room temperature. Olive, canola, safflower, and peanut oils contain mostly monounsaturated fatty acids. Soybean, corn, and cottonseed oils contain mostly polyunsaturated fatty acids. (See Table 9.2.)

Table 9.2 — Types of Fatty Acids

TYPE OF FATTY ACID	FOUND IN*
Saturated	• Animal fats (especially fatty meats and poultry fat and skin) • Butter, cheese, and other high-fat dairy products • Palm and coconut oils
Trans	• Some frozen pizza • Some types of popcorn • Deep-fried fast foods • Stick margarines, shortening • Packaged cookies and crackers • Processed snacks and sweets
Monounsaturated	• Olive, canola, and safflower oils • Avocados, olives • Peanut butter (without added fat) • Many nuts, including almonds, cashews, pecans, and pistachios
Polyunsaturated—omega-3[†]	• Fatty fish, including salmon, white albacore tuna, mackerel, anchovies, and sardines • Compared to fish, lesser amounts are found in canola and soybean oils; tofu; walnuts; flaxseeds; and dark green leafy vegetables
Polyunsaturated—omega-6[†]	• Corn, soybean, and cottonseed oils (often used in margarine, mayonnaise, and salad dressings)

*Food fats contain a combination of types of fatty acids in various proportions. For example, canola oil is composed mainly of monounsaturated fatty acids (62%) but also contains polyunsaturated (32%) and saturated (6%) fatty acids.

[†]The essential fatty acids are polyunsaturated: Linoleic acid is an omega-6 fatty acid and alpha-linolenic acid is an omega-3 fatty acid.

Hydrogenation and Trans Fats   When unsaturated vegetable oils undergo the chemical process known as partial **hydrogenation,** the result is a more solid fat that contains a mixture of saturated and unsaturated fatty acids. Hydrogenation also changes some unsaturated fatty acids to **trans fatty acids**—unsaturated fatty acids with an atypical shape that affects their behavior in the body. In some studies, trans fats are associated with an increase in **low-density lipoprotein (LDL) cholesterol,** or "bad" cholesterol, and a lowering of **high-density lipoprotein (HDL) cholesterol,** or "good" cholesterol. These attributes are part of a dietary pattern that correlates with heart disease.

Food manufacturers used hydrogenation to increase the stability of an oil so that it could be reused for deep frying, to improve the texture of certain foods (to make pie crusts flakier, for example), and to extend the shelf life of foods made with oil. Hydrogenation is also used to transform liquid oil into margarine or vegetable shortening.

Recommended Fat Intake   To meet the body's demand for essential fats, adult men need about 17 grams per day of linoleic acid and 1.6 grams per day of alpha-linolenic acid; adult women need 12 grams of linoleic acid and 1.1 grams of alpha-linolenic acid. It takes only 3–4 teaspoons (15–20 grams) of vegetable oil per day incorporated into your diet to supply these essential fats. Most Americans consume sufficient amounts of the essential fats; limiting unhealthy fats is a much greater health concern.

Limits for total fat, saturated fat, and trans fat intake have been set by a number of government and research organizations. As with protein, a range of levels of fat consumption is associated with good health. The AMDR for total fat is 20–35% of total daily calories. Although more difficult for consumers to monitor, AMDRs have also been set for omega-6 fatty acids (5–10% of total calories) and omega-3 fatty acids (0.6–1.2% of total calories) as part of total daily fat intake.

TERMS

hydrogenation   A chemical process by which hydrogen atoms are added to molecules of unsaturated fats, increasing the degree of saturation and turning liquid oils into solid fats. Hydrogenation produces a mixture of saturated fatty acids, and *cis* (standard) and *trans* forms of unsaturated fatty acids.

trans fatty acid   A type of unsaturated fatty acid produced during the process of hydrogenation; trans fats have an atypical shape that affects their chemical activity. Trans fats are associated with an increase in LDL cholesterol and a lowering of HDL cholesterol, attributes associated with risk of heart disease.

cholesterol   A waxy substance in the blood and cells, needed for synthesis of cell membranes, vitamin D, and hormones.

low-density lipoprotein (LDL)   Blood fat that transports cholesterol to organs and tissues; excess amounts result in the accumulation of deposits in artery walls, causing hardening of the arteries and potentially cardiovascular disease.

high-density lipoprotein (HDL)   Blood fat that helps transport cholesterol out of the arteries, thereby protecting against cardiovascular disease.

The latest federal guidelines place greater emphasis on the types of fats consumed than on the overall amount of fat in the diet; the guidelines suggest choosing healthy unsaturated fats in place of saturated and trans fats. Avoid highly processed reduced-fat foods that substitute refined carbohydrates and added sugars for fats. Information about the types of fats present in a food can be found on the food label or, for unlabeled products, in nutrition guides and online (see "For More Information" at the end of the chapter).

Look at your choices in the overall context of your diet. For example, peanut butter eaten on whole-wheat bread and served with a banana, carrot sticks, and a glass of reduced-fat milk makes a nutritious lunch. In comparison, peanut butter on high-fat crackers with potato chips, cookies, and whole milk is a less healthy combination.

Carbohydrates—An Ideal Source of Energy

Carbohydrates are needed in the diet primarily to supply energy for body cells. Some cells, such as those found in the brain and other parts of the nervous system and in blood, use only the carbohydrate glucose for fuel. During high-intensity exercise, muscles also use energy from carbohydrates as their primary fuel source.

Simple and Complex Carbohydrates
Carbohydrates are classified into two groups: simple and complex. *Simple carbohydrates* include single sugar molecules (monosaccharides) and double sugar molecules (disaccharides). The monosaccharides are glucose, fructose, and galactose. Glucose is the most common sugar and is used by both animals and plants for energy. The disaccharides are pairs of single sugars; they include sucrose or table sugar (fructose + glucose), maltose or malt sugar (glucose + glucose), and lactose or milk sugar (galactose + glucose). Simple carbohydrates add sweetness to foods; they are found naturally in fruits and milk and are added to soft drinks, fruit drinks, candy, sweet desserts,

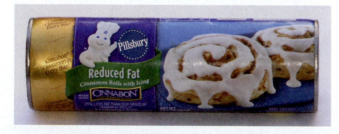

An isolated focus on reducing dietary fat intake contributed to an explosion in the availability of processed foods promoted as being low in fat, such as the reduced fat cinnamon rolls shown here. Many of these choices, however, are high in refined grains and added sugars and are not healthy choices. Focus on your overall dietary pattern and limit your intake of saturated fats, processed grains, *and* added sugars. Choose unsaturated fats in place of saturated fats in a dietary pattern also rich in whole grains, fruits, and vegetables.

© Diana Haronis/Moment Mobile/Getty Images

and a variety of other processed foods. As described below, diets high in added sugars are linked to obesity.

Complex carbohydrates include starches and most types of dietary fiber. Starches are found in a variety of plants, especially grains (wheat, rye, rice, oats, barley, and millet), legumes (dry beans, peas, and lentils), and tubers (potatoes and yams). Most other vegetables contain a mixture of complex and simple carbohydrates. Fiber, discussed in the next section, is found in grains, fruits, and vegetables.

During digestion, your body breaks down carbohydrates into simple sugar molecules, such as **glucose,** for absorption. Once glucose is in the bloodstream, the pancreas releases the hormone insulin, which allows cells to take up glucose and use it for energy. The liver and muscles take up glucose to provide carbohydrate storage in the form of a starch called **glycogen.** Some people have problems controlling their blood glucose levels, a disorder called *diabetes mellitus* (Chapter 11).

Refined versus Whole Grains
Complex carbohydrates from grains can be further divided into refined or processed carbohydrates and unrefined carbohydrates or whole grains. Before they are processed, all grains are **whole grains,** consisting of an inner layer, the germ; a middle layer, the endosperm; and an outer layer, the bran. During processing, the germ and bran are often removed, leaving just the starchy endosperm. The refinement of whole grains transforms whole-wheat flour into white flour, brown rice into white rice, and so on.

Refined grains usually retain all the calories of their unrefined counterparts, but they tend to be much lower in fiber, vitamins, minerals, and other beneficial compounds—less nutrient dense. Many refined grain products are enriched or fortified with vitamins and minerals, but not all of the nutrients lost in processing are replaced.

Whole grains tend to take longer to chew and digest than refined ones; they also enter the bloodstream more slowly. This slower digestive pace tends to make people feel full sooner and for a longer period. Also, a slower rise in blood glucose levels following the consumption of unrefined complex carbohydrates may help in the management of diabetes. Whole grains are also high in dietary fiber and so have all the benefits of fiber (discussed later).

Consumption of whole grains has been linked to a reduced risk of heart disease, diabetes, and cancer and

> **TERMS**
>
> **carbohydrate**   An essential nutrient, required for energy for cells; sugars, starches, and dietary fiber are all carbohydrates.
>
> **glucose**   A simple sugar that is the body's basic fuel.
>
> **glycogen**   A starch stored in the liver and muscles.
>
> **whole grain**   The entire edible portion of a grain (such as wheat, rice, or oats), consisting of the germ, endosperm, and bran; processing removes parts of the grain, often leaving just the endosperm.

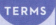

Because whole-grain foods offer so many health benefits, federal dietary guidelines recommend six or more servings of grain products every day, with at least half of those servings from whole grains. Currently, however, Americans average less than one serving of whole grains per day.

What Are Whole Grains?

The first step in increasing your intake of whole grains is to correctly identify them. The following are whole grains:

Whole wheat	Whole-grain corn
Whole rye	Popcorn
Whole oats	Brown rice
Oatmeal	Whole-grain barley

More unusual choices include bulgur (cracked wheat), millet, kasha (roasted buckwheat kernels), quinoa, wheat and rye berries, amaranth, wild rice, graham flour, whole-grain kamut, whole-grain spelt, and whole-grain triticale.

Wheat flour, unbleached flour, enriched flour, and degerminated corn meal are not whole grains. Wheat germ and wheat bran are also not whole grains, but they are the constituents of wheat typically left out when wheat is processed and so are healthier choices than regular wheat flour, which typically contains just the grain's endosperm.

Checking Packages for Whole Grains

To find packaged foods—such as bread or pasta—that are rich in whole grains, read the list of ingredients and check for special health claims related to whole grains. The *first* item on the list of ingredients should be one of the whole grains in the preceding list. Product names and food color can be misleading. *When in doubt, always check the list of ingredients and make sure "whole" is the first word on the list.* The word "enriched" means that it is white flour to which some of the nutrients that were removed in the milling process have been added back.

The U.S. Food and Drug Administration (FDA) allows manufacturers to include special health claims for foods that contain 51% or more whole-grain ingredients. Such products may display a statement such as the following on their packaging:

"Rich in whole grain."
"Made with 100% whole grain."
"Diets rich in whole-grain foods may help reduce the risk of heart disease and certain cancers."

However, many whole-grain products do not carry such claims. This is one more reason to check the ingredient list to make sure you're buying a product made from one or more whole grains.

---

plays an important role in gastrointestinal health and body weight management. For all these reasons, whole grains are recommended over those that have been refined. See the box "Choosing More Whole-Grain Foods" for tips on increasing your intake of whole grains.

Glycemic Index   Insulin and glucose levels rise and fall following a meal or snack containing any type of carbohydrate. Some foods such as table sugar cause a quick and dramatic rise in glucose and insulin levels, whereas others have a slower, more moderate effect. A food that has a rapid effect on blood glucose levels is said to have a high **glycemic index.** Whole grains, high-fiber foods, and high-fat foods generally tend to have a lower glycemic index, but patterns are less clear for other types of foods. The body's response to carbohydrates also depends on other factors, such as how much carbohydrate is consumed, what other foods are consumed at the same time, and the individual's fitness status. For people with particular health concerns, such as obesity and diabetes, glycemic index may be an important consideration in choosing specific foods. But for most people, the best bet is to choose an overall dietary pattern that includes a variety of whole grains and vegetables daily and limits foods that are high in refined grains and added sugars.

Added Sugars   Food manufacturers or individuals sometimes add sugars to foods. The term *added sugars* refers to white sugar, brown sugar, high-fructose corn syrup, and other sweeteners added to most processed foods. Naturally occurring sugars in fruit and milk are not considered added sugars. Foods high in added sugar are generally high in calories and low in essential nutrients and fiber, thus providing "empty calories." High intake of added sugars from foods and sugar-sweetened beverages is associated with dental caries (cavities), excess body weight, and increased risk of type 2 diabetes, and it may also increase risk for hypertension, stroke, and heart disease.

Added sugars currently contribute about 250–300 calories in the typical daily American diet, representing about 13–17% of total energy intake. A limit of 10% is suggested by the U.S. Department of Agriculture (USDA) and other organizations; even lower intakes may meet all nutrient needs at a given level of calorie intake. Major sources of added sugar in the U.S. diet are sugar-sweetened beverages, snacks, and sweets. Beginning in 2018, amounts of added sugars will appear on food labels.

glycemic index   A measure of how a particular food affects blood glucose levels.   **TERMS**

The sugars in your diet should come mainly from whole fruits, which are excellent sources of vitamins and minerals, and from low-fat milk and other dairy products, which are high in protein and calcium. Dietary patterns low in added sugars are described in detail later in the chapter.

Recommended Carbohydrate Intake On average, Americans consume 200–300 grams of carbohydrate per day—well above the 130 grams needed to meet the body's requirement for essential carbohydrate. A range of intakes is associated with good health; the AMDR for carbohydrates is 45–65% of total daily calories. That's about 225–325 grams of carbohydrate for someone who consumes 2000 calories per day. The focus should be on consuming a variety of foods rich in complex carbohydrates, especially whole grains.

Athletes in training can especially benefit from high-carbohydrate diets (60–70% of total daily calories), which enhance the amount of carbohydrates stored in their muscles and therefore provide more fuel for use during endurance events or long workouts. Carbohydrates consumed during prolonged athletic events (e.g., low-sugar sports beverages and gels) can provide fluid, electrolytes, and glucose to help fuel muscles and extend the availability of glycogen stored in muscles. Caution is in order, however, because over-consumption of carbohydrates can lead to fatigue and under-consumption of other nutrients.

Fiber—A Closer Look

Fiber is the term given to nondigestible carbohydrates naturally present in plants such as whole grains, fruits, legumes, and vegetables. Instead of being digested, like starch, fiber moves through the intestinal tract and provides bulk for feces in the large intestine, which in turn facilitates elimination. In the large intestine, bacteria break down some types of fiber into acids and gases, which explains why consuming too much fiber can lead to intestinal gas. Even though humans don't digest fiber, they need it for good health.

Types of Fiber The Food and Nutrition Board has defined two types of fiber:

• **Dietary fiber** refers to the nondigestible carbohydrates (and the noncarbohydrate substance *lignin*) that are naturally present in plants such as grains, fruits, legumes, and vegetables. There are two types of dietary fiber: soluble and insoluble. Both types are important for health. **Soluble (viscous) fiber** such as that found in oat bran or legumes can delay stomach emptying, slow the movement of glucose into the blood after eating, and reduce absorption of cholesterol. **Insoluble fiber**, such as that found in wheat bran or psyllium seed, increases fecal bulk and helps prevent constipation, hemorrhoids, and other digestive disorders.

• **Functional fiber** refers to nondigestible carbohydrates that have been either isolated from natural sources or synthesized in a laboratory and then added to a food product or dietary supplement.

Total fiber refers to the sum of dietary and functional fiber in your diet. A high-fiber diet can help reduce the risk of type 2 diabetes, heart disease, and pulmonary disease, as well as improve gastrointestinal health and aid in the management of metabolic syndrome and body weight. Some studies have linked high-fiber diets with a reduced risk of colon and rectal cancer. Other studies have suggested that it is the total dietary pattern—one rich in fruits, vegetables, and whole grains—that may be responsible for this reduction in risk (see Chapter 12).

Sources of Fiber All plant foods contain some dietary fiber. Fruits, legumes, oats (especially oat bran), and barley all contain the viscous types of fiber that help lower blood glucose and cholesterol levels. Wheat (especially wheat bran), other grains and cereals, and vegetables are good sources of cellulose and other fibers that help prevent constipation. Psyllium, which is often added to cereals or used in fiber supplements and laxatives, improves intestinal health and also helps control glucose and cholesterol levels. The processing of packaged foods can remove fiber, so it is important to rely on fresh fruits and vegetables and foods made from whole grains as your main sources of fiber.

Recommended Fiber Intake To reduce the risk of chronic disease and maintain intestinal health, the Food and Nutrition Board recommends a daily fiber intake of 38 grams for adult men and 25 grams for adult women. Americans currently consume about half this amount. Fiber should come from foods, not supplements, which should be used only under medical supervision.

TERMS

dietary fiber Nondigestible carbohydrates and lignin that are intact in plants.

soluble (viscous) fiber Fiber that dissolves in water or is broken down by bacteria in the large intestine.

insoluble fiber Fiber that does not dissolve in water and is not broken down by bacteria in the large intestine.

functional fiber Nondigestible carbohydrates either isolated from natural sources or synthesized; these may be added to foods and dietary supplements.

total fiber The total amount of dietary fiber and functional fiber in the diet.

Ask Yourself **?**

QUESTIONS FOR CRITICAL THINKING AND REFLECTION

Experts say that two of the most important factors in a healthy diet are eating the "right" kinds of carbohydrates and eating the "right" kinds of fats. Based on what you've read so far in this chapter, which are the "right" carbohydrates and fats? How would you say your own diet stacks up when it comes to carbohydrates and fats?

Vitamins—Organic Micronutrients

Vitamins are organic (carbon-containing) substances required in small amounts to regulate various processes within living cells (Table 9.3). Humans need 13 vitamins; of these, 4 are fat-soluble (A, D, E, and K), and 9 are water-soluble (C, and the B vitamins thiamin, riboflavin, niacin, vitamin B-6, folate, vitamin B-12, biotin, and pantothenic acid).

Functions of Vitamins   Many vitamins help chemical reactions take place. They provide no energy to the body directly but help unleash the energy stored in carbohydrates, proteins, and fats. Other vitamins are critical in the production of red blood cells and the maintenance of the nervous, skeletal, and immune systems. Some vitamins act as **antioxidants,** which help preserve the health of cells.

Sources of Vitamins   The human body does not manufacture most of the vitamins it requires and must obtain them from foods. Vitamins are abundant in fruits, vegetables, and grains. In addition, many processed foods, such as flour and breakfast cereals, contain added vitamins. A few vitamins are made in certain parts of the body: The skin makes vitamin D when it is exposed to sunlight, and intestinal bacteria make vitamin K. Nonetheless, we still need vitamin D and vitamin K from foods. Table 9.3 lists good food sources of vitamins.

Vitamin Deficiencies   If your diet lacks a particular vitamin, characteristic symptoms of deficiency can develop (see Table 9.3). Physicians have known about some common deficiency-related ailments for generations. For example, *scurvy* is a potentially fatal illness caused by a long-term lack of vitamin C. Children who do not get enough vitamin D can develop *rickets,* which leads to potentially disabling bone deformations. Vitamin A deficiency may cause blindness, and anemia can develop in people whose diet lacks vitamin B-12, folate, or B-6. Although the data are not conclusive, low levels of folate and vitamins B-6 and B-12 have been linked to an increased risk of heart disease and stroke. Plant foods are not a source of B-12. Vegetarians must rely on fortified cereals or supplements for B-12.

New research connects vitamin deficiencies with other health risks, as well. For example, experts once thought that vitamin D was the only vitamin that played a role in bone health. Now scientists know that vitamins C, A, and K, as well as several B vitamins, are also important in the prevention of osteoporosis. A great deal of recent research has focused on vitamin D, with inconsistent results for conditions such as cardiovascular disease and cancers. And although vitamin A plays an important role in bone growth, too much vitamin A can trigger bone loss and increase the risk of fracture.

Overall, vitamin-deficiency diseases are common in rural areas of developing countries; they are relatively rare in the United States because vitamins are readily available from our fortified food supply. Still, many Americans consume lower-than-recommended amounts of several vitamins. Even in the face of new findings, there is not enough evidence to suggest that the majority of the population begin taking vitamin supplements. Supplementation is discussed in detail later in this chapter.

Vitamin Excesses   Extra vitamins in the diet can also be harmful, especially when taken as supplements for an extended period of time. Megadoses of fat-soluble vitamins are particularly dangerous because the excess is stored in the body rather than excreted, increasing the risk of toxicity. Even when vitamins are not taken in excess, relying on supplements for an adequate intake of vitamins can be a problem because many health benefits from other, nonvitamin ingredients in foods are likely to be missed.

Minerals—Inorganic Micronutrients

Minerals are inorganic (non-carbon-containing) elements you need in relatively small amounts to help regulate body functions, aid in the growth and maintenance of body tissues, and help release energy (Table 9.4). There are about 17 essential minerals. The major minerals, which the body needs in amounts exceeding 100 milligrams per day, include calcium, phosphorus, magnesium, sodium, potassium, and chloride. The essential trace minerals, which you need in minute amounts, include copper, fluoride, iodide, iron, selenium, and zinc.

Characteristic symptoms develop if an essential mineral is consumed in a quantity too large or too small for good health. The minerals commonly lacking in the American diet are iron, calcium, potassium, and magnesium. Iron-deficiency **anemia** is a problem in some age groups, but particularly among menstruating women and among women who have had multiple pregnancies. Researchers fear that poor calcium intakes in childhood are sowing the seeds for future **osteoporosis,** especially in women. The box "Eating for Healthy Bones," which has tips for building and maintaining bone density. Low potassium intake is considered a public health concern because it is linked to high blood pressure and heart disease.

Water—Vital but Often Ignored

Water is the major component in both foods and the human body: We are composed of about 50–60% water. Our need

Table 9.3 Facts about Vitamins

VITAMIN AND RECOMMENDED INTAKES*	IMPORTANT DIETARY SOURCES	MAJOR FUNCTIONS	SIGNS OF PROLONGED DEFICIENCY	TOXIC EFFECTS OF MEGADOSES
Fat-soluble				
Vitamin A Men: 900 µg Women: 700 µg	Liver, milk, butter, cheese, fortified margarine, carrots, spinach, orange and deep green vegetables and fruits	Immune function and maintenance of vision; skin; and linings of the nose, mouth, and digestive and urinary tracts	Night blindness, scaling skin, increased susceptibility to infection, loss of appetite, anemia, kidney stones	Liver damage, miscarriage, birth defects, headache, vomiting, diarrhea, vertigo, double vision, bone abnormalities
Vitamin D Men: 15 µg Women: 15 µg	Fortified milk and margarine, fish oils, butter, egg yolks; sunlight on skin also produces vitamin D	Development and maintenance of bones and teeth, promotion of calcium absorption	Rickets (bone deformities) in children; bone softening, loss, and fractures in adults	Kidney damage, calcium deposits in soft tissues, depression, death
Vitamin E Men: 15 mg Women: 15 mg	Vegetable oils, whole grains, nuts and seeds, green leafy vegetables, asparagus, peaches	Protection and maintenance of cellular membranes	Red blood cell breakage and anemia, weakness, neurological problems, muscle cramps	Relatively nontoxic, but may cause excess bleeding or formation of blood clots
Vitamin K Men: 120 µg Women: 90 µg	Green leafy vegetables; smaller amounts widespread in other foods	Production of factors essential for blood clotting and bone metabolism	Hemorrhaging	None reported
Water-soluble				
Biotin Men: 30 µg Women: 30 µg	Cereals, yeast, egg yolks, soy flour, liver; widespread in foods	Synthesis of fats, glycogen, and amino acids	Rash, nausea, vomiting, weight loss, depression, fatigue, hair loss	None reported
Folate Men: 400 µg Women: 400 µg	Green leafy vegetables, yeast, oranges, whole grains, legumes, liver	Amino acid metabolism, synthesis of RNA and DNA, new cell synthesis	Anemia, weakness, fatigue, irritability, shortness of breath, swollen tongue	Masking of vitamin B-12 deficiency
Niacin Men: 16 mg Women: 14 mg	Eggs, poultry, fish, milk, whole grains, nuts, enriched breads and cereals, meats, legumes	Conversion of carbohydrates, fats, and proteins into usable forms of energy	Pellagra (symptoms include diarrhea, dermatitis, inflammation of mucous membranes, dementia)	Flushing of the skin, nausea, vomiting, diarrhea, liver dysfunction, glucose intolerance
Pantothenic acid Men: 5 mg Women: 5 mg	Animal foods, whole grains, broccoli, potatoes; widespread in foods	Metabolism of fats, carbohydrates, and proteins	Fatigue, numbness and tingling of hands and feet, gastrointestinal disturbances	None reported
Riboflavin Men: 1.3 mg Women: 1.1 mg	Dairy products, enriched breads and cereals, lean meats, poultry, fish, green vegetables	Energy metabolism; maintenance of skin, mucous membranes, and nervous system structures	Cracks at corners of mouth, sore throat, skin rash, hypersensitivity to light, purple tongue	None reported
Thiamin Men: 1.2 mg Women: 1.1 mg	Whole-grain and enriched breads and cereals, organ meats, lean pork, nuts, legumes	Conversion of carbohydrates into usable forms of energy, maintenance of appetite and nervous system function	Beriberi (symptoms include muscle wasting, mental confusion, anorexia, enlarged heart, nerve changes)	None reported
Vitamin B-6 Men: 1.3 mg Women: 1.3 mg	Eggs, poultry, fish, whole grains, nuts, soybeans, liver, kidney, pork	Metabolism of amino acids and glycogen	Anemia, convulsions, cracks at corners of mouth, dermatitis, nausea, confusion	Neurological abnormalities and damage
Vitamin B-12 Men: 2.4 µg Women: 2.4 µg	Meat, fish, poultry, fortified cereals	Synthesis of blood cells, other metabolic reactions	Anemia, fatigue, nervous system damage, sore tongue	None reported
Vitamin C Men: 90 mg Women: 75 mg	Peppers, broccoli, spinach, brussels sprouts, citrus fruits, strawberries, tomatoes, potatoes, cabbage, other fruits and vegetables	Maintenance and repair of connective tissue, bones, teeth, and cartilage; promotion of healing; absorption of iron	Scurvy, anemia, reduced resistance to infection, loosened teeth, joint pain, poor wound healing, hair loss, poor iron absorption	Urinary stones in some people, acid stomach from ingesting supplements in pill form, nausea, diarrhea, headache, fatigue

*Recommended intakes for adults aged 19–30; to calculate your personal Dietary Reference Intakes (DRIs) based on age, sex, and other factors, visit the Interactive DRI website (http://fnic.nal.usda .gov/fnic/interactiveDRI).

SOURCES: The following reports may be accessed via www.nap.edu: *Dietary Reference Intakes for Thiamin, Riboflavin, Niacin, Vitamin B6, Folate, Vitamin B12, Pantothenic Acid, Biotin and Choline* (1998); *Dietary Reference Intakes for Vitamin C, Vitamin E, Selenium, and Carotenoids* (2000); *Dietary Reference Intakes for Vitamin A, Vitamin K, Arsenic, Boron, Chromium, Copper, Iodine, Iron, Manganese, Molybdenum, Nickel, Silicon, Vanadium, and Zinc* (2001); and *Dietary Reference Intakes for Calcium and Vitamin D* (2011); Ross, A. C., et al., eds. 2014. *Modern Nutrition in Health and Disease,* 11th ed. Baltimore, MD: Lippincott Williams & Wilkins.

Table 9.4	Facts about Selected Minerals

MINERAL AND RECOMMENDED INTAKES*	IMPORTANT DIETARY SOURCES	MAJOR FUNCTIONS	SIGNS OF PROLONGED DEFICIENCY	TOXIC EFFECTS OF MEGADOSES
Calcium Men: 1000 mg Women: 1000 mg	Milk and milk products, tofu, fortified orange juice and bread, green leafy vegetables, bones in fish	Formation of bones and teeth, control of nerve impulses, muscle contraction, blood clotting	Stunted growth in children, bone mineral loss in adults, urinary stones	Kidney stones, calcium deposits in soft tissues, inhibition of mineral absorption, constipation
Fluoride Men: 4 mg Women: 3 mg	Fluoridated water, tea, marine fish eaten with bones	Maintenance of tooth and bone structure	Higher frequency of tooth decay	Increased bone density, mottling of teeth, impaired kidney function
Iodine Men: 150 µg Women: 150 µg	Iodized salt, seafood, processed foods	Essential part of thyroid hormones, regulation of body metabolism	Goiter (enlarged thyroid), cretinism (birth defect)	Depression of thyroid activity, hyperthyroidism in susceptible people
Iron Men: 8 mg Women: 18 mg	Meat and poultry, fortified grain products, dark green vegetables, dried fruit	Component of hemoglobin, myoglobin, and enzymes	Iron-deficiency anemia, weakness, impaired immune function, gastrointestinal distress	Nausea, diarrhea, liver and kidney damage, joint pains, sterility, disruption of cardiac function, death
Magnesium Men: 400 mg Women: 310 mg	Widespread in foods and water (except soft water); especially found in grains, legumes, nuts, seeds, green vegetables, milk	Transmission of nerve impulses, energy transfer, activation of many enzymes	Neurological disturbances, cardiovascular problems, kidney disorders, nausea, growth failure in children	Nausea, vomiting, diarrhea, central nervous system depression, coma; death in people with impaired kidney function
Phosphorus Men: 700 mg Women: 700 mg	Present in nearly all foods, especially milk, cereal, peas, eggs, meat	Bone growth and maintenance, energy transfer in cells	Impaired growth, weakness, kidney disorders, cardiorespiratory and nervous system dysfunction	Drop in blood calcium levels, calcium deposits in soft tissues, bone loss
Potassium Men: 4700 mg Women: 4700 mg	Meats, milk, fruits, vegetables, grains, legumes	Nerve function, body water balance	Muscular weakness, nausea, drowsiness, paralysis, confusion, disruption of cardiac rhythm	Cardiac arrest
Selenium Men: 55 µg Women: 55 µg	Seafood, meat, eggs, whole grains	Defense against oxidative stress, regulation of thyroid hormone action	Muscle pain and weakness, heart disorders	Hair and nail loss, nausea and vomiting, weakness, irritability
Sodium Men: 1500 mg Women: 1500 mg	Salt, soy sauce, salted foods, tomato juice	Body water balance, acid–base balance, nerve function	Muscle weakness, loss of appetite, nausea, vomiting; deficiency is rarely seen	Edema (excess fluid buildup), hypertension in sensitive people
Zinc Men: 11 mg Women: 8 mg	Whole grains, meat, eggs, liver, seafood (especially oysters)	Synthesis of proteins, RNA, and DNA; wound healing; immune response; ability to taste	Growth failure, loss of appetite, impaired taste acuity, skin rash, impaired immune function, poor wound healing	Vomiting, impaired immune function, decline in blood HDL levels, impaired copper absorption

*Recommended intakes for adults aged 19–30; to calculate your personal DRIs based on age, sex, and other factors, visit the Interactive DRI website (http://fnic.nal.usda.gov/fnic/interactiveDRI).

SOURCES: The following reports may be accessed via www.nap.edu: *Dietary Reference Intakes for Calcium, Phosphorous, Magnesium, Vitamin D, and Fluoride* (1997); *Dietary Reference Intakes for Vitamin A, Vitamin K, Arsenic, Boron, Chromium, Copper, Iodine, Iron, Manganese, Molybdenum, Nickel, Silicon, Vanadium, and Zinc* (2001); *Dietary Reference Intakes for Water, Potassium, Sodium, Chloride, and Sulfate* (2005); and *Dietary Reference Intakes for Calcium and Vitamin D* (2011). Ross, A. C., et al., eds. 2014. *Modern Nutrition in Health and Disease*, 11th ed. Baltimore, MD: Lippincott Williams & Wilkins.

for other nutrients, in terms of weight, is much less than our need for water. We can live up to 50 days without food but only a few days without water.

Water is distributed all over the body, among lean and other tissues and in blood and other body fluids. Water is used in the digestion and absorption of food and is the medium in which most of the chemical reactions take place within the body. Some water-based fluids, like blood, transport substances around the body, whereas other fluids serve as lubricants or cushions. Water also helps regulate body temperature.

Water is contained in almost all foods, particularly in liquids, fruits, and vegetables. The foods and beverages you consume provide 80–90% of your daily water intake; the remainder is generated through metabolism. You lose water each day in urine, feces, and sweat and through evaporation from your lungs.

Most people can maintain a healthy water balance by consuming beverages at meals and drinking fluids in response to thirst. The Food and Nutrition Board has set levels of adequate water intake to maintain hydration. Under these guidelines, men need about 3.7 total liters of water daily, with 3.0 liters (about 13 cups) coming from beverages; women need 2.7 total liters, with 2.2 liters (about 9 cups) coming from beverages. All fluids, including those containing

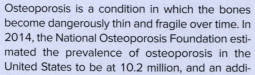

Osteoporosis is a condition in which the bones become dangerously thin and fragile over time. In 2014, the National Osteoporosis Foundation estimated the prevalence of osteoporosis in the United States to be at 10.2 million, and an additional 43.4 million adults over age 50 have low bone mass. Women account for about 80% of osteoporosis cases. Most of our adult bone mass is built by age 18 in girls and age 20 in boys. After bone density peaks between ages 25 and 35, bone mass is lost slowly over time and then at an increasing rate after menopause. To prevent osteoporosis, the best strategy is to build as much bone as possible during your youth and do everything you can to maintain it as you age. Up to 50% of bone loss is determined by controllable lifestyle factors such as resistance training and diet. Key nutrients for bone health include the following:

- **Calcium.** Getting enough calcium is important throughout life to build and maintain bone mass. Milk, yogurt, and calcium-fortified orange juice, bread, and cereals are all good sources.

- **Vitamin D.** Vitamin D is necessary for bones to absorb calcium. The Institute of Medicine recommends a daily intake of 600 IU (15 μg) of vitamin D for most adults and 800 IU (20 μg) of vitamin D for men and women over the age of 70 years. Vitamin D can be obtained from foods and is manufactured by the skin when exposed to sunlight. Candidates for vitamin D supplements include people who don't eat many foods rich in vitamin D; those who don't expose their faces, arms, and hands to the sun (without sunscreen) for

5–15 minutes a few times each week; and people who live north of an imaginary line roughly between Boston and the Oregon–California border (where the sun is weaker).

- **Vitamin K.** Vitamin K promotes the synthesis of proteins that help keep bones strong. Broccoli and leafy green vegetables are rich in vitamin K.

- **Other nutrients.** Other nutrients that may play an important role in bone health include vitamin C, vitamin A, magnesium, potassium, phosphorus, fluoride, manganese, zinc, copper, and boron.

Several dietary substances may have a *negative* effect on bone health, especially if consumed in excess. These include alcohol, sodium, caffeine, and retinol (a form of vitamin A). Drinking lots of soda, which often replaces milk in the diet, has been shown to increase the risk of bone fractures in teenage girls.

The effect of protein intake on bone mass depends on other nutrients. Protein helps build bone as long as calcium and vitamin D intake are adequate. But if intake of calcium and vitamin D is low, high protein intake can lead to bone loss.

Weight-bearing aerobic exercise helps maintain bone mass throughout life, and strength training improves bone density, muscle mass, strength, and balance. Drinking alcohol only in moderation, refraining from smoking, and managing depression and stress are also important for maintaining strong bones. For people who develop osteoporosis, a variety of medications are available to treat the condition.

caffeine, can count toward your total daily fluid intake. If you exercise vigorously or live in a hot climate, you need to consume additional fluids to maintain a balance between water consumed and water lost. Severe dehydration causes weakness and can lead to death.

Other Substances in Food

Many substances in food are not essential nutrients but may influence health.

Antioxidants   When the body uses oxygen or breaks down certain fats or proteins as a normal part of metabolism, it gives rise to substances called **free radicals.** Environmental factors such as cigarette smoke, exhaust fumes, radiation, excessive sunlight, certain drugs, and stress can increase free radical production. A free radical is a chemically unstable molecule that reacts with fats, proteins, and DNA, damaging cell membranes and mutating genes. Free radicals have been implicated in aging, cancer, cardiovascular disease, and other degenerative diseases like arthritis.

Antioxidants found in foods can help protect the body from damage by free radicals in several ways. Some prevent or reduce the formation of free radicals; others remove free radicals from the body; still others repair some types of free radical

damage after it occurs. Some antioxidants, such as vitamin C, vitamin E, and selenium, are also essential nutrients. Others—such as the carotenoids found in yellow, orange, and deep green vegetables—are not. Some of the top antioxidant-containing foods and beverages include blackberries, walnuts, strawberries, artichokes, cranberries, brewed coffee, raspberries, pecans, blueberries, cloves, grape juice, baking chocolate, sour cherries, and red wine. Also high in antioxidants are brussels sprouts, kale, cauliflower, and pomegranates.

Phytochemicals   Antioxidants fall into the broader category of **phytochemicals,** which are substances found in plant foods that may help prevent chronic disease. In just the past 30 years, researchers have identified and studied hundreds of compounds found in foods, and many findings are promising.

free radical   An electron-seeking compound that **TERMS** can react with fats, proteins, and DNA, damaging cell membranes and mutating genes in its search for electrons; produced through chemical reactions in the body and by exposure to environmental factors such as sunlight and tobacco smoke.

phytochemical   A naturally occurring substance found in plant foods that may help prevent and treat chronic diseases like cancer and heart disease; *phyto* means plant.

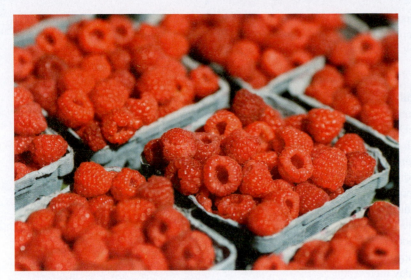

Berries are rich in antioxidants, vitamins, and dietary fiber.
© Nash Photos/Getty Images RF

Dietary Reference Intakes (DRIs)

The Food and Nutrition Board of the Institute of Medicine establishes dietary standards, or recommended intake levels, for Americans of all ages. The current set of standards, the Dietary Reference Intakes (DRIs), was introduced in 1997. The DRIs are reviewed frequently and are updated as new nutrition-related information becomes available. The DRIs have a broad focus, being based on research that looks not just at the prevention of nutrient deficiencies but also at the role of nutrients in promoting health and preventing chronic diseases such as cancer, osteoporosis, and heart disease.

The DRIs include a set of four reference values used as standards for both recommended intakes and maximum safe intakes. The recommended intake of each nutrient is expressed as either a *Recommended Dietary Allowance (RDA)* or an *Adequate Intake (AI)*. An AI is set when there is not enough information available to set an RDA value; regardless of the type of standard used, however, the DRI represents the best available estimate of intake for optimal health.

Used primarily in nutrition policy and research, the *Estimated Average Requirement (EAR)* is the average daily nutrient intake level estimated to meet the requirement of half the healthy individuals in a given gender and life stage. The *Tolerable Upper Intake Level (UL)* is the maximum daily intake that is unlikely to cause health problems in a healthy person. For example, the RDA for calcium for an 18-year-old female is 1300 mg per day; the UL is 3000 mg per day.

Because of lack of data, ULs have not been set for all nutrients. The absence of ULs does not mean that people can tolerate chronic intakes of these vitamins and minerals above

For example, certain substances found in soy foods may help lower cholesterol levels. Sulforaphane, a compound isolated from broccoli and other **cruciferous vegetables,** may render some carcinogenic compounds harmless. Allyl sulfides, a group of chemicals found in garlic and onions, appear to boost the activity of immune cells and lower total cholesterol concentrations. Carotenoids found in green vegetables may help preserve eyesight with age. Further research on phytochemicals may extend the role of nutrition to the prevention and treatment of many chronic diseases.

If you want to increase your intake of phytochemicals, eat a variety of fruits, vegetables, and unprocessed grains rather than relying on supplements. Like many vitamins and minerals, isolated phytochemicals may be harmful if taken in high doses. Another reason to get your phytochemicals from foods is that their health benefits could be the result of many chemical substances working in combination. Eating more fruits and vegetables is a smart alternative to less healthy foods. In contrast, people who rely more on supplements may take them and eat large portions of unhealthy foods.

NUTRITIONAL GUIDELINES: PLANNING YOUR DIET

Scientific and government groups have created a variety of tools to help people design healthy diets: **Dietary Reference Intakes (DRIs)** are standards for nutrient intake designed to prevent nutritional deficiencies and reduce the risk of chronic diseases; **Dietary Guidelines for Americans** were established to promote health and reduce the risk of major chronic diseases through diet and physical activity; and **MyPlate** provides a food guidance system to help people apply the Dietary Guidelines for Americans to their own diets.

TERMS

cruciferous vegetables   Vegetables of the cabbage family, including cabbage, broccoli, brussels sprouts, kale, and cauliflower; the flower petals of these plants form the shape of a cross, hence, the name.

Dietary Reference Intakes (DRIs)   An umbrella term for four types of nutrient standards designed to prevent nutritional deficiencies and reduce the risk of chronic diseases. Estimated Average Requirement (EAR) is the amount estimated to meet the nutrient needs of half the individuals in a population group; Adequate Intake (AI) and Recommended Dietary Allowance (RDA) are levels of intake considered adequate to prevent nutrient deficiencies and reduce the risk of chronic disease for most individuals in a population group; and Tolerable Upper Intake Level (UL) is the maximum daily intake that is unlikely to cause health problems.

Dietary Guidelines for Americans   National nutritional recommendations issued jointly by the U.S. Department of Agriculture and the U.S. Department of Health and Human Services every five years; designed to promote health and reduce the risk of chronic diseases.

MyPlate   The USDA food guidance system designed to help Americans make healthy food choices.

recommended levels. Like all chemical agents, nutrients can produce adverse effects if intakes are excessive. There is no established benefit from consuming nutrients at levels above the RDA or AI.

The DRIs for many nutrients are found in Tables 9.1, 9.3, and 9.4. For a personalized DRI report for all nutrients, appropriate for your sex and life stage, visit the Interactive DRI website (https://fnic.nal.usda.gov/fnic/interactiveDRI).

Because the DRIs are too cumbersome to use as a basis for food labels, the FDA uses another set of dietary standards, the **Daily Values.** The Daily Values are based on several different sets of guidelines and include standards for fat, cholesterol, carbohydrate, dietary fiber, and selected vitamins and minerals. The Daily Values represent appropriate intake levels for a 2000-calorie diet. The Daily Value percentage on a food label shows how well that food contributes to your recommended daily intake, assuming you follow a 2000-calorie-per-day diet. Food labels are described in detail later in this chapter.

Dietary Guidelines for Americans

To provide general guidance for choosing a healthy diet and reducing the risk of chronic diseases, the USDA and the U.S. Department of Health and Human Services issue the *Dietary Guidelines for Americans,* revising them every five years. These guidelines are intended for all healthy Americans, including children age 2 years and over. The information in the Dietary Guidelines is used in developing federal food, nutrition, and health policies and programs and also serves as the basis for federal nutrition education materials.

The Dietary Guidelines are designed to help Americans make healthy and informed food choices. The main objective of the 2015–2020 Dietary Guidelines is to encourage healthy eating patterns and regular physical activity among Americans, two-thirds of whom are overweight or obese and yet at the same time undernourished in several key nutrients. The guidelines focus on the total diet and offer practical tips for how people can make *shifts* in their diet to integrate healthier choices. And they include findings on the broader environmental and societal aspects of the American diet—that is, the "food environment."

Earlier versions of the Dietary Guidelines focused more on individual dietary components such as food groups and nutrients. However, people do not eat individual nutrients or single foods but rather foods in combination, to form an overall eating pattern that has cumulative effects on health. The 2015–2020 Dietary Guidelines point out the large discrepancy between the recommendations and the actual American diet, which includes too much added sugar, solid fat, refined grain, and sodium and not enough vegetables, fruits, high-fiber whole grains, low-fat milk and milk products, and seafood.

> **Daily Values**   A simplified version of the RDAs used on food labels; also included are values for nutrients with no RDA per se.
>
> **eating pattern**   The result of choices on multiple eating occasions over time, both at home and away from home.
>
> **TERMS**

Eating patterns and their food and nutrient characteristics are the focus of the recommendations and are based on the growing body of research that has examined the relationship between overall eating patterns, health, and risk of chronic disease. Following these guidelines promotes health and reduces risk of diseases such as heart disease, cancer, diabetes, stroke, osteoporosis, and obesity. Each of the guidelines is supported by an extensive review of scientific and medical evidence.

General Recommendations   The Dietary Guidelines offer five overarching recommendations:

1. **Follow a healthy eating pattern across the lifespan.** All food and beverage choices matter. Choose a healthy eating pattern at an appropriate calorie level to help achieve and maintain a healthy body weight, support nutrient adequacy, and reduce the risk of chronic disease.

2. **Focus on variety, nutrient density, and amount.** To meet nutrient needs within calorie limits, choose a variety of nutrient-dense foods across and within all food groups in recommended amounts.

3. **Limit calories from added sugars and saturated fats and reduce sodium intake.** Consume an eating pattern low in added sugars, saturated fats, and sodium. Cut back on foods and beverages higher in these components to amounts that fit within healthy eating patterns.

4. **Shift to healthier food and beverage choices**. Choose nutrient-dense foods and beverages across and within all food groups in place of less healthy choices. Consider cultural and personal preferences to make these shifts easier to accomplish and maintain.

5. **Support healthy eating patterns for all.** Everyone has a role in helping to create and support healthy eating patterns in multiple settings nationwide, from home to school to work to communities.

The report recognizes the challenges that make it difficult for Americans to reach their food and fitness goals. It acknowledges that all segments of our society, from families to food producers and restaurants to policymakers, have a responsibility in supporting healthy choices. The Dietary Guidelines emphasize that a healthy eating pattern is not a rigid prescription, but rather an adaptable framework in which individuals can enjoy foods that meet their personal, cultural, and traditional preferences and fit within their budget and lifestyle. Adopting a healthy eating pattern and engaging in regular physical activity will go a long way toward improving health and reducing the risk of chronic disease in every life stage.

Building Healthy Eating Patterns   The first three guidelines focus on healthy eating and physical activity patterns. A healthy eating pattern is one that meets nutrient needs while not exceeding calorie requirements and while staying within limits for dietary components that are typically overconsumed. The Dietary Guidelines highlight three healthy eating patterns:

- **Healthy U.S.-Style Pattern.** Based on the types and proportions of foods Americans typically consume, but in nutrient-dense forms and appropriate amounts.

- **Healthy Vegetarian Pattern.** Includes more legumes, processed soy products, nuts and seeds, and whole grains; it contains no meat, poultry, or seafood but is close to the Healthy U.S.-Style Pattern in amounts of all other food groups. Dairy and eggs are still included because the majority of vegetarians eat them; however, the plan can be vegan with plant-based substitutions.

- **Healthy Mediterranean-Style Pattern.** Reflecting a dietary pattern associated with many cultures bordering the Mediterranean Sea, which includes more fruit and seafood and less dairy than the Healthy U.S.-Style Pattern. (The Mediterranean diet has been associated with positive health outcomes such as lower rates of heart disease and lower total mortality.)

All three patterns are based on amounts of food from different food groups (and subgroups) according to overall energy intake. They share an emphasis on whole fruits, vegetables, whole grains, beans and peas, fat-free and low-fat milk and milk products, and healthy oils; they include less red meat and more seafood than the typical American diet. Healthy dietary patterns include oils, but they limit the amount of energy that people should consume from solid fats.

A fundamental principle of all healthy dietary patterns is that people should eat nutrient-dense foods—foods with little or no solid fats, added sugars, and added refined starches—so that they can obtain all the needed nutrients without exceeding their daily energy requirements. In addition, people should strive to get their nutrients from foods rather than from dietary supplements, although supplements or fortification may be helpful for certain populations.

Following a healthy pattern allows you to meet all the DRIs for essential nutrients and stay within the AMDRs established by the Food and Nutrition Board for nutrients that supply energy. Table 9.5 compares the three patterns for

Table 9.5	USDA Healthy Food Patterns at the 2000-Calorie Level		
FOOD GROUP	HEALTHY U.S.-STYLE PATTERN	HEALTHY VEGETARIAN PATTERN	HEALTHY MEDITERRANEAN-STYLE PATTERN
Vegetables	**2½ c-eq/day**	**2½ c-eq/day**	**2½ c-eq/day**
Dark green	1½ c-eq/wk	1½ c-eq/wk	1½ c-eq/wk
Red and orange	5½ c-eq/wk	5½ c-eq/wk	5½ c-eq/wk
Legumes (beans and peas)	1½ c-eq/wk	3 c-eq/wk*	1½ c-eq/wk
Starchy	5 c-eq/wk	5 c-eq/wk	5 c-eq/wk
Other	4 c-eq/wk	4 c-eq/wk	4 c-eq/wk
Fruit	**2 c-eq/day**	**2 c-eq/day**	**2½ c-eq/day**
Grains	**6 oz-eq/day**	**6½ oz-eq/day**	**6 oz-eq/day**
Whole grains	3 oz-eq/day	3½ oz-eq/day	3 oz-eq/day
Refined grains	3 oz-eq/day	3 oz-eq/day	3 oz-eq/day
Dairy	**3 c-eq/day**	**3 c-eq per day**	**2 c-eq per day**
Protein Foods	**5½ oz-eq/day**	**3½ oz-eq/day**	**6½ oz-eq/day**
Seafood	8 oz-eq/wk	N/A	15 oz-eq/wk
Meat, poultry, eggs	26 oz-eq/wk	3 oz-eq/wk (eggs)	26 oz-eq/wk
Nuts, seeds, soy products	5 oz-eq/wk	15 oz-eq/wk	5 oz-eq/wk
Oils	**27 g/day**	**27 g/day**	**27 g/day**
Limit on calories for other uses (% of total calories) **	270 cal/day (14%)	290 cal/day (15%)	260 cal/day (13%)

NOTE: c-eq = cup-equivalent, the amount of a food or beverage product that is considered equal to 1 cup from the vegetables, fruits, or dairy food groups; oz-eq = ounce-equivalent, the amount of a food product that is considered equal to 1 ounce from the grain or protein food groups; N/A = not applicable.

*For the Vegetarian Pattern, half of total legume intake counts as vegetables and half as protein foods.

**If all food choices to meet food group recommendations are in nutrient-dense forms, a small number of calories remain within the overall calorie limit of the pattern (i.e., limit on calories for other uses). Calories up to the specified limit can be used to consume added sugars, added refined starches, solid fats, or alcohol, or to eat more than the recommended amount of food in a food group.

SOURCE: U.S Department of Health and Human Services and U.S. Department of Agriculture. 2015. *2015–2020 Dietary Guidelines for Americans,* 8th ed. (http://health.gov/dietaryguidelines/2015/guidelines/).

a 2000-calorie diet. To see recommendations for calorie levels in all three food patterns, visit the Dietary Guidelines website (https://health.gov/dietaryguidelines/2015). Food groups, subgroups, and servings sizes are described in detail in the next section.

Although the greatest emphasis of the Dietary Guidelines is on consuming an overall healthy eating pattern, specific recommendations have been set for dietary components of particular public health concern. Sticking to these limits can help individuals stay within calorie limits while achieving a healthy eating pattern:

- Consume less than 10% of calories per day from added sugars.
- Consume less than 10% of calories per day from saturated fats.
- Consume less than 2300 mg per day of sodium.
- If you consume alcohol, do so in moderation—up to one drink per day for women and two drinks per day for men—and only if you are of legal drinking age.

In addition, all Americans should strive to meet the federal physical activity guidelines (described in detail in Chapter 10) and aim to achieve and maintain a healthy body weight.

Making Shifts to Align with Healthy Eating Patterns

The eating patterns of the U.S. population are low in vegetables, fruits, whole grains, dairy, seafood, and oil, while they are high in refined grains, added sugars, saturated fats, sodium, as well as meats, poultry, and eggs. Additionally, most Americans consume too many calories, and only 20%

meet the Physical Activity guidelines. For many individuals, achieving a healthy eating pattern will require changes to their current food and beverage choices. Figure 9.2 shows the lack of alignment between the typical eating patterns currently in the United States and those in the Dietary Guidelines.

Most of us would benefit from shifting food choices both within and across food groups. Some shifts can be minor and accomplished by making simple substitutions, while others may require greater determination. Every food choice is an opportunity to move toward a healthy eating pattern. Making small positive dietary changes over time can cumulatively make a big difference and support your efforts at maintaining a healthy body weight, meeting nutrient needs, and reducing your risk for chronic disease. See the box "Positive Changes to Meet the Dietary Guidelines" for some strategies to get you started.

People have many options for incorporating the recommendations of the Dietary Guidelines into healthy eating patterns that (1) meet nutrient needs; (2) stay within calorie limits; (3) accommodate cultural, ethnic, traditional, and personal preferences; and (4) take into account food cost and availability.

Supporting Healthy Eating Patterns Making healthy choices can be challenging, but ultimately each person makes decisions about what, where, when, and how much to eat. Individuals are more likely to shift their eating patterns toward the guidelines if we make a collaborative effort across all segments of society. By doing so, we create a culture in which healthy lifestyle choices at home, school, work, and everywhere else are easy, accessible, affordable, and normative.

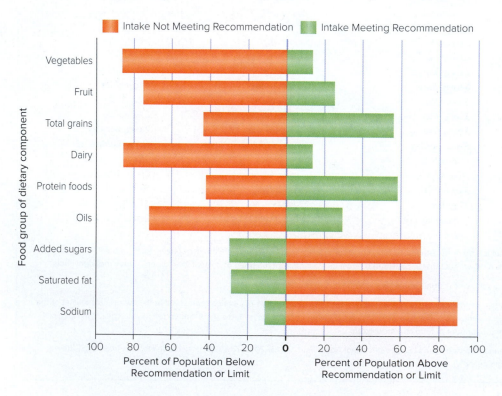

FIGURE 9.2 Dietary intakes compared to recommendations. The bars show the percentages of the U.S. population age 1 year and over who are below, at, or above each dietary goal or limit. The center (0) line is the goal or limit. For most people, meaning those represented by the red sections of the bars, shifting toward the center line will improve eating patterns. For example, over 80% of people do not eat enough vegetables—they fall below the recommendation. Within the area of the graph demonstrating our consumption of foods we should limit—added sugars, saturated fat, and sodium—the red bars show that over 80% of people exceed the recommended limit for sodium intake.

SOURCES: What We Eat in America, NHANES 2007–2010 for average intakes by age-sex group. Healthy U.S.-Style Food Patterns, which vary based on age, sex, and activity level, for recommended intakes and limits. (see 2015–2020 Dietary Guidelines, https://health.gov/dietaryguidelines/2015/guidelines/chapter-2/current-eating-patterns-in-the-united-states/)

Positive Changes to Meet the Dietary Guidelines

Remember to focus on nutrient-dense options for the majority of your food choices: Use your calorie budget wisely. The tips here focus on the types of changes and swaps needed for the majority of Americans to move toward the dietary pattern recommended in the Dietary Guidelines.

Vegetables: Consume More Vegetables from All Subgroups

- Increase the vegetable content of mixed dishes while decreasing the amounts of other food components that you may overconsume—for example, cut the meat or cheese in half and double the vegetables in a soup, stew, or casserole.
- Always choose a green salad or a vegetable as a side dish.
- Incorporate vegetables into most meals and snacks.
- Replace foods high in calories, saturated fat, or sodium, such as some meats, poultry, cheeses, and snack foods, with vegetables.

Fruits: Increase Fruit Intake, Especially from Whole Fruits

- Choose more fruits as snacks, in salads, as side dishes, and as desserts in place of foods with added sugars such as cookies, pies, cakes, and ice cream.

Grains: Swap Whole Grains for Refined

- Shift from refined to whole-grain versions of commonly eaten foods—from white to 100% whole-wheat breads, white to whole-grain pasta, and white to brown rice (see the section on whole grains earlier in the chapter for more information on using food labels to identify whole grains).
- Cut back on refined-grain desserts and sweet snacks that are high in added sugars, solid fats, or both. Choose smaller portions and eat them less often. For healthy swaps, try plain popcorn instead of buttered and bread instead of a croissant or biscuit, for example.

Dairy: Increase Intake

- Drink fat-free or low-fat milk (or soy beverage) with meals, choose yogurt as a snack, or use yogurt as an ingredient in salad dressings, spreads, and other prepared dishes.
- Favor milk and yogurt for additional dairy servings; cheese has more sodium and saturated fat and less potassium, vitamin A, and vitamin D than milk and yogurt.

Protein: Add Variety and Make More Nutrient-dense Choices

- Increase seafood intake if yours is low: Try seafood as the protein choice in meals twice per week in place of meat, poultry, or eggs—for example, a tuna sandwich or a salmon steak.
- Use legumes or nuts and seeds in mixed dishes instead of some meat or poultry—for example, bean chili instead of a mixed-meat dish or almonds instead of ham on a main-dish salad.

Oils: Increase Intake as You Reduce Solid Fats

- Use oils rather than solid fats in food preparation where possible—for example, vegetable oil in place of butter, stick margarine, shortening, lard, or coconut oils when cooking.
- Increase intake of foods that naturally contain oils, such as seafood and nuts, in place of some meat and poultry.
- Choose options for salad dressings and spreads made with oils instead of solid fats.

Saturated Fats: Reduce to Less Than 10% of Calories Per Day

- Substitute foods high in unsaturated fats for foods high in saturated fats; for example, use oils rather than solid fats for food preparation.
- Read food labels to identify the types of fats in prepared foods; compare and choose lower-fat forms of foods and beverages that contain solid fats (e.g., fat-free milk instead of 2% or whole).
- Adjust proportions of ingredients in mixed dishes to increase vegetables, whole grains, lean meat, and lower-fat cheeses in place of some of the fatty meat or regular cheeses.
- Consume foods higher in solid fats less often and in smaller portions.

Added Sugars: Reduce to Less Than 10% of Calories Per Day

- Choose beverages with no added sugars, such as water, in place of sugar-sweetened beverages.
- Reduce portion sizes of sugar-sweetened beverages, and choose them less often.
- Limit servings and decrease portion sizes of grain-based and dairy desserts and sweet snacks.
- Choose unsweetened or no-sugar-added versions of canned fruit, fruit sauces, and yogurt.

Sodium: Reduce Intake

- Read food labels to compare sodium content, choosing products with less sodium.
- Choose fresh, plain frozen, or no-salt-added canned vegetables and fresh protein sources rather than processed meat and poultry.
- Eat at home more often; cooking from scratch allows you to control the sodium content.
- Limit sauces, mixes, and "instant" flavoring packs that come with rice and noodles; use your own flavorings based on herbs and spices rather than salt.

Physical Activity: Do More!

- Increase weekly physical activity; target transportation and leisure activities.
- Reduce sedentary time; take frequent breaks during sedentary activities.

SOURCE: U.S. Department of Health and Human Services and U.S. Department of Agriculture. 2015. *2015–2020 Dietary Guidelines for Americans,* 8th ed. (http://health.gov/dietaryguidelines/2015/guidelines/).

The Dietary Guidelines offer the Social-Ecological Model (SEM) as a way to understand and address these complex problems. The SEM is defined by the Centers for Disease Control and Prevention (CDC) as a theoretical framework for understanding the factors that influence health and wellness at varying levels surrounding individuals, groups, and populations. The Dietary Guidelines SEM considers how interaction among factors influences eating and physical activity behaviors and their associated health outcomes:

- Individual factors, such as age, sex, socioeconomic status, race/ethnicity, disability, knowledge and skills, and food preferences
- Environmental settings, such as home, schools, workplaces, recreational facilities, and restaurants
- Sectors of influence, such as government, education, health care, public health and community organizations, agriculture, marketing and media, food and beverage industries, and retail
- Social and cultural norms and values, such as belief systems, traditions, heritage, religion, priorities, body image, and lifestyle

How do these factors stack up in your life? Are healthy food options available and affordable at your school and worksite? How far is it from your home to the nearest place to purchase fruits and vegetables? How many food advertisements are you exposed to daily, and what are they for? Factors such as these can have an enormous influence on individual behavior—both positive and negative—sometimes without our awareness. If the environment supports public health guidelines, individuals are more likely to attain fitness, nutritional, health, and body weight goals. Although societal policies can promote health at all stages of the life cycle, managing health, chronic diseases, body weight, and physical activity still remains a personal responsibility.

The guidelines call on all elements of society, ranging from educators to communities to government policymakers, to implement strategies aimed at improving the food and activity environment in the United States. Examples of such strategies are expanding access to grocery stores, farmers' markets, and other sources of healthy food; ensuring that meals and snacks served in schools are consistent with the Dietary Guidelines; encouraging physical activity in schools; developing policies to limit food and beverage marketing to children; supporting sustainable agricultural practices; and providing nutrition assistance programs. Such measures have the potential to improve the health of current and future generations by making healthy physical activity and eating choices the norm.

USDA's MyPlate

To further help consumers put the Dietary Guidelines for Americans into practice, the USDA issues the food-guidance system known as MyPlate. MyPlate provides a simple graphic showing how to use the five good groups to build a healthy plate at each meal (Figure 9.3). If you need to make changes in your dietary pattern, use MyPlate to build a healthy eating style by focusing on variety, amount of food consumed, and nutrition. Follow the recommendations in the Dietary Guidelines to limit saturated fat, added sugars, and sodium. Start with small changes; they will add up over time.

You can get a personalized version of MyPlate recommendations by visiting ChooseMyPlate.gov. Using the daily food plan feature, you can determine the amount of each food group you need daily based on your calorie allowance. Your plan is personalized based on your age, gender, weight, height, and level of physical activity. Another feature available at ChooseMyPlate.gov is the SuperTracker, which helps consumers create a personalized food and activity plan, look up and track individual foods, compare food choices to recommendations, and get suggestions and support to make healthier choices. MyPlate is available in Spanish, and it offers special recommendations for dieters, preschoolers aged 2–5, children aged 6–11, and pregnant and breastfeeding women.

Energy Intake and Portion Sizes To build a healthy eating style, your food group goals should be based on an appropriate level of energy intake. Table 9.6 provides ranges for calorie intake for weight maintenance. Everyone is different, however, and the number of calories you need will vary depending on multiple factors. If your weight is stable,

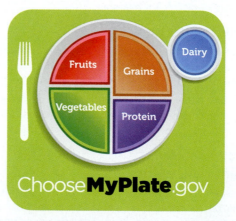

FIGURE 9.3 MyPlate. The USDA's MyPlate is designed as a simple graphic to help Americans apply the Dietary Guidelines to their own diets.

SOURCE: U.S. Department of Agriculture. Accessed July 2016. *Choose MyPlate* (http://www.choosemyplate.gov).

© USDA

Table 9.6 — Estimated Daily Calorie Needs

AGE (years)	SEDENTARY*	MODERATELY ACTIVE**	ACTIVE***
Females**			
16–18	1800	2000	2400
19–25	2000	2200	2400
26–30	1800	2000	2400
31–50	1800	2000	2200
51–60	1600	1800	2200
61 & up	1600	1800	2000
Males			
16–18	2400	2800	3200
19–20	2600	2800	3000
21–25	2400	2800	3000
26–35	2400	2600	3000
36–40	2400	2600	2800
41–45	2200	2600	2800
46–55	2200	2400	2800
56–60	2200	2400	2600
61–65	2000	2400	2600
66–75	2000	2200	2600
76 & up	2000	2200	2400

*Sedentary means a lifestyle that includes only the physical activity of independent living.

**Moderately active means a lifestyle that includes physical activity equivalent to walking about 1.5–3 miles per day at 3–4 miles per hour, in addition to the activities of independent living.

***Active means a lifestyle that includes physical activity equivalent to walking more than 3 miles per day at 3–4 miles per hour, in addition to the activities of independent living.

****Estimates for females do not include women who are pregnant or breastfeeding.

SOURCES: U.S. Department of Health and Human Services and U.S. Department of Agriculture. 2015. *2015–2020 Dietary Guidelines for Americans*, 8th ed. (http://health.gov/dietaryguidelines/2015/guidelines/); Food and Nutrition Board, Institute of Medicine. 2002. *Dietary Reference Intakes for Energy, Carbohydrate, Fiber, Fat, Fatty Acids, Cholesterol, Protein, and Amino Acids*. Washington, DC: National Academies Press.

Most people underestimate the number of calories they consume and the size of their portions. See the box "Judging Portion Sizes" for strategies to improve the accuracy of your estimates. MyPlate doesn't use number of portions as the basis of recommendations; instead, amounts are listed in terms of cup-equivalents and ounce-equivalents. These units of measurement allow for the alignment of servings of foods that differ—those that are concentrated versus those that are more airy or contain more water. For example, ½ cup of blueberries and ¼ cup of raisins both count as ½ cup-equivalent of fruit.

Next, let's take a brief look at each food group.

Fruits: Focus on Whole Fruits People who eat more vegetables and fruits as part of an overall healthy diet are likely to have a reduced risk of some chronic diseases. Fruits are rich in carbohydrates, dietary fiber, and many vitamins, especially vitamin C. A 2000-calorie diet should include 2 cups of fruit daily. Each of the following counts as 1 cup-equivalent from the fruit group:

- 1 cup fresh, canned, or frozen fruit
- 1 cup fruit juice (100% juice)
- 1 small whole fruit
- ½ cup dried fruit

Choose whole fruits often; they are higher in fiber and often lower in energy than fruit juices. Fruit *juices* typically contain more nutrients and less added sugar than fruit *drinks*. When buying canned fruits, choose those packed in 100% fruit juice or water rather than in syrup.

Vegetables: Vary Your Veggies Together, fruits and vegetables should make up half your plate. Vegetables contain carbohydrates, dietary fiber, carotenoids, vitamin C, folate, potassium, and other nutrients. They are naturally low in calories and fat and contain no cholesterol. A 2000-calorie diet should include 2½ cups of vegetables daily. Each of the following counts as 1 cup-equivalent from the vegetable group:

- 1 cup raw or cooked vegetables
- 2 cups raw leafy salad greens
- 1 cup vegetable juice

Because vegetables vary in the nutrients they provide, eat a variety to obtain maximum nutrition. MyPlate recommends weekly servings from the five subgroups within the vegetables group (see Table 9.5). Eat vegetables from several subgroups each day.

- Dark green vegetables (e.g., broccoli, bok choy, romaine lettuce, spinach, collards, kale)
- Red and orange vegetables (e.g., tomatoes, carrots, sweet potatoes, red peppers, winter squash)
- Beans and peas (e.g., split and black-eyed peas; lentils; soybeans; black, kidney, navy, pinto, and white beans)

your current energy intake is in balance with calories expended; you can set a more personal calorie goal by carefully tracking your food intake for several days to determine your current calorie intake. Once you select a calorie level for your eating plan, monitor your body weight and adjust calorie intake and physical activity based on changes in weight over time.

The Dietary Guidelines recommend that adults who are obese change their eating and physical-activity behaviors to prevent additional weight gain and/or promote weight loss. Adults who are overweight should not gain additional weight, and weight loss is recommended for people who are overweight and have one or more risk factors for cardiovascular disease. To lose weight, most people need to reduce the number of calories they get from foods and beverages and increase physical activity.

Studies have shown that most people underestimate the size of their food portions, in many cases by as much as 50%. If you need to retrain your eye, try using measuring cups and spoons and an inexpensive kitchen scale when you eat at home. With a little practice, you'll learn the difference between 3 and 8 ounces of chicken or meat and what a half-cup of rice really looks like. For quick estimates, use the following equivalents:

• 1 teaspoon margarine = the tip of your thumb

• 1 ounce cheese = your thumb, four dice stacked together, or an ice cube

• 3 ounces chicken or meat = a deck of cards

• 1 cup pasta = a small fist or a tennis ball

• ½ cup rice or cooked vegetables = an ice cream scoop or one-third of a can of soda

• 2 tablespoons peanut butter = a ping pong ball or a large marshmallow

• 1 medium potato = a computer mouse

• 2-ounce muffin or roll = a plum or a large egg

• 2-ounce bagel = a hockey puck or a yo-yo

• 1 medium fruit (apple or orange) = a baseball

• ¼ cup nuts = a golf ball

• small cookie or cracker = a poker chip

• Starchy vegetables (e.g., corn, potatoes, green peas)
• Other vegetables (e.g., artichokes, asparagus, beets, cauliflower, green beans, head lettuce, onions, mushrooms, zucchini)

Grains: Make Half Your Grains Whole Grains   Foods from this group are usually low in fat and rich in complex carbohydrates, dietary fiber (if grains are unrefined), and vitamins and minerals, including thiamin, riboflavin, iron, niacin, folic acid (if enriched or fortified), and zinc. A 2000-calorie diet should include 6 ounce-equivalents each day, with half of those servings from whole grains. The following items count as 1 ounce-equivalent:

• 1 slice of bread
• 1 small (2½-inch diameter) muffin
• 1 cup ready-to-eat cereal flakes
• ½ cup cooked cereal, rice, grains, or pasta
• 1 6-inch tortilla

Choose foods that are typically made with little fat or sugar (bread, rice, pasta) over those that are high in fat and sugar (croissants, chips, cookies).

Protein Foods: Vary Your Protein Routine   This group includes meat, poultry, fish, dried beans and peas, eggs, nuts and seeds, and processed soy foods. These foods provide protein, niacin, iron, vitamin B-6, zinc, and thiamin. The animal foods in this group also provide vitamin B-12. A 2000-calorie diet should include

---

QUICK STATS

Top sources of calories in the U.S. diet are snacks and sweets (**16%** of total calories); burgers, sandwiches, and tacos (**14%**); and beverages other than milk or 100% fruit juice (**12%**).

—U.S. Department of Health and Human Services and U.S. Department of Agriculture, 2015b

---

5½ ounce-equivalents daily. Each of the following counts as 1 ounce-equivalent:

• 1 ounce cooked lean meat, poultry, or fish
• ¼ cup cooked dried beans (legumes) or tofu
• 1 egg
• 1 tablespoon peanut butter
• ½ ounce nuts or seeds

Choose a variety of lean meats and skinless poultry, select a variety of protein foods, and watch serving sizes carefully. Choose at least one serving of plant proteins, such as black beans, lentils, or tofu, every day, and include at least 8 ounces of cooked seafood per week. Vegetarian options in the protein foods group include beans and peas, processed soy products, and nuts and seeds.

Dairy: Move to Low-Fat and Fat-Free Dairy   This group includes milk and milk products, such as yogurt and cheeses that retain their calcium, as well as calcium-fortified soy milk. Foods from this group are high in protein, carbohydrate, calcium, potassium, riboflavin, and vitamin D (if fortified). Dairy choices should be fat-free or low-fat as much as possible to reduce energy intake. A 2000-calorie diet should include 3 cups of milk or the equivalent daily. Each of the following counts as 1 cup-equivalent:

• 1 cup milk
• 1 cup yogurt
• ½ cup ricotta cheese
• 1½ ounces natural cheese
• 2 ounces processed cheese

Cottage cheese is lower in calcium than most other cheeses; ½ cup is equivalent to ¼ cup milk. Ice cream is also lower in calcium and higher in sugar and fat than many other dairy products; one scoop counts as ⅓ cup milk.

Oils Included in this category are oils and fats that are liquid at room temperature; they come mostly from plant and fish sources. Also included are soft margarines, soft vegetable oil table spreads, mayonnaise, and some salad dressings that have no trans fats. Oils are major sources of vitamin E and unsaturated fatty acids, including essential fatty acids, but they are *not a food group.* A 2000-calorie diet should include 6 teaspoons (27 g) of oils per day. A 1-teaspoon serving is the equivalent of the following:

- 1 teaspoon vegetable oil or soft margarine
- 1 tablespoon mayonnaise-type salad dressing

Foods that are mostly oils include nuts, olives, avocados, and some fish. The following portions include about 1 teaspoon of oil: 8 large olives, ⅙ medium avocado, ½ tablespoon peanut butter, and ⅓ ounce roasted nuts. Food labels can help you identify the types and amounts of fat in various foods.

Solid Fats and Added Sugars If you choose nutrient-dense foods from all food groups, you will have a small proportion of your daily calorie budget left to "spend." For those wanting to maintain weight, these calories may be used to increase the amount of food from a food group, to consume foods that contain solid fats or added sugars, or to consume alcohol. People who are trying to lose weight and improve their health should limit solid fats and added sugars. The average American consumes nearly 800 calories daily from solid fats and added sugars—far higher than the recommended limits.

Physical Activity The Dietary Guidelines for Americans and MyPlate strongly encourage all Americans to be physically active as much as possible. Daily physical activity improves health, reduces the risk of chronic diseases, and helps people manage body weight. The MyPlate recommendation for adults is 2½ hours of moderate physical activity or 1¼ hours of vigorous physical activity per week, equivalent to the 150 minutes of moderate activity or 75 minutes of vigorous activity recommended in the 2008 Physical Activity Guidelines for Americans.

See Figure 9.4 for a summary of the MyPlate recommendations for a 2000-calorie diet. To see recommendations for calorie levels in all three food patterns, visit the Dietary Guidelines website (https://health.gov/dietaryguidelines/2015).

DASH Eating Plan

Other food-group plans have been proposed by a variety of experts and organizations, some to address the needs of special populations. One well-studied alternative is DASH, which stands for Dietary Approaches to Stop Hypertension. As its name suggests, the DASH eating plan was developed to help people control high blood pressure, and it is tailored with special attention to sodium, potassium, and other nutrients of concern for blood pressure. For details on following the DASH Eating Plan, visit the National Institutes of Health website at https://www.nhlbi.nih.gov/health/health-topics/topics/dash/followdash.

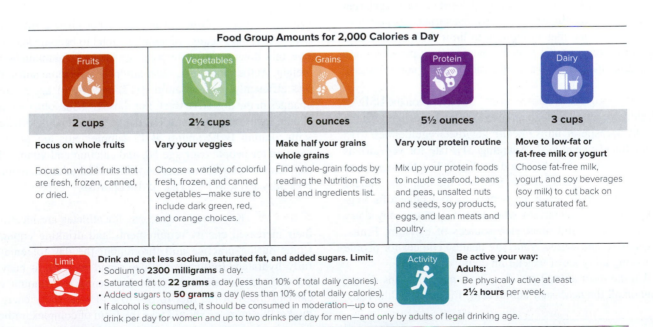

FIGURE 9.4 MyPlate food group amounts and recommendations for a 2000-calorie diet.

SOURCE: MyPlate.gov. 2016. *MyPlate Daily Checklist for 2,000 Calories* (http://www.choosemyplate.gov/MyPlate-Daily-Checklist).

The Vegetarian Alternative

Vegetarians choose a diet with one basic difference from the diets described previously—they restrict or exclude foods of animal origin (meat, poultry, fish, eggs, and milk). Vegetarian diets tend to be lower in total fat, saturated fat, cholesterol, and animal protein while being higher in complex carbohydrates, dietary fiber, magnesium, folate, vitamins C and E, carotenoids, and phytochemicals. Individuals who follow a vegetarian diet generally have a lower body mass index than do nonvegetarians. Vegetarian-style diet patterns are associated with lower mortality rates. Many people adopt a vegetarian diet for health reasons, whereas others do so out of concern for the environment, financial reasons, or reasons related to ethics or religion. Whatever the reason, vegetarians should carefully choose foods so as to meet requirements for all nutrients, especially those that are predominantly from animal sources, for example, vitamin B-12 and highly bioavailable iron.

Types of Vegetarian Diets

There are various vegetarian styles. The wider the variety of the diet eaten, the easier it is to meet nutritional needs. What type of vegetarian might you be? *Vegans* eat only plant foods. *Lacto-vegetarians* eat plant foods and dairy products. *Lacto-ovo-vegetarians* eat plant foods, dairy products, and eggs. Others can be categorized as partial vegetarians, semivegetarians, or pesco-vegetarians. The latter—also called pescatarians or pescetarians—have diets that are mainly plant-based but also include fish and other seafood. Partial vegetarians generally eat plant foods, dairy products, eggs, and usually a small selection of poultry, fish, and other seafood. Many other people choose vegetarian meals frequently but are not strictly vegetarians. A quarter of Americans make dietary choices to limit their meat intake. Including some animal protein (such as dairy products) in a vegetarian diet makes planning easier, but it is not necessary.

A Food Plan for Vegetarians

For details on the USDA's Healthy Vegetarian diet plan for a 2000-calorie diet, visit the USDA website at https://health.gov/dietaryguidelines/2015/guidelines/appendix-5/. Adapting MyPlate for vegetarians requires only a few key modifications: For the meat and beans group, vegetarians can focus on the nonmeat choices of dry beans, nuts, seeds, eggs, and soy foods like tofu. Vegans and other vegetarians who do not consume any dairy products must find other rich sources of calcium. Fruits, vegetables, and whole grains are healthy choices for people following all types of vegetarian diets.

Unlike most animal proteins, most plant proteins do not contain all the necessary amino acids for good health. Thus,

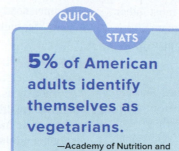

QUICK STATS

5% of American adults identify themselves as vegetarians.

—Academy of Nutrition and Dietetics, 2015

a healthy vegetarian diet must emphasize a wide variety of plant foods in order to include all the necessary a-mino acids. Choosing minimally processed and unrefined foods will maximize nutrient value and provide ample dietary fiber. Daily consumption of a variety of plant foods in amounts that meet total energy needs can provide all needed nutrients, except vitamin B-12 and possibly calcium, iron, zinc, and vitamin D.

Dietary Challenges for Various Population Groups

The Dietary Guidelines for Americans and MyPlate can help nearly anyone create a healthy diet. However, some population groups face special dietary challenges.

College Students   Convenient foods are not always the healthiest choices. Students who eat in buffet-style dining halls can easily overeat, and the foods offered are not necessarily high in nutrients or low in fat, sodium, and added sugars. The same is true of meals at fast-food restaurants. See the box "Eating Strategies for College Students" for tips on making healthy eating convenient and affordable.

Pregnant and Breastfeeding Women   Good nutrition is essential to a healthy pregnancy. Before conception, nutrition counseling can help a woman establish a balanced eating plan and healthy body weight for pregnancy. During pregnancy and while breastfeeding, women have special nutritional needs and are often advised to take nutrient supplements (see Chapter 5).

Older Adults   Nutrient needs do not change much as people age, but because older adults tend to become less active, they don't need as much energy intake to maintain body weight. At the same time, older adults absorb some nutrients less efficiently (e.g., vitamin B-12) because of age-related changes in the digestive tract. For these reasons, older adults should focus on eating nutrient-dense foods. Foods fortified with vitamin B-12 and/or B-12 supplements are recommended for people over age 50, and calcium and vitamin D supplements may be recommended for older adults to reduce bone loss and lower the risk of osteoporosis.

Athletes   Key dietary concerns for athletes are meeting their increased energy requirements and drinking enough fluids during practice and throughout the day to remain fully hydrated. Endurance athletes and athletes in heavy training may also benefit from increasing the amount of carbohydrates in the diet to 60–70% of total daily energy intake; this increase should take the form of complex, rather than simple, carbohydrates. Athletes who need to maintain a low body weight—such as skaters, gymnasts, and wrestlers—must avoid unhealthy eating patterns, which can

vegetarian   Someone who follows a diet that restricts or eliminates foods of animal origin.

TERMS

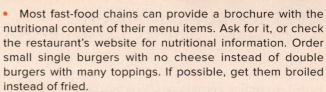

All the Time

- Eat a colorful, varied diet. The more colorful your diet is, the more varied and rich in fruits and vegetables it will be. Fruits and vegetables are typically inexpensive, delicious, and nutrient-dense.

- Eat breakfast. You'll have more energy in the morning and be less likely to grab an unhealthy snack later on.

- Choose healthy snacks—fruits, vegetables, whole grains, and cereals.

- Drink nonfat milk, water, mineral water, or 100% fruit juice more often than soft drinks or sweetened beverages.

- Pay attention to portion sizes. Enjoy your food, but eat less.

- Plan to eat meals with friends and family members who choose healthy foods and can provide support and inspiration.

- Combine physical activity with healthy eating.

Eating in the Dining Hall

- Choose a meal plan that includes breakfast.

- Decide what you want to eat before you get in line, and stick to your choices.

- Build your meals around whole grains and vegetables. Ask for small servings of meat and high-fat main dishes.

- Choose leaner poultry, fish, or bean dishes without added sugar or high sodium rather than high-fat meats and fried entrees.

- Ask that gravies and sauces be served on the side; limit your intake.

- Choose broth-based or vegetable soups, not cream soups.

- At the salad bar, load up on leafy greens, beans, and fresh vegetables. Avoid mayonnaise-coated salads, bacon, croutons, and high-fat dressings. Put dressing on the side, and dip your fork into it rather than pouring it over the salad.

- Choose fruit for dessert rather than baked goods.

Eating in Fast-Food Restaurants

- Most fast-food chains can provide a brochure with the nutritional content of their menu items. Ask for it, or check the restaurant's website for nutritional information. Order small single burgers with no cheese instead of double burgers with many toppings. If possible, get them broiled instead of fried.

- Ask for items to be prepared without mayonnaise, tartar sauce, sour cream, or other high-fat sauces. Ketchup, mustard, and fat-free mayonnaise or sour cream are better choices and are available at many fast-food restaurants.

- Choose whole-grain bread for burgers and sandwiches.

- Choose chicken items made from chicken breast, not processed chicken.

- Order vegetable pizzas without extra cheese.

- Try a salad or fruit as a side item. If you can't resist french fries or onion rings, get the smallest size.

- For food truck meals, use the same strategies suggested for fast-food restaurants: Choose lean proteins and ask for condiments on the side. If your favorite food truck doesn't have healthy options, ask that they be added to the menu.

Eating on the Run

- When you need to eat in a hurry, remember that you can carry healthy foods in your backpack or a small insulated lunch sack (with a frozen gel pack to keep fresh food from spoiling).

- Carry items that are small and convenient but nutritious, such as fresh fruits or vegetables, whole-wheat buns or muffins, snack-size cereal boxes, and water.

- When buying beverages from vending machines, choose water or 100% fruit juice. When buying snacks, choose whole-grain crackers, pretzels, nuts or seeds, baked chips, low-fat popcorn, or low-fat granola bars.

lead to eating disorders. Eating for exercise is discussed in more detail in Chapter 10; see Chapter 11 for information about eating disorders.

People with Special Health Concerns People with diabetes benefit from a well-balanced diet that is low in simple sugars and high in complex carbohydrates. People with high blood pressure need to control their weight and limit their sodium consumption. If you have a health concern that requires a special diet, discuss your situation with a physician or registered dietitian.

Global Nutrition Transitions

No population seems to be isolated from the effects of a *nutrition transition*, in which the quality and quantity of our diet is changing with globalization: that is, an increased availability of cheap foods, urbanization, and increased sedentary activities. In the United States, as our incomes increase, we eat fewer starches and more meats, vegetable oils, animal fats, and added sugars. The increases in fats and sugars are implicated in cardiovascular disease, obesity, and diabetes. The increases in animal protein and energy-dense foods are advantageous for undernourished people (in 2014, some 95 million children worldwide were underweight) but problematic for overweight people (in the same year, the number of overweight children worldwide rose to 42 million).

A PERSONAL PLAN: MAKING INFORMED CHOICES ABOUT FOOD

Understanding the basics of good nutrition should get you started on creating a healthy diet that works for you. But eating for health involves other skills, including how to interpret the labels on food products and dietary supplements, knowing how to handle and prepare food safely, understanding the nutritional content of foods and the various ways foods can be processed before going to market.

Reading Food Labels

All processed foods regulated by either the FDA or the USDA include standardized nutrition information on their labels. Every food label shows serving sizes and the amounts of fat, saturated fat, trans fat, cholesterol, sodium, total carbohydrate, dietary fiber, sugars, and protein in each serving. To make informed choices about food, learn to read and *understand* food labels (see the box "Using Food Labels").

Food label regulations also require that foods meet strict definitions if their packaging includes terms such as *light, low-fat,* or *high-fiber* (Table 9.7). Health claims such as "good source of dietary fiber" or "low in saturated fat" on packages are also regulated and can be signals that a product can be wisely included in your diet. Overall, the food label is an important tool to help you choose a healthy dietary pattern.

Calorie Labeling: Restaurants and Vending Machines

In 2014, the FDA issued new regulations requiring that calorie information be provided on restaurant menus and vending machines; these new rules were required as part of the 2010 Affordable Care Act. As of May 2017, calorie information is required on menus and menu boards in chain restaurants and similar retail food establishments (those with 20 or more locations). If no menus or boards are available, calories must be shown on signs near the foods. In addition, chain restaurants are also required to provide more detailed nutrition information on their menu items—on posters, tray liners, signs, handouts, or other similar locations—so look for it!

Calorie labels are also now required (by July 2018) for vending machine operators who own or operate 20 or more machines. Calories will be shown on a sign or digital display near the food items or selection button. Use the information as you consider your options and monitor your calorie intake.

Table 9.7	Food Package Nutrient Claims
TERM	**DEFINITION**
Healthy*	A food that is low in total fat, is low in saturated fat; has no more than 360–480 mg sodium and 60 mg cholesterol; and provides 10% or more of the Daily Value for vitamin A, vitamin C, protein, calcium, iron, or dietary fiber
Light or lite	33% fewer calories or 50% less fat than a similar product
Reduced or fewer	At least 25% less of a nutrient than a similar product; can be applied to fat ("reduced fat"), saturated fat, cholesterol, sodium, and calories
Extra or added	10% or more of the Daily Value per serving when compared to a similar product
Good source	10–19% of the Daily Value for a particular nutrient per serving
High, rich in, or excellent source of	20% or more of the Daily Value for a particular nutrient per serving
Low calorie	40 calories or less per serving
High fiber	5 grams or more of fiber per serving
Good source of fiber	2.5–4.9 grams of fiber per serving
Fat-free	Less than 0.5 gram of fat per serving
Low-fat	3 grams or less of fat per serving
Saturated- or trans-fat-free	Less than 0.5 gram of saturated fat and 0.5 gram of trans fatty acids per serving
Low saturated fat	1 gram or less of saturated fat per serving and no more than 15% of total calories
Low sodium	140 mg or less of sodium per serving
Very low sodium	35 mg or less of sodium per serving
Lean	Cooked seafood, meat, or poultry with less than 10 grams of fat, 4.5 grams or less of saturated fat, and less than 95 mg of cholesterol per serving
Extra lean	Cooked seafood, meat, or poultry with less than 5 grams of fat, 2 grams of saturated fat, and 95 mg of cholesterol per serving

NOTE: The FDA has not yet defined nutrient claims relating to carbohydrates, so foods labeled low- or reduced-carbohydrate do not conform to any approved standard.

*In mid-2016, the FDA began the process of redefining the "healthy" nutrient content claim.

SOURCE: U.S. Food and Drug Administration. 2013. *Food Labeling Guide* (http://www.fda.gov/Food/Guidance Regulation/GuidanceDocumentsRegulatoryInformation/LabelingNutrition/ucm2006828.htm).

The Nutrition Facts panel on a food label is designed to help consumers make food choices based on the nutrients that are most important to good health. In addition to listing nutrient content by weight, the label puts the information in the context of a daily diet of 2000 calories that includes no more than 65 grams of fat (approximately 30% of total calories). For example, if a serving of a particular product has 13 grams of fat, the label will show that the serving represents 20% (13/65) of the daily fat allowance. If your daily diet contains fewer or more than 2000 calories, you need to adjust these calculations accordingly.

Food labels contain uniform serving sizes. This means that if you look at different brands of salad dressing, for example, you can compare calories and fat content based on the serving amount. Keep in mind, however, that food label serving sizes may be larger or smaller than MyPlate serving-size equivalents.

The Nutrition Facts label had been in use without major changes since the 1990s. Based on research into how consumers use food labels as well as changes to the nutrients of most concern to Americans, the FDA announced changes to the look and content of the label in 2016. Most food manufacturers have until July 2018 to adopt the new style of label, although smaller manufacturers have an additional year. Here are some of the key changes:

- Adding added sugars, vitamin D, and potassium to all labels; Vitamins A and C will no longer be required

- Removing the listing for "Calories from Fat" because research shows the type of fat is more important than the amount

- Revising Daily Values for certain nutrients to reflect the latest recommendations

- Updating serving-size labeling for certain packages to be more realistic and to reflect amounts typically eaten at one time

- Refreshing the design to highlight calorie content and serving size and to make other parts of the label easier to read

SOURCE: U.S. Food and Drug Administration. 2016. *Changes to the Nutrition Facts Label* (http://www.fda.gov/Food/GuidanceRegulation/GuidanceDocumentsRegulatoryInformation/LabelingNutrition/ucm385663.htm).

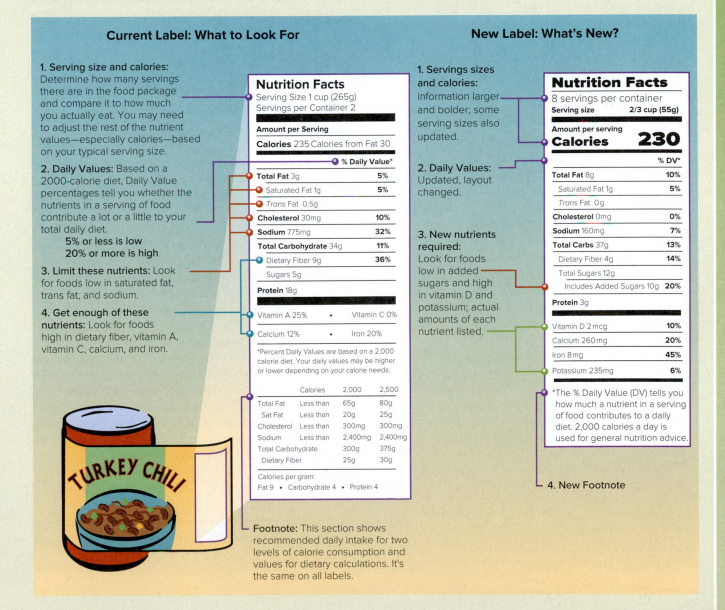

Current Label: What to Look For

1. Serving size and calories: Determine how many servings there are in the food package and compare it to how much you actually eat. You may need to adjust the rest of the nutrient values—especially calories—based on your typical serving size.

2. Daily Values: Based on a 2000-calorie diet, Daily Value percentages tell you whether the nutrients in a serving of food contribute a lot or a little to your total daily diet.
> 5% or less is low
> 20% or more is high

3. Limit these nutrients: Look for foods low in saturated fat, trans fat, and sodium.

4. Get enough of these nutrients: Look for foods high in dietary fiber, vitamin A, vitamin C, calcium, and iron.

Nutrition Facts
Serving Size 1 cup (265g)
Servings per Container 2

Amount per Serving

Calories 235 Calories from Fat 30

	% Daily Value*
Total Fat 3g	**5%**
Saturated Fat 1g	**5%**
Trans Fat 0.5g	
Cholesterol 30mg	**10%**
Sodium 775mg	**32%**
Total Carbohydrate 34g	**11%**
Dietary Fiber 9g	**36%**
Sugars 5g	
Protein 18g	

Vitamin A 25%	•	Vitamin C 0%	
Calcium 12%	•	Iron 20%	

*Percent Daily Values are based on a 2,000 calorie diet. Your daily values may be higher or lower depending on your calorie needs:

		Calories	2,000	2,500
Total Fat	Less than		65g	80g
Sat Fat	Less than		20g	25g
Cholesterol	Less than		300mg	300mg
Sodium	Less than		2,400mg	2,400mg
Total Carbohydrate			300g	375g
Dietary Fiber			25g	30g

Calories per gram:
Fat 9 • Carbohydrate 4 • Protein 4

Footnote: This section shows recommended daily intake for two levels of calorie consumption and values for dietary calculations. It's the same on all labels.

New Label: What's New?

1. Servings sizes and calories: Information larger and bolder; some serving sizes also updated.

2. Daily Values: Updated, layout changed.

3. New nutrients required: Look for foods low in added sugars and high in vitamin D and potassium; actual amounts of each nutrient listed.

Nutrition Facts
8 servings per container
Serving size	2/3 cup (55g)

Amount per serving

Calories **230**

	% DV*
Total Fat 8g	**10%**
Saturated Fat 1g	**5%**
Trans Fat 0g	
Cholesterol 0mg	**0%**
Sodium 160mg	**7%**
Total Carbs 37g	**13%**
Dietary Fiber 4g	**14%**
Total Sugars 12g	
Includes Added Sugars 10g	**20%**
Protein 3g	

Vitamin D 2mcg	**10%**
Calcium 260mg	**20%**
Iron 8mg	**45%**
Potassium 235mg	**6%**

*The % Daily Value (DV) tells you how much a nutrient in a serving of food contributes to a daily diet. 2,000 calories a day is used for general nutrition advice.

4. New Footnote

Dietary Supplements

All government food guidance systems encourage people to meet their nutritional needs with a nutritionally balanced diet of whole foods rather than with vitamin and mineral supplements. The use of supplements to reduce heart disease or cancer risk remains controversial, so experts suggest that you avoid taking any nutrient at a level exceeding the Tolerable Upper Intake Level (UL). Although dietary supplements are sold over the counter, they are not necessarily safe, especially when consumed over a long period of time. Some vitamins and minerals are dangerous when taken in excess. Large doses of particular nutrients can also cause health problems by affecting the absorption of certain vitamins or minerals or interacting with medications. For this reason, ask your doctor, your pharmacist, or a dietician before taking any high-dosage supplement.

People Who Benefit from Supplements
In establishing the DRIs, the Food and Nutrition Board recommended supplements of particular nutrients for specific groups:

• Women who are capable of getting pregnant should get 400 µg per day of folic acid (the synthetic form of the vitamin folate) from fortified foods and supplements in addition to folate from a varied diet. This level of folate can reduce the risk of neural tube defects in a developing fetus. Enriched breads, flours, cornmeal, rice, noodles, and other grain products are fortified with folic acid. Folate is found naturally in leafy green vegetables, legumes, oranges, and strawberries.

• As noted earlier, people over age 50 should eat foods fortified with vitamin B-12, take a B-12 supplement, or combine the two to meet the RDA of 2.4 µg daily. Up to 30% of people over age 50 may have trouble absorbing protein-bound B-12 in foods.

• Because of the oxidative stress caused by smoking, smokers should get 35 mg more vitamin C per day than the RDA set for their age and sex. Supplements aren't usually necessary, however, because this extra vitamin C can easily be found in foods. For example, an 8-ounce glass of orange juice has about 100 mg of vitamin C.

Supplements may be recommended in other cases. Women with heavy menstrual flows, for example, may need extra iron. Older adults, people with dark skin, and people exposed to little sunlight may need extra vitamin D. Other people may benefit from supplementation based on their physical condition, the medicines they take, or their dietary habits.

Before deciding whether to take a vitamin or mineral supplement, consider whether you already eat a fortified breakfast cereal every day. Many breakfast cereals contain almost as many nutrients as a multivitamin pill. If you elect to take a supplement, choose one that contains 50–100% of the Daily Values for vitamins and minerals. Avoid supplements containing large doses of particular nutrients.

Reading Supplement Labels
Dietary supplements include vitamins, minerals, amino acids, herbs, carotenoids, enzymes, and other compounds. They are available as tablets, capsules, liquids, and powders. Although dietary supplements are often thought to be safe and sometimes labeled "natural," they can contain powerful bioactive chemicals that have the potential for harm.

In the United States, dietary supplements are not legally considered drugs and are not regulated the same way drugs are. The FDA does not authorize or test dietary supplements, and supplement manufacturers are not required to demonstrate either safety or effectiveness prior to marketing. Although dosage guidelines exist for some of the compounds in dietary supplements, dosages for many are not well established and purity can vary widely.

Dietary supplement manufacture is not as closely regulated, and there is no guarantee that a product even contains a given ingredient, let alone in the appropriate amount. In addition, herbs can be contaminated or misidentified at any stage from harvest to packaging.

To provide consumers with more reliable and consistent information about supplements, the FDA requires supplements to have labels similar to those found on foods (see the box "Using Dietary Supplement Labels" for more information). Label statements and claims about supplements are also regulated.

Protecting Yourself against Foodborne Illness

The CDC estimates that about 1000 reported disease outbreaks and approximately 48 million illnesses, 128,000 hospitalizations, and 3000 deaths occur each year in the United States due to foodborne illnesses. Symptoms include diarrhea, vomiting, fever, pain, headache, and weakness. Although the effects of foodborne illnesses are usually not serious, some groups, such as children, pregnant women, individuals with immune deficits and the elderly, are more at risk for severe complications such as rheumatic diseases, seizures, blood poisoning, hemolytic uremic syndrome, and death.

Most cases of foodborne illness are caused by **pathogens**—disease-causing microorganisms. Food can be contaminated with pathogens through improper handling, and pathogens can grow if food is prepared or stored improperly. According to the CDC, eight known pathogens contribute to the vast majority of illnesses, hospitalizations, and deaths related to foodborne illnesses: *Salmonella* (most often found in eggs, on vegetables, and on poultry); *Norovirus* (most often found in salad ingredients and shellfish); *Campylobacter jejuni* (most often found in meat and poultry); *Toxoplasma* (most often found in meat); *Escherichia coli (E. coli)* O157:H7 (most often found in meat

pathogen A microorganism that causes disease. **TERMS**

Since 1999, specific types of information have been required on the labels of dietary supplements. In addition to basic information about the product, labels include a "Supplement Facts" panel, modeled after the "Nutrition Facts" panel used on food labels (see the label illustrated in this box). Under the Dietary Supplement Health and Education Act (DSHEA) and food labeling laws, supplement labels can make three types of health-related claims:

- **Nutrient content claims,** such as "high in calcium," "excellent source of vitamin C," or "high potency." The claims "high in" and "excellent source of" mean the same as they do on food labels. A "high-potency" single-ingredient supplement must contain 100% of that nutrient's Daily Value; a "high-potency" multi-ingredient product must contain 100% or more of the Daily Value of at least two-thirds of the nutrients present for which Daily Values have been established.

- **Health claims,** if they have been authorized by the FDA or another authoritative scientific body. The association between adequate calcium intake and lower risk of osteoporosis is an example of an approved health claim. Since 2003, the FDA has also allowed so-called *qualified* health claims for situations in which there is emerging but as yet inconclusive evidence for a particular claim. These claims must include qualifying language such as "scientific evidence suggests but does not prove [the claim]."

- **Structure–function claims,** such as "antioxidants maintain cellular integrity" or "this product enhances energy levels." Because these claims are not reviewed by the FDA, they must carry a disclaimer (see the sample label).

Tips for Choosing and Using Dietary Supplements

- Check with your physician before taking a supplement. Many are not meant for children, older adults, women who are pregnant or breastfeeding, people with chronic illnesses or upcoming surgery, or people taking prescription or over-the-counter medications. When you visit your doctor, bring a list of all dietary supplements you are taking. Do not take megadoses (more than double the DRI levels) without your doctor's approval.

- Choose brands made by nationally known food and drug manufacturers or house brands from large retail chains. Due to their size and visibility, such sources are likely to have high manufacturing standards.

- Look for the "USP" (United States Pharmacopeial Convention) verification mark on the label, indicating that the product meets minimum safety and purity standards developed under the USP Dietary Supplement Verification Program. The USP mark means that the product (1) contains the listed ingredients, (2) has the declared amount and strength of ingredients, (3) will dissolve effectively, (4) has been screened for harmful contaminants, and (5) has been manufactured using safe, sanitary, and well-controlled procedures. The National Nutritional Foods Association (NNFA) has a self-regulatory testing program for its members; other associations and laboratories, including ConsumerLab.com, also test and rate dietary supplements.

- Follow the label's cautions, directions for use, and dosage.

- If you experience side effects, stop using the product and contact your physician. Report any serious reactions to the FDA's MedWatch monitoring program (800-FDA-1088 or online at http://www.fda.gov/Safety/MedWatch/default.htm).

For More Information about Dietary Supplements

NIH Office of Dietary Supplements (http://ods.od.nih.gov)
FDA (http://www.fda.gov/food/dietarysupplements)
USDA (http://fnic.nal.usda.gov/dietary-supplements)

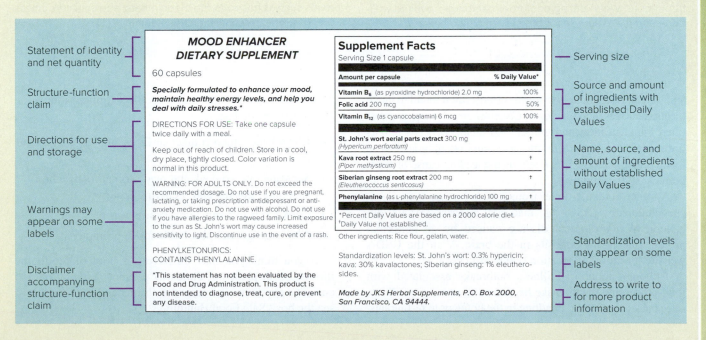

Statement of identity and net quantity	**MOOD ENHANCER DIETARY SUPPLEMENT** 60 capsules	Serving size
Structure-function claim	*Specially formulated to enhance your mood, maintain healthy energy levels, and help you deal with daily stresses.**	Source and amount of ingredients with established Daily Values
Directions for use and storage	DIRECTIONS FOR USE: Take one capsule twice daily with a meal. Keep out of reach of children. Store in a cool, dry place, tightly closed. Color variation is normal in this product.	Name, source, and amount of ingredients without established Daily Values
Warnings may appear on some labels	WARNING: FOR ADULTS ONLY. Do not exceed the recommended dosage. Do not use if you are pregnant, lactating, or taking prescription antidepressant or anti-anxiety medication. Do not use with alcohol. Do not use if you have allergies to the ragweed family. Limit exposure to the sun as St. John's wort may cause increased sensitivity to light. Discontinue use in the event of a rash. PHENYLKETONURICS: CONTAINS PHENYLALANINE.	Standardization levels may appear on some labels
Disclaimer accompanying structure-function claim	*This statement has not been evaluated by the Food and Drug Administration. This product is not intended to diagnose, treat, cure, or prevent any disease.	Address to write to for more product information

Supplement Facts
Serving Size 1 capsule

Amount per capsule	% Daily Value*
Vitamin B₆ (as pyroxidine hydrochloride) 2.0 mg	100%
Folic acid 200 mcg	50%
Vitamin B₁₂ (as cyanocobalamin) 6 mcg	100%
St. John's wort aerial parts extract 300 mg (*Hypericum perforatum*)	†
Kava root extract 250 mg (*Piper methysticum*)	†
Siberian ginseng root extract 200 mg (*Eleutherococcus senticosus*)	†
Phenylalanine (as L-phenylalanine hydrochloride) 100 mg	†

*Percent Daily Values are based on a 2000 calorie diet.
†Daily Value not established.

Other ingredients: Rice flour, gelatin, water.

Standardization levels: St. John's wort: 0.3% hypericin; kava: 30% kavalactones; Siberian ginseng: 1% eleutherosides.

Made by JKS Herbal Supplements, P.O. Box 2000, San Francisco, CA 94444.

- Don't buy food in containers that leak, bulge, or are severely dented. Refrigerated foods should be cold, and frozen foods should be solid when you buy them.

- Refrigerate perishable items as soon as possible after purchase. Use or freeze fresh meats within 3–5 days and fresh poultry, fish, and ground meat within 1–2 days.

- Store raw meat, poultry, fish, and shellfish in containers in the refrigerator so that the juices don't drip onto other foods. Keep these items away from other foods, surfaces, utensils, or serving dishes to prevent cross-contamination.

- Thaw frozen food in the refrigerator or in the microwave oven, not on the kitchen counter. Cook foods immediately after thawing.

- Thoroughly wash your hands with warm, soapy water for 20 seconds before and after handling food, especially raw meat, fish, shellfish, poultry, or eggs.

- Make sure counters, cutting boards, dishes, utensils, and other equipment are cleaned thoroughly with hot, soapy water before and after use. Wash dishcloths frequently.

- If possible, use separate cutting boards for meat, poultry, and seafood and for foods that will be eaten raw. Replace cutting boards once they become worn or develop hard-to-clean grooves.

- Thoroughly rinse and scrub fruits and vegetables with a brush, if possible, or peel off the skin.

- Cook foods thoroughly, especially beef, poultry, fish, pork, wild game, and eggs; cooking kills most microorganisms. Use a food thermometer to ensure that foods are cooked to a safe temperature. Hamburgers should be cooked to at least 160°F. Turn or stir microwaved food to make sure it is heated evenly throughout. When eating out, order hamburger cooked well-done and make sure foods are served piping hot.

- Keep hot foods hot (140°F or above) and cold foods cold (40°F or below). Harmful bacteria can grow rapidly between these two temperatures. Refrigerate foods within two hours of purchase or preparation, and within one hour if the air temperature is above 90°F. Refrigerate foods at or below 40°F and freeze at or below 0°F. Use refrigerated leftovers within 3–4 days.

- Don't eat raw animal products, including raw eggs in homemade hollandaise sauce or eggnog. Use only pasteurized milk and juice, and look for pasteurized eggs, which are now available in some states.

- Cook eggs until they're firm, and fully cook foods containing eggs. Store eggs in the cooler parts of the refrigerator, not in the door, and use them within 3–5 weeks.

- Avoid raw sprouts. Even sprouts grown under clean conditions in the home can be risky because bacteria may be present in the seeds. Cook sprouts before eating them.

- Read the food label and package information, and follow safety instructions such as "Keep Refrigerated" and the "Safe Handling Instructions."

- According to the USDA, "When in doubt, throw it out." Even if a food looks and smells fine, it may not be safe. If you aren't sure that a food has been prepared, served, and stored safely, don't eat it.

Additional precautions are recommended for people at particularly high risk for foodborne illness—pregnant women, very young children, older people, and people with weakened immune systems or certain chronic illnesses. If you are a member of one of these groups, don't eat or drink any of the following products: unpasteurized juices; raw sprouts; unpasteurized (raw) milk and products made from unpasteurized milk; raw or undercooked meat, poultry, eggs, fish, or shellfish; and soft cheeses such as feta, Brie, Camembert, or blue-veined cheeses. To protect against *Listeria,* avoid ready-to-eat foods such as hot dogs, luncheon meats, and cold cuts unless they are reheated until they are steaming hot.

and water); *Listeria monocytogenes* (most often found in lunch meats, sausages, and hot dogs); *Clostridium perfringens* (most often found in meat and gravy); and *Staphylococcus aureus* (most often resulting from improper hand washing leading to food contamination). *Salmonella* is the leading cause of foodborne hospitalizations.

Another potential threat from food is bovine spongiform encephalopathy (BSE), or "mad cow disease"—a fatal degenerative neurological disease caused by an abnormal protein that forms deposits in the brain. Visit the USDA website for more information (www.usda.gov).

Although foodborne illness outbreaks associated with food-processing plants make headlines, most cases of illness trace back to poor food handling in the home or in restaurants.

Food safety experts encourage people to follow four basic food safety principles:

- *Clean* hands, food contact surfaces, and vegetables and fruits.
- *Separate* raw, cooked, and ready-to-eat foods while shopping, storing, and preparing foods.
- *Cook* foods to a safe temperature.
- *Chill* (refrigerate) perishable foods promptly.

If you think you may be having a bout of foodborne illness, drink plenty of fluids to prevent dehydration and consult a physician. For more details on handling food safely, see the box "Safe Food Handling."

Although pathogens are usually destroyed during cooking, the U.S. government has taken steps to bring down levels of contamination by improving national surveillance and testing. Careful food handling greatly reduces the risk of foodborne illness. Raw meat and poultry products are now sold with safe handling and safe cooking instructions, and all packaged, unpasteurized fresh fruit and vegetable juices carry warnings about potential contamination. In 2011, the Food Safety Modernization Act (FSMA) was signed into law to reform the food safety system in the United States and further ensure the safety of the U.S. food supply. The FSMA allows the FDA to focus more on preventing food safety problems than on reacting to problems after they occur.

Organic Foods

Some people who are concerned about pesticides and other environmental contaminants choose to buy foods that are **organic.** To be certified as organic by the USDA, foods must meet strict production, processing, handling, and labeling criteria. Organic crops must meet limits on pesticide residues. For meat, milk, eggs, and other animal products to be certified organic, animals must be given organic feed and access to the outdoors and may not be given antibiotics or growth hormones. The use of genetic engineering, ionizing radiation, and sewage sludge is prohibited. Products can be labeled "100% organic" if they contain all organic ingredients and "organic" if they contain at least 95% organic ingredients; all such products may carry the USDA organic seal. A product with at least 70% organic ingredients can be labeled "made with organic ingredients" but cannot use the USDA seal.

Some experts recommend that consumers who want to buy organic produce spend their money on those fruits and vegetables that have the highest levels of pesticide residue when grown conventionally (the "dirty dozen"): apples, bell peppers, celery, cherries, imported grapes, nectarines, peaches, pears, potatoes, red raspberries, spinach, and strawberries. Experts also recommend buying organic beef, poultry, eggs, dairy products, and baby food. Fruits and vegetables that carry little pesticide residue whether grown conventionally or organically include asparagus, avocados, bananas, broccoli, cauliflower, corn, kiwi, mangoes, onions, papaya, pineapples, and peas. All foods are subject to strict pesticide limits; the debate about the health effects of small amounts of residue is ongoing.

Whether organic foods are better for your health or not, organic farming is better for the environment. Benefits include sustainable farming practices, preservation of biodiversity, healthier soil, protection of water supplies, reduced use of fossil fuels, improved animal welfare, protection of ecosystems, and safer conditions for farmworkers. Buying organic food, buying locally grown foods, and participating in a community garden are ways to support food production that benefits and sustains the environment.

Guidelines for Fish Consumption

A specific area of concern has been mercury contamination in fish. Overall, fish and shellfish are healthy sources of protein, omega-3 fats, and other nutrients. Prudent choices can minimize the risk of any possible negative health effects.

According to FDA and Environmental Protection Agency (EPA) guidelines, women who are or may become pregnant and nursing mothers should follow these guidelines to minimize their exposure to mercury:

- Do not eat shark, swordfish, king mackerel, or tilefish.
- Eat 8–12 ounces a week of a variety of fish and shellfish that are lower in mercury, such as shrimp, canned light tuna, salmon, pollock, and catfish. Limit consumption of albacore tuna to 6 ounces per week.
- Check advisories about the safety of recreationally caught fish from local lakes, rivers, and coastal areas; if no information is available, limit consumption to 6 ounces per week.

The same FDA/EPA guidelines apply to children, although they should consume smaller servings.

Additives in Food

According to the FDA's "Everything Added to Food in the United States (EAFUS)" database, approximately 3000 substances are intentionally added to foods to maintain or improve nutritional quality, maintain freshness, help in processing or preparation, or alter taste or appearance. The most widely used food additives are sugar, salt, and corn syrup; these three plus citric acid, baking soda, vegetable colors, mustard, and pepper account for 98% by weight of all food additives used in the United States.

Additives having potential health concerns include nitrates and nitrites, used in processed meats and associated with the synthesis of cancer-causing agents in the stomach; BHA (butylated hydroxyanisole) and BHT (butylated hydroxytoluene), used to maintain freshness and possibly associated with an increased risk of some cancers; sulfites, used to keep vegetables from turning brown and associated with severe reactions in sensitive people; and monosodium glutamate (MSG), used as a flavor enhancer and associated with episodes of increased blood pressure and sweating in sensitive people. If you are sensitive to an additive, check food labels when you shop and ask questions when you eat out.

Food Biotechnology

Modern biotechnology tools, such as genetic engineering and cloning, allow for more precise, productive, and efficient

organic   A designation applied to foods grown and produced according to strict guidelines limiting the use of pesticides, nonorganic ingredients, hormones, antibiotics, irradiation, genetic engineering, and other practices.   **TERMS**

development of crops and livestock. Internationally, 28 countries planted biotech crops grown by more than 17 million farmers. In the United States, biotechnology is used in about 90% of the current soybean, cotton, and corn crops. The USDA, FDA, and EPA are the three federal agencies in charge of the regulatory oversight of biotechnology.

Food irradiation is the treatment of foods with gamma rays, X-rays, or high-voltage electrons to kill potentially harmful pathogens, including bacteria, parasites, insects, and fungi that cause foodborne illness. Irradiation also reduces spoilage and extends a product's shelf life.

Even though irradiation has been generally endorsed by agencies such as the World Health Organization (WHO), the CDC, and the American Medical Association (AMA), few irradiated foods are currently on the market due to consumer resistance and skepticism. Studies indicate that when consumers are given information about the process of irradiation and the benefits of irradiated foods, most want to purchase them. All primary irradiated foods (meat, vegetables, and so on) are labeled with the flowerlike Radura symbol and a brief information label; spices and foods that are merely ingredients do not have to be so labeled.

Genetic engineering involves altering the characteristics of a plant, animal, or microorganism by adding, rearranging, or replacing genes in its DNA; the result is a **genetically modified organism (GMO).** New DNA may come from related species or from entirely different types of organisms. Many GM crops are already grown in the United States. Products made with GMOs include juice, soda, nuts, tuna, frozen pizza, spaghetti sauce, canola oil, chips, salad dressings, and soup.

The potential benefits of GM foods cited by supporters include improved yields overall and in difficult growing conditions, increased disease resistance, improved nutritional content, lower prices, and less pesticide use. Critics of biotechnology argue that unexpected harmful effects may occur: Gene manipulation could elevate levels of naturally occurring toxins or allergens, permanently change the gene pool, reduce biodiversity, and produce pesticide-resistant insects. Experience has shown that GM products are difficult to keep separate from non-GM products. Animal escapes, cross-pollination, and contamination during processing are just a few ways in which GMOs could potentially appear unexpectedly in the food supply or the environment.

Food Allergies and Food Intolerances

For some people, consuming a particular food causes symptoms such as itchiness, swollen lips, or abdominal pain. Adverse reactions like these may be due to a food allergy or a food intolerance, and symptoms may range from annoying to life-threatening.

A true **food allergy** is a reaction of the body's immune system to a food or food ingredient, usually a protein. The immune system perceives the reaction-provoking substance, or allergen, as foreign and acts to destroy it. This immune reaction can occur within minutes of ingesting the food, resulting in symptoms that affect the skin (hives),

gastrointestinal tract (cramps or diarrhea), respiratory tract (asthma), or mouth (swelling of the lips or tongue). The most severe response is a systemic reaction called *anaphylaxis,* which involves a potentially life-threatening drop in blood pressure and narrowing of airways blocking normal breathing. Repeated exposure to the allergen may result in more severe symptoms.

Although numerous food allergens have been identified, just eight foods account for more than 90% of the food allergies in the United States: cow's milk, eggs, peanuts, tree nuts (walnuts, cashews, and so on), soy, wheat, fish, and shellfish. Food labels are now required to state the presence of the eight most common allergens in plain language in the ingredient list.

Many people who believe they have food allergies may actually suffer from a much more common source of adverse food reactions—a **food intolerance.** In the case of a food intolerance, the problem usually lies with metabolism rather than with the immune system. Typically the body cannot adequately digest a food or food component, often because of some type of chemical deficiency; in other cases, the body reacts to a particular compound in a food. Lactose intolerance is a fairly common food intolerance.

A more serious condition may be intolerance of gluten, a protein component of some grains. In recent decades, the prevalence of celiac disease has risen in Western populations. Currently, almost 1% of Americans have a problem that causes the body to attack the small intestine when gluten is ingested and can lead to other debilitating medical problems. An additional 18 million people, or about 6% of the population, is believed to have gluten sensitivity, a less severe problem with the protein in wheat, barley, and rye and other foods that gives elasticity to dough and stability to the shape of baked goods. Sulfite, a common food additive, can produce severe asthmatic reactions in sensitive individuals.

Food intolerance reactions often produce symptoms similar to those of food allergies, such as diarrhea or cramps, but reactions are typically localized and not life-threatening. Exceptions are gluten and sulfite, which must be avoided by sensitive individuals. Through trial and error, most people with food intolerances can adjust their intake of the trigger food to an appropriate level.

TERMS

food irradiation The treatment of foods with gamma rays, X-rays, or high-voltage electrons to kill potentially harmful pathogens and increase shelf life.

genetically modified organism (GMO) A plant, animal, or microorganism in which genes have been added, rearranged, or replaced through genetic engineering.

food allergy An adverse reaction to a food or food ingredient in which the immune system perceives a particular substance (allergen) as foreign and acts to destroy it.

food intolerance An adverse reaction to a food or food ingredient that doesn't involve the immune system; intolerances are often due to a problem with metabolism.

Ask Yourself ?

QUESTIONS FOR CRITICAL THINKING AND REFLECTION

What is the least healthy food you eat every day (either during meals or as a snack)? Identify at least one substitute that would be healthier but just as satisfying.

TIPS FOR TODAY AND THE FUTURE ✳

Opportunities to improve your diet present themselves every day, and small changes add up.

RIGHT NOW YOU CAN:

- Substitute a healthy snack for an unhealthy one.
- Drink a glass of water and put a reusable water bottle in your backpack for tomorrow.
- Plan to make healthy selections when you eat out, such as steamed vegetables instead of french fries, or salmon instead of steak.

IN THE FUTURE YOU CAN:

- Visit the MyPlate website at ChooseMyPlate.gov and use the online tools to create a personalized nutrition plan and begin tracking your eating habits.
- Learn to cook healthier meals. Hundreds of free websites and low-cost cookbooks provide recipes for healthy dishes.

SUMMARY

- To function at its best, the human body requires about 45 essential nutrients in certain relative proportions. People get these nutrients from foods; the body cannot synthesize most of them.

- Proteins, made up of amino acids, form muscles and bones and help make up blood, enzymes, hormones, and cell membranes. Foods from animal sources provide complete proteins; plants provide incomplete proteins and must be combined in order to attain the right balance of amino acids, especially if no or limited animal protein is in the diet. Protein intake should be 10–35% of total daily energy intake.

- Fats, a concentrated source of energy, also help to insulate the body and cushion the organs; 3–4 teaspoons of vegetable oil per day supplies the essential fats. Dietary fat intake should be 20–35% of total daily energy intake. In general, you can still eat high-fat foods, but avoid trans fats and limit the size of your portions and balance your intake with low-fat foods.

- Carbohydrates supply energy to the brain and other parts of the nervous system as well as to red blood cells. The body needs about 130 grams of carbohydrates a day, but more is recommended. Carbohydrates should make up 45–65% of total daily energy intake.

- Fiber includes nondigestible carbohydrates provided mainly by plants. A high-fiber diet can help people manage diabetes and high cholesterol levels and improve intestinal health.

- The 13 vitamins needed in the diet are organic substances that regulate various processes within living cells and promote specific chemical reactions. Deficiencies or excesses can cause serious illnesses and even death.

- The approximately 17 minerals needed in the diet are inorganic substances that regulate body functions, aid in the growth and maintenance of body tissues, and help in the release of energy from foods.

- Water is used to digest and absorb food, transport substances around the body, and regulate body temperature.

- Foods contain other substances such as phytochemicals, which may not be essential nutrients but may help reduce chronic disease risk.

- Dietary Reference Intakes (DRIs) are standards for nutrient intake designed to prevent nutritional deficiencies and reduce the risk of chronic diseases.

- The Dietary Guidelines for Americans are designed to help people make healthy and informed food choices. Following the guidelines promotes health and reduces the risk of chronic disease. The *2015–2020 Dietary Guidelines for Americans* presents five guidelines in several areas: (1) Follow a healthy eating pattern across the lifespan; (2) focus on variety, nutrient density, and amount; (3) limit calories from added sugars and saturated fats and reduce sodium intake; (4) shift to healthier food and beverage choices; and (5) support healthy eating patterns for all.

- Choosing the right amount of foods from each food group in MyPlate every day ensures that you get enough necessary nutrients without overconsuming calories.

- A vegetarian diet can meet human nutritional needs but must be planned carefully to prevent potential micronutrient deficiencies, especially of vitamin B-12 and readily bioavailable iron.

- Almost all foods have labels that show how much fat, cholesterol, protein, fiber, and sodium they contain. Serving sizes are standardized, and health claims are regulated carefully. Dietary supplements also have uniform labels that provide supplement facts.

- Food additives, environmental containments, and foodborne illnesses from *Salmonella, E. coli, Norovirus*, and other microorganisms can pose threats to health. Other dietary issues of concern to some people include food irradiation, genetic modification of foods, and food allergies and intolerances.

American Diabetes Association. An organization with the aim of leading the fight against the deadly consequences of diabetes and fighting for those affected by diabetes.

http://www.diabetes.org

*Academy of Nutrition and Dietetics (*formerly the *American Dietetic Association).* Provides a variety of nutrition-related educational materials.

http://www.eatright.org

The Dietary Guidelines. The official site for the Dietary Guidelines for Americans, 2015.

http://health.gov/dietaryguidelines/2015/guidelines/

FDA Center for Food Safety and Applied Nutrition. Offers information about topics such as food labeling, food additives, dietary supplements, and foodborne illness.

http://www.fda.gov/food

Food Safety Hotlines. Provide information on safe purchase, handling, cooking, and storage of food.

888-SAFEFOOD (FDA)

800-535-4555 (USDA)

Fruit and Veggies: More Matters. A nonprofit organization designed to increase consumption of fruits and vegetables to five or more servings a day to improve the health of Americans.

http://www.fruitsandveggiesmorematters.org

Gateways to Government Nutrition Information. Provides access to government resources relating to food safety and nutrition.

http://www.foodsafety.gov

http://www.nutrition.gov

Harvard School of Public Health: The Nutrition Source. Provides recent key research findings, an overview of the Healthy Eating Plate, and suggestions for building a healthful diet.

http://www.hsph.harvard.edu/nutritionsource

MyPlate. Provides personalized dietary plans and interactive food and activity tracking tools.

http://www.ChooseMyPlate.gov

National Academies' Food and Nutrition Board. Provides information about the Dietary Reference Intakes and related guidelines.

http://www.nap.edu/read/11537/chapter/1

USDA Center for Nutrition Policy and Promotion. Established in 1994 to improve the nutrition and well-being of Americans. Includes information about the Dietary Guidelines and MyPlate.

http://www.choosemyplate.gov/

USDA Food and Nutrition Information Center. Provides a variety of materials and extensive links relating to the Dietary Guidelines, food labels, MyPlate, and many other topics.

https://fnic.nal.usda.gov

SELECTED BIBLIOGRAPHY

Academy of Nutrition and Dietetics. 2013. Position of the Academy of Nutrition and Dietetics: Functional foods. *Journal of the Academy of Nutrition and Dietetics* 113(8): 1096–1103.

Academy of Nutrition and Dietetics. 2015. Position of the Academy of Nutrition and Dietetics: Vegetarian diets. *Journal of the Academy of Nutrition and Dietetics* 115: 801–810.

American Heart Association. 2012. *Diet and Lifestyle Recommendations* (http://www.heart.org/HEARTORG/GettingHealthy/Diet-and-Lifestyle-Recommendations_UCM_305855_Article.jsp).

American Heart Association. 2012. *Fish and Omega-3 Fatty Acids* (http://www.heart.org/HEARTORG/GettingHealthy/NutritionCenter/HealthyDietGoals/Fish-and-Omega-3-Fatty-Acids_UCM_303248_Article.jsp).

American Heart Association. 2015. *Saturated Fats* (http://www.heart.org/HEARTORG/GettingHealthy/NutritionCenter/HealthyEating/Saturated-Fats_UCM_301110_Article.jsp#).

Bellavia, A., F. Stilling, and A. Wolk. 2016. High red meat intake and all-cause cardiovascular and cancer mortality: Is the risk modified by fruit and vegetable intake? *American Journal of Clinical Nutrition*, 24 August (epub ahead of print).

Centers for Disease Control and Prevention. 2012. *CDC and the Food Safety Modernization Act* (http://www.cdc.gov/foodsafety/fsma.html).

Centers for Disease Control and Prevention. 2012. Vital signs: Food categories contributing the most to sodium consumption—United States, 2007–2008. *MMWR* 61(5): 92–98.

Centers for Disease Control and Prevention. 2014. *Estimates of Foodborne Illness in the United States* (http://www.cdc.gov/foodborneburden/2011-foodborne-estimates.html).

Centers for Disease Control and Prevention. 2014. Sugar-sweetened beverage consumption among adults—18 states, 2012. *MMWR* 63(32): 686–690.

Centers for Disease Control and Prevention. 2015. *Foodborne Germs and Illnesses* (http://www.cdc.gov/foodsafety/foodborne-germs.html).

Centers for Disease Control and Prevention. 2015. Percentage of Adults Aged 65 and Over With Osteoporosis or Low Bone Mass at the Femur Neck or Lumbar Spine: United States, 2005–2010 (http://www.cdc.gov/nchs/data/hestat/osteoporsis/osteoporosis2005_2010.pdf).

Centers for Disease Control and Prevention. Office of Public Health Genomics. 2016. *Does Osteoporosis Run in Your Family?* (http://www.cdc.gov/features/osteoporosis/).

Centers for Disease Control and Prevention. 2016. *Sodium: The Facts* (http://www.cdc.gov/salt/pdfs/Sodium_Fact_Sheet.pdf).

Centers for Disease Control and Prevention. National Center for Health Statistics. What We Eat in America, Data Tables (http://www.ars.usda.gov/Services/docs.htm?docid=18349)

Chowdhury, R., et al. 2014. Association of dietary, circulating, and supplement fatty acids with coronary risk: A systematic review and meta-analysis. *Annals of Internal Medicine* 160(6): 398–406.

Dahl, W. J., and M. L. Steward. 2015. Position of the Academy of Nutrition and Dietetics: Health implications of dietary fiber. *Journal of the Academy of Nutrition and Dietetics* 115(11): 1861–1870.

Eckel, R., et al. 2013. AHA/ACC guideline on lifestyle management to reduce cardiovascular risk: A report of the American College of Cardiology/American Heart Association task force on practice guidelines. *Circulation.* DOI: 10.1161/01.cir.0000437740.48606.d1.

FAO, IFAD, and WFP. 2015. *The State of Food Insecurity in the World 2015. Meeting the 2015 International Hunger Targets: Taking Stock of Uneven Progress* (http://www.fao.org/3/a4ef2d16-70a7-460a-a9ac-2a65a533269a/i4646e.pdf).

Fink, S. W. 2012. Key articles of dietary interventions that influence cardiovascular mortality. *Pharmacotherapy* 32(4): e54–87.

Finkelstein, E. A., et al. 2012. Obesity and severe obesity forecasts through 2030. *American Journal of Preventive Medicine Online* (http://www.ajpmonline.org/webfiles/images/journals/amepre/AMEPRE_33853stamped2.pdf).

Food and Nutrition Board, Institute of Medicine. 2005. *Dietary Reference Intakes for Energy, Carbohydrate, Fiber, Fat, Fatty Acids, Cholesterol, Protein, and Amino Acids.* Washington, DC: National Academies Press.

Food and Nutrition Board, Institute of Medicine. 2005. *Dietary Reference Intakes for Water, Potassium, Sodium, Chloride, and Sulfate.* Washington, DC: National Academies Press.

Food and Nutrition Board, Institute of Medicine. 2011. *Dietary Reference Intakes for Calcium and Vitamin D.* Washington, DC: National Academies Press.

Freeland-Graves, J. H., and S. Nitzke. 2013. Position of the Academy of Nutrition and Dietetics: Total diet approach to healthy eating. *Journal of the Academy of Nutrition and Dietetics* 113(2): 307–317.

Harvard Medical School. 2015. *The Truth about Fats: The Good, the Bad, and the In-Between* (http://www.health.harvard.edu/staying-healthy /the-truth-about-fats-bad-and-good).

Harvard School of Public Health, Department of Nutrition. 2010. *The Nutrition Source: Knowledge for Healthy Eating* (http://www.hsph .harvard.edu/nutritionsource).

Insel, P., et al. 2016. *Nutrition,* 6th ed. Burlington, MA: Jones & Bartlett Learning.

Jackson, S. L., et al. 2016. Prevalence of excess sodium intake in the United States—NHANES, 2009–2012. *MMWR* 64(52); 1393–1397.

Jesri, M., W. Y. Lou, and M. R. L'Abbé. 2016. 2015 Dietary Guidelines for Americans is associated with a more nutrient-dense diet and lower risk of obesity. *American Journal of Clinical Nutrition*, 28 September (epub ahead of print).

Johnson, R. K., et al. 2009. Dietary sugars intake and cardiovascular health: A scientific statement from the American Heart Association. *Circulation* 120(11): 1011–1020.

Jonnalagadda, S. S., et al. 2011. Putting the whole grain puzzle together: Health benefits associated with whole grains—Summary of American Society for Nutrition 2010 Satellite Symposium. *Journal of Nutrition* 14(5): 1011S–1022S.

Kiage, J. N., et al. 2013. Trans fat intake and all-cause mortality in the Reasons for Geographical and Racial Differences in Stroke (REGARDS) cohort. *American Journal of Clinical Nutrition* 97: 1121–1128.

Lebwohl, B., J. F. Ludvigsson, and P. H. Green. 2015. Celiac disease and non-celiac gluten sensitivity. *BMJ* 351: h4347. DOI: 10.1136/bmj.h4347.

Maki, K. C., et al. 2010. Whole-grain ready-to-eat oat cereal, as part of a dietary program for weight loss, reduces low-density lipoprotein cholesterol in adults with overweight and obesity more than a dietary program including low-fiber control foods. *Journal of the American Dietetic Association* 110(2): 205–214.

National Institutes of Health. Osteoporosis and Related Bone Diseases. National Resource Center. 2015. *Vitamin A and Bone Health* (http://www .niams.nih.gov/Health_Info/Bone/Bone_Health/Nutrition/vitamin_a.asp).

National Osteoporosis Foundation. 2014. 54 Million Americans affected by osteoporosis and low bone mass. National Osteoporosis Foundation online news, June 2 (http://nof.org/news/2948).

Ng, M., et al. 2014. Global, regional, and national prevalence of overweight and obesity in children and adults during 1980–2013: A systematic analysis for the Global Burden of Disease Study 2013. *Lancet* 384(9945): 766–781.

Nowak, V., J. Du, and R. Charrondière. 2016. Assessment of the nutritional composition of quinoa (*Chenopodium quinoa* Willd.) *Food Chemistry* 193:47–54.

Orlich, M. J., et al. 2013. Vegetarian Dietary patterns and mortality in Adventist Health Study 2. *JAMA Intern Medicine* 173(13): 1230–1238.

Rodriguez, L. A., et al. 2016. Added sugar intake and metabolic syndrome in U.S. adolescents. *Public Health Nutrition* 19(13): 2424–2434.

Siri-Tarino, P. W., et al. 2010. Meta-analysis of prospective cohort studies evaluating the association of saturated fat with cardiovascular disease. *American Journal of Clinical Nutrition* 91(3): 535–546.

Teicholz, N. 2014. *The Big Fat Surprise: Why Butter, Meat & Cheese Belong in a Healthy Diet.* New York: Simon & Schuster.

Tucker, K. L. 2009. Osteoporosis prevention and nutrition. *Current Osteoporosis Reports* 7(4): 111–117.

U.S. Department of Agriculture. 2011. *ChooseMyPlate* (http://www .choosemyplate.gov).

U.S. Department of Agriculture. 2013. *Household Food Security in the United States in 2012* (Economic Research Report No. ERR-155) (http://www.ers.usda.gov/publications/err-economic-research -report/err155.aspx).

U.S. Department of Agriculture, 2016. *Biotechnology. Frequently Asked Questions. (FAQs).* (http://www.usda.gov/wps/portal/usda/usdahome?n avid=AGRICULTURE&contentid=BiotechnologyFAQs.xml).

U.S. Department of Agriculture, Agricultural Research Service, Nutrient Data Laboratory. 2015. *USDA National Nutrient Database for Standard Reference, Release 28* (http://www.ars.usda.gov/nea/bhnrc/ndl).

U.S. Department of Health and Human Services and U.S. Department of Agriculture. 2015a. *2015–2020 Dietary Guidelines for Americans*, 8th ed. (http://health.gov/dietaryguidelines/2015/guidelines/).

U.S. Department of Health and Human Services and U.S. Department of Agriculture. 2015b. *Scientific Report of the 2015 Dietary Guidelines Advisory Committee,* Figure D1.33 (http://www.health .gov/dietaryguidelines/2015-scientific-report).

U.S. Department of Health and Human Services and U.S. Food and Drug Administration. 2014. *Everything Added to Food in the United States (EAFUS)* (http://www.fda.gov/Food/IngredientsPackagingLabeling/ FoodAdditivesIngredients/ucm115326.htm).

U.S. Department of Health and Human Services and U.S. Food and Drug Administration. 2015. *FDA Takes Step to Remove Artificial Trans Fats from Processed Foods* (http://www.fda.gov/food/newsevents/ constituentupdates/ucm449145.htm).

U.S. Environmental Protection Agency. 2012. *Fish Consumption Advisories* (http://www.epa.gov/hg/advisories.htm).

U.S. Food and Drug Administration. 2012. *Food Allergies: What You Need to Know* (http://www.fda.gov/food/resourcesforyou/consumers/ ucm079311.htm).

U.S. Food and Drug Administration. 2016. *"Healthy" on Food Labeling* (http://www.fda.gov/Food/GuidanceRegulation/GuidanceDocuments- RegulatoryInformation/LabelingNutrition/ucm520695.htm).

Vos, M. S., et al. 2016. Added sugars and cardiovascular risk in children: A scientific statement from the American Heart Association. *Circulation*, 22 August (epub ahead of print).

Wang, D. D., et al. 2016. Association of specific dietary fats with total and cause-specific mortality. *JAMA Internal Medicine* 176(8): 1134–1145.

World Health Organization. 2016. *Global Health Observatory Data: Underweight in Children* (http://www.who.int/gho/mdg/poverty _hunger/underweight_text/en/).

World Health Organization. 2016. *Global Strategy on Diet, Physical Activity, and Health: Child Overweight and Obesity* (http://www.who .int/dietphysicalactivity/childhood/en/).

BEHAVIOR CHANGE STRATEGY
Improving Your Diet by Choosing Healthy Beverages

After reading this chapter and completing the dietary assessment, you can probably identify several ways to improve your diet. As an example here, we focus on choosing healthy beverages to increase intake of nutrients and decrease intake of empty calories from added sugars and fat. This model can be applied to any change you want to make to your diet.

Gather Data and Establish a Baseline

Begin by tracking your beverage consumption in a journal. Write down the types and amounts of beverages you drink, including water. Also note where you were at the time and whether you got the beverage there or brought it with you. At the same time, investigate your options. Find out what other beverages you can easily find during your daily routine. This information will help you put together a successful plan for change.

Analyze Your Data and Set Goals

Evaluate your beverage consumption by dividing your typical daily consumption between healthy and less healthy choices. Use the following guide as a basis, and add other beverages to the lists as needed:

Choose More Often	Servings Daily	Choose Less Often	Servings Daily
Water: plain, mineral, sparkling		Regular soda	
Low-fat or fat-free milk		Whole milk	
Fruit juice (100%)		Fruit beverages made with little fruit juice	
Unsweetened or noncaloric sweetened herbal tea		Sugar-sweetened beverages such as iced tea and sports drinks	
Others		Others	

How many beverages do you consume daily from each category? What would be a healthy and realistic goal for change? For example, if your beverage consumption is currently evenly divided between the "choose more often" and "choose less often" categories (four from each list), you might set a final goal for your behavior change program of increasing your healthy choices by two (to six from the "more often" list and two from the "less often" list).

Develop a Plan for Change

Once you've set your goal, you need to develop strategies that will help you choose healthy beverages more often. Consider the following possibilities:

- Keep healthy beverages on hand. If you live in a dorm, rent a small refrigerator or keep water in a reusable bottle and other healthy choices in the dorm kitchen's refrigerator.
- Plan ahead, and carry a reusable bottle with water or 100% juice in your backpack every day.
- Check food labels on beverages for serving sizes, energy content, and nutrients; compare products to find the healthiest choices; and watch your serving sizes. Use this information to make your "choose more often" list longer and more specific.
- If you eat out frequently, examine all the beverages available at the places you typically eat your meals. You'll probably find that plain water or other healthy choices are available.

You may also need to make changes in your routine to decrease the likelihood that you'll make unhealthy choices. For example, your journal might reveal that you always buy a soda after class when you pass a particular vending machine. If this is the case, try another route that bypasses the machine. Guard against impulse buying by carrying water or a healthy snack with you every day.

To complete your plan, try some of the other behavior change strategies described in Chapter 1: Develop and sign a contract, set up a system of rewards, involve other people in your program, and develop strategies for challenging situations. Once your plan is complete, take action. Keep track of your progress by continuing to monitor and evaluate your beverage consumption.

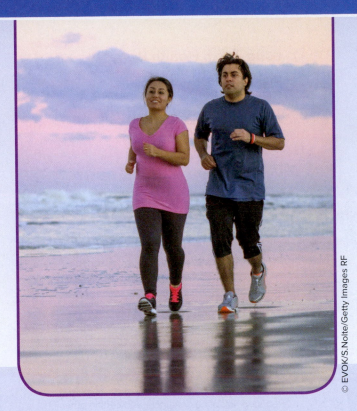

© EVOK/S.Nolte/Getty Images RF

CHAPTER OBJECTIVES

- Describe the benefits of exercise
- Define physical fitness
- Explain the components of an active lifestyle
- Put together a personalized exercise program
- Explain strategies for staying on track with an exercise program

CHAPTER 10

Exercise for Health and Fitness

Your body is a wonderful moving machine made to work best when it is physically active. It readily adapts to practically any level of activity and exercise: The more you ask of your body, the stronger and more fit it becomes. The opposite is also true. Left unchallenged, bones lose their density, joints stiffen, muscles weaken, and the body's energy systems degenerate. To be truly healthy, human beings must be active.

This chapter gives you the basic information you need to put together a physical fitness program that will work for you. If approached correctly, physical activity and exercise can contribute immeasurably to overall wellness, add fun and joy to life, and provide the foundation for a lifetime of fitness.

THE BENEFITS OF EXERCISE

The human body is adaptable. The greater the demands, the more it adjusts and the more fit it becomes. Over time, immediate, short-term adjustments translate into long-term changes and improvements (Figure 10.1).

Reduced Risk of Premature Death

Physically active people have a reduced risk of dying prematurely from all causes; the most active people experience the greatest health benefits (Figure 10.2).

Improved Cardiorespiratory Functioning

During exercise, the cardiorespiratory system (heart, lungs, and circulatory system) must work harder to meet the body's increased demand for oxygen. Regular cardiorespiratory endurance exercise improves the functioning of the heart and the ability of the cardiorespiratory system to carry oxygen to body tissues. Exercise directly affects the health of your arteries, keeping them from stiffening or clogging with plaque and reducing the risk of cardiovascular disease. Exercise also improves sexual function and general vitality.

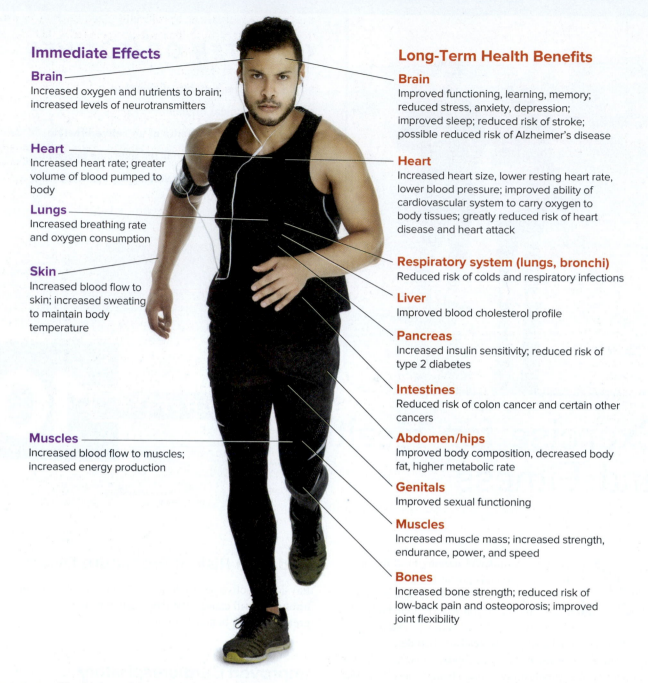

Immediate Effects

Brain
Increased oxygen and nutrients to brain; increased levels of neurotransmitters

Heart
Increased heart rate; greater volume of blood pumped to body

Lungs
Increased breathing rate and oxygen consumption

Skin
Increased blood flow to skin; increased sweating to maintain body temperature

Muscles
Increased blood flow to muscles; increased energy production

Long-Term Health Benefits

Brain
Improved functioning, learning, memory; reduced stress, anxiety, depression; improved sleep; reduced risk of stroke; possible reduced risk of Alzheimer's disease

Heart
Increased heart size, lower resting heart rate, lower blood pressure; improved ability of cardiovascular system to carry oxygen to body tissues; greatly reduced risk of heart disease and heart attack

Respiratory system (lungs, bronchi)
Reduced risk of colds and respiratory infections

Liver
Improved blood cholesterol profile

Pancreas
Increased insulin sensitivity; reduced risk of type 2 diabetes

Intestines
Reduced risk of colon cancer and certain other cancers

Abdomen/hips
Improved body composition, decreased body fat, higher metabolic rate

Genitals
Improved sexual functioning

Muscles
Increased muscle mass; increased strength, endurance, power, and speed

Bones
Increased bone strength; reduced risk of low-back pain and osteoporosis; improved joint flexibility

FIGURE 10.1 Health benefits of exercise.
© PeopleImages/Getty Images RF

More Efficient Metabolism and Improved Cell Health

Endurance exercise improves metabolism—the process that converts food to energy and builds tissue. This process involves oxygen, nutrients, hormones, and enzymes. A physically fit person's body can more efficiently use energy from carbohydrates and fats and better regulate hormones. Exercise may also protect cells from damage from free radicals, which are destructive chemicals produced normally during metabolism (see Chapter 9), and from inflammation caused by obesity, high blood pressure or cholesterol, nicotine, and overeating.

Training activates antioxidants that prevent free radical damage and maintain cell health. Regular physical activity prevents the deterioration of telomeres, which form the protective ends of chromosomes that are vital for cell health and repair.

Improved Body Composition

Exercise can improve body composition in several ways. Endurance exercise significantly increases daily calorie expenditure. It can also slightly raise *metabolic rate,* the rate at which the body burns calories, for several hours after an exercise session. Strength training increases muscle mass,

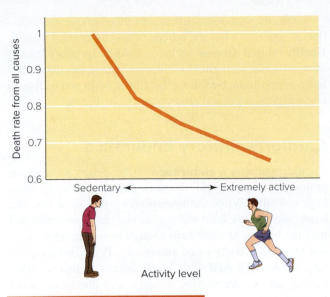

FIGURE 10.2 **Exercise promotes longevity.** Poor muscle strength increases the risk of premature death.

SOURCES: Adapted from a composite of 13 studies involving more than 200,000 men and women. Arem, H., et al. 2015. Leisure time physical activity and mortality: A detailed pooled analysis of the dose-response relationship. *JAMA* 175(6): 959–967; Physical Activity Guidelines Advisory Committee. 2008. *Physical Activity Guidelines Advisory Committee Report, 2008.* Washington, DC: U.S. Department of Health and Human Services.

thereby tipping the body composition ratio toward fat-free mass and away from fat. It can also help with losing fat because metabolic rate is directly proportional to fat-free mass: The more muscle mass, the higher the metabolic rate.

Disease Prevention and Management

Regular physical activity lowers your risk of many chronic, disabling diseases.

Cardiovascular Disease   A sedentary lifestyle is one of six major risk factors for cardiovascular disease (CVD), including heart attack and stroke. Sedentary people have CVD death rates significantly higher than those of fit individuals. Physical inactivity increases the risk of CVD by as much as 240%.

The benefits of physical activity begin at moderate levels of exercise and increase as the amount and intensity of activity rise. Exercise positively affects the risk factors for CVD, including cholesterol levels, insulin resistance, and blood pressure. Exercise also directly interferes with the disease process itself, lowering the risk of heart disease and stroke.

Cancer   Studies have shown a relationship between increased physical activity and a reduced risk of cancer. Specifically, a new analysis of data from studies of 1.44 million subjects concludes that higher levels of leisure-time physical activity were associated with lower risks for 13 of 26 types of cancer, including kidney, colon, head and neck, bladder, rectal, and liver cancer. Most of these associations applied whether or not the participants were overweight/obese or had a history of smoking. Exercise may decrease the risk of colon cancer by speeding the movement of food through the gastrointestinal tract (quickly eliminating potential carcinogens), lowering blood-insulin levels, enhancing immune function, and reducing blood fats. Physical activity during high school and college years may be particularly important for preventing breast cancer later in life.

Osteoporosis   A special benefit of exercise, especially for women, is protection against osteoporosis, a disease that results in loss of bone density and poor bone strength. Weight-bearing exercise, which includes almost everything except swimming, helps build bone during childhood and the teens and twenties. Older people with denser bones can better endure the bone loss that occurs with aging. Strength training and impact exercises such as jumping rope help maintain bone and muscle health throughout life. With stronger bones and muscles and better balance, fit people are less likely to experience debilitating falls and bone fractures.

Type 2 Diabetes   People with diabetes are prone to heart disease, blindness, and severe problems of the nervous and circulatory systems. Exercise prevents type 2 diabetes, the most common form of the disease. Exercise burns excess sugar and makes cells more sensitive to insulin. Exercise also helps keep body fat at healthy levels, which is important because obesity is a key risk factor for type 2 diabetes. For people who have diabetes, physical activity is an important part of treatment.

Improved Psychological and Emotional Wellness

Physically active people enjoy many social, psychological, and emotional benefits, including the following:

- *Reduced anxiety and depression.* Exercise reduces symptoms of anxiety, such as worry and self-doubt and is associated with a lower risk for panic. Exercise also relieves feelings of sadness and hopelessness and can be as effective as psychotherapy in treating mild to moderate cases of depression.

- *Improved sleep.* Regular physical activity helps people fall asleep more easily; it also improves sleep quality.

- *Reduced stress.* Exercise reduces the body's overall response to all forms of stressors and helps people deal more effectively with stress.

QUICK STATS

75,578 Americans died from diabetes in 2014, making it the seventh leading cause of death that year.

—Centers for Disease Control and Prevention, 2016

- *Enhanced self-esteem, self-confidence, and self-efficacy.* Exercise can boost self-esteem and self-confidence by providing opportunities for people to succeed and excel. Exercise also improves body image. Sticking with an exercise program increases people's belief in their ability to be active, thereby boosting self-efficacy.

- *Enhanced creativity and intellectual functioning.* In studies of people of all ages, physically active people score higher than sedentary people on tests of creativity and mental function. Exercise improves alertness and memory in the short term. Over time, exercise helps maintain reaction time, short-term memory, and nonverbal reasoning skills and enhances brain metabolism.

- *Increased opportunities for social interaction.* Exercise provides many chances for people to have positive interactions with other people.

Improved Immune Function

Exercise can have either positive or negative effects on the immune system—the physiological processes that protect us from disease. Moderate endurance exercise boosts immune function, whereas excessive training depresses it. Physically fit people get fewer colds and upper respiratory tract infections than people who are not fit.

Prevention of Injuries and Low-Back Pain

Increased muscle strength and endurance provide protection against injury because they help people maintain spinal stability, good posture, and appropriate body mechanics when performing everyday activities such as walking, lifting, and carrying. Good muscle endurance in the abdomen, hips, lower back, and legs supports the back in proper alignment and helps prevent low-back pain, which afflicts more than 85% of Americans at some time in their lives.

Improved Wellness for Life

Although people differ in the maximum levels of fitness they can achieve through exercise, the wellness benefits of exercise are available to everyone. Exercising regularly may be the single most important thing you can do now to improve the quality of your life in the future.

WHAT IS PHYSICAL FITNESS?

Physical fitness is a set of physical attributes that allow the body to respond or adapt to the demands and stress of physical effort—to perform moderate to vigorous levels of physical activity without becoming overly tired.

Some components of fitness are related to specific activities or sports, whereas others relate to general health. **Health-related fitness** includes cardiorespiratory endurance, muscular strength, muscular endurance, flexibility, and body composition. Health-related fitness helps you withstand physical challenges and protects you from diseases.

Cardiorespiratory Endurance

Cardiorespiratory endurance is the ability to perform prolonged, large-muscle, dynamic exercise at moderate to high intensity. When cardiorespiratory fitness is low, the heart has to work hard during normal daily activities and may not be able to work hard enough to sustain high-intensity physical activity in an emergency. Poor cardiorespiratory fitness is linked with heart disease, diabetes, colon cancer, stroke, depression, anxiety, and premature death from all causes.

Regular **cardiorespiratory endurance training,** however, conditions the heart and metabolism. Endurance training makes the heart stronger and improves the function of the entire cardiorespiratory system. As cardiorespiratory fitness improves, related physical functions also improve. The heart pumps more blood per heartbeat, resting heart rate slows and resting blood pressure decreases, blood volume increases, blood supply to tissues improves, the body can cool itself better, and metabolic health improves, which helps the body process fuels and regulate cell function.

A healthy heart can better withstand the strains of daily life, the stress of occasional emergencies, and the wear and tear of time. You can develop cardiorespiratory endurance through activities that involve continuous, rhythmic movements of large muscle groups, such as the legs. Such activities include walking, jogging, cycling, and aerobic dancing.

Muscular Strength

Muscular strength is the amount of force a muscle can produce with a single maximum effort. It depends on factors such as the size of muscle cells and the ability of nerves to activate muscle cells. Strong muscles are important for

> **TERMS**
>
> **physical fitness** The body's ability to respond or adapt to the demands and stress of physical effort.
>
> **health-related fitness** Physical capabilities that contribute to health, including cardiorespiratory endurance, muscular strength, muscular endurance, flexibility, and body composition.
>
> **cardiorespiratory endurance** The ability of the body to perform prolonged, large-muscle, dynamic exercise at moderate to high levels of intensity.
>
> **cardiorespiratory endurance training** Exercise intended to improve cardiorespiratory endurance.
>
> **muscular strength** The amount of force a muscle can produce with a single maximum effort.

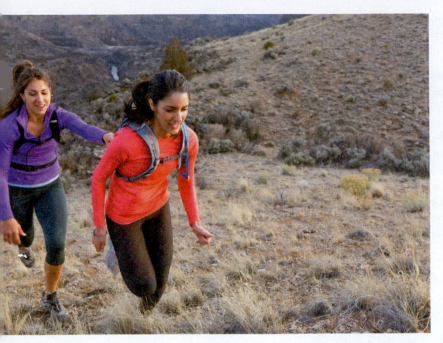

Cardiorespiratory endurance is a critical component of fitness.

© Blend Images/Michael DeYoung/Getty Images RF

accustomed to develops muscle endurance as well as muscular strength. The degree to which strength or endurance develops depends on the type and amount of stress that is applied.

Flexibility

Flexibility is the ability of joints to move through their full range of motion. It depends on joint structure, the length and elasticity of connective tissue, and nervous system activity. Flexible, pain-free joints are important for good health and well-being. Inactivity causes the joints to become stiffer with age. Stiffness, in turn, often causes older people to assume unnatural body postures that can stress joints and muscles. Stretching exercises can help ensure a healthy range of motion for all major joints.

Body Composition

Body composition refers to the proportion of fat and **fat-free mass** (muscle, bone, and water) in the body. Healthy body composition involves a high proportion of fat-free mass and an acceptably low level of body fat, adjusted for age and sex. The best way to lose fat is through a lifestyle that includes a sensible diet and exercise. The best way to add muscle mass is through resistance training such as weight training.

Skill-Related Components of Fitness

In addition to the five health-related components of physical fitness, the ability to perform a particular sport or activity may depend on **skill-related fitness** components such as speed, power, agility, balance, coordination, and reaction time.

Skill-related fitness is sport specific and is best developed through practice. Playing a sport can be fun, can help build fitness, and may contribute to other areas of wellness.

everyday activities, such as climbing stairs, as well as for emergencies. Strong muscles help keep the skeleton in proper alignment, preventing back and leg pain and providing the support necessary for good posture. Recreational activities also require muscular strength: Strong people can hit a tennis ball harder, kick a soccer ball farther, and ride a bicycle uphill more easily.

Muscle tissue is an important element of overall body composition. Greater muscle mass makes possible a higher rate of metabolism and faster energy use, which help people to maintain a healthy body weight.

Strength training helps maintain muscle mass, function, and balance in older people, which greatly enhances their quality of life and prevents injuries. Strength training promotes cardiovascular health, reduces the risk of osteoporosis (bone loss), and prevents premature death from all causes. Muscular strength can be developed by training with weights or by using the weight of the body for resistance during calisthenic exercises such as push-ups and curl-ups.

Muscular Endurance

Muscular endurance is the ability to resist fatigue and sustain a given level of muscle tension—that is, to hold a muscle contraction for a long time or to contract a muscle over and over again.

Muscular endurance is important for good posture and for injury prevention. Muscular endurance helps people cope with the physical demands of everyday life and enhances performance in sports and work. Stressing the muscles with a greater load (weight) than they are

> **TERMS**
>
> **muscular endurance**   The ability of a muscle or group of muscles to remain contracted or to contract repeatedly for a long period of time.
>
> **flexibility**   The joints' ability to move through their full range of motion.
>
> **body composition**   The proportion of fat and fat-free mass (muscle, bone, and water) in the body.
>
> **fat-free mass**   The nonfat components of the human body, consisting of skeletal muscle, bone, and water.
>
> **skill-related fitness**   Physical abilities that contribute to performance in a sport or activity, including speed, power, agility, balance, coordination, and reaction time.

COMPONENTS OF AN ACTIVE LIFESTYLE

Despite the many benefits of an active lifestyle, levels of physical activity remain low for all populations of Americans. **Physical activity** is any body movement carried out by the skeletal muscles that requires energy. Different types of physical activity can be arranged on a continuum based on the amount of energy they require. Quick, easy movements such as standing up or walking down a hallway require little energy or effort. More intense, sustained activities such as cycling five miles or running in a race require considerably more.

Exercise refers to a subset of physical activity—planned, structured, repetitive movement of the body intended specifically to improve or maintain physical fitness. To develop fitness, a person must perform enough physical activity to stress the body and cause long-term physiological changes.

Moderate-intensity physical activity is essential to health and confers wide-ranging health benefits, but more intense exercise is necessary to improve physical fitness. This important distinction between physical activity and exercise is a key concept in understanding the guidelines discussed in this chapter.

Increasing Physical Activity

In 2011, the American College of Sports Medicine (ACSM) released the newest version of its exercise guidelines for healthy adults. This update followed the 2010 U.S. Surgeon General's report on overweight and obesity in American children and adults, *The Surgeon General's Vision for a Healthy and Fit Nation,* and the landmark 2008 report from the U.S. Department of Health and Human Services, *Physical Activity Guidelines for Americans.* Although each of these reports has a somewhat different focus, they all stress the importance of regular physical activity for health, wellness, and the prevention of chronic diseases and premature death. The 2011 guidelines include the following key recommendations for adults:

- For substantial health benefits, adults should do at least 150 minutes (2.5 hours) a week of moderate-intensity aerobic physical activity, or 75 minutes (1 hour and 15 minutes) a week of vigorous-intensity aerobic physical activity, or an equivalent combination of moderate- and vigorous-intensity aerobic activity. Activity should preferably be spread throughout the week.

- For additional and more extensive health benefits, adults should increase their aerobic physical activity to 300 minutes (5 hours) a week of moderate-intensity activity, or 150 minutes (2.5 hours) a week of vigorous-intensity activity, or an equivalent combination of moderate- and vigorous-intensity activity.

- Adults should also do muscle-strengthening activities that are moderate or high intensity and involve all major muscle groups on two or more days a week.

- Everyone should avoid inactivity.

These levels of physical activity promote health and wellness by lowering the risk of high blood pressure, stroke, heart disease, type 2 diabetes, colon cancer, and osteoporosis and by reducing feelings of mild to moderate depression and anxiety. What's the difference between moderate- and vigorous-intensity physical activity? *2008 Physical Activity Guidelines for Americans* defines moderate-intensity physical activity as activity that causes a noticeable increase in heart rate, such as brisk walking. Vigorous-intensity physical activity is activity that causes rapid breathing and a substantial increase in heart rate, such as jogging. Brisk walking, dancing, swimming, cycling, and yardwork can all help you meet the physical activity recommendations. You can burn the same number of calories by doing a moderate-intensity activity for a longer time or higher-intensity activity for a shorter time.

The daily total of physical activity can be accumulated in multiple bouts of 10 or more minutes—for example, two 10-minute bike rides to and from class and a brisk 10-minute walk to the store. In this lifestyle approach to physical activity, people can choose activities that they find enjoyable and that fit into their daily routine. Everyday tasks at school, work, and home can be structured to contribute to the daily activity total (see the box "Making Time for Physical Activity").

Ask Yourself

QUESTIONS FOR CRITICAL THINKING AND REFLECTION
When you think about exercise, do you think of only one or two of the five components of health-related fitness, such as muscular strength or body composition? If so, where do you think your ideas come from? What role do the media play in shaping your ideas about fitness?

Reducing Sedentary Time

Researchers have found that too much sedentary time—sitting too much—is detrimental to health regardless of whether an individual meets the physical activity goals for health or exercise. A 2015 review found that sedentary

TERMS

physical activity   Any body movement carried out by the skeletal muscles that requires energy.

exercise   Planned, structured, repetitive movement of the body intended to improve or maintain physical fitness.

"Too little time" is a common excuse for not being physically active. Learning to manage your time successfully is crucial if you are to maintain a wellness lifestyle. Begin by keeping a record of how you currently spend your time. List each type of activity and the total time you engaged in it on a given day—for example, sleeping, 7 hours; eating, 1.5 hours; studying, 3 hours; and so on. Prioritize your activities according to how important they are to you, from essential to somewhat important to not important at all.

Make changes in your daily schedule by subtracting time from some activities in order to make time for physical activity. Look carefully at your leisure-time activities and your methods of transportation—these are areas where it is easy to build in physical activity. For example, you may choose to reduce the total amount of time you spend playing computer games to make time for an after-dinner bike ride or a walk with a friend. You may decide to watch 10 fewer minutes of television in the morning to change your 5-minute drive to class into a 15-minute walk.

Here are just a few ways to incorporate more physical activity into your daily routine:

- Take the stairs instead of the elevator or escalator.

- Walk to the mailbox, post office, store, bank, or library whenever possible.

- Do at least one chore every day that requires physical activity: Wash the windows or your car, clean your room or house, mow the lawn, or rake the leaves.

- Take study or work breaks to avoid sitting for more than 30 minutes at a time. Get up and walk around the library, your office, or your home or dorm; go up and down a flight of stairs.

- When you take public transportation, get off one stop early and walk to your destination.

- Take the dog for a walk every day.

- If weather or neighborhood safety rule out walking outside, look for alternative locations—an indoor track, an enclosed shopping mall, or even a long hallway.

- Seize every opportunity to get up and walk around. Move more and sit less.

---

time was associated with increased risk of disease and death independent of activity level. The risk of negative outcomes from sedentary time was lower among people with higher levels of physical activity, but they were not eliminated.

How does sedentary time affect health? Although not completely understood, sedentary time is associated with markers of poor metabolic functioning, including unhealthy levels of blood glucose, insulin, and blood fats, as well as a large waist circumference. A study that looked at the impact of increased sedentary time in moderately active individuals found that sitting for more than 30 or 60 minutes at a time resulted in significantly elevated glucose and insulin levels. Sedentary time also affects blood fats and markers for inflammation. All these factors can contribute to the development of type 2 diabetes, metabolic syndrome, heart disease, and cancer.

What does this mean for an individual? Studies have found that the average American adult spends more than half her or his waking day in sedentary activities, such as using a computer, studying, or watching television. Luckily, evidence so far suggests that frequent breaks from sedentary time—2 minutes every 20 or 30 minutes, for example—protect against some impacts of sedentary time. So, take frequent breaks when you are engaged in sedentary activities, whether at work or school or during leisure time. Try the strategies suggested in the box "Move More, Sit Less" and invent your own.

Ask Yourself

QUESTIONS FOR CRITICAL THINKING AND REFLECTION

Does your current lifestyle include enough physical activity—150 minutes of moderate-intensity activity a week—to support health and wellness? Do you go beyond this level to include enough vigorous activity and exercise to build physical fitness? What changes could you make in your lifestyle to start developing physical fitness?

DESIGNING YOUR EXERCISE PROGRAM

The best exercise program has two primary characteristics: It promotes your health, and it's fun for you to do. Exercise can provide some of the most pleasurable moments of your day, once you make it a habit. A little thought and planning will help you achieve these goals.

Figure 10.3 shows a physical activity pyramid. At the top, the small triangle represents what you should limit: sedentary activities. The wide section at the bottom of the pyramid shows activities that you should engage in more frequently throughout the day: walking, climbing stairs, doing yardwork, and sweeping the floor. From there, work up to

TAKE CHARGE
Move More, Sit Less

Regular exercise provides huge wellness benefits, but it does not cancel out all the negative effects of too much sitting during the day. Advances in technology promote sedentary behavior: We can now work or study at a desk, watch TV or play video games in our leisure time, order take-out and delivery for meals, and shop and bank online. To avoid the negative health effects of too little daily activity, try some of the following strategies:

• Stand up and/or walk when you are at work or making personal phone calls.

• Take the stairs whenever and wherever you can; walk up and down escalators instead of riding them.

• At work, walk to a coworker's desk rather than e-mailing or calling, take the long route to the restroom, and take a walk break whenever you take a coffee or snack break. Drink plenty of water so that you'll have to take frequent restroom breaks.

• Set reminders to get up and move: Use commercial breaks while watching TV to remind yourself to move or stretch. At work or while using a digital device, set the clock function on your computer or phone to remind you to get up at least every hour. Moving every 20 or 30 minutes is even better.

• Engage in active chores and leisure activities.

• Track your sedentary time to get a baseline, and then continue monitoring to note any improvements. You can also use a step counter to track your general activity level and movement patterns.

meeting the goal of 150 minutes of moderate-intensity exercise per week. Choose to be active whenever you can. If weight management is a concern for you, begin by achieving the goal of 150 minutes per week and then gradually increase your activity level to 300 minutes per week while reducing caloric intake, especially from added sugars and other empty calories (see Chapter 9).

For even greater benefits, move up to the next two levels of the pyramid, which illustrate parts of a formal exercise program. They take up less of your time than the activities on the lower two levels of the pyramid, but they will develop all the health-related components of physical fitness. New research shows that high-intensity interval training—repetitions of high-intensity exercise followed by rest—builds fitness rapidly in less time

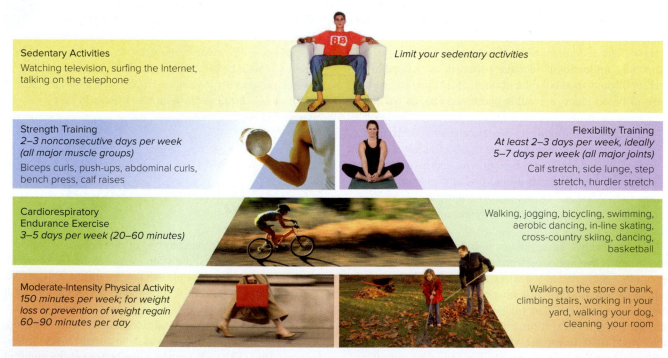

Sedentary Activities
Watching television, surfing the Internet, talking on the telephone

Limit your sedentary activities

Strength Training
2–3 nonconsecutive days per week (all major muscle groups)
Biceps curls, push-ups, abdominal curls, bench press, calf raises

Flexibility Training
At least 2–3 days per week, ideally 5–7 days per week (all major joints)
Calf stretch, side lunge, step stretch, hurdler stretch

Cardiorespiratory Endurance Exercise
3–5 days per week (20–60 minutes)
Walking, jogging, bicycling, swimming, aerobic dancing, in-line skating, cross-country skiing, dancing, basketball

Moderate-Intensity Physical Activity
150 minutes per week; for weight loss or prevention of weight regain 60–90 minutes per day
Walking to the store or bank, climbing stairs, working in your yard, walking your dog, cleaning your room

FIGURE 10.3 **Physical activity pyramid.** Make activities at the base of the pyramid part of your everyday life; limit the amount of time you spend in the sedentary activities listed at the top.

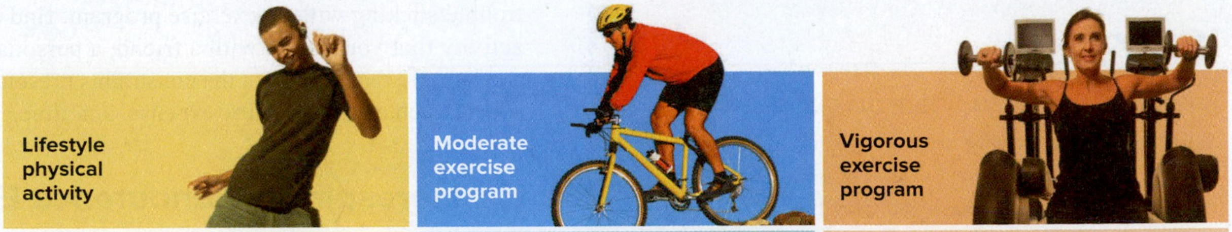

	Lifestyle physical activity	Moderate exercise program	Vigorous exercise program
Description	Moderate physical activity (150 minutes per week; muscle-strengthening exercises 2 or more days per week)	Cardiorespiratory endurance exercise (20–60 minutes, 3–5 days per week); strength training (2–3 nonconsecutive days per week); and stretching exercises (2 or more days per week)	Cardiorespiratory endurance exercise (20–60 minutes, 3–5 days per week); interval training; strength training (3–4 nonconsecutive days per week); and stretching exercises (5–7 days per week)
Sample activities or program	*One of the following:* • Walking to and from work, 15 minutes each way • Cycling to and from class, 10 minutes each way • Yard work for 30 minutes • Dancing (fast) for 30 minutes • Playing basketball for 20 minutes	• Jogging for 30 minutes, 3 days per week • Weight training, 1 set of 8 exercises, 2 days per week • Stretching exercises, 3 days per week	• Running for 45 minutes, 3 days per week • Intervals: running 400 m at high effort, 4 sets, 2 days per week • Weight training, 3 sets of 10 exercises, 3 days per week • Stretching exercises, 6 days per week
Health and fitness benefits	Better blood cholesterol levels, reduced body fat, better control of blood pressure, improved metabolic health, and enhanced glucose metabolism; improved quality of life; reduced risk of some chronic diseases. Greater amounts of activity can help prevent weight gain and promote weight loss.	All the benefits of lifestyle physical activity, plus improved physical fitness (increased cardiorespiratory endurance, muscular strength and endurance, and flexibility) and even greater improvements in health and quality of life and reductions in chronic disease risk.	All the benefits of lifestyle physical activity and a moderate exercise program, with greater increases in fitness and somewhat greater reductions in chronic disease risk. Participating in a vigorous exercise program may increase risk of injury and overtraining.

FIGURE 10.4 **Health and fitness benefits of different amounts of physical activity and exercise.**

© RubberBall Productions; © Royalty-Free/CORBIS; © Thinkstock Images/Jupiter Images RF

than traditional aerobic training. The remaining sections of this chapter will show you how to develop a personalized exercise program. For a summary of the health and fitness benefits of different levels of physical activity, see Figure 10.4.

First Steps

Are you thinking about starting a formal exercise program? A little planning can help make it a success.

Medical Clearance Previously inactive men over 40 and women over 50 should get a medical examination before beginning an exercise program. Diabetes, asthma, heart disease, and extreme obesity are conditions that may call for a modified program. If you have an increased risk of heart disease because of smoking, high blood pressure, or obesity, get a physical checkup, including an **electrocardiogram (ECG *or* EKG),** before beginning an exercise program.

Basic Principles of Physical Training To put together an effective exercise program, you should first understand the basic principles of physical training.

SPECIFICITY To develop a fitness component, you must perform exercises that are specifically designed for that component. This is the principle of **specificity.** Weight training, for example, develops muscular strength but is less effective for developing flexibility or cardiorespiratory endurance. Specificity also applies to the skill-related fitness components and to the different parts of the body. A well-rounded exercise program includes exercises geared to each component of fitness, to different parts of the body, and to specific activities or sports.

PROGRESSIVE OVERLOAD Your body adapts to the demands of exercise by improving its functioning. When the amount of exercise, or overload, is increased progressively,

electrocardiogram (ECG or EKG) A recording of the changes in electrical activity of the heart. **TERMS**

specificity The training principle that the body adapts to the particular type and amount of stress placed on it.

Ask Yourself

QUESTIONS FOR CRITICAL THINKING AND REFLECTION
Which benefits of exercise are most important to you, and why? For example, is there a history of heart disease or diabetes in your family? Have you thought about how regular exercise could reduce your risks for specific diseases?

?

fitness continues to improve. This training principle is called **progressive overload.** Too little exercise has no effect on fitness; too much may cause injury. The appropriate amount depends on your current level of fitness, your genetic capacity to adapt to exercise, your fitness goals, and the fitness components being developed.

The amount of overload needed to maintain or improve a particular level of fitness is determined in four dimensions, represented by the acronym FITT: Frequency, Intensity, Time, and Type.

REST AND RECUPERATION Fitness gains occur following exercise as the body adapts to the stress of training. Adequate rest is as important to this process as training. Overtraining—an imbalance between training and recovery—leads to injury, illness, and excessive fatigue.

REVERSIBILITY The body adjusts to lower levels of physical activity the same way it adjusts to higher levels—this is the principle of **reversibility.** When you stop exercising, you can lose up to 50% of fitness improvements within two months. Try to exercise consistently, and don't quit if you miss a few workouts.

INDIVIDUAL DIFFERENCES There are genetic limits to how much a person can improve fitness, as well as large individual differences between people in their ability to improve fitness, achieve a desirable body composition, and perform and learn sports skills. In studies, some people on a diet and exercise program improve fitness by 50%, whereas others on the same program improve by only 2–3%. It is more difficult for those whose bodies don't respond as well to exercise to make changes in fitness or body fat levels. Elite athletes start out with a genetic advantage over the average person. However, everyone has the capacity to improve fitness and reap the health benefits of exercise.

Selecting Activities If you have been inactive, begin by gradually increasing the amount of moderate physical activity in your life (the bottom of the activity pyramid shown in Figure 10.3). Once your body adjusts to your new level of activity, you can choose additional activities for your exercise program.

Be sure the activities you choose contribute to your overall wellness and make sense for you. Are you competitive? If so, try racquetball, basketball, or squash. Do you prefer to exercise alone? Then consider cross-country skiing or road running. Have you been sedentary? A walking program may be a good place to start. If you think you may have trouble sticking with an exercise program, find a structured activity that you can do with a friend, a personal trainer, or a group. Be realistic about the constraints presented by some sports, such as accessibility, expense, and time.

Cardiorespiratory Endurance Exercise

Exercises that condition your heart and lungs and improve your metabolism should have a central role in your fitness program.

Frequency The optimal workout schedule for endurance training is 3–5 days per week. Beginners should start with 3 days and work up to 5 days. Training more than 5 days a week often leads to injury for recreational athletes. Although you get health benefits from exercising vigorously only 1 or 2 days per week, you risk injury because your body never gets a chance to adapt fully to regular exercise training.

Intensity The most misunderstood aspect of conditioning, even among experienced athletes, is training intensity. Intensity is the crucial factor in attaining a significant training effect—that is, in increasing the body's cardiorespiratory capacity. A primary purpose of endurance training is to increase **maximal oxygen consumption** ($\dot{V}O_{2max}$). $\dot{V}O_{2max}$ represents the cells' maximum ability to use oxygen and is considered the best measure of cardiorespiratory capacity. Intensity of training is the crucial factor in improving $\dot{V}O_{2max}$.

One of the easiest ways to determine exactly how intensely you should work involves measuring your heart rate. It is not necessary or desirable to exercise at your maximum heart rate—the fastest heart rate possible before exhaustion sets in—to improve your cardiorespiratory capacity. Beneficial effects occur at lower heart rates with a much lower risk of injury. Your **target heart rate zone** is the range of rates within which you should exercise to obtain cardiorespiratory benefits. To determine the intensity at which you should exercise, see the box "Determine Your Target Heart Rate".

If you have been sedentary, start by exercising at the lower end of your target heart rate range (65% of maximum heart rate) for at least 4–6 weeks. For people with a very low initial level of fitness, a lower training intensity may be sufficient to achieve improvements in maximal oxygen consumption, especially at the start of an

---

TERMS

progressive overload The training principle that placing increasing amounts of stress (in the form of exercise) on the body causes adaptations that improve fitness.

reversibility The training principle that fitness improvements are lost when demands on the body are lowered.

maximal oxygen consumption ($\dot{V}O_{2max}$) The body's maximum ability to transport and use oxygen.

target heart rate zone The range of heart rates that should be reached and maintained during cardiorespiratory endurance exercise to obtain benefits.

Determine Your Target Heart Rate

One of the best ways to monitor the intensity of cardiorespiratory endurance exercise is to measure your heart rate. It isn't necessary to exercise at your maximum heart rate to improve maximal oxygen consumption. Fitness adaptations occur at lower heart rates with a much lower risk of injury.

According to the American College of Sports Medicine, your target heart rate zone—rates at which you should exercise to experience cardiorespiratory benefits—is between 65% and 90% of your maximum heart rate. To calculate your target heart rate zone, follow these steps:

1. Estimate your maximum heart rate (MHR) by subtracting your age from 220, or have it measured precisely by undergoing an exercise stress test in a doctor's office, hospital, or sports medicine lab. (*Note:* The formula to estimate MHR carries an error of about ±10–15 beats per minute [bpm] and can be very inaccurate for some people, particularly older adults and young children.)

2. Multiply your MHR by 65% and 90% to calculate your target heart rate zone. Very unfit people should use 55% of MHR for their training threshold.

For example, a 19-year-old would calculate her target heart rate zone as follows:

MHR = 220 − 19 = 201

65% training intensity = 0.65 × 201 = 131 bpm

90% training intensity = 0.90 × 201 = 181 bpm

To gain fitness benefits, the young woman in our example would have to exercise at an intensity that raises her heart rate to between 131 and 181 bpm.

An alternative method for calculating target heart rate range uses heart rate reserve, the difference between maximum heart rate and resting heart rate. With this method, target heart rate is equal to resting heart rate plus between 50% (40% for very unfit people) and 85% of heart rate reserve. Although some people (particularly those with very low levels of fitness) will obtain more accurate results using this more complex method, both methods provide reasonable estimates of an appropriate target heart rate zone.

exercise program. Heart rate monitors are useful if close tracking of heart rate is important in your program. Heart rate can be integrated into workout information provided by smartphone apps such as Cyclemeter, Strava, Spotify, and Garmin Connect.

Another way scientists describe fitness is in terms of the capacity to increase metabolism (energy usage level) above rest. Scientists use METs to measure the *metabolic cost* of an exercise. One **MET** represents the body's resting metabolic rate—that is, the energy or calorie requirement of the body at rest. Exercise intensity is expressed in multiples of resting metabolic rate. Activities that increase metabolism by 6–8 METs are classified as moderate-intensity exercises and are suitable for most people beginning an exercise program.

Time (Duration)   A total time of 20–60 minutes per workout is recommended for cardiorespiratory endurance training. Exercise can be done in a single session or several sessions lasting 10 or more minutes. The total duration of exercise depends on its intensity. To improve cardiorespiratory endurance during a moderate-intensity activity such as

walking or slow swimming, you should exercise for 45–60 minutes. For high-intensity exercise performed at the top of your target heart rate zone, a duration of 20 minutes is sufficient. Start with less vigorous activities and gradually increase intensity.

Type   The best exercises for developing cardiorespiratory endurance stress a large portion of the body's muscle mass for a prolonged period of time. These include walking, jogging, running, swimming, bicycling, and aerobic dance. Many popular sports and recreational activities, such as racquetball, tennis, basketball, and soccer, are also good if the skill level and intensity of the game are sufficient to provide a vigorous workout.

The Warm-Up and Cool-Down   It is always important to warm up before you exercise and to cool down afterward. Warming up enhances your performance and decreases your chances of injury.

A warm-up session should include low-intensity movements similar to those in the activity that will follow. For example, hit forehands and backhands before a tennis game or jog slowly for 400 meters before progressing to an 8-minute mile. Some people like to include stretching exercises in their warm-up, but experts recommend stretching *after* the active part of your warm-up, when your body temperature is elevated. Studies have found that stretching prior to exercise can temporarily decrease muscle strength and power.

> **MET**   A measure of the metabolic cost of an exercise. One MET represents the body's resting metabolic rate—the energy or calorie requirement of the body at rest; exercise intensity is expressed in multiples of resting metabolic rate.   **TERMS**

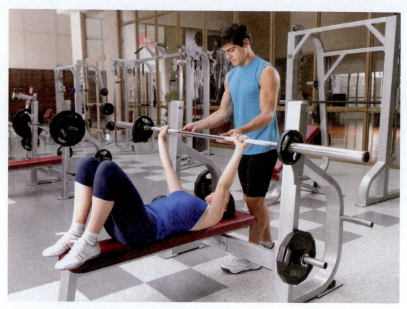

Weight training exercises are isotonic (dynamic) exercises that involve applying force with movement.

© Glow Wellness/Alamy

Isometric (static) exercises involve applying force without movement, such as when you contract your abdominal muscles. This type of exercise is valuable for toning and strengthening muscles. Isometrics can be practiced anywhere and do not require any equipment. For maximum strength gains, hold an isometric contraction maximally for 6 seconds, and do 3–10 repetitions. Don't hold your breath: Doing so can restrict blood flow to your heart and brain. Within a few weeks, you will notice the effect of this exercise. Isometrics are particularly useful when recovering from an injury.

Isotonic (dynamic) exercises involve applying force with movement, as in weight training exercises such as the bench press. These types of exercises are the most popular for increasing muscle strength and seem to be most valuable for developing strength that can be transferred to other forms of physical activity. They include exercises using barbells, dumbbells, kettlebells, weight machines, and body weight (as in push-ups or pull-ups).

Cooling down after exercise is important to restore the body's circulation to its normal resting condition. When you are at rest, a relatively small percentage of your total blood volume is directed to muscles, but during exercise, as much as 90% of the heart's output is directed to them. During recovery from exercise, continuing to exercise at a low level is important to provide a smooth transition to the resting state. Cooling down helps regulate the return of blood to your heart. After exercising, avoid taking a hot shower until you have cooled down.

> **QUICK STATS**
>
> **5–10 minutes**
> of warming up and cooling down are adequate for a 30-minute workout of brisk walking.
>
> —Centers for Disease Control and Prevention, 2016

Core Training The core muscles include those in the abdomen, pelvic floor, sides of the trunk, back, buttocks, hips, and pelvis. They stabilize the midsection when you sit, stand, reach, walk, jump, twist, squat, throw, or bend. During any dynamic movement, the core muscles and active muscles work together. Some shorten to cause movement, whereas others contract and hold to provide stability, lengthen to brake the movement, or send signals to the brain about the movements and positions of the muscles, joints, and bones. When specific core muscles are weak or tired, the nervous system steps in and uses other muscles. This substitution causes abnormal stress on the joints, decreases power, and increases the risk of injury.

Spinal stability and stiffness are more important for health and performance than core movement strength. Isometric core exercises like side bridges build core stiffness, which strengthens core muscles and improves their endurance, reduces low back pain, and boosts sports performance. Greater core stiffness transfers strength and

Exercises for Muscular Strength and Endurance

Any program designed to promote health should include exercises that develop muscular strength and endurance.

Types of Strength Training Exercises Muscular strength and endurance can be developed in many ways, from weight training to calisthenics. Common exercises such as curl-ups, push-ups, pull-ups, and nonweighted squats maintain the muscular strength of most people if they practice them several times a week. To condition and tone your whole body, choose exercises that work the major muscles of the shoulders, chest, back, arms, abdomen, and legs.

To increase muscular strength and endurance, you must do **resistance exercise**—exercises in which your muscles must exert force against a significant amount of resistance. Resistance can be provided by weights, exercise machines, your own body weight, or even objects such as rocks.

> **TERMS**
>
> **resistance exercise**   Exercise that forces muscles to contract against increased resistance; also called *strength training.*
>
> **isometric (static) exercise**   The application of force without movement.
>
> **isotonic (dynamic) exercise**   The application of force with movement.

speed to the limbs, increases the load-bearing capacity of the spine, and protects the internal organs during sports movements.

The best exercises for low-back health are whole-body exercises that force the core muscles to stabilize the spine in many different directions. Exercises that focus on the core muscles include the lunge, side bridges, stir-the-pot, and bird dogs. These exercises are generally safe for beginning exercisers and, with physician approval, people with back pain.

Sex Differences in Muscular Strength

Within a given genetic population, men are generally stronger than women because their bodies are typically larger overall and a larger proportion of their total body mass is made up of muscle. But when strength is expressed per unit of muscle tissue, men are only 1–2% stronger than women in the upper body and about equal to women in the lower body.

Three factors that help explain the strength disparities between men and women are testosterone levels, skeletal size, and nerve-conduction velocity. Testosterone promotes the growth of muscle tissue in both males and females, but testosterone levels are about 6–10 times higher in men than in women, so men develop larger muscles. Also, men are usually bigger than women, which gives them more leverage. Nerve-conduction velocity in the brain is about 4% faster in men than women, which provides a slight advantage in muscle activation speed.

Most women will not develop large muscles from strength training. Resistance exercise helps women reduce their overall body fat levels and reduce fat in the midsection. It also helps them preserve muscle mass as they age. Because men start out with more muscle when they are young and don't lose power as quickly as women, older women often have greater impairment of muscle function than older men.

Choosing Equipment

Many people prefer weight machines to free weights because they are safe, convenient, and easy to use. You set the resistance, sit down at the machine, and start working. Free weights require more care, balance, and coordination to use, but they strengthen your body in ways that are more adaptable to real life.

Choosing Exercises

A complete weight training program works all the major muscle groups: neck, upper back, shoulders, arms, chest, core, thighs, buttocks, and calves. Different exercises work different muscles, so it usually takes about 8–10 exercises to get a complete workout for general fitness. For example, you can do bench presses to develop the chest, shoulders, and upper arms; pull-ups to work the biceps and upper back; squats to develop the legs and buttocks; toe raises to work the calves; and so on.

Frequency

For general fitness, the American College of Sports Medicine (ACSM) recommends a strength workout frequency of at least 2 nonconsecutive days per week. This schedule allows your muscles one or more days of rest between workouts to avoid soreness and injury. If you enjoy weight training and would like to train more often, try working different muscle groups on alternate days.

Intensity and Time

The amount of weight (resistance) you lift in weight training exercises is equivalent to intensity in cardiorespiratory endurance training, and the number of repetitions of each exercise is equivalent to time. To improve fitness, you must do enough repetitions of each exercise to temporarily fatigue your muscles. The number of repetitions needed to cause fatigue depends on the amount of resistance: The heavier the weight, the fewer repetitions to reach fatigue. In general, a heavy weight and a low number of repetitions (1–5) build strength, whereas a light weight and a high number of repetitions (10–25) build endurance. For a general fitness program to build both strength and endurance, try to do 8–12 repetitions of each exercise. For people who are over 50 years of age, 10–15 repetitions of each exercise using a lighter weight is recommended.

To start, choose a weight that you can move easily through 8–12 repetitions. Add weight when you can do more than 12 repetitions of an exercise. If adding weight means you can do only 7 or 8 repetitions before your muscles fatigue, stay with that weight until you can again complete 12 repetitions. If you can do only 4–6 repetitions after adding weight, or if you can't maintain good form, you've added too much and should take some off. As a general guideline, try increases of approximately a half-pound of additional weight for each 10 pounds you are currently lifting.

For developing strength and endurance for general fitness, a single set (a group of repetitions) of each exercise is sufficient, provided you use enough weight to fatigue your muscles. Doing more than one set of each exercise may increase strength development further, and most serious weight trainers do at least three sets of each exercise. If you do more than one set of an exercise, rest long enough between sets (1–5 minutes) to allow your muscles to recover. You should warm up before every weight training session and cool down afterward.

A Caution about Supplements

No nutritional supplement or drug will change a weak person into a strong person. Those changes require regular training that stresses the body and causes physiological adaptations. Supplements or drugs that promise quick, large gains in strength usually don't work and are often dangerous, expensive, or illegal. Over-the-counter supplements are not regulated carefully, and their long-term effects have not been studied systematically.

Flexibility Exercises

Flexibility, or stretching, exercises are important for maintaining the normal range of motion in the major joints of the body. Some exercises, such as running, can decrease flexibility because they require only a partial range of motion. Like a good weight training program, a good stretching program includes exercises for all the major muscle groups and joints of the body: neck, shoulders, back, hips, thighs, hamstrings, and calves. In tandem with core training, flexibility training is important for preventing low-back injuries and maintaining low-back health.

Proper Stretching Technique Timing determines the best stretching technique: In general, do static stretching after a workout and dynamic or active stretching before a workout. *Static stretching* involves extending to a certain position and then holding it. *Dynamic stretching* is done by actively moving through the joints' ranges of motion. *Ballistic stretching* (known as "bouncing") is dangerous and counterproductive. The safest and most convenient technique for increasing flexibility may be active static stretching with a passive assist. For example, you might do a seated stretch of your calf muscles by contracting the muscles on the top of your shin and by grabbing your feet and pulling them toward you.

Frequency Do stretching exercises at least 2 or 3 days per week (but 5–7 days is optimal). If you stretch during your cool-down after cardiorespiratory endurance exercise or strength training, you may develop more flexibility because your muscles are warmer then and can be stretched farther.

Intensity and Time Do stretching exercises statically. Stretch to the point of mild discomfort, hold the position for 10–30 seconds, rest for 30–60 seconds, and then repeat, trying to stretch a bit farther. Stretch each muscle group for a total of 60 seconds. Older adults might benefit more from holding a stretch for 30–60 seconds.

Increase your intensity gradually over time. Improved flexibility takes many months to develop. There are large individual differences in joint flexibility. Don't feel you have to compete with others during stretching workouts.

Training in Specific Skills

The final component in your fitness program is learning the skills required for the sports or activities in which you choose to participate. By taking the time and effort to acquire competence, you can achieve a sense of mastery and add a new physical activity to your repertoire.

The first step in learning a new skill is getting help. Sports like tennis, golf, and skiing require mastery of basic movements and techniques, so instruction from a qualified teacher or coach can save you hours of frustration and increase your enjoyment. Skill is also important in conditioning activities such as jogging, swimming, and cycling. Even if you learned a sport as a child, additional instruction now can help you refine your technique, get over stumbling blocks, and relearn skills that you may have learned incorrectly.

Putting It All Together

Now that you know the basic components of a fitness program, you can put them all together in a program that works for you. See Figure 10.5 for a summary of the FITT principle for the health-related components of fitness.

GETTING STARTED AND STAYING ON TRACK

Once you have a program that fulfills your basic fitness needs and suits your personal tastes, adhering to a few basic principles will help you improve quickly, have fun, and minimize the risk of injury.

Selecting Instructors, Equipment, and Facilities

Once you've chosen the activities for your program, you may need to look for the appropriate information, instruction, and equipment or find an appropriate facility.

One of the best places to get help is an exercise class, where an expert instructor can teach you the basics of training and answer your questions. A qualified personal trainer can also get you started on an exercise program or a new form of training. Make sure that your instructor or trainer has proper qualifications, such as a college degree in exercise physiology, kinesiology, or physical education and certification by the American College of Sports Medicine, National

	Cardiorespiratory Endurance Training	Strength Training	Flexibility Training
Frequency	3–5 days per week	2–3 nonconsecutive days per week	2–3 days per week (minimum); 5–7 days per week (ideal)
Intensity	55/65–90% of maximum heart rate	Sufficient resistance to fatigue muscles	Stretch to the point of tension
Time	20–60 minutes in sessions lasting 10 minutes or more	8–12 repetitions of each exercise, 1 or more sets	2–4 repetitions held for 10–30 seconds, for a total of 60 seconds per exercise
Type	Continuous rhythmic activities using large muscle groups	Resistance exercises for all major muscle groups	Stretching exercises for all major joints

FIGURE 10.5 **A summary of the FITT principle for the health-related components of fitness.**

Strength and Conditioning Association, International Sports Science Association, or another professional organization.

Many websites provide fitness programs, including ongoing support and feedback via e-mail. Many of these sites charge fees, so it is important to review the sites, decide which ones seem most appropriate, and if possible go through a free trial period before subscribing. Also remember to consider the reliability of the information at fitness websites, especially those that also advertise or sell products.

Good equipment will enhance your enjoyment and decrease your risk of injury. Appropriate safety equipment, such as pads and helmets for skateboarding, is particularly important. If you shop around, you can often find bargains through mail-order companies and discount or used equipment stores.

Before you invest in a new piece of equipment, investigate it. Try it out at a local gym to make sure that you'll use it regularly. Footwear is an important piece of equipment for almost any activity; see the box "What to Wear" for shopping strategies.

If you are thinking of joining a health club or fitness center, be sure to choose one that has the right programs and equipment available at the times you will use them. Also make sure the facility is certified. Look for the displayed names American College of Sports Medicine, National Strength and Conditioning Association, American Council on Exercise, or Aerobics and Fitness Association of America. These trade associations have established standards to help protect consumer health, safety, and rights.

Ask Yourself

QUESTIONS FOR CRITICAL THINKING AND REFLECTION

Think of a few physical activities and sports that you would like to do, but haven't. Given your current fitness and skill level, which ones could you reasonably incorporate into your exercise program?

Eating and Drinking for Exercise

Most people do not need to change their eating habits when they begin a fitness program. In most cases a well-balanced diet contains all the energy and nutrients needed to sustain an exercise program (see Chapter 9).

A balanced diet is also the key to improving body composition when you begin to exercise more. One of the promises of a fitness program is a decrease in body fat and an increase in muscle mass. As a general rule, if you consume more calories than you expend through metabolism and exercise, fat increases. However, the control of body fat is determined by the amount and kind of calories you consume. Reduce your intake of added sugars and trans fats, and be physically active.

One of the most important principles to follow when exercising is to keep your body well hydrated by drinking enough fluids. Your body depends on water to sustain many chemical reactions and to maintain correct body temperature. Sweating during exercise depletes the body's water supply and can lead to dehydration if fluids are not replaced. Serious dehydration can cause reduced blood volume, accelerated heart rate, elevated body temperature, muscle cramps, heat stroke, and other serious problems.

Drinking fluids before and during exercise is important to prevent dehydration and enhance performance. Thirst receptors in the brain make you want to drink fluids, but during heavy or prolonged exercise or exercise in hot weather, thirst alone isn't a good indication of how much fluid you need to drink. As a rule of thumb, drink at least 16 ounces of fluid two to four hours before exercise and then drink enough during exercise to prevent significant fluid loss in sweat. Don't drink more than one quart per hour during exercise. After exercise, let thirst be your guide to your fluid needs. You can also check your weight before and after an exercise session; any weight loss is due to fluid loss that needs to be replaced.

Carry fluids when you exercise so that you can replace your fluids when they're depleted. For exercise sessions lasting less than 60–90 minutes, cool water is an excellent fluid replacement. For longer workouts, ACSM recommends a sports drink that contains water and small amounts of electrolytes (sodium, potassium, and magnesium) and simple carbohydrates (sugar, usually in the form of sucrose or glucose). After your workout, replace any lost fluids. Nonfat or low-fat milk, for those who can tolerate dairy products, are excellent post-exercise fluid replacement beverages because they promote long-term hydration. Milk is digested more slowly than water or sports beverages and also contains electrolytes.

Managing Your Fitness Program

How can you tell when you're in shape? When do you stop improving and start maintaining? How can you stay motivated? For your program to become an integral part of your life, these questions are key.

Starting Slowly, Getting in Shape Gradually As Table 10.1 shows, an exercise program can be divided into three phases:

- *Initial phase.* The body adjusts to the new type and level of activity.
- *Improvement phase.* Fitness increases.
- *Maintenance phase.* The targeted level of fitness is sustained over the long term.

Clothing

Modern exercise clothing is attractive, comfortable, and functional. Shorts made of elastic material, such as spandex, hug the body, supplying support. If you prefer, you can wear running shorts and a T-shirt. The main requirement for workout clothes is that they let you move easily but are not so loose that they get caught in the exercise machines or on fences when running outside. Don't wear street clothes when exercising because they can interfere with movement, and sweat, oil, and dirt can ruin them. If you run or cycle on the street, wear bright-colored clothing so that motorists can see you, and cyclists should wear a helmet to prevent head injury in case of an accident.

Specifics for Women and Men

- **For women.** Wear a good sports bra whenever you exercise. Breast support is important when running, playing volleyball, or weight training, The breasts can be injured if barbells press too firmly against them when you are weight-training or if they aren't properly supported when you run. A good sports bra should support the breasts in all directions, contain minimal elastic material, absorb moisture freely, and be easily laundered. Seams, hooks, and catches should not irritate the skin. You might consider buying a bra with an underwire for added support and a pocket in which to insert padding if you do exercises that could cause injury.

- **For men.** Wear a protective cup and jockstrap when participating in contact sports, such as football, baseball, cricket, hockey, wrestling, and karate. These protections can help guard against male infertility.

Footwear

Footwear is perhaps the most important item of equipment for almost any activity. Shoes protect and support your feet and improve traction. When you jump or run, you place as much as six times more force on your feet than when you stand still. Shoes can help cushion against the stress that this additional force places on your lower legs, thereby preventing injuries. Some athletic shoes are also designed to help prevent ankle rollover, another common source of injury.

When choosing athletic shoes, first consider the activity you've chosen for your exercise program. Shoes appropriate for different activities have different characteristics. Foot type is another important consideration. If your feet tend to roll inward excessively, you may need additional stability features on the inner side of the shoe to counteract this movement. If your feet tend to roll outward excessively, you may need highly flexible and cushioned shoes that promote foot motion. Most women will get a better fit if they choose shoes that are specially designed for women's feet rather than downsized versions of men's shoes.

Barefoot Shoes or Minimalist Footwear

Two-thirds of runners experience an injury every year. Humans have evolved to run, so some scientists blame running shoes for the high injury rate. Most runners strike heel first when using

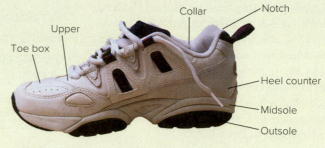

© Photodisc

heavily padded running shoes. Barefoot runners strike the ground with their forefoot (at least they're supposed to), which better uses the shock absorbing capacity of the skeleton. Some researchers speculated that using "minimalist" footwear allows people to run more naturally, which should cut down on the injury rate. Other research suggests that traditional running shoes provide a physiological advantage that makes running easier. We need more research to determine whether barefoot running is safe and viable or just the latest running fad.

Successful Shopping

For successful shoe shopping, keep the following strategies in mind:

- Shop late in the day or, ideally, following a workout. Your foot size increases during the day and after exercise.

- Wear socks like those you plan to wear during exercise.

- Try on both shoes and wear them around for 10 minutes or more. Try walking on an uncarpeted surface. Approximate the movements of your activity: walk, jog, run, jump, and so on.

- Check the fit and style carefully:

  - Is the toe box roomy enough? Your toes will spread out when your foot hits the ground or you push off. There should be at least one thumb's width of space from the longest toe to the end of the toe box.

  - Do the shoes have enough cushioning? Do your feet feel supported when you bounce up and down? Try bouncing on your toes and on your heels.

  - Do your heels fit snugly in the shoe? Do they stay put when you walk, or do they slide up?

  - Are the arches of your feet on top of the shoes' arch supports?

  - Do the shoes feel stable when you twist and turn on the balls of your feet? Try twisting from side to side while standing on one foot.

  - Do you feel any pressure points?

- If you exercise at dawn or dusk, choose shoes with reflective sections for added visibility and safety.

- Replace athletic shoes about every three months or 300–500 miles of jogging or walking.

Table 10.1 — Sample Progression for an Endurance Program

STAGE/WEEK	FREQUENCY (days/week)	INTENSITY* (beats/minute)	TIME (duration in minutes)
Initial stage			
1	3	120–130	15–20
2	3	120–130	20–25
3	4	130–145	20–25
4	4	130–145	25–30
Improvement stage			
5–7	3–4	145–160	25–30
8–10	3–4	145–160	30–35
11–13	3–4	150–165	30–35
14–16	4–5	150–165	30–35
17–20	4–5	160–180	35–40
21–24	4–5	160–180	35–40
Maintenance stage			
25+	3–5	160–180	20–60

*The target heart rates shown here are based on calculations for a healthy 20-year-old. The program progresses from an initial target heart rate of 50% to a maintenance range of 70–90% of maximum heart rate.

SOURCE: Adapted from American College of Sports Medicine. 2013. *ACSM's Guidelines for Exercise Testing and Prescription*, 9th ed. Philadelphia: Wolters Kluwer/Lippincott Williams & Wilkins Health.

When beginning a program, start slowly to give your body time to adapt to the stress of exercise. Choose activities carefully according to your fitness status.

Exercising Consistently Steady fitness improvement comes when you overload your body consistently over time. The best way to ensure consistency is to record the details of your workouts in a journal: how far you ran, how much weight you lifted, and so on. This record will help you evaluate your progress and plan workout sessions intelligently. Don't increase your exercise volume by more than 5–10% per week. Table 10.1 shows how to increase the amount of overload.

Assessing Your Fitness When are you in shape? It depends. One person may be out of shape running a mile in 5 minutes, but another may be in shape running a mile in 12 minutes. As mentioned earlier, your ultimate level of fitness depends on your goals, your program, and your natural ability. The important thing is to set goals that make sense for you.

Preventing and Managing Athletic Injuries If you learn how to deal with injuries, they won't derail your fitness program (Table 10.2). Some injuries require medical attention. See a physician right away if you suffer a head or eye injury, a possible ligament injury, a broken bone,

Table 10.2 — Care of Common Exercise Injuries and Discomforts

INJURY	SYMPTOMS	TREATMENT
Blister	Accumulation of fluid in one spot under the skin	Don't pop or drain it unless it interferes too much with your daily activities. If it does pop, clean the area with antiseptic and cover with a bandage. Do not remove the skin covering the blister.
Bruise (contusion)	Pain, swelling, and discoloration	R-I-C-E: rest, ice, compression, elevation.
Fracture and/or dislocation	Pain, swelling, tenderness, loss of function, and deformity	Seek medical attention, immobilize the affected area, and apply cold.
Joint sprain	Pain, tenderness, swelling, discoloration, and loss of function	R-I-C-E. Apply heat about 2 days after injury. Stretch and strengthen affected area.
Muscle cramp	Painful, spasmodic muscle contractions	Gently stretch for 15–30 seconds at a time and/or massage the cramped area. Drink fluids and increase dietary salt intake if exercising in hot weather.
Muscle soreness or stiffness	Pain and tenderness in the affected muscle	Stretch the affected muscle gently; exercise at a low intensity; apply heat.
Muscle strain	Pain, tenderness, swelling, and loss of strength in the affected muscle	R-I-C-E. Apply heat about 2 days after injury. Stretch and strengthen the affected area.
Plantar fasciitis	Pain and tenderness in the connective tissue on the bottom of the foot	Apply ice and stretch. Wear night splints when sleeping.
Shin splint	Pain and tenderness on the front of the lower leg; sometimes also pain in the calf muscle	Rest. Apply ice or heat to the affected area several times a day and before exercise; wrap with tape for support. Stretch and strengthen muscles in the lower legs. Purchase good-quality footwear and run on soft surfaces.
Side stitch	Pain on the side of the abdomen	Stretch the arm on the affected side as high as possible; if that doesn't help, try bending forward while tightening the abdominal muscles.
Tendinitis	Pain, swelling, and tenderness of the affected area	R-I-C-E. Apply heat about 2 days after injury. Stretch and strengthen the affected area.

SOURCE: Fahey, T. D., et al. 2017. *Fit and Well: Core Concepts and Labs in Physical Fitness and Wellness*, 12th ed. New York: McGraw-Hill. Copyright © 2017 The McGraw-Hill Companies, Inc.

or an internal disorder such as chest pain, fainting, or intolerance to heat. Also seek medical attention for apparently minor injuries that do not get better within a reasonable amount of time.

For minor cuts and scrapes, stop the bleeding and clean the wound with soap and water. Treat soft tissue injuries (muscles and joints) with the R-I-C-E principle: rest, ice, compress, and elevate the injured area.

After 36–48 hours, if the swelling has disappeared, apply heat to relieve pain, relax muscles, and reduce stiffness. Immerse the affected area in warm water or apply warm compresses, a hot water bottle, or a heating pad.

To prevent injuries, follow six basic guidelines:

1. Stay in condition: Haphazard exercise programs invite injury.

2. Warm up thoroughly before exercising.

3. Use proper body mechanics when lifting objects or executing sports skills.

4. Don't exercise when you're ill or overtrained (experiencing extreme fatigue due to overexercising).

5. Use the proper equipment.

6. Don't return to your normal exercise program until athletic injuries have healed.

You can minimize the risk of injury by following safety guidelines, respecting signals from your body that something may be wrong, and treating injuries promptly. Use special caution in heat or humidity (over 80°F and over 60% humidity): Exercise slowly, rest frequently in the shade, wear clothing that breathes, and drink plenty of fluids. Slow down or stop if you begin to feel uncomfortable. During hot weather, exercise in the early morning or evening when temperatures are lowest.

Staying with Your Program Once you have attained your desired level of fitness, you can maintain it by exercising regularly at a consistent intensity, 3–5 days a week. In general, if you exercise at the same intensity over a long period, your fitness will level out and can be maintained easily.

Adapt your program to changes in environment or schedule. Don't use wet weather or a new job as an excuse to give up your fitness program. If you walk in the summer, dress appropriately and walk in the winter as well. If you can't go out because of darkness or an unsafe neighborhood, walk in a local shopping mall or on campus or join a gym and walk on a treadmill.

What if you run out of steam? Although good health is an important *reason* to exercise, it's a poor *motivator*. You'll find specific suggestions for staying with your program in the Behavior Change Strategy box at the end of the chapter.

Cross-training can add variety to your workouts. Cross-training emphasizes whole-body, high-intensity training using exercises such as deadlifts, cleans, squats, presses, jerks, kettlebell exercises, snatches, plyometrics, sled pulls, and weight carrying. They also do aerobics such as running,

cycling, rope skipping, and rowing, but the emphasis is on speed and intensity. Cross-training programs, such as Cross-Fit, attempt to develop well-rounded fitness by including exercises that build cardiovascular and respiratory endurance, stamina, strength, flexibility, power, speed, coordination, agility, balance, and accuracy.

> **cross-training** Participating in two or more activities to develop a variety of fitness components. **TERMS**

TIPS FOR TODAY AND THE FUTURE

Physical activity and exercise offer benefits in nearly every area of wellness. Even a low to moderate level of activity provides valuable health benefits.

RIGHT NOW YOU CAN:

- Go outside and take a brisk 15-minute walk.
- Look at your calendar for the rest of the week and write in some physical activity—such as walking, running, or playing Frisbee—on as many days as you can. Schedule the activity for a specific time and stick to it.
- Call a friend and invite him or her to start planning a regular exercise program with you.

IN THE FUTURE YOU CAN:

- Schedule a session with a qualified personal trainer who can evaluate your current fitness level and help you set personalized fitness goals.
- Create seasonal workout programs for the summer, spring, fall, and winter. Develop programs that are varied but consistent with your overall fitness goals.

SUMMARY

- Exercise improves the functioning of the heart and the ability of the cardiorespiratory system to carry oxygen to the body's tissues. It also increases metabolic efficiency and improves body composition.

- Exercise lowers the risk of cardiovascular disease by improving blood fat levels, reducing high blood pressure, and interfering with the disease process that causes coronary artery blockage.

- Exercise reduces the risk of cancer, osteoporosis, and diabetes. It improves immune function and psychological health and helps prevent injuries and low-back pain.

- The five components of physical fitness most important to health are cardiorespiratory endurance, muscular strength, muscular endurance, flexibility, and body composition.

- Most people should accumulate at least 150 minutes of moderate-intensity or 75 minutes of vigorous-intensity physical activity each week. Longer-duration or more vigorous activity produces additional health and fitness benefits.

- Cardiorespiratory endurance exercises stress a large portion of the body's muscle mass. Endurance exercise should be performed 3–5 days per week for a total of 20–60 minutes per day. Intensity can be evaluated by measuring the heart rate.

- Warming up before exercising and cooling down afterward improve your performance and decrease your chances of injury.

- Exercises that develop muscular strength and endurance involve exerting force against a significant resistance. A strength training program for general fitness typically involves one or more sets of 8–12 repetitions of 8–10 exercises performed on at least 2 nonconsecutive days per week.

- A good stretching program includes exercises for all the major muscle groups and joints of the body. Do a series of active, static stretches at least 2– or 3 days per week. Hold each stretch for 10–30 seconds and do 2–4 repetitions. Stretch when muscles are warm.

- Individuals should choose instructors, equipment, and facilities carefully to enhance enjoyment and prevent injuries.

- A well-balanced diet contains all the energy and nutrients needed to sustain a fitness program. When exercising, remember to drink enough fluids.

- Rest, ice, compression, and elevation (R-I-C-E) are treatments for minor muscle and joint injuries.

- People can maintain a desired level of fitness by exercising 3–5 days a week at a consistent intensity.

- Strategies for maintaining an exercise program over the long term include having meaningful goals, varying the program, and trying new activities.

FOR MORE INFORMATION

American Alliance for Health, Physical Education, Recreation, and Dance (AAHPERD). A professional organization dedicated to promoting quality health and physical education programs.

http://www.aahperd.org

American College of Sports Medicine (ACSM). The principal professional organization for sports medicine and exercise science. Provides brochures, publications, and audio- and videotapes.

http://www.acsm.org

American Council on Exercise (ACE). Promotes exercise and fitness; the website features fact sheets on many consumer topics, including choosing shoes, cross-training, and steroids.

http://www.acefitness.org

CDC Physical Activity Information. Provides information about the benefits of physical activity and suggestions for incorporating moderate physical activity into daily life.

http://www.cdc.gov/physicalactivity/

Disabled Sports USA. Provides sports and recreation services to people with physical or mobility disorders.

http://www.disabledsportsusa.org

International Health, Racquet, & Sportsclub Association (IHRSA): Health Clubs. Provides guidelines for choosing a health or fitness facility and links to clubs that belong to IHRSA.

http://www.healthclubs.com

International Sports Sciences Association (ISSA). Trains and certifies personal trainers.

www.issaonline.com

MedlinePlus: Exercise and Physical Fitness. Provides links to news and reliable information about fitness and exercise from government agencies and professional associations.

http://www.nlm.nih.gov/medlineplus
/exerciseandphysicalfitness.html

President's Council on Physical Fitness and Sports (PCPFS). Provides information about PCPFS programs and publications, including fitness guides and fact sheets.

http://www.fitness.gov

http://www.presidentschallenge.org

Shape Up America! A nonprofit organization that provides information and resources for exercise, nutrition, and weight loss.

http://www.shapeup.org

SELECTED BIBLIOGRAPHY

American College of Sports Medicine. 2013. *ACSM's Guidelines for Exercise Testing and Prescription*, 9th ed. Philadelphia, PA: Wolters Kluwer/Lippincott Williams & Wilkins Health.

American College of Sports Medicine. 2013. Exercise and fluid replacement. *ACSM's Health & Fitness Journal* 17(4): 3.

Arem, H., et al. 2015. Leisure time physical activity and mortality: A detailed pooled analysis of the dose-response relationship. *JAMA Internal Medicine* 175(6): 959–967.

Bajer, B., et al. 2015. Exercise associated hormonal signals as powerful determinants of an effective fat mass loss. *Endocrine Regulations* 49(3): 151–163.

Biswas, A., et al. 2015. Sedentary time and its association with risk for disease incidence, mortality, and hospitalization in adults: A systematic review and meta-analysis. *Annals of Internal Medicine* 162: 123–132.

Burfoot, A., 2016. Milk and other surprising ways to stay hydrated. *New York Times*, June 30.

Centers for Disease Control and Prevention. 2016. Deaths: Final data for 2014. *National Vital Statistics Reports* 65(4).

Centers for Disease Control and Prevention. 2016. Physical Activity Basics, http://www.cdc.gov/physicalactivity/basics.

Centers for Disease Control and Prevention. 2013. Adult participation in aerobic and muscle-strengthening physical activities—United States, 2011. *MMWR* 62(17): 326–330.

Clark, J. E. 2015. Diet, exercise or diet with exercise: Comparing the effectiveness of treatment options for weight-loss and changes in fitness for adults (18–65 years old) who are overfat, or obese; systematic review and meta-analysis. *Journal of Diabetes & Metabolic Disorders* 14: 31.

Dankel, S. J., et al. 2016. Does the fat-but-fit paradigm hold true for all-cause mortality when considering the duration of overweight/obesity? Analyzing the WATCH (Weight, Activity and Time Contributes to Health) paradigm. *Preventive Medicine* 83: 37–40.

Demark-Wahnefried, W., et al. 2015. Quality of life outcomes from the Exercise and Nutrition Enhance Recovery and Good Health for You (ENERGY)-randomized weight loss trial among breast cancer survivors. *Breast Cancer Research and Treatment* 154(2): 329–337.

Dorneles, G. P., et al. 2016. High intensity interval exercise decreases IL-8 and enhances the immunomodulatory cytokine interleukin-10 in lean and overweight-obese individuals. *Cytokine* 77: 1–9.

Fahey, T. D., et al. 2017. *Fit & Well: Core Concepts and Labs in Physical Fitness and Wellness,* 12th ed. New York: McGraw-Hill.

Garber, C. E., et al. 2011. Quantity and quality of exercise for developing and maintaining cardiorespiratory, musculoskeletal, and neuromotor fitness in apparently healthy adults: Guidance for prescribing exercise. *Medicine & Science in Sports & Exercise* 43(7): 1334–1359.

Hogstom, G., et al. 2015. Aerobic fitness in late adolescence and the risk of early death: A prospective cohort study of 1.3 million Swedish men. *International Journal of Epidemiology* DOI: 10.1093/ije/dyv321.

Hunter, G. R., et al. 2015. Exercise training and energy expenditure following weight loss. *Medicine & Science in Sports & Exercise* 47(9): 1950–1957.

International Health, Racquet & Sportsclub Association. 2015. Health Club Industry Continues Impressive Growth, http://www.ihrsa.org/news/2015/4/22/health-club-industry-continues-impressive-growth.html.

Keadle, S. K., et al. 2015. Impact of changes in television viewing time and physical activity on longevity: A prospective cohort study. *International Journal of Behavioral Nutrition and Physical Activity* 12(1): 156.

Klos, L. A., et al. 2015. Losing weight on reality TV: A content analysis of the weight loss behaviors and practices portrayed on The Biggest Loser. *Journal of Health Communication* 20(6): 639–646.

Kyu, H. H., et al. 2016. Physical activity and risk of breast cancer, colon cancer, diabetes, ischemic heart disease, and ischemic stroke events: systematic review and dose-response meta-analysis for the Global Burden of Disease Study 2013. *BMJ* doi: 10.1136/bmj.i3857.

Lee, B. C. Y., and S. M. McGill. 2015. Effect of long-term isometric training on core/torso stiffness. *Journal of Strength & Conditioning Research* 29(6): 1515–1526.

Lyden, K., et al. 2015. Discrete features of sedentary behaviors impact cardiometabolic risk factors. *Medicine & Science in Sports & Exercise* 47(5): 1079–1086.

Maughan, R. J., et al. 2016. A randomized trial to assess the potential of different beverages to affect hydration status: development of a beverage hydration index. *American Journal of Clinical Nutrition, 103*: 717–723.

Moore, S. C., et al. 2016. Association of leisure-time physical activity with risk of 26 types of cancer in 1.44 million adults. *JAMA Internal Medicine.* DOI: 10.1001/jamainternmed.2016.1548.

Physical Activity Guidelines Advisory Committee. 2008. *Physical Activity Guidelines Advisory Committee Report, 2008.* Washington, DC: U.S. Department of Health and Human Services.

President's Council on Fitness, Sports & Nutrition. 2012. Too much sitting: Health risks of sedentary behavior and opportunities for change. *Research Digest* Series 13, Number 3.

Schnohr, P., et al. 2013. Longevity in male and female joggers: The Copenhagen City Heart Study. *American Journal of Epidemiology* 177(7): 683–689.

Stephens, J., et al. 2015. Young adults, technology, and weight loss: A focus group study. *Journal of Obesity* 2015: 379769.

Stubbs, B., et al. 2016. Exercise improves cardiorespiratory fitness in people with depression: A meta-analysis of randomized control trials. *Journal of Affective Disorders* 190: 249–253.

Swain, D. P. 2013. *ACSM's Resource Manual for Guidelines for Exercise Testing and Prescription,* 7th ed. Philadelphia, PA: Lippincott Williams and Wilkins.

U.S. Department of Health and Human Services. 2008. *2008 Physical Activity Guidelines for Americans.* Hyattsville, MD: U.S. Department of Health and Human Services.

U.S. Department of Health and Human Services. 2010. *Healthy People 2020.* Washington, DC: U.S. Department of Health and Human Services (http://www.healthypeople.gov).

Williams, B. M., and R. R. Kraemer. 2015. Comparison of cardiorespiratory and metabolic responses in kettlebell high-intensity interval training versus sprint interval cycling. *Journal of Strength & Conditioning Research* 29(12): 3317–3325.

Young, D. R., et al. 2016. Sedentary behavior and cardiovascular morbidity and mortality. A science advisory from the American Heart Association. *Circulation* 134(13): e262-e279.

Although most people recognize the importance of incorporating exercise into their lives, many find it difficult to do. No single strategy will work for everyone, but the general steps outlined here should help you create an exercise program that fits your goals, preferences, and lifestyle. A carefully designed contract and program plan can help you convert your vague wishes into a detailed plan of action. And the strategies for program compliance outlined here and in Chapter 1 can help you enjoy and stick with your program for the rest of your life.

Step 1: Set Goals

Setting specific goals is an important first step in a successful fitness program because it establishes the direction you want to take. Your goals might be specifically related to health, such as lowering your blood pressure and risk of heart disease, or they might relate to other aspects of your life, such as improving your tennis game or the fit of your clothes. If you can decide why you're starting to exercise, it can help you keep going. Make sure your goals meet the SMART criteria described in Chapter 1.

Step 2: Select Activities

The success of your fitness program depends on the consistency of your involvement. Select activities that encourage your commitment: The right program will be its own incentive to continue, but poor activity choices provide obstacles and can turn exercise into a chore. When choosing activities for your fitness program, consider the following:

- Is this activity fun? Will it hold my interest over time?
- Will this activity help me reach the goals I have set?
- Will my current fitness and skill level enable me to participate fully in this activity?
- Can I easily fit this activity into my daily schedule? Are there any special requirements (e.g., facilities, partners, equipment) that I must plan for?
- Can I afford any special costs required for equipment or facilities?

- If I have special exercise needs due to a particular health problem, does this activity conform to those exercise needs? Will it enhance my ability to cope with my specific health problem?

Using these guidelines listed, select a number of sports and activities, and apply the FITT principle. Review your program plan and confirm that it meets the criteria of a complete fitness program.

Step 3: Make a Commitment

By completing a contract, you make a firm commitment and will be more likely to follow through until you meet your goals.

Step 4: Begin and Maintain Your Program

Start slowly and increase your intensity and duration gradually to allow your body time to adjust. Be realistic and patient—meeting your goals will take time. The important first step is to break your established pattern of inactivity. The following guidelines may help you start and stick with your program:

- **Set aside regular periods for exercise.** Choose times that fit in best with your schedule, and stick to them. Allow an adequate amount of time for warm-up, cool-down, and a shower.
- **Take advantage of any opportunity for exercise that presents itself.** For example, walk to class or take stairs instead of an elevator.
- **Do what you can to make your program fun and avoid boredom.** Do stretching exercises or jumping jacks to music.
- **Exercise with a group that shares your goals and general level of competence.** The social side of exercise is an important motivator for many people.
- **Vary the program.** Change your activities periodically. Alter your route or distance if biking or jogging.
- **Establish mini-goals or a point system, and work rewards into your program.** Until you reach your main goals, a series of small rewards will help you stick with your program.

- **Focus on the positive.** Concentrate on the improvements you get from your program, and how good you feel during and after exercise. Visualize what it will be like to reach your goals.
- **Revisit and revise.** If your program turns out to be unrealistic, revise it. Expect to make many adjustments in your program along the way.
- **Expect fluctuation and lapses.** Don't let lapses discourage you or make you feel guilty. Instead make a renewed commitment to your exercise program.
- **Plan ahead for difficult situations.** Think about what circumstances might make it tough to keep up with your fitness routine, and develop strategies for sticking with your program. For example, devise a plan for your program during vacation, travel, bad weather, and so on.
- **Renew your attitude.** If you notice you're slacking off, try to list the negative thoughts and behaviors that are causing you to lose interest. Devise a strategy to reduce negative thoughts and behaviors. Make changes in your program plan and reward system to help renew your enthusiasm and commitment.

Step 5: Record and Assess Your Progress

Keeping a record that notes the daily results of your program will help remind you of your ongoing commitment to your program and give you a sense of accomplishment. It can also help you identify problems. Create daily and weekly program logs or use one of the many available apps for exercise tracking. Record the activity frequency, intensity, time, and type. Post or check your log frequently to remind you of your activity schedule and to provide incentive for improvement.

SOURCE: Adapted from Kusinitz, I., and M. Fine. 1995. *Your Guide to Getting Fit,* 3rd ed. Mountain View, CA: Mayfield.

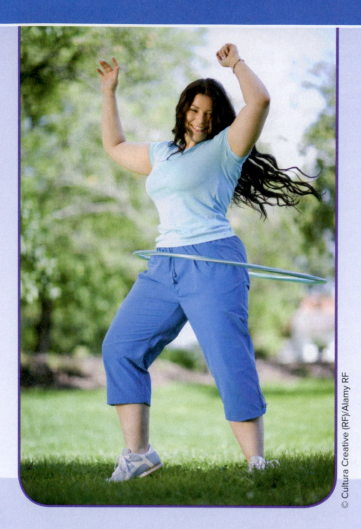

CHAPTER OBJECTIVES

- Discuss methods for assessing body weight and body composition
- Explain the effects of body fat on wellness
- Explain factors that contribute to excess body fat
- Describe lifestyle factors associated with successful weight management
- Name and describe approaches to overcoming a weight problem
- Explain the relationship between body image and eating disorders and the associated health risks

CHAPTER 11

Weight Management

Achieving and maintaining a healthy body weight is a public health priority and a serious challenge for many Americans. According to standards developed by the National Institutes of Health (NIH), the prevalence of obesity among Americans is just over 36% in adults and 17% in youth (Table 11.1 and Figure 11.1). Of adolescents aged 12–19, about 20.5% are obese. Of adult men, an estimated 34.3% are obese, and of adult women, an estimated 38.3% are obese. One study predicted that if current rates continue, 42% of Americans will be obese by the year 2050. As millions struggle to lose weight, others fall into dangerous eating patterns such as binge eating or self-starvation.

This chapter explores body composition and the problems associated with excess body fat. It also explores factors that contribute to the development of overweight and suggests strategies for reaching and maintaining a healthy weight. Finally, we will look at body image and the development and treatment of eating disorders.

EVALUATING BODY WEIGHT AND BODY COMPOSITION

There are different methods for measuring and evaluating the health risks associated with body weight and body composition. First, let's look at the concept of body composition in more detail.

Body Composition

The human body can be divided into fat-free mass and body fat. Fat-free mass is composed of all the body's nonfat tissues: bone, water, muscle, connective tissue, organ tissues, and teeth.

Table 11.1	Weight of Americans Aged 20 and Older, 2011–2014

GROUP	PERCENT OBESE
Both sexes	37.8*
All races, male	34.3
All races, female	38.3
Non-Hispanic white, male	33.6
Non-Hispanic white, female	35.5
Non-Hispanic black, male	37.5
Non-Hispanic black, female	56.9
Hispanic, male	39.0
Hispanic, female	45.7

*Data from 2013–2014 only.

SOURCES: National Center for Health Statistics. 2016. *Health, United States, 2015: With Special Feature on Racial and Ethnic Health Disparities.* Hyattsville, MD: National Center for Health Statistics. Ogden, C., et al. 2015. *Prevalence of Obesity Among Adults and Youth: United States, 2011–2014.* NCHS Data Brief No. 219. (http://www.cdc.gov/nchs/products/databriefs/db219.htm).

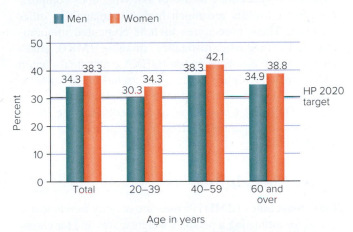

FIGURE 11.1 **Prevalence of obesity in American adults, by sex and age, 2011–2014.** The government's Healthy People 2020 initiative has set a target to reduce the proportion of adults who are obese from current levels down to 30.5%.

SOURCE: Ogden, C., et al. 2015. *Prevalence of Obesity Among Adults and Youth: United States, 2011–2014.* NCHS Data Brief No. 219. (http://www.cdc.gov/nchs/products/databriefs/db219.htm).

A certain amount of body fat is necessary for the body to function. Fat is incorporated into the nerves, brain, heart, lungs, liver, mammary glands, and other body organs and tissues. It is the main source of stored energy in the body. It also cushions body organs and helps regulate body temperature. This **essential fat** makes up about 3–5% of total body weight in men and about 8–12% in women. The percentage is higher in women due to such factors as fat deposits in the breasts and uterus.

Most of the fat in the body is stored in fat cells, or **adipose tissue,** located under the skin (**subcutaneous fat**) and around major organs (**visceral fat** or *intra-abdominal fat*). People have a genetically determined number of fat cells, but these cells can increase or decrease in size depending on how much fat is being stored. The amount of stored fat depends on several factors, including age, sex, metabolism, diet, and activity level. The primary source of stored body fat comes from excess calories consumed in the diet—that is, calories consumed in excess of calories expended in metabolism, physical activity, and exercise.

When looking at body composition, one important consideration is the proportion of the body's total weight that is fat—the **percent body fat.** For example, two women may both be 5 feet, 5 inches tall and weigh 130 pounds. But one woman may have only 15% of her body weight as fat, whereas the other woman could have 34% body fat. Although neither woman is overweight by most standards, the second woman is considered overfat.

Defining Healthy Weight, Overweight, and Obesity

For a variety of reasons, many people struggle with body dissatisfaction and are concerned about their weight. But how do you decide if you are at a healthy weight? How thin is too thin, and at what point does being overweight present a health risk?

Overweight is defined as total body weight above the recommended range for good health, as determined by large-scale population surveys. **Obesity** is defined as a more serious degree of overweight that carries multiple health risks. Both terms are used to identify weight ranges that are associated with increased likelihood of certain diseases and health problems.

Several methods can be used to measure and evaluate body weight and percent body fat. These assessments can give you information about the health risks associated with your current body weight and body composition. They can also help you establish reasonable goals and set a starting point for current and future decisions about weight loss and weight gain. These methods are body composition, body mass index (BMI), and body fat distribution.

essential fat Fat incorporated in various tissues of the body; critical for normal body functioning. **TERMS**

adipose tissue Connective tissue in which fat is stored.

subcutaneous fat Fat located under the skin.

visceral fat Fat located around major organs; also called *intra-abdominal fat.*

percent body fat The percentage of total body weight that is composed of fat.

overweight Body weight above the recommended range for good health.

obesity Severe overweight, characterized by an excessive accumulation of body fat; may also be defined in terms of some measure of total body weight.

Estimating Body Composition

Methods for determining percent body fat provide only an estimate of the amount of body fat (or adipose tissue) and the amount of lean body mass (or lean tissue) you have. A healthy body fat range for men is considered to be about 12–20%, and for women, about 20–30%. Men with more than 25% body fat are considered obese, as are women with more than 33% body fat.

Bioelectrical Impedance Analysis (BIA)

In this method, a person stands barefoot on a machine that resembles a scale, uses a handheld machine, or lies down with spot electrodes attached at various points on the body that are also connected to a bioelectrical machine. A very low level of electrical current is sent between electrodes through the body, transmitting current from one point to another. The electrical conduction through the body favors the path of the fat-free tissues over the fat tissues, so the amount of resistance to the current is related to the amount of fat-free tissue in the body. Percent body fat is then calculated from the measurements of resistance to the current. BIA can estimate your body fat within a margin of error of about 3–4%.

Skinfold Measurement

Skinfold measurement is a simple and practical way to assess body composition based on the amount of subcutaneous fat. A technician measures the thickness of skinfolds at several different sites on the body with a device, called calipers, that painlessly "pinches" the folds of skin and its underlying fat. The measurements are used in formulas that calculate body fat percentages. When performed by a skilled technician, this method can estimate body fat within a 3–4% margin of error.

Hydrostatic Weighing

In hydrostatic (underwater) weighing, a person is first weighed on a traditional scale.

Then the person is submerged and weighed under water. Muscle has a higher density than water, and fat has a lower density than water, so people with more fat tend to "float" and weigh less under water, whereas lean people tend to "sink" and weigh more under water. The amount of water displaced is used to calculate percent body fat. Under the best circumstances, underwater weighing can estimate body fat within a 2–3% margin of error.

The Bod Pod

The Bod Pod is a specialized body composition analysis device that uses air displacement instead of water. A person sits in a chamber for about 5 minutes, and computerized pressure sensors determine the amount of air displaced by the person's body to determine percentage of body fat. The Bod Pod machine costs more than other methods. It is accurate to within 1–2.7 percentage points.

Scanning Procedures

High-tech scanning procedures are very accurate means of assessing body composition, but the costs are much higher compared to other methods. These procedures include computed tomography (CT), magnetic resonance imaging (MRI), dual-energy X-ray absorptiometry (DEXA), and dual-photon absorptiometry. Other procedures include near infrared reactance (Futrex 1100) and total body electrical conductivity (TOBEC). Considered to be very accurate, these techniques are generally offered only at medical or research facilities.

Body Mass Index

Body mass index (BMI) is a measure of body weight that is useful for estimating a person's weight status and for classifying the health risks of body weight if more sophisticated methods aren't available. BMI is based on the concept that weight should be proportional to height. Easy to calculate and rate, BMI is a fairly accurate measure of the health risks related to body weight for most average (nonathletic) people. BMI is correlated with body fat, but it does not directly measure body fat.

Calculating Your BMI

BMI is calculated by dividing your body weight (expressed in kilograms or pounds) by the square of your height (expressed in meters or inches). You can look up your BMI in the chart in Figure 11.2, or

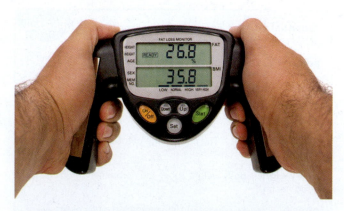

Bioelectrical impedance analysis calculates percent body fat by measuring resistance to a low level of electrical current.

© Murat Sen/Getty Images RF

	<18.5 Underweight		18.5–24.9 Normal						25–29.9 Overweight					30–34.9 Obesity (Class I)					35–39.9 Obesity (Class II)					≥40 Extreme obesity
BMI	17	18	19	20	21	22	23	24	25	26	27	28	29	30	31	32	33	34	35	36	37	38	39	40
Height												Body Weight (pounds)												
4' 10"	81	86	91	96	101	105	110	115	120	124	129	134	139	144	148	153	158	163	168	172	177	182	187	192
4' 11"	84	89	94	99	104	109	114	119	124	129	134	139	144	149	154	159	163	168	173	178	183	188	193	198
5'	87	92	97	102	108	113	118	123	128	133	138	143	149	154	159	164	169	174	179	184	190	195	200	205
5' 1"	90	95	101	106	111	117	122	127	132	138	143	148	154	159	164	169	175	180	185	191	196	201	207	212
5' 2"	93	98	104	109	115	120	126	131	137	142	148	153	159	164	170	175	181	186	191	197	202	208	213	219
5' 3"	96	102	107	113	119	124	130	136	141	147	153	158	164	169	175	181	186	192	198	203	209	215	220	226
5' 4"	99	105	111	117	122	128	134	140	146	152	157	163	169	175	181	187	192	198	204	210	216	222	227	233
5' 5"	102	108	114	120	126	132	138	144	150	156	162	168	174	180	186	192	198	204	210	216	222	229	235	241
5' 6"	105	112	118	124	130	136	143	149	155	161	167	174	180	186	192	198	205	211	217	223	229	236	242	248
5' 7"	109	115	121	128	134	141	147	153	160	166	173	179	185	192	198	204	211	217	224	230	236	243	249	256
5' 8"	112	118	125	132	138	145	151	158	165	171	178	184	191	197	204	211	217	224	230	237	244	250	257	263
5' 9"	115	122	129	136	142	149	156	163	169	176	183	190	197	203	210	217	224	230	237	244	251	258	264	271
5' 10"	119	126	133	139	146	153	160	167	174	181	188	195	202	209	216	223	230	237	244	251	258	265	272	279
5' 11"	122	129	136	143	151	158	165	172	179	187	194	201	208	215	222	230	237	244	251	258	265	273	280	287
6'	125	133	140	148	155	162	170	177	184	192	199	207	214	221	229	236	243	251	258	266	273	280	288	295
6' 1"	129	137	144	152	159	167	174	182	190	197	205	212	220	228	235	243	250	258	265	273	281	288	296	303
6' 2"	132	140	148	156	164	171	179	187	195	203	210	218	226	234	242	249	257	265	273	281	288	296	304	312
6' 3"	136	144	152	160	168	176	184	192	200	208	216	224	232	240	248	256	264	272	280	288	296	304	312	320
6' 4"	140	148	156	164	173	181	189	197	206	214	222	230	238	247	255	263	271	280	288	296	304	312	321	329

FIGURE 11.2 Body mass index (BMI). To determine your BMI, find your height in the left column. Move across the appropriate row until you find the weight closest to your own. The number at the top of the column is the BMI at that height and weight.

SOURCES: U.S. Department of Health and Human Services and U.S. Department of Agriculture. 2015. *2015–2020 Dietary Guidelines for Americans,* 8th ed. (http://health.gov/dietaryguidelines/2015/guidelines).

you can use the following formula to calculate it more precisely:

$$BMI = \frac{\text{weight in kg}}{(\text{height in meters})^2}$$

or $\dfrac{\text{weight in pounds}}{(\text{height in inches})^2} \times 703$ (conversion factor)

Body weight status is categorized as underweight, healthy weight, overweight, or obese in comparison with what is considered healthy for a given height. Under standards issued by the National Institutes of Health and adopted by the Dietary Guidelines for Americans, a BMI between 18.5 and 24.9 is considered healthy, a BMI of 25 or above is classified as overweight, and a BMI of 30 or above is classified as obese. A person with a BMI below 18.5 is classified as underweight, although low BMI values may be healthy in some cases if they are not the result of smoking, an eating disorder, or an underlying disease. For a more accurate assessment of health status, BMI is often combined with waist measurement; as described in the next section, waist measurement provides an assessment of body fat distribution.

Limitations of BMI BMI is a valuable tool for assessing weight status, but it is not intended to determine body composition or track changes in body weight in relation to gains in muscle mass and loss of fat. BMI does not distinguish between fat weight and fat-free weight. It can also be inaccurate for some groups, including people shorter than 5 feet tall, muscular athletes, and older adults with little muscle mass due to inactivity or an underlying disease.

Body Fat Distribution

To complete the assessment and evaluation of your current body weight, it is important to consider how fat is distributed throughout your body. The location of fat on your body is an important indicator of health, as it is known to affect your risk for various diseases.

Two of the simplest methods for measuring body fat distribution are waist circumference measurement and waist-to-hip ratio calculation. In the first method, waist circumference is measured using a tape measure placed around your abdomen at the top of your hip bone. A waist circumference of greater than 40 inches (102 cm) for men or greater than 35 in (88 cm) for women is associated with an increased risk for chronic disease for most adults. In the second method, a mathematic formula (waist circumference divided by hip circumference) is used to find your waist-to-hip ratio. A waist-to-hip ratio above 0.94 for young men and above 0.82 for young women is associated with an increased risk of heart disease and diabetes. More research is needed to determine the precise degree of risk associated with specific values for these two assessments of body fat distribution.

Men and postmenopausal women tend to store fat in the upper regions of their bodies, particularly in the abdominal area, as visceral fat. People with this *android* pattern of fat distribution are said to be apple shaped. Premenopausal women usually store fat in the hips, buttocks, and thighs, as subcutaneous fat. People with this *gynoid* pattern are said to be pear shaped.

Abdominal obesity increases the risk of high blood pressure, diabetes, early-onset heart disease, stroke, certain types of cancer, and mortality. This risk is independent of a person's BMI. The reason for the increased risk associated with abdominal obesity appears to be that visceral fat is more easily mobilized and sent into the bloodstream, increasing disease-related blood fat levels. Visceral fat contains many biologically active substances such as inflammatory chemicals and growth factors, which can adhere to the lining of blood vessels, cause insulin resistance, and have a negative influence on cardiovascular health.

What Is the Right Weight for You?

There are limits to the changes you can make to body weight and body shape, both of which are influenced by heredity. The changes that can and should be made are lifestyle changes, as described throughout this chapter.

To answer the question of what you should weigh, assess your health and body composition status and let your lifestyle be your guide. As described in Chapter 9, the *Dietary Guidelines for Americans 2015–2020* recommends that adults who are obese and adults who are overweight and have additional CVD risk factors should change their eating and physical activity behaviors to prevent additional weight gain and/or to promote weight loss. Instead of focusing on a particular weight, focus on living a lifestyle that includes following a healthy dietary pattern, getting plenty of exercise, thinking positively, and learning to cope with stress. Then let the pounds fall where they may. For many people, the result will be close to recommended weight ranges. For some, their weight will be somewhat higher than societal standards—but right for them. By letting a healthy lifestyle determine your weight, you can avoid developing unhealthy patterns of eating and a negative body image. Later in the chapter, we'll take a closer look at lifestyle recommendations for healthy weight management.

BODY FAT AND WELLNESS

The amount and distribution of fat in the body—both too much and too little—can have profound effects on health. Obesity doubles mortality rates and can reduce life expectancy by 10–20 years. Obese people have an increased risk of death from all causes compared with people of normal weight. Obesity is associated with a number of chronic conditions such as diabetes, CVD, many kinds of cancer, impaired immune function, gallbladder and kidney diseases, skin problems, impotence, sleep and breathing disorders, back

pain, arthritis, and other bone and joint disorders. Obesity is also associated with complications of pregnancy, menstrual irregularities, urine leakage (stress incontinence), increased surgical risk, and psychological disorders and problems (such as depression, low self-esteem, and body dissatisfaction). Research has found that nearly one in five U.S. deaths is associated with being overweight.

In addition, studies show a decrease in the quality of life (measured by such things as self-image, bullying, bodily pain, quality of food intake, physical activity, and screen time) in overweight and obese children and adolescents compared to those of normal weight. It is also important to realize that small weight losses—5–10% of total body weight—can lead to significant health improvements.

There is debate over the health risks for people who are overweight but not obese (BMI of 25–29), particularly for people who are overweight and physically active. These risks depend in part on an individual's overall health and other risk factors, such as high blood pressure, unhealthy cholesterol levels, body fat distribution, tobacco use, and level of physical activity.

The health consequences of obesity may affect racial and ethnic populations in different ways. For example, at a given level of BMI, Hispanics are significantly more likely to have type 2 diabetes than are non-Hispanic whites. For Asian Americans or people of Asian descent, waist circumference is a better indicator of relative disease risk than BMI, and disease risk goes up at a lower level of BMI than for individuals of other groups. For Asian populations, World Health Organization guidelines have a lower BMI cutoff for defining overweight (BMI 23 or more, compared to the general suggested cutoff of 25; the same lower cutoff is recommended for people of Asian descent for diabetes screening by the American Diabetes Association.

Diabetes

According to the American Diabetes Association, an estimated 29.1 million Americans have one of the two major types of **diabetes mellitus,** a disease that disrupts normal metabolism. An estimated 1.4 million Americans are diagnosed with diabetes every year, and an estimated 8.1 million people are believed to have undiagnosed diabetes. It is projected that by the year 2050 as many as one out of every three adults in the United States could have diabetes.

Even mild to moderate overweight is associated with a substantial increase in the risk of the most common form of diabetes. Obese people are more than three times as likely as nonobese people to develop type 2 diabetes, and the incidence of this disease among Americans has increased dramatically as the rate of obesity has climbed.

diabetes mellitus A disease that disrupts normal metabolism, interfering with cells' ability to take in glucose for energy production. **TERMS**

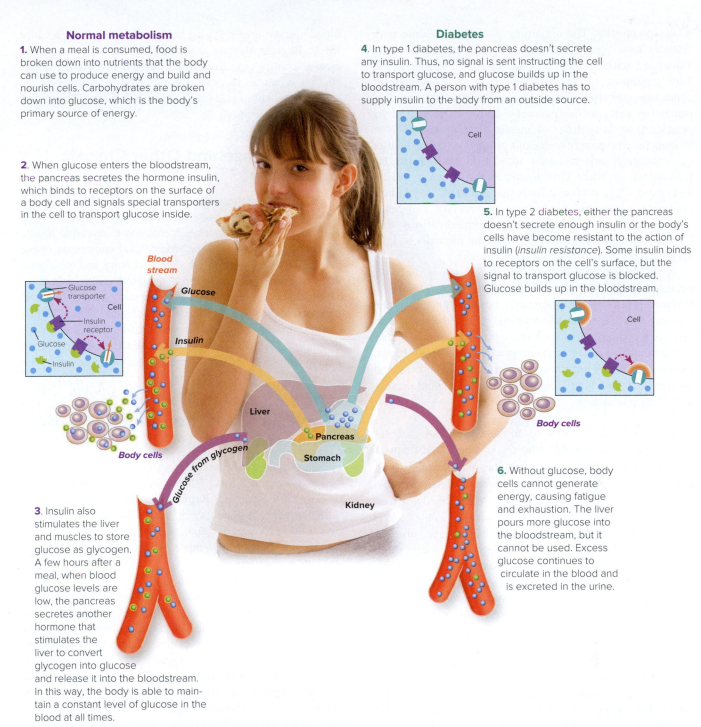

Normal metabolism

1. When a meal is consumed, food is broken down into nutrients that the body can use to produce energy and build and nourish cells. Carbohydrates are broken down into glucose, which is the body's primary source of energy.

2. When glucose enters the bloodstream, the pancreas secretes the hormone insulin, which binds to receptors on the surface of a body cell and signals special transporters in the cell to transport glucose inside.

Blood stream

Glucose transporter
Cell
Insulin receptor
Glucose
Insulin

Glucose

Insulin

Body cells

Glucose from glycogen

Liver

Pancreas

Stomach

Kidney

3. Insulin also stimulates the liver and muscles to store glucose as glycogen. A few hours after a meal, when blood glucose levels are low, the pancreas secretes another hormone that stimulates the liver to convert glycogen into glucose and release it into the bloodstream. In this way, the body is able to maintain a constant level of glucose in the blood at all times.

Diabetes

4. In type 1 diabetes, the pancreas doesn't secrete any insulin. Thus, no signal is sent instructing the cell to transport glucose, and glucose builds up in the bloodstream. A person with type 1 diabetes has to supply insulin to the body from an outside source.

Cell

5. In type 2 diabetes, either the pancreas doesn't secrete enough insulin or the body's cells have become resistant to the action of insulin (*insulin resistance*). Some insulin binds to receptors on the cell's surface, but the signal to transport glucose is blocked. Glucose builds up in the bloodstream.

Cell

Body cells

6. Without glucose, body cells cannot generate energy, causing fatigue and exhaustion. The liver pours more glucose into the bloodstream, but it cannot be used. Excess glucose continues to circulate in the blood and is excreted in the urine.

FIGURE 11.3 **Diabetes mellitus.** During digestion, carbohydrates are broken down in the small intestine into glucose, a simple sugar that enters the bloodstream. The presence of glucose signals the pancreas to release insulin, a hormone that helps cells take up glucose; once inside a cell, glucose can be converted to energy. In diabetes, this process is disrupted, resulting in a buildup of glucose in the bloodstream.
© webphotographeer/Getty Images RF

Diabetes involves a disruption in the process of metabolism. In normal metabolism, the pancreas secretes insulin, which stimulates cells to take up blood sugar (glucose) to produce energy (Figure 11.3). In diabetes, this process is disrupted, causing a buildup of glucose in the bloodstream. Diabetes is associated with kidney failure; nerve damage; circulation problems and amputations; retinal damage and blindness; and increased rates of heart attack, stroke, and hypertension. Diabetes is currently the seventh leading cause of death in the United States.

Types of Diabetes About 5–10% of people with diabetes have a form known as type 1 diabetes, a disease that usually begins in childhood or adolescence and is not related to obesity. The remaining 90–95% of people with diabetes have type 2 diabetes, a disease that is strongly associated with excess body fat. In type 1 diabetes, the body's immune system, triggered by a viral infection or some other environmental factor, destroys the insulin-producing cells in the pancreas. Little or no insulin is produced, so daily doses of insulin are required. In type 2 diabetes, the pancreas doesn't produce enough insulin, or body cells are resistant to insulin (called *insulin resistance*), or both. This condition can develop slowly, and about 25% of type 2 diabetics are unaware of their condition. About one-third of people with type 2 diabetes must take insulin; others may take medications that increase insulin production or stimulate the cells to take up glucose.

A third type of diabetes, called *gestational diabetes,* occurs in about 7% of women during pregnancy. The condition usually resolves after pregnancy, but about half of women who experience it eventually develop type 2 diabetes. *Prediabetes* is a condition in which blood sugar levels are higher than normal but not high enough for a diagnosis of full-blown diabetes. About 79 million Americans have prediabetes, and most will develop type 2 diabetes unless they adopt preventive lifestyle measures.

Stages and Risk Factors

In the early stages, diabetes has no symptoms; possible warning signs include: frequent urination, extreme hunger or thirst, unexplained weight loss, extreme fatigue, blurred vision, frequent infections, slow wound healing, tingling or numbness in the hands or feet, and generalized dry skin and itching with no rash.

The major risk factors for diabetes are age, obesity, physical inactivity, a family history of diabetes, and lifestyle. Race and ethnicity also play a role, with Native Americans, Alaska Natives, African Americans, and Hispanics having higher rates than Asian Americans and white Americans. Excess body fat reduces cell sensitivity to insulin, and insulin resistance is almost always a precursor of type 2 diabetes. Nearly 90% of people with type 2 diabetes are overweight when diagnosed, including 55% who are obese.

Screening involves a blood test to check glucose levels after either a period of fasting or the administration of a set dose of glucose. A fasting glucose level of 126 mg/dl or higher indicates diabetes; a level of 100–125 mg/dl indicates prediabetes. If you are concerned about your risk for diabetes, talk with your physician about being tested.

It is estimated that 90% of cases of type 2 diabetes could be prevented if people adopted healthy lifestyle behaviors, including regular physical activity, a moderate diet to control body fat, and modest weight loss. Even a small amount of weight loss can be beneficial. For people with prediabetes, lifestyle measures are more effective than medication for delaying or preventing the development of diabetes. Exercise (endurance and/or strength training) makes cells more sensitive to insulin and helps stabilize blood glucose levels; it also helps keep body fat at healthy levels. Regular exercise and a healthy diet are often sufficient to control type 2 diabetes. There is no cure for diabetes, but it can be successfully managed by keeping blood sugar levels within safe limits through diet, exercise, and, if necessary, medication.

Heart Disease and Other Chronic Conditions

Obesity is one of the six major controllable risk factors for heart disease. Excess body fat is strongly associated with hypertension, unhealthy cholesterol and triglyceride levels, and impaired heart function. Many overweight and obese people—especially those who are sedentary and eat a poor diet—also suffer from a group of symptoms called *metabolic syndrome*. Symptoms include insulin resistance, high blood pressure, high blood glucose, unhealthy cholesterol levels, chronic inflammation, and abdominal fat. Metabolic syndrome increases the risk of heart disease, more so in men than in women. Obesity is also a risk factor for certain types of cancer.

Problems Associated with Very Low Levels of Body Fat

Health experts have generally viewed very low levels of body fat—less than 8–12% for women and 3–5% for men—as a threat to wellness. Extreme leanness has been linked with reproductive, circulatory, and immune system disorders. Extremely lean people may experience muscle wasting and fatigue. They are also more likely to suffer from dangerous eating disorders.

In physically active women and girls, particularly those involved in sports where weight and appearance are important (ballet, gymnastics, skating, and distance running, for example), a condition called the **female athlete triad** may develop. The triad consists of three interrelated disorders: abnormal eating patterns (and excessive exercising), followed by **amenorrhea** (absence of menstruation), followed by decreased bone density (premature osteoporosis). Prolonged amenorrhea can cause bone density to erode to a point that a woman in her twenties will have the bone density of a woman in her sixties. Left untreated, the triad can lead to decreased physical performance, increased incidence of bone fractures, disturbances of heart rhythm and metabolism, and even death.

---

female athlete triad A condition consisting of three interrelated disorders: abnormal eating patterns (and excessive exercising) followed by lack of menstrual periods (amenorrhea) and decreased bone density (premature osteoporosis).

amenorrhea The absence of menstruation.

TERMS

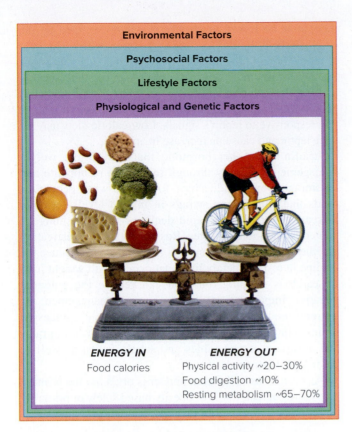

Environmental Factors

Psychosocial Factors

Lifestyle Factors

Physiological and Genetic Factors

ENERGY IN
Food calories

ENERGY OUT
Physical activity ~20–30%
Food digestion ~10%
Resting metabolism ~65–70%

FIGURE 11.4 **The energy balance equation.** Body weight remains constant if the number of calories consumed equals the number of calories expended. Many factors influence components of the energy balance equation, some of which are out of an individual's control.

© Ryan McVay/Getty Images RF; © Royalty-Free/CORBIS; © Brand X Pictures/PunchStock; © Stockdisc/PunchStock; © Stockdisc/PunchStock; © C Squared Studios/Getty Images RF; © Comstock/Jupiter Images; © Photodisc/PunchStock

FACTORS CONTRIBUTING TO EXCESS BODY FAT

Body weight and body composition may be determined by multiple factors that vary with each individual.

Energy Balance

The key to maintaining a healthy body weight and keeping a healthy ratio of fat to fat-free mass across the lifespan is **energy balance** (Figure 11.4). In general terms, energy balance is the relationship between the amount of energy (calories) taken into the body through food and drink (energy in), and the amount of calories expended (energy out). If we look at the energy balance equation today for

> **energy balance** A condition that occurs when energy intake equals energy expenditure; the key to achieving and maintaining a healthy body weight.
>
> **TERMS**

many Americans, it is tipped toward the energy-in side—a *positive energy balance* that promotes weight gain. This means that many people take in more calories than they expend. A *negative energy balance* is the opposite condition, which occurs when energy intake is less than energy use.

This relatively simple equation, however, doesn't reflect the many factors that influence what and how much we eat, how much physical activity we engage in, and how our bodies process energy and respond to changes in diet and exercise patterns. Factors that influence the components of energy balance can be grouped into genetic, physiological, lifestyle, psychosocial, and environmental factors. Although some of the factors are outside your control, the good news is that you can control key aspects of the energy balance equation through choices you make every day. Specific strategies for altering energy balance are discussed throughout this chapter.

Genetic Factors

Estimates of the genetic contribution to obesity vary widely, from about 25% to 40% of an individual's body fat. Scientists have so far identified more than 600 genes associated with obesity. Genes influence body size and shape, body fat distribution, and metabolic rate. Genetic factors also affect the ease with which weight is gained as a result of overeating and where on the body extra weight is added.

If both parents are obese, their children have an 80% risk of being obese; children with only one obese parent face a 50% risk of becoming obese. In studies that compared adoptees and their biological parents, the weights of the adoptees were found to be more like those of the biological parents than those of the adoptive parents, again indicating a strong genetic link.

Hereditary influences, however, must be balanced against the contribution of environmental factors. Not all children of obese parents become obese, and normal-weight parents may have overweight children. Environmental factors like diet and exercise are probably responsible for such differences. Thus the tendency to develop obesity may be inherited, but the expression of this tendency is affected by environmental influences.

The *set-point theory* suggests that our bodies are designed to maintain a normal and generally stable weight within a narrow range, or at a "set point," despite the variability in energy intake and expenditure. This theory is based on the idea that the rate at which our body burns calories adjusts according to the amount of food that we eat, but it does not imply that we cannot maintain weight loss.

It is true that some people have a harder time losing weight and maintaining weight loss than others. However, with increased exercise and attention to diet, even those with a genetic tendency toward obesity can maintain a healthy body weight. And regardless of genetic factors, lifestyle choices remain the cornerstone of successful weight management.

Physiological Factors

Metabolism is a key physiological factor in the regulation of body fat and body weight. Hormones, fat cell types, and possibly gut flora also play roles.

Metabolism   Metabolism is the sum of all the vital processes by which food energy and nutrients are made available to and used by the body. The largest component of metabolism, **resting metabolic rate (RMR),** is the energy required to maintain vital body functions, including respiration, heart rate, body temperature, and blood pressure, while the body is at rest. As shown in Figure 11.4, RMR accounts for about 65–70% of daily energy expenditure. The energy required to digest food accounts for as much as 10% of daily energy expenditure. The remaining 20–30% is expended during physical activity.

Both genetics and behavior affect metabolic rate. Men, who have a higher proportion of muscle mass than women do, have a higher RMR because muscle tissue is more metabolically active than fat. A higher RMR means that a person burns more calories while at rest and can therefore take in more calories without gaining weight.

A number of factors reduce metabolic rate, making weight management more challenging. Low-calorie intake and weight loss reduce RMR. When energy intake declines and weight is lost, the body responds by trying to conserve energy, reducing both RMR and the energy required to perform physical tasks. In essence, the body "defends" the original starting weight. For example, consider two people of the same size and activity level who both currently weigh 150 pounds, but one of whom used to weigh 170 pounds; the individual who lost weight will need to consume fewer calories to maintain the 150-pound weight than the person who had always been at that weight. This physiological response of the body points to the importance of preventing weight gain in the first place.

RMR also tends to decline with age, possibly the result of a decline in lean body mass. Weight loss also involves loss of lean muscle mass (along with fat mass). One reason why exercise is so important throughout life and during a weight loss program is that exercise can help maintain muscle mass and metabolic rate.

Hormones   Hormones clearly play a role in the accumulation of body fat, especially for females. Hormonal changes at puberty, during pregnancy, and at menopause contribute to the amount and location of fat accumulation. One hormone thought to be linked to obesity is *leptin*. Secreted by the body's fat cells, leptin is carried to the brain, where it appears to let the brain know how big or small the body's fat stores are. With this information, the brain can regulate appetite and metabolic rate accordingly. Leptin levels are higher in people who are obese, but obesity may cause the body to be less responsive to leptin's signals. Low-calorie diets may reduce leptin and cause an increase in appetite.

Insulin is another hormone that may affect weight management, possibly through regulation of appetite and fat storage. Some studies have found that when people eat foods that cause large swings in insulin levels—a rapid increase followed by a rapid decline—they feel hungrier and consume more calories. Researchers are investigating whether limiting insulin swings might also help reduce the decline in resting metabolism that occurs with weight loss. Research is ongoing, but you can reduce the potential negative impact of insulin on weight management by limiting foods high in added sugars and highly processed grains; consume a diet rich in unprocessed whole grains and a variety of vegetables and whole fruits, as well as other high-fiber foods.

As most of us will admit, hunger is often *not* the primary reason we overeat. Cases of obesity based solely or primarily on hormone abnormalities do exist, but they are rare.

Fat Cells   The amount of fat (adipose tissue) the body can store is a function of the number and size of fat (adipose) cells. Some people are born with an above-average number of fat cells and thus have the potential for storing more energy as body fat. Overeating at critical times, such as in childhood, can cause the body to create more fat cells. If a person loses weight, fat cell content is depleted, but it is unclear whether the number of fat cells can be decreased. Fat tissue is not a passive form of energy storage; fat cells send out chemical signals that affect multiple organs and systems, including those controlling appetite, metabolism, and immunity.

Gut Microbiota   The human intestine houses millions of bacteria that form the intestinal flora (gut flora). These bacteria help digest the foods you eat and they produce some vitamins. Studies show that lean and overweight humans may differ in the composition of their intestinal flora, suggesting that intestinal flora may be involved in the development of obesity. Although the general composition of intestinal microbiota is similar in most healthy people, the species composition is highly personalized and largely determined by environment and diet. Diets high in processed foods have been linked to less diverse intestinal microbiota and to a higher proportion of bacteria types that are associated with increased energy absorption and hormonal changes that increase appetite—both factors that can contribute to obesity. More research is needed into the precise impact of gut microbiota and on how changes to the bacterial balance might help individuals lose weight and maintain weight loss.

resting metabolic rate (RMR)   The energy required to maintain vital body functions, including respiration, heart rate, body temperature, and blood pressure, while the body is at rest.   **TERMS**

Lifestyle Factors

Although genetic and physiological factors may increase the risk for excess body fat, they are not sufficient to explain the increasingly high rate of obesity seen in the United States. The gene pool has not changed dramatically in the past 60 years, but the rate of obesity among Americans has more than doubled. Clearly other factors are at work—particularly lifestyle factors such as increased energy intake, especially in the form of processed low-nutrient foods, and decreased physical activity.

Energy Intake and Dietary Patterns Americans today consume more calories overall than in the past—up nearly 20% since 1983—and more of those calories come from low-quality foods. Americans now eat out more frequently and rely more heavily on fast food and packaged convenience foods. Restaurant and packaged food portions sizes tend to be large; the foods themselves are often low in essential nutrients and high in empty calories from added sugars, processed carbohydrates, and solid fats. As described in Chapter 9, the typical American diet is far from the pattern recommended in the Dietary Guidelines for Americans.

Physical Activity Activity levels among Americans are declining, beginning in childhood and continuing throughout life. Many schools have cut back on physical education classes and recess. Most adults drive to work, sit all day, and then relax in front of the television at night. Incidence of overweight is consistently linked to excessive screen time—whether the time is spent watching television, playing video games, or using computers. Additionally, fewer than half of all adults meet the current Physical Activity Guidelines for Americans.

Sleep Short sleep duration and sleep debt are associated with increased BMI and abdominal obesity, but researchers are still investigating how they might be linked. Lack of sleep may affect hormone levels (for example, increases in ghrelin), appetite regulation, and metabolism. Short sleep duration is also associated with increased snacking and overall energy intake. Use of multimedia may contribute to sleep deprivation and increase both energy intake and sedentary time. Getting adequate sleep is critical for overall wellness; see Chapter 2 for more on sleep.

Psychosocial Factors

Many people have learned to use food as a means of coping with stress and negative emotions. When food and eating become the primary means of regulating emotions, binge eating or other disturbed eating patterns can develop.

Obesity is strongly associated with socioeconomic status. The prevalence of obesity in women and children tends to decrease as income level goes up, though it stays the same in men. These differences may reflect the greater sensitivity and concern for a slim physical appearance among upper-income women, as well as greater access to information about nutrition, to unprocessed and low-calorie foods, and to opportunities for physical activity. It may also reflect the greater acceptance of obesity among certain ethnic groups, as well as different cultural values related to food choices.

In many families and cultures, food is used as a symbol of love and caring. It is an integral part of social gatherings and celebrations. In such cases, it may be difficult to change established eating patterns because they are linked to cultural and family values.

Environmental Factors

The environment in which most Americans live and work is "obesogenic"—meaning it promotes overconsumption of calories while discouraging physical activity, thereby promoting weight gain rather than weight maintenance or loss.

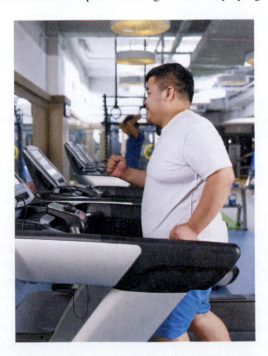

Regular physical activity is a key lifestyle strategy for weight loss and maintenance.

© imtmphoto/Alamy RF

Ask Yourself

QUESTIONS FOR CRITICAL THINKING AND REFLECTION

How do you view your own body composition? Where do you think you've gotten your ideas about how your body should look and perform? In light of what you've read in this chapter, do the ideals and images promoted in our culture seem reasonable? Do they seem healthy?

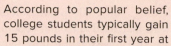

WELLNESS ON CAMPUS
The Freshman 15: Fact or Myth?

According to popular belief, college students typically gain 15 pounds in their first year at school—the infamous "freshman 15." Is this the fate of all college students, or is it a myth that adds stress for body-conscious young adults?

Research indicates that the truth lies somewhere between these two scenarios. Although many people do gain weight in the first year at college, the amount of weight gain varies. A study that looked at a group of male and female students during their first three years of college found significant three-year gains for weight, BMI, percent body fat, and fat mass, with weight gain highest during freshman and junior years. Studies find that about 60% of students gain weight in their freshman year and they gain, on average, 7.5 pounds. Comparatively, those in the same age group who are not attending college tend to gain 3–4 pounds during this time of life. Reasons for the weight gain include newfound food independence, changes in eating habits, stress, and social comparison and the influence of roommates and friends. Another study evaluating how snacks and stress contribute to weight gain for many college freshmen demonstrated an increased demand for unhealthy snack foods as the college semester progressed and in particular at the very end of the semester.

Even small weight increases can pose a health risk or contribute to lower self-esteem. Changes in body composition—specifically, increased body fat—can become a troublesome pattern for students. Even if they don't have a spike in weight during their first year, college-educated individuals tend to experience a moderate but steady weight gain during and after college.

More important, whether the weight gain is 5 pounds, 15 pounds, or even more, freshman weight gain is avoidable! In addition to the healthy eating strategies for college students described in Chapter 9, follow these tips and guidelines for avoiding freshman weight gain:

- Listen to your hunger cues, eating when you are hungry (and not for emotional reasons) and stopping when you are satisfied.

- Watch portion sizes, and avoid second and third servings; many people underestimate portion sizes by up to 25%.

- Avoid getting "too hungry"; don't go longer than 3–4 hours without eating. This means don't skip meals—especially breakfast.

- Plan ahead so that you have healthy snacks handy.

- Avoid late-night eating.

- Be more physically active: Walk to and from class, use the campus fitness facility, and consider taking a sports class for credit (e.g., tennis, dance, aerobics, weight training).

SOURCES: Vadeboncoeur, C., N. Townsend, and C. Foster. 2015. A meta-analysis of weight gain in first year university students: is freshman 15 a myth? *BMC Obesity* 2: 22; Smith-Jackson, T., and J. J. Reed. 2012. Freshman women and the "Freshman 15": Perspectives on prevalence and causes of college weight gain. *Journal of American College Health,* 60(1): 14–20; Wansink, B., et al. 2013. College cafeteria snack food purchases become less healthy with each passing week of the semester. *Public Health Nutrition* 16(7): 1291–1295; Gropper, S. S., et al. 2012. Weight and body composition changes during the first three years of college. *Journal of Obesity,* September 25; Gillen, M. M., and E. S. Lefkowitz. 2011. The "freshman 15": Trends and predictors in a sample of multiethnic men and women. *Eating Behaviors* 12(4): 261–266.

The food industry promotes the sale of high-calorie processed foods at every turn (for example, vending machines that offer mainly chocolate bars and unhealthy snacks, airlines that offer complimentary soft drinks, and restaurants that provide all-you-can-eat fried food buffets). People living in areas with limited access to healthy foods and opportunities for physical activity may suffer consequences of this obesogenic environment more so than those who live in more enriched environments where healthier choices exist.

Many experts observe that U.S. agricultural policy encourages farmers to produce corn and its byproduct, high fructose corn syrup, at the expense of fruits and vegetables. As a result, over the past 30 years, the price of fruits and vegetables rose much faster than the prices of other consumer goods, while the price of sugar, sweets, and carbonated drinks declined. Experts recommend shifts in federal policy to promote increased consumption of unprocessed whole grains, whole fruits, legumes and a variety of other nonstarchy vegetables, nuts, fish, and vegetable oils, as well as decreased consumption of red meat, processed meats, and processed foods high in added sugars, refined grains, solid fats, and sodium.

Issues of price and availability of healthy food can have a profound impact on food choices. It is estimated that more than 2 million U.S. households have no access to a supermarket. Low-income neighborhoods often have only fast-food venues or convenience stores offering high-calorie, highly processed foods. Public policies can also have a positive influence. For example, the new regulations requiring chain restaurants and vending machine operators to post calorie information should help consumers make more informed choices.

Designing healthy communities can help the United States to combat obesity by encouraging increased physical activity and healthier food choices. Look around your community, school, and workplace: What aspects of the environment make it easier or more difficult to make healthy choices?

What foods are available for purchase—and where and at what cost? Does the community environment and transportations system support walking? Are there safe spaces to engage in physical activity?

ADOPTING A HEALTHY LIFESTYLE FOR SUCCESSFUL WEIGHT MANAGEMENT

Slow weight gain—just one or two pounds per year—is a major cause of overweight and obesity, so weight management is important for everyone, not just for people who are currently overweight (see the box, "The Freshman 15: Fact of Myth"?). A good time to develop a lifestyle for successful weight management is during your teens and early adulthood, when many behavior patterns form.

Dietary Patterns and Eating Habits

In contrast to *dieting,* which may involve some form of food restriction, a *diet* or *dietary pattern* refers to your daily food choices over the long term. Everyone has a diet, but not everyone is dieting. You need to develop a way of eating that you enjoy and that enables you to maintain a healthy body composition. Use the healthy dietary patterns recommended by the Dietary Guidelines for Americans, MyPlate, or the DASH Eating Plan as the basis for a healthy diet (see Chapter 9). For weight management, pay special attention to total calories, especially sugars, portion sizes, energy and nutrient density, and eating habits.

Total Calories MyPlate suggests approximate daily energy needs based on gender, age, and activity level. However, individual energy balance may be a more important consideration for weight management than total calories consumed (refer back to Figure 11.4). To maintain your current weight, the calories you eat must equal the number you burn, based on your personal energy balance. To lose weight, you must reduce your energy intake and/or increase the number of calories you burn; to gain weight, the reverse is true. If you choose to track calories, keep in mind that most people underestimate their energy intake and that energy needs change as body weight changes.

If weight loss is your goal, most experts recommend an increase in physical activity with moderate calorie reduction targeting added sugars, refined carbohydrates and other processed foods, and solid fats. A focus on calorie sources can be just as

important as total energy intake for successful weight loss. To maintain weight loss, you will need to maintain some degree of the calorie restriction you used to lose the weight. Therefore, you need to adopt a practical level of food intake that provides all the essential nutrients and that you can live with over the long term. For many people, maintaining weight loss is more difficult than losing the weight in the first place.

Portion Sizes Overconsumption of total calories is tied closely to portion sizes. Many Americans are unaware that the portions of packaged foods and of foods served at restaurants have increased in size, and most of us significantly underestimate the amount of food we eat (Figure 11.5). Studies have found that the larger the meal, the more calories people tend to eat. Portion size is associated with body weight, so limiting portion sizes is critical for maintaining a healthy body weight.

Quality of Food Choices: Energy (Calorie) Density and Nutrient Density Experts recommend that you pay attention to *energy density*—the number of calories per ounce or gram of weight in a food. Ice cream, potato chips, croissants, crackers, and cakes and cookies are examples of foods high in energy density; in general, diets high in energy density are associated with higher rates of obesity. Foods that are low in energy density have more volume and bulk—that is, they are relatively heavy but have few calories, often due

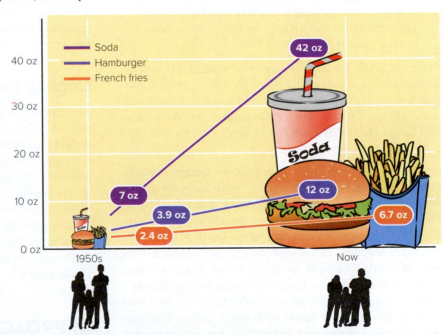

FIGURE 11.5 The new (ab)normal. Portion sizes have been growing. So have we. The average restaurant meal today is more than four times larger than in the 1950s. Adults today are, on average, 26 pounds heavier. To become healthier eaters, there are things we can do for ourselves and our community. Order the smaller meals on the menu, split a meal with a friend, or eat half and take the rest home. Ask the managers at favorite restaurants to offer smaller meals.

SOURCE: Centers for Disease Control and Prevention; for more information, visit http://MakingHealthEasier.org/TimeToScaleBack.

...gh water and fiber content. Examples include air-popped popcorn, fat-free yogurt with fruit, and fresh fruits and vegetables.

As you decrease consumption of foods high in energy density, choose foods high in nutrient density—foods that are relatively low in calories but high in nutrients. Strategies for lowering the energy density of your diet while at the same time increasing its nutrient density include the following:

- Eat whole fruit with breakfast and for dessert.
- Add extra vegetables to sandwiches, casseroles, stir-fry dishes, pizza, pasta dishes, and fajitas.
- Start meals with a bowl of broth-based soup; include a green salad or fruit salad.
- Snack on fresh fruits and vegetables rather than crackers, chips, or other processed snack foods.
- Limit serving sizes of energy-dense foods such as butter, mayonnaise, cheese, fatty meats, croissants, and other sources of solid fats.
- Pay special attention to your beverage choices—many sweetened drinks are low in nutrients and high in calories from added sugar; for example, a can of regular soda may have more than 35 grams of added sugar but no other nutrients, while the same amount of low-fat milk has no added sugars and is rich in many essential nutrients.
- Limit processed foods, especially those high in added sugars and refined carbohydrates; these are usually energy dense, nutrient poor, and also high on the glycemic index, which may increase rather than reduce your appetite.

Processed foods labeled "fat-free" or "reduced fat" may be high in calories as well as high-glycemic-index refined carbohydrates; stick to the calorie and food pattern recommendations offered by the Dietary Guidelines for Americans, MyPlate, or the DASH Eating Plan (see Chapter 9).

Eating Habits Equally important to weight management is the habit of eating regular meals daily, including breakfast and snacks. Eating every 3–4 hours can help to fuel healthy metabolism, maintain muscle mass, and prevent between-meal hunger that often leads to unhealthy snacking. Skipping meals leads to excessive hunger, feelings of deprivation, and increased vulnerability to binge eating or unhealthy snacking. In addition to establishing a regular pattern of eating, set some rules to govern your food choices. Balance your meals with whole grains, lean protein, fiber-rich fruits and vegetables, low-fat dairy, and moderate amounts of healthy fats. Rules for breakfast might be these, for example: Choose a high-fiber cereal that is low in added sugar with low-fat milk on most days; save pancakes and waffles for special occasions unless they are whole grain. A good goal is to eat in moderation; no foods need to be entirely off-limits, though some should be eaten judiciously.

Physical Activity and Exercise

Physical activity and exercise burn calories and keep the metabolism geared to using food for energy instead of storing it as fat. Exercise has a positive effect on metabolism. When people exercise, they increase the number of calories their bodies burn at rest (resting metabolic rate). Regular physical activity also improves cardiovascular and respiratory health, enhances mood, results in a higher quality of sleep, increases self-esteem, and gives us a sense of accomplishment. All these changes enhance our ability to engage in long-term healthful lifestyle behaviors.

Thinking and Emotions

The way you think about yourself influences, and is influenced by, how you feel and how you act. In fact, research on people who struggle with their weight indicates that many of these individuals suffer from low self-esteem and the negative emotions that accompany it. Often people with low self-esteem mentally compare the actual self to an internally held picture of an "ideal self," an image based on perfectionistic goals and beliefs about how they and others should be. The more these two pictures differ, the larger the negative impact on self-esteem and the more likely the presence of negative emotions.

Besides the internal picture of ourselves, we all carry on an internal dialogue about events happening to us and around us. This *self-talk* can be self-deprecating or positively motivating, depending on our beliefs and attitudes. Having realistic beliefs and goals and practicing positive self-talk and problem solving support a healthy lifestyle.

Coping Strategies

Appropriate coping strategies help you deal with the stresses of life. They are also an important lifestyle factor in weight management. Those who overeat might use food to alleviate loneliness or to serve as a pickup for fatigue, as an antidote to boredom, or as a distraction from problems.

Those who recognize that they are misusing food in such ways can analyze their eating habits with fresh eyes. They can consciously attempt to find new coping strategies and begin to use food appropriately—to fuel life's activities, to foster growth, and to bring pleasure, but *not* as a way to manage stress.

APPROACHES TO OVERCOMING A WEIGHT PROBLEM

Americans spend approximately $60 billion on weight loss efforts every year, including diet plans, diet products, and health club memberships. If you are overweight, you may already be creating a plan to lose weight and keep it off. You have many options.

Doing It Yourself

If you need to lose weight, focus on adopting the healthy lifestyle described throughout this book. The right weight for you will evolve naturally, and you won't have to diet. Combine modest cuts in energy intake with exercise, and avoid very-low-calorie diets.

According to the Centers for Disease Control and Prevention, reasonable weight loss for someone who is obese is 5–10% of body weight over six months. For example, for someone who weighs 200 pounds, a 5% weight loss equals 10 pounds, or reducing weight to 190 pounds. The person in this example may still be in the "overweight" or "obese" range, but this degree of weight loss can reduce the chronic disease risks related to obesity. Modest weight loss can also be easier to maintain. American Heart Association guidelines state that even smaller weight loss, in the 3–5% range, is beneficial if maintained.

Don't try to lose weight more rapidly than 0.5–2.0 pounds per week, which will require a negative energy balance of at least 250–1000 calories per day. A pound of body fat represents 3500 calories, meaning a negative energy balance of that amount over time that should in theory result in a loss of 1 pound of body weight. Although that may be true at the start of a diet, as described earlier in the chapter, because of physiological changes, as you reduce energy intake and lose weight, a greater negative calorie balance is needed to compensate for reductions in metabolism. In general, a low-calorie diet should provide at least 1200–1500 calories per day.

Most low-calorie diets cause a rapid loss of body water at first. When this phase passes, weight loss declines. As a result, dieters are often misled into believing that their efforts are not working. They then give up, not realizing that smaller, mostly fat, losses later in the diet are actually better than the initial larger, mostly fluid losses.

For many Americans, maintaining weight loss is a bigger challenge than losing weight. Weight management is a life-long project. A registered dietitian or nutritionist can recommend an appropriate plan for you when you want to lose weight on your own. For more tips, refer to the Behavior Change Strategy section at the end of the chapter.

Diet Books

Many people who try to lose weight by themselves fall prey to one or more of the dozens of diet books on the market. Although some contain useful advice and motivational tips, most make empty promises. Accept books that advocate a balanced approach to diet plus exercise and sound nutritional advice, but reject any book that advocates an unbalanced way of eating; claims to be based on a "scientific breakthrough" or to have the "secret to success;" uses gimmicks, such as matching eating to blood type; or promises quick weight loss or severely limits food choices.

Many diets can cause weight loss in the short term; however, the real difficulty is finding a safe and healthy pattern of food choices and physical activity that results in long-term maintenance of a healthy body weight and reduced risk of chronic disease (see the box "Are All Calories and Dietary Patterns Equal for Weight Loss?")

Dietary Supplements and Diet Aids

Dietary supplements marketed for weight loss are subject to fewer regulations than over-the-counter (OTC) medications. According to the Federal Trade Commission, more than half of advertisements for weight loss products make representations that are likely to be false. And although the FTC will order companies to stop making baseless and bogus product claims when monitors become aware of them, consumers are urged to critically evaluate any product that sounds too good to be true.

Formula Drinks and Food Bars
Canned diet drinks, powders used to make shakes, and diet food bars and snacks are designed to achieve weight loss by substituting for some or all of a person's daily food intake. However, most people find it difficult to use these products for long periods, and muscle loss and other serious health problems may result if they are used as the sole source of nutrition for an extended period. Use of such products sometimes results in rapid short-term weight loss, but the weight is typically regained because users don't learn to change their eating and lifestyle behaviors.

Herbal Supplements
Most herbal weight loss products work by increasing urination (causing water loss); by stimulating the central nervous system (causing the body's activities to speed up or increasing metabolism); or by affecting levels of brain chemicals (causing appetite suppression). As described in Chapter 9, herbs are marketed as dietary supplements, so little information is available about

CRITICAL CONSUMER
Are All Calories and Dietary Patterns Equal for Weight Loss?

Many popular diets are promoted as the weight loss answer for all, but researchers continue to investigate the complex web of factors that influence the success or failure of efforts to lose weight and maintain that loss over time. Most researchers agree that total calorie intake is important, but preliminary evidence suggests some specific foods and eating patterns may help improve the odds for people trying to manage their weight.

Dietary Composition: Balance of Protein, Carbohydrates, and Fats

Scientists are investigating whether particular patterns of macronutrient intake (e.g., higher protein, lower fat, or lower carbohydrate) are better for weight loss, for weight loss maintenance, and/or for improving health markers such as blood fat levels. How might macronutrient balance impact weight management? Two possible areas of influence are appetite and resting metabolic rate (RMR).

Eating foods high in protein tends to make people feel fuller than eating foods high in fat or carbohydrate. This increase in satiety may help people refrain from overeating, thereby managing overall energy intake. On the flip side, foods high in simple sugars and refined carbohydrates may cause an increase in appetite (and eating) due to swings in the level of insulin.

As described in the chapter, one of the key challenges for weight loss maintenance is the drop in RMR that follows weight loss. In some small, short-term studies, researchers compared the impact on RMR following weight loss associated with low-fat, low-glycemic-index, and low-carbohydrate dietary patterns. On average, the low-carbohydrate dietary pattern showed the smallest reduction in RMR. However, additional studies are needed to confirm the findings and determine their importance over a longer time period. An additional challenge is that extreme shifts in macronutrient balance are difficult for people to maintain over time.

How do diets measure up over months and years? Researchers studying the impact of dietary composition over the long term have not found significant differences. A study comparing weight loss among adults assigned to one of four reduced-calorie diets differing in percentages of protein, carbohydrate, and fat found that weight loss at two years was similar for all four diets (about nine pounds). Weight loss was strongly associated with attendance at group sessions. Other studies have also found little difference in weight loss among popular reduced-calorie diets; most resulted in modest weight loss and reduced heart disease risk factors. The more closely people adhered to each diet, the more weight they lost. The American Heart Association notes that many dietary patterns can produce weight loss, and their latest guidelines list more than 15 dietary approaches that can lead to weight loss if calories are reduced.

An interesting finding of multiple weight-loss and weight-maintenance studies is that different people seem to respond differently to different diets. So, for example, on a diet with a given balance of protein, carbohydrates, and fats, some people experience much greater weight loss than others. Similarly, changes in RMR after weight loss on different diets also vary. These findings point to individual differences in the factors affecting weight management—genetics, metabolism, hormones, intestinal flora. Thus, there is no single best diet for everyone. Researchers are looking to identify methods of matching people to an approach likely to be effective, but in the meantime, people can experiment with different dietary patterns to see what seems to work best for them.

---

effectiveness, proper dosage, drug interactions, or side effects. In addition, labels may not accurately reflect the ingredients and dosages present, and safe manufacturing practices are not guaranteed. Weight loss occurs only while the product is being taken.

Other Supplements Fiber is another common ingredient in OTC diet aids, promoted for appetite control. Many diet aids contain only 3 or fewer grams of fiber, which does not contribute much toward the recommended daily intake of 25–38 grams. Other popular dietary supplements include chitosan, chromium picolinate, conjugated linoleic acid, glucomannan, carnitine, green tea extract, pyruvate, calcium, B vitamins, and a number of products labeled "fat absorbers," "fat blockers," and "starch blockers." Research has not found these products to be effective, and many have potentially adverse side effects.

Weight Loss Programs

Weight loss programs come in a variety of types, including noncommercial support organizations, commercial programs, websites, and clinical programs. According to the NIH, safe and effective weight loss programs should include the following:

- Healthy eating plans that reduce calories but do not exclude specific foods or food groups
- Tips on ways to increase moderate-intensity physical activity
- Tips on healthy habits that also keep your cultural needs in mind, such as lower-fat versions of your favorite foods
- Slow and steady weight loss; depending on your starting weight, experts recommend losing weight at a rate of 0.5–2.0 pounds per week

Quality Food Choices in Healthy Dietary Patterns

The typical American dietary pattern—high in sugary beverages, refined carbohydrates, red meat, and solid fats—is associated with obesity. For weight loss, choose high-quality calorie sources in a healthier dietary pattern; refer back to the patterns and food choices recommended in Chapter 9. Remember that there is more to foods than just energy! Focus on consuming high-quality calorie sources, whatever dietary composition you choose. Nutrient-dense foods can help with both weight management and chronic disease prevention:

- **Choose often:** unprocessed whole grains; a variety of vegetables from different MyPlate subgroups (e.g., don't overconsume potatoes, which have a high glycemic index); whole fruits; beans, fish, nuts, seeds, and other healthy protein sources; and plant oils.

- **Limit:** sugar-sweetened beverages, refined grains and sweets, red and processed meats, and solid fats (replace with plant oils and not with processed grains).

To reduce calorie intake, start by cutting empty calories from sugar-sweetened beverages and the processed foods that many Americans typically overeat. For some people, reducing sugar may be more effective than focusing on fats.

Weight Loss Maintenance: Clues from the National Weight Control Registry

Important lessons can be drawn from the National Weight Control Registry—an ongoing study of people who have lost significant amounts of weight and kept it off. The average participant in the registry has lost 71 pounds and kept the weight off for more than five years. Nearly all participants use a combination of diet and exercise to manage their weight. Common strategies include eating breakfast, self-monitoring weight and food intake, and getting regular exercise of about one hour per day. The most common dietary pattern used by registry participants was low-fat/high-carbohydrate. Greater weight regain in this group of individuals comes as a result of decreases in physical activity, having less dietary restraint, less individual monitoring of body weight, and increases in percentage of energy intake from fat. This study illustrates that to lose weight and keep it off, you must decrease daily calorie intake and/or increase daily physical activity—and continue to do so over your lifetime. Whatever dietary pattern you choose, make sure it contains high-quality, nutrient-dense foods and that it is a pattern that you can maintain over the long term.

SOURCES: Hall, K. D., et al. 2016. Energy expenditure and body composition changes after an isocaloric ketogenic diet in overweight and obese men. *American Journal of Clinical Nutrition* 104(2): 324-333; Ebeling, C. B., et al. 2012. Effects of dietary composition on energy expenditure during weight-loss maintenance. *Journal of the American Medical Association* 307(24): 2627–2634; M. D. Jensen, et al. 2014. AHA/ACC/TOC guideline for the management of overweight and obesity in adults: A report of the American College of Cardiology/American Heart Association Task Force on Practice Guidelines and the Obesity Society. *Circulation* 129(25 Suppl. 2): S102–S138; Thomas, J.G., et al. 2014. Weight-loss maintenance for 10 years in the National Weight Control Registry. *American Journal of Preventive Medicine* 46(1): 17–23; U.S. Department of Health and Human Services and U.S. Department of Agriculture. 2015. *2015–2020 Dietary Guidelines for Americans,* 8th ed. (http://health.gov/dietaryguidelines/2015/guidelines); Sacks, F. M., et al. 2009. Comparison of weight-loss diets with different compositions of fat, protein, and carbohydrate. *New England Journal of Medicine* 360(9): 859–873.

- A recommendation for medical evaluation and care if you have health problems, are taking medication, or are planning to follow a special formula diet that requires monitoring by a doctor

- A plan to keep the weight off after you have lost it

Noncommercial Weight Loss Programs Noncommercial programs such as TOPS (Take Off Pounds Sensibly) and Overeaters Anonymous (OA) mainly provide group support. They do not advocate any particular diet but do recommend seeking professional advice for creating an individualized plan. These types of programs are generally free. Your physician or a registered dietitian can also provide information and support for weight loss.

Commercial Weight Loss Programs Commercial weight loss programs typically provide group support, nutrition education, physical activity recommendations, and behavior modification advice. Some also make available packaged foods to assist in following dietary advice.

In addition to the features of a safe and effective program outlined earlier, commercial weight loss programs should provide information about all fees and costs, including those of supplements and prepackaged foods, as well as data on risks and expected outcomes of participating in the program. They should also have a registered dietitian on staff along with qualified counselors and health professionals.

A strong commitment and a plan for maintenance are especially important because only about 10–15% of program participants maintain their weight loss—the rest gain back all or more than they had lost. One study found that important predictors of weight loss and maintenance of weight loss in commercial programs include daily self-monitoring; an increased intake of vegetables, fruit, and low-fat dairy products;

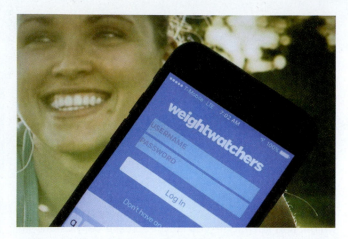

Weight Watchers is one of the best-known commercial weight loss programs. It offers plans that include in-person meetings as well as fully online options.

© Bloomberg/Getty Images

decreased intake of sweets; regular exercise; and adequate water consumption. A strong predictor of weight gain was frequent television viewing.

Online Weight Loss Programs   Online diet websites have millions of subscribers worldwide. Most weight loss websites combine self-help with group support through chat rooms, bulletin boards, and e-newsletters. Many sites offer online self-assessment for diet and physical activity habits as well as a meal plan; some provide access to a staff professional for individualized help. Many are free, but some charge a weekly or monthly fee. Research suggests that this type of program provides an alternative to in-person diet counseling and can lead to weight loss for some people.

Clinical Weight Loss Programs   Medically supervised clinical programs are usually located in a hospital or other medical setting. Designed to help those who are severely obese, these programs typically involve a closely monitored, very-low-calorie diet. The cost of a clinical program is usually high, but insurance may cover part of the fee for those with obesity-related health problems.

QUICK STATS

On average, bariatric surgery patients lose about **15%** to **30%** of their starting weight.
—National Institutes of Health, 2016

Ask Yourself

QUESTIONS FOR CRITICAL THINKING AND REFLECTION

Why do you think people continue to buy into fad diets and weight loss gimmicks, even though they are constantly reminded that the key to weight management is lifestyle change? Have you ever tried a fad diet or weight loss supplement? If so, what were your reasons for trying it? What were the results?

Prescription Drugs

The medications most often prescribed for weight loss are appetite suppressants that reduce feelings of hunger or increase feelings of fullness. Appetite suppressants usually work by increasing levels of catecholamine or serotonin—two brain chemicals that affect mood and appetite.

Appetite suppressants approved for long-term use include Belviq (lorcaserin), Qsymia (phentermine and topiramate extended-release), Contrave (bupropion and naltrexone), and Saxenda (liraglutide). All prescription weight-loss drugs have potential side effects: Reported side effects include sleeplessness, nervousness, and euphoria, as well as increases in blood pressure and heart rate. Headaches, constipation or diarrhea, dry mouth, and insomnia are other side effects.

The other prescription medication approved for long-term use is Xenical (orlistat). This medication works differently: It is a lipid inhibitor that blocks fat absorption in the intestines. Orlistat prevents about 30% of the fat in food from being digested. Similar to the fat substitute olestra, orlistat reduces the absorption of fat-soluble vitamins and antioxidants. Therefore, taking a vitamin supplement is highly recommended for people taking orlistat. Side effects include diarrhea, cramping, and other gastrointestinal problems if users do not follow a low-fat diet. Alli is an FDA-approved, lower-dose version of orlistat that is sold over the counter.

Prescription medications work best in conjunction with behavior modification. Studies have generally found that appetite suppressants produce modest weight loss above the loss expected with nondrug obesity treatments. Unfortunately, weight loss tends to level off or reverse after four to six months on a medication, and many people regain the weight they've lost when they stop taking the medication.

Prescription weight loss drugs are not for people who want to lose only a few pounds. The latest federal guidelines advise people to try lifestyle modification for at least six months before trying drug therapy. Prescription drugs are recommended only in certain cases: for people who have been unable to lose weight with nondrug options and who have a BMI over 30 (or over 27 if two or more additional risk factors such as diabetes and high blood pressure are present).

Surgery

The National Health and Nutrition Examination Survey (NHANES) estimates that 6.3% of adult Americans age 20 years and over have a BMI greater than 40, qualifying them as extremely or "morbidly" obese. The number of severely obese people has nearly doubled in the past two decades. Extreme obesity is a serious medical condition that is often complicated by other health problems such as diabetes, heart disease, arthritis, and sleep disorders. Surgical intervention may be necessary as a treatment of last resort. According to the NIH, weight loss (bariatric) surgery is recommended for patients with a BMI greater than 40, or greater than 35 with obesity-related illnesses.

Bariatric surgery modifies the gastrointestinal tract by changing either the size of the stomach or how the intestine drains, thereby reducing food intake. The keys to success with surgical weight loss procedures are adequate follow-up and continued motivation to permanently change eating patterns and lifestyle behaviors.

BODY IMAGE AND EATING DISORDERS

The collective picture of the body as seen through the mind's eye, **body image** consists of perceptions, images, thoughts, attitudes, and emotions. A negative body image is characterized by dissatisfaction with the body in general or some part of the body in particular. Recent surveys indicate that the majority of Americans, many of whom are not overweight, are unhappy with their body weight or with some aspect of their appearance. People may be dissatisfied with their bodies for a variety of reasons, including sociocultural forces and factors that are specific to life stages.

Losing weight or getting cosmetic surgery does not necessarily improve body image. In fact, improvements in body image may occur in the absence of changes in weight or appearance. Many experts now believe that body image issues must be dealt with as part of treating obesity and eating disorders. Developing a positive body image is an important aspect of psychological wellness and an important component of successful weight management.

Severe Body Image Problems

Poor body image can cause significant psychological distress. A person can become preoccupied with a perceived defect in appearance, thereby damaging self-esteem and interfering with relationships. Adolescents and adults who have a negative body image are more likely to diet restrictively, eat compulsively, or develop some other form of disordered eating.

When a person's dissatisfaction with his or her own body image becomes extreme, the condition is called *body dysmorphic disorder* (BDD). Although many people are dissatisfied with some part of their body or their appearance,

these concerns usually do not constantly occupy their thoughts. Individuals with BDD are constantly preoccupied and upset about body imperfections, such as thinking their nose is too big or that their hair is never right. They cannot seem to stop checking or obsessing about their appearance, often focusing on perceived flaws that are not obvious to others. Low self-esteem is common. Individuals with BDD may spend hours every day thinking about their flaws and looking at themselves in mirrors; they may desire and seek repeated cosmetic surgeries. BDD affects about 2% of Americans, males and females in equal numbers. It usually begins before age 18 but can begin in adulthood.

This condition is related to obsessive-compulsive disorder and can lead to depression, social phobia, and suicide if left untreated. An individual with BDD needs to get professional evaluation and treatment. Medication and therapy can help people with BDD.

In some cases, body image may bear little resemblance to fact. People suffering from the eating disorder anorexia nervosa typically have a severely distorted body image—they believe themselves to be fat even when they have become emaciated. Distorted body image is also a hallmark of *muscle dysmorphia,* a disorder experienced by some bodybuilders and other active people who see themselves as small and out of shape despite being very muscular. Those who suffer from muscle dysmorphia may let obsessive exercise—particularly muscle-building exercise, such as weight training—interfere with their work and relationships. They may also use steroids and other potentially dangerous muscle-building drugs.

Eating Disorders

Problems with body weight and weight control are not limited to excessive body fat. A growing number of people, especially adolescent girls and young women, experience **eating disorders**—psychological disorders characterized by

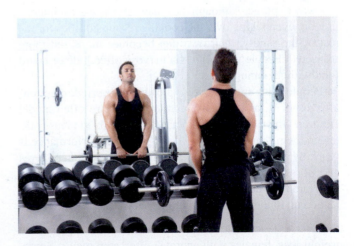

Exercise is a healthy practice, but people with muscle dysmorphia sometimes exercise compulsively, building their lives around their workouts. Compulsive exercise can lead to injuries and problems with work and relationships.
© Antonio Balaguer Soler/123RF

Ask Yourself

QUESTIONS FOR CRITICAL THINKING AND REFLECTION
Describe your own body image in the fewest words possible. What satisfies you most and least about your body? Do you think your self-image is in line with the way others see you?

?

severe disturbances in body image, eating patterns, and eating-related behaviors. The main categories of eating disorders include anorexia nervosa, bulimia nervosa, and binge-eating disorder. In the United States, it is estimated that 20 million women and 10 million men suffer from an eating disorder some time in their lives. Many more people have abnormal eating habits and attitudes about food that disrupt their lives, even though these habits do not meet the criteria for a major eating disorder.

Anorexia Nervosa

A person with **anorexia nervosa** does not eat enough food to maintain a reasonable body weight. An estimated 0.5–3.7% of women suffer from anorexia nervosa in their lifetimes. Although it can occur earlier or later, anorexia typically develops during puberty and the late teenage years, with an average age of onset of about 19 years.

CHARACTERISTICS OF ANOREXIA NERVOSA People with anorexia have an intense fear of gaining weight or becoming fat. Their body image is so distorted that even when emaciated they think they are fat. People with anorexia may engage in compulsive behaviors or rituals that help keep them from eating, though some may also binge and **purge.** A purge occurs when a person uses vomiting, laxatives, excessive exercise, restrictive dieting, enemas, diuretics, or diet pills to compensate for food that she or he has eaten and that the person fears will produce weight gain. Some people also use vigorous and prolonged exercise to reduce body weight as a way to purge. Although they may express a great interest in food, even taking over the cooking responsibilities for the rest of the family, their own diet becomes more and more restricted. People with anorexia nervosa often hide or hoard food without eating it.

People with anorexia are typically introverted, emotionally reserved, and socially insecure. They are often model children who rarely complain and are anxious to please others and win their approval. Although school performance is typically above average, they are often critical of themselves and not satisfied with their accomplishments. For people with anorexia nervosa, their entire sense of self-esteem may be tied up in their evaluation of their body shape and weight.

HEALTH RISKS OF ANOREXIA NERVOSA Because of extreme weight loss, females with anorexia often stop menstruating, become intolerant of cold, and develop low blood pressure and heart rate. They develop dry skin that is often covered by fine body hair like that of a newborn. Their hands and feet may swell and take on a blue tinge.

Anorexia nervosa has been linked to a variety of medical complications, including disorders of the cardiovascular, gastrointestinal, endocrine, and skeletal systems. When body fat is virtually gone and muscles are severely wasted, the body turns to its own organs in a desperate search for protein. Death can occur from heart failure caused by electrolyte imbalances. About 1 in 10 women with anorexia dies of starvation, cardiac arrest, or other medical complications—the highest death rate for any psychiatric disorder. Depression is also a serious risk: About half the fatalities related to anorexia are suicides.

Bulimia Nervosa

A person suffering from **bulimia nervosa** engages in recurrent episodes of binge eating followed by purging. Bulimia is often difficult to recognize because sufferers conceal their eating habits and usually maintain a normal weight, although they may experience weight fluctuations of 10–15 pounds. Although bulimia usually begins in adolescence or young adulthood, it has begun to emerge at increasingly younger (11–12 years) and older (40–60 years) ages; the average age of onset is about 20 years.

CHARACTERISTICS OF BULIMIA NERVOSA During a binge, a bulimic person may rapidly consume thousands of calories. This is followed by an attempt to get rid of the food by purging, usually by vomiting or using laxatives or diuretics. During a binge, bulimics feel as though they have lost control and cannot stop or limit how much they eat. Some binge and purge only occasionally; others do so many times every day.

People with bulimia may appear to eat normally, but they are rarely comfortable around food. Binges usually occur in secret and can become nightmarish—uncontrollably raiding the kitchen for food, going from one grocery store to another to buy food, or stealing food. During the binge, food acts as an anesthetic, blocking out feelings. Afterward, bulimics feel physically drained and emotionally spent. They usually feel deeply ashamed and disgusted with both themselves and their behavior and terrified that they will gain weight from the binge.

Major life changes such as leaving for college, getting married, having a baby, or losing a job can trigger a

TERMS

anorexia nervosa An eating disorder characterized by a refusal to maintain body weight at a minimally healthy level and an intense fear of gaining weight or becoming fat; self-starvation.

purge The use of vomiting, laxatives, excessive exercise, restrictive dieting, enemas, diuretics, or diet pills to compensate for food that has been eaten and that the person fears will produce weight gain.

bulimia nervosa An eating disorder characterized by recurrent episodes of binge eating and purging—overeating and then using compensatory behaviors such as vomiting, laxatives, and excessive exercise to prevent weight gain.

binge-purge cycle. At such times, stress is high and the person may have no good outlet for emotional conflict or tension. As with anorexia nervosa, bulimia sufferers are often insecure and depend on others for approval and self-esteem. They may hide difficult emotions such as anger and disappointment from themselves and others. Binge eating and purging become a way of dealing with feelings.

HEALTH RISKS OF BULIMIA NERVOSA The binge-purge cycle of bulimia places a tremendous strain on the body and can have serious health effects. Contact with vomited stomach acids erodes tooth enamel. Bulimic people often develop tooth decay because they binge on foods that are high in simple sugars. Repeated vomiting or the use of laxatives, in combination with deficient calorie intake, can damage the liver and kidneys and cause cardiac arrhythmia. Chronic hoarseness and esophageal tearing with bleeding may also result from vomiting. More rarely, binge eating can lead to rupture of the stomach. Although many bulimic women maintain normal weight, even a small weight loss to lower-than-normal weight can cause menstrual problems. And although less often associated with suicide or premature death than anorexia, bulimia is associated with increased depression, excessive preoccupation with food and body image, and sometimes disturbances in cognitive functioning.

Binge-Eating Disorder

Binge-eating disorder affects 3–5% of American women and 2% of men. It is characterized by uncontrollable eating, usually followed by feelings of guilt and shame about weight gain. Common eating patterns are eating more rapidly than normal, eating until uncomfortably full, eating when not hungry, and preferring to eat alone. Binge eaters may eat large amounts of food throughout the day, with no planned mealtimes. Many people with binge-eating disorder mistakenly see rigid dieting as the only solution to their problem. However, rigid dieting usually causes feelings of deprivation and a return to overeating.

Compulsive overeaters rarely eat because of hunger. Instead food is used as a means of coping with stress, conflict, and other difficult emotions or to provide solace and entertainment. People who do not have the resources to deal effectively with stress may be more vulnerable to binge-eating disorder. Inappropriate overeating often begins during childhood. In some families, eating may be used as an activity to fill otherwise empty time. Parents may reward children with food for good behavior or withhold food as a means of punishment, thereby creating distorted feelings about the experience of eating.

Binge eaters are almost always obese, so they face all the health risks associated with obesity. In addition, binge eaters may have higher rates of depression and anxiety. To overcome binge eating, a person must learn to put food and eating into proper perspective and develop other ways of coping with stress and painful emotions.

Other Patterns of Disordered Eating

Eating habits and body image run along a continuum from healthy to seriously disordered. Where an individual falls along that continuum can change depending on life stresses, illnesses, and many other factors. People who have feeding or eating disorders that can cause significant distress or impairment, but who do not meet the criteria for another feeding or eating disorder, may be classified as having **other specified feeding or eating disorders (OSFED),** according to the American Psychiatric Association's *Diagnostic and Statistical Manual of Mental Disorders*. Examples of OSFED include atypical anorexia nervosa, a condition in which weight is not below normal; bulimia nervosa, a condition with less frequent bulimic episodes; purging disorder, a condition without binge eating; and night eating syndrome, in which the individual engages in excessive nighttime food consumption.

If you suspect you have an eating problem, don't go it alone or delay getting help because disordered eating habits can develop into a full-blown eating disorder. Check with your student health or counseling center—nearly all colleges have counselors and medical personnel who can help you or refer you to a specialist if needed.

Treating Eating Disorders

Anorexia nervosa treatment first involves averting a medical crisis by restoring adequate body weight; then the psychological aspects of the disorder can be addressed. The treatment of bulimia nervosa or binge-eating disorder involves first stabilizing the eating patterns, then identifying and changing the patterns of thinking that led to disordered eating, and then improving coping skills. Concurrent problems, such as depression, anxiety, and other mental disorders may be present and must also be addressed.

Treatment of eating disorders usually involves a combination of psychotherapy and medical management. The therapy may be done individually or in a group; sessions involving the entire family may be recommended. A support or self-help group can be a useful adjunct to such treatment.

TERMS

binge-eating disorder An eating disorder characterized by episodes of binge eating and a lack of control over eating behavior in general.

other specified feeding or eating disorders (OSFED) A feeding or eating disorder that causes significant distress or impairment but does not meet the criteria for another feeding or eating disorder.

Ask Yourself

?

QUESTIONS FOR CRITICAL THINKING AND REFLECTION

Do you know someone you suspect may suffer from an eating disorder? Have you ever experienced disordered eating patterns yourself? If so, can you identify the reasons for them?

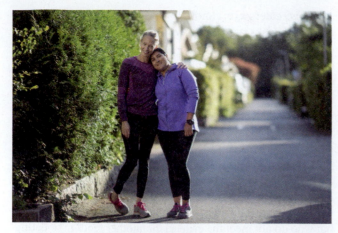

A balanced, realistic attitude toward weight management is part of overall wellness. Many healthy people do not fit society's image of ideal body size and shape.

© Zing Images/Getty Images RF

Positive Body Image: Finding Balance

Knowing when you've reached the limits of healthy change—and learning to accept those limits—is crucial for overall wellness. People who view their bodies positively tend to be more intuitive eaters, relying on internal hunger and fullness cues to regulate what and how much they eat. They think more about how their bodies feel and function than how they appear to others. Many healthy people do not fit society's image of ideal body size and shape. To minimize your risk of developing a body image problem, keep the following strategies in mind:

- Focus on healthy habits and good physical health.

- Put concerns about physical appearance in perspective. Your worth as a human being does not depend on how you look.

- Practice body acceptance. You can influence your body size and type through lifestyle to some degree, but the fact is that some people are genetically designed to be bigger or heavier than others.

- Find things to appreciate in yourself besides an idealized body image. People who can learn to value other aspects of themselves are more accepting of the physical changes that occur naturally with age.

- View eating as a morally neutral activity—eating dessert isn't "bad" and doesn't make you a bad person.

- See the beauty and fitness industries for what they are. Realize that their goal is to prompt you to feel dissatisfaction with yourself so that you will buy their products.

Weight management needs to take place in a positive and realistic atmosphere. A reasonable weight must take into account a person's weight history, social circumstances, metabolic profile, and psychological well-being.

SUMMARY

- Body composition is the relative amounts of fat-free mass and fat in the body. *Overweight* and *obesity* refer to body weight or the percentage of body fat that exceeds what is associated with good health.

- Standards for assessing body weight and body composition include body mass index (BMI) and percent body fat.

- Too much or too little body fat is linked to health problems; the distribution of body fat can also be a significant risk factor for many kinds of health problems.

- Genetic factors help determine a person's weight, but the influence of heredity can be overcome with attention to lifestyle factors.

- Physiological factors involved in the regulation of body weight and body fat include metabolic rate, hormonal influences, and the size and number of fat cells.

- Nutritional guidelines for weight management include consuming a moderate number of calories; limiting portion sizes, energy density, and the intake of simple sugars, refined carbohydrates, and solid fats; and developing an eating schedule and rules for food choices.

- Activity guidelines for weight management emphasize daily physical activity and regular sessions of cardiorespiratory endurance exercise and strength training.

- Weight management requires developing positive self-talk and self-esteem, realistic weight and body composition goals, and a repertoire of appropriate techniques for handling stress and other emotional and physical challenges.

• People can be successful at long-term weight loss on their own by combining diet and exercise.

• Diet books, over-the-counter diet aids and supplements, and formal weight loss programs should be assessed for safety and efficacy.

• Professional help is needed in cases of severe obesity; medical treatments include prescription drugs and surgery.

• An inaccurate or negative body image is common and can lead to psychological distress.

• Dissatisfaction with weight and shape are common to all eating disorders. Anorexia nervosa is characterized by self-starvation, distorted body image, and an intense fear of gaining weight. Bulimia nervosa is characterized by recurrent episodes of uncontrolled binge eating and frequent purging. Binge-eating disorder involves binge eating without regular use of compensatory purging. People with other patterns of disordered eating have some symptoms of eating disorders but do not meet the full diagnostic criteria for anorexia, bulimia, or binge-eating disorder.

FOR MORE INFORMATION

American Diabetes Association. Provides information, a free newsletter, and referrals to local support groups; the website includes an online diabetes risk assessment.

http://www.diabetes.org

Calorie Control Council. Includes a variety of interactive calculators, including an Exercise Calculator that estimates the calories burned from various forms of physical activity.

http://www.caloriecontrol.org

Centers for Disease Control and Prevention: Obesity. The home page for accessing all the CDC's information about overweight and obesity, their health risks, statistics, and diet and exercise.

http://www.cdc.gov/obesity/index.html

FDA Center for Food Safety and Applied Nutrition: Dietary Supplements. Provides background facts and information on the current regulatory status of dietary supplements, including compounds marketed for weight loss.

http://www.fda.gov/Food/DietarySupplements/default.htm

National Heart, Lung, and Blood Institute (NHLBI): *Aim for a Healthy Weight.* Provides information and tips on diet and physical activity, as well as a BMI calculator.

http://www.nhlbi.nih.gov/health/educational/lose_wt/

National Institute of Diabetes and Digestive and Kidney Diseases (NIDDK): *Weight-Control Information Network.* Provides information and referrals for problems related to obesity, weight control, and nutritional disorders.

http://win.niddk.nih.gov

Resources for People Concerned About Eating Disorders:

Eating Disorder Referral and Information Center
http://www.edreferral.com

Eating Disorders Coalition for Research, Policy and Action
http://www.eatingdisorderscoalition.org

MedlinePlus: Eating Disorders
http://www.nlm.nih.gov/medlineplus/eatingdisorders.html

National Association of Anorexia Nervosa and Associated Disorders
630-577-1330 (help line)
http://www.anad.org

National Eating Disorders Association
800-931-2237
http://www.nationaleatingdisorders.org

National Institute of Mental Health: Eating Disorders
http://www.nimh.nih.gov/health/topics/eating-disorders/index.shtml

SELECTED BIBLIOGRAPHY

Andreyeva, T., A. S. Tripp, and M. B. Schwartz. 2015. Dietary quality of Americans by Supplemental Nutrition Assistance Program participation status: A systematic review. *American Journal of Preventive Medicine* 49(4): 594–604.

Boulangé, C. L., et al. 2016. Impact of the gut microbiota on inflammation, obesity, and metabolic disease. *Genome Medicine.* DOI: 10.1186/s13073-016-0303-2.

Bray, M. S., et al. 2016. NIH working group report—using genomic information to guide weight management: from universal to precision treatment. *Obesity* 24(1): 14–22.

Brown, P. 2016. Carbohydrate study leaves diet researchers divided. *MedPageToday*, 11 July 2016 (http://www.medpagetoday.com/primarycare/dietnutrition/59012).

Buttitta, M., et al. 2014. Quality of life in overweight and obese children and adolescents: A literature review. *Quality of Life Research* 23(4): 1117–1139.

Center for Disease Control and Prevention. 2014a. *Diabetes 2014 Report Card* (http://www.cdc.gov/diabetes/pdfs/library/diabetesreportcard2014.pdf).

Center for Disease Control and Prevention 2014b. *Facts about Physical Activity* (http://www.cdc.gov/physicalactivity/data/facts.html).

Centers for Disease Control and Prevention. 2014. *FastStats: Obesity and Overweight, 2014* (http://www.cdc.gov/nchs/fastats/obesity-overweight.htm).

Centers for Disease Control and Prevention 2015a. *About Child & Teen BMI* (http://www.cdc.gov/healthyweight/assessing/bmi/childrens_bmi/about_childrens_bmi.html).

Centers for Disease Control and Prevention. 2015b. *How Much Physical Activity Do Adults Need?* (http://www.cdc.gov/physicalactivity/basics/adults/).

Centers for Disease Control and Prevention. 2015c. *Public Health Genomics. Obesity* (http://www.cdc.gov/genomics/public/features/obesity.htm).

Centers for Disease Control and Prevention. 2015d. *Rethink Your Drink. Healthy Weight: It's Not a Diet, It's a Lifestyle* (http://www.cdc.gov/healthyweight/healthy_eating/drinks.html).

Champagne, C. M., et al. 2011. Dietary intakes associated with successful weight loss and maintenance during the Weight Loss Maintenance trial. *Journal of the American Dietetic Association* 111(12): 1826–1835.

Cheung, P. C., et al. 2016. Childhood obesity incidence in the United States: A systematic review. *Childhood Obesity* 12(1): 1–11.

Diabetes Prevention Program Research Group. 2015. Long-term effects of lifestyle intervention or metformin on diabetes development and microvascular complications over 15-year follow-up: the Diabetes Prevention Program Outcomes Study. *Lancet: Diabetes & Endocrinology* 3(11): 866–875.

Dyson, P. 2015. Low carbohydrate diets and type 2 diabetes: what is the latest evidence? *Diabetes Therapy* 6(4): 411–424.

Fothergill, E., et al. 2016. Persistent metabolic adaptation 6 years after "The Biggest Loser" competition. *Obesity* 24(8): 1612–1619.

Freedhoff, Y., and K. D. Hall. 2016. Weight loss diet studies: we need help not hype. *Lancet* 388(10047): 849–851.

Global BMI Mortality Collaboration. 2016. Body-mass index and all-cause mortality: individual-participant-data meta-analysis of 239 prospective studies in four continents. *Lancet* 388(10046): 776–786.

Hall, K. D., et al. 2016. Energy expenditure and body composition changes after an isocaloric ketogenic diet in overweight and obese men. *American Journal of Clinical Nutrition* 104(2): 324–333.

Healthy People 2020. 2015. Nutrition, Physical Activity, and Obesity. Office of Disease Prevention and Health Promotion, Centers for Disease Control and Prevention (https://www.healthypeople.gov/2020/leading-health-indicators/2020-lhi-topics/Nutrition-Physical-Activity-and-Obesity/data).

Hutchesson, M. J., et al. 2014. Changes to dietary intake during a 12-week commercial web-based weight loss program: A randomized controlled trial. *European Journal of Clinical Nutrition* 68(1): 64–70.

Karl, J. P., et al. 2015. Effects of carbohydrate quantity and glycemic index on resting metabolic rate and body composition during weight loss. *Obesity* 23(11): 2190–2198.

Khera, R., et al. 2016. Association of pharmacological treatments for obesity with weight loss and adverse events: A systematic review and meta-analysis. *Journal of the American Medical Association* 315(22): 2424–2434.

Kiviruusu, O., et al. 2016. Self-esteem and body mass index from adolescence to mid-adulthood. A 26-year follow-up. *International Journal of Behavioral Medicine* 23(3): 355–363.

Lasikiewicz, N., et al. 2014. Psychological benefits of weight loss following behavioural and/or dietary weight loss interventions. A systematic research review. *Appetite* 72:123–137.

Levis, L. 2016. Are all calories equal? *Harvard Magazine*, May–June, 2016.

Ludwig, D. 2016. Lifespan weighed down by diet. *Journal of the American Medical Association* 315(21): 2269–2270.

MacLean, P. S., et al. 2015. NIH working group report: innovative research to improve maintenance of weight loss. *Obesity* 23(1): 7–15.

Marketdata Enterprises, Inc. 2015. *The U.S. Weight Loss Market: 2015 Status Report & Forecast.* January 29.

Masters, E., et al. 2013. The impact of obesity on US mortality levels: The importance of age and cohort factors in population estimates. *American Journal of Public Health* 103(10): 1895–1901.

Mazidi, M., et al. 2016. Gut microbiome and metabolic syndrome. *Diabetes and Metabolic Syndrome.* DOI: 10.1016/j.dsx.2016.01.024.

Micali, N., et al. 2014. Frequency and patterns of eating disorder symptoms in early adolescence. *Journal of Adolescent Health* 54(5): 574–581.

Mozzafarian, D. 2016. Dietary and policy priorities for cardiovascular disease, diabetes, and obesity: A comprehensive review. *Circulation* 133(2): 187–225.

National Center for Health Statistics. 2016. *Health, United States, 2015: With Special Feature on Racial and Ethnic Health Disparities.* Hyattsville, MD: National Center for Health Statistics.

National Eating Disorder Association. n.d. *Get the Facts on Eating Disorders. What Are Eating Disorders?* (https://www.nationaleatingdisorders.org/get-facts-eating-disorders).

National Eating Disorders Association. n.d. *Other Specified Feeding or Eating Disorders* (https://www.nationaleatingdisorders.org/other-specified-feeding-or-eating-disorder).

National Institutes of Health, National Institute of Diabetes and Digestive and Kidney Disorders. 2016. Definition and Facts for Bariatric Surgery (https://www.niddk.nih.gov/health-information/health-topics/weight-control/bariatric-surgery/Pages/definition-facts.aspx).

Ogden, C., et al. 2015. *Prevalence of Obesity Among Adults and Youth: United States, 2011–2014.* NCHS Data Brief No. 219. (http://www.cdc.gov/nchs/products/databriefs/db219.htm).

Ogilvie, R. P., et al. 2016. Actigraphy measured sleep indices and adiposity: The Multi-Ethnic Study of Atherosclerosis (MESA). *Sleep* 39(9): 1701–1708.

Pedersen, E., et al. 2014. High protein weight loss diets in obese subjects with type 2 diabetes mellitus. *Nutrition, Metabolism & Cardiovascular Diseases* 24(5): 554–562.

Postrach, E., et al. 2013. Determinants of successful weight loss after using a commercial web-based weight reduction program for six months: Cohort study. *Journal of Medical Internet Research* 15(10).

Prevention Program Research Group. 2015. Long-term effects of lifestyle intervention or metformin on diabetes development and microvascular complications over 15-year follow-up: the Diabetes Prevention Program Outcomes Study. *Lancet: Diabetes & Endocrinology* 3(11): 866–875.

Pritchard, S. J., et al. 2014. A randomised trial of the impact of energy density and texture of a meal on food and energy intake, satiation, satiety, appetite and palatability responses in healthy adults. *Clinical Nutrition* 33(5): 768–775.

Rouhani, M. H., et al. 2016. Associations between dietary energy density and obesity: A systematic review and meta-analysis of observational studies. *Nutrition.* DOI: 10.1016/j.nut.2016.03.017.

Siegel, K.R., et al. 2016. Association of higher consumption of foods derived from subsidized commodities with adverse cardiometabolic risk among US adults. *JAMA Internal Medicine* 176(8): 1124–1132.

Sheikh, V. K., and H. A. Raynor. 2016. Decreases in high-fat and/or high-added-sugar food group intake occur when a hypocaloric, low-fat diet is prescribed within a lifestyle intervention: a secondary cohort analysis. *Journal of the Academy of Nutrition and Dietetics* 116(10): 1599–1605.

Tsukumo, D. M., et al. 2015. Translational research into gut microbiota: New horizons on obesity treatment: Updated 2014. *Archives of Endocrinology and Metabolism* 59(2): 154–160.

U.S. Department of Health and Human Services and U.S. Department of Agriculture. 2015. *2015-2020 Dietary Guidelines for Americans,* 8th ed. (http://health.gov/dietaryguidelines/2015/guidelines).

Whitham, C., et al. 2013. Weight maintenance over 12 months after weight loss resulting from participation in a 12-week randomized controlled trial comparing all meal provision to self-directed diet in overweight adults. *Journal of Human Nutrition and Dietetics* 27(4): 384–390.

Williams, R. A., et al. 2013. Assessment of satiety depends on the energy density and portion size of the test meal. *Obesity* 22(2): 318–324.

Zheng, H., et al. 2013. Obesity and mortality risk: New findings from body mass index trajectories. *American Journal of Epidemiology* 178(11): 1591–1599.

The behavior management plan described in Chapter 1 provides an excellent framework for a weight management program. Following are some suggestions about specific ways you can adapt that general plan to control your weight.

Motivation and Commitment

Make sure you are motivated and committed before you begin. Failure at weight loss is a frustrating experience that can make it more difficult to lose weight in the future. Think about why you want to lose weight. Make a list of your reasons for wanting to lose weight, and post it in a prominent place.

Setting Goals

Choose a reasonable weight you think you would like to reach over the long term, and be willing to renegotiate it as you get further along. Break down your long-term weight and behavioral goals into a series of short-term action-oriented goals.

Creating a Negative Energy Balance

When your weight is constant, you are burning approximately the same number of calories as you are taking in. To tip the energy balance toward weight loss, you must consume fewer calories, or burn more calories through physical activity, or both. To generate a negative energy balance, it's usually best to begin by increasing activity level rather than decreasing your calorie consumption.

Physical Activity

Consider how you can increase your energy output simply by increasing routine physical activity, such as walking or taking the stairs. (Chapter 10 lists activities that use about 150 calories.) If you are not already involved in a regular exercise routine aimed at increasing endurance and building or maintaining muscle mass, seek help from someone who is competent to help you plan and start an appropriate exercise routine. If you are already doing regular physical exercise, evaluate your program according to the guidelines in Chapter 10.

Diet and Eating Habits

If you can't generate a large enough negative energy balance solely by increasing physical activity, you may want to supplement exercise with modest cuts in your calorie intake. Your goal is to make small changes in your diet that you can maintain for a lifetime. Focus on cutting your intake of added sugars, refined carbohydrates, and solid fats and on eating a variety of nutritious foods in moderation. Don't skip meals, fast, or go on a very-low-calorie diet or a diet that is unbalanced.

Self-Monitoring

Keep a record of your weight and behavior change progress. Try keeping a record of everything you eat. Record what you plan to eat, in what quantity, *before* you eat. You'll find that just having to record something that is not okay to eat is likely to stop you from eating it. Also, keep track of your daily activities and your formal exercise program so that you can monitor increases in physical activity.

Putting Your Plan into Action

- Examine the environmental cues that trigger poor eating and exercise habits, and devise strategies for dealing with them. Anticipate problem situations, and plan ways to handle them more effectively.

- Create new environmental cues that will support your new healthy behaviors. Move fruits and vegetables to the front of the refrigerator.

- Get others to help. Talk to friends and family members about what they can do to support your efforts. Find a buddy to join you in your exercise program.

- Give yourself lots of praise and rewards. Focus attention on your accomplishments and achievements and congratulate yourself. Plan special nonfood treats for yourself, such as a walk or a movie. Reward yourself often and for anything that counts toward success.

- If you slip, don't waste time on self-criticism. Think positively instead of getting into a cycle of guilt and self-blame.

- Don't get discouraged. Be aware that, although weight loss is bound to slow down after the first loss of body fluid, the weight loss at this slower rate is more permanent than earlier, more dramatic, losses.

- Remember that weight management is a lifelong project. You need to adopt reasonable goals and strategies that you can maintain over the long term.

CHAPTER 12

CHAPTER OBJECTIVES

- Identify the major components of the cardiovascular system
- Describe the risk factors associated with cardiovascular disease
- Discuss the major forms of cardiovascular disease
- List the steps you can take to protect yourself against cardiovascular disease
- Explain the basic facts about cancer
- Discuss causes of cancer and how to avoid or minimize them
- Describe how cancer can be detected, diagnosed, and treated
- Describe common cancers as well as detection and treatment options for each

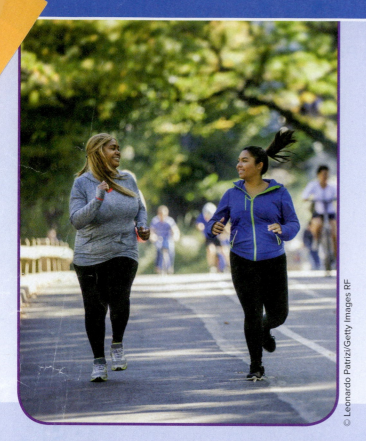

© Leonardo Patrizi/Getty Images RF

Cardiovascular Health and Cancer

Cardiovascular disease (CVD) affects more than 85 million Americans and is the leading cause of death in the United States, claiming one life every 40 seconds—more than 2200 Americans every day. Heart disease and stroke are the number-one and number-five causes of death, respectively, making them the most common life-threatening manifestations of CVD. Cancer is the second leading cause of human death in the United States, and is responsible for nearly one in four deaths, claiming over 595,000 lives annually—more than 1600 each day.

Although genes, age, and environmental factors play roles in the development of these diseases, CVD and cancer are also lifestyle diseases, linked to many lifestyle factors. The following sections provide information that can help you maintain a healthy heart for life and reduces your risks of developing cancer.

THE CARDIOVASCULAR SYSTEM

The **cardiovascular system (CVS)** consists of the heart and blood vessels, which includes both arteries and veins. Together they transport blood throughout the body (Figure 12.1). When the lungs are included, the system is known as the *cardiorespiratory* or *cardiopulmonary system*.

The heart is a four-chambered, fist-sized muscle located just beneath the sternum (breastbone). It pumps deoxygenated (oxygen-poor) blood to the lungs and delivers oxygenated (oxygen-rich) blood to the rest of the body. Blood actually

cardiovascular disease (CVD) The collective term for various diseases of the heart and blood vessels.

cardiovascular system (CVS) The system that circulates blood through the body; consists of the heart and blood vessels.

TERMS

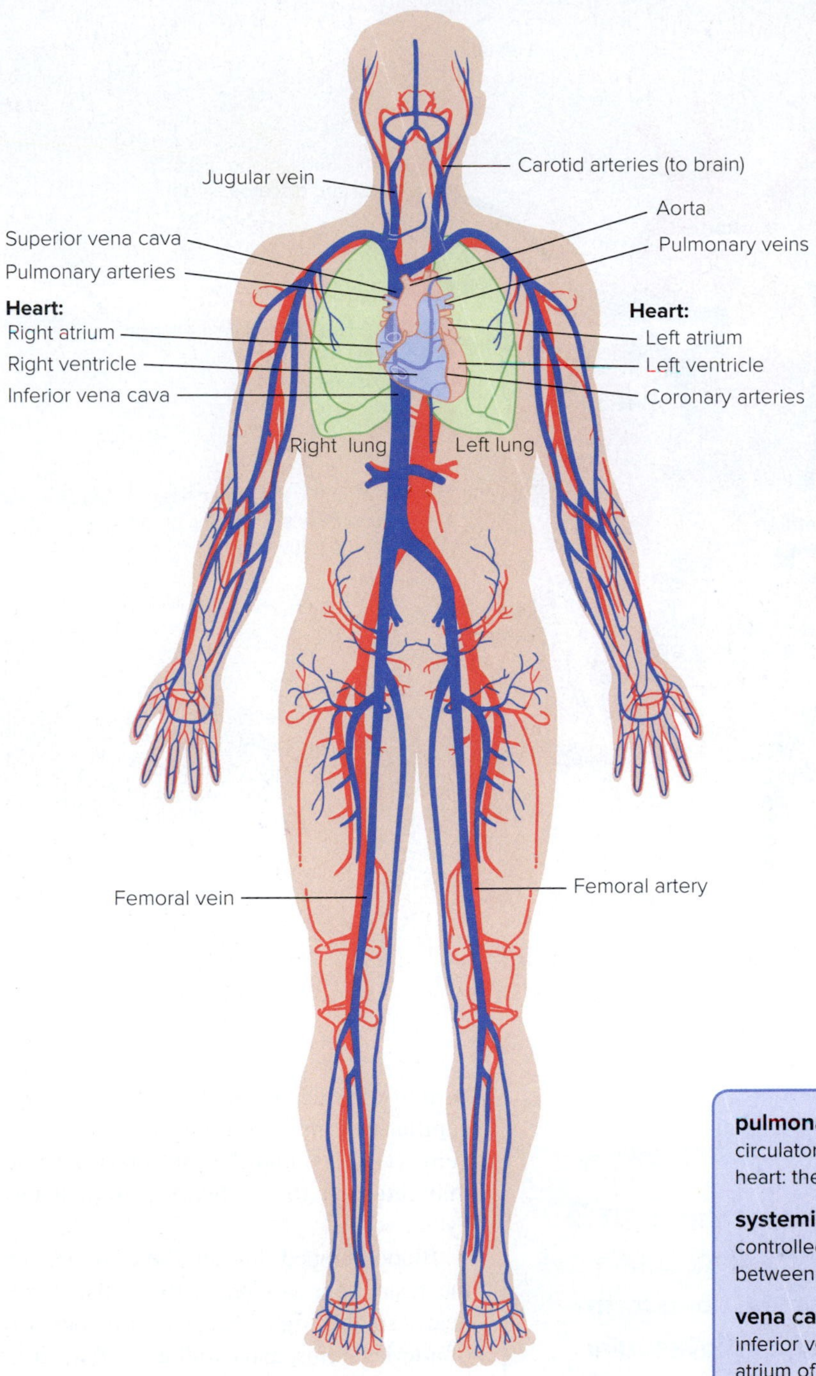

Jugular vein
Carotid arteries (to brain)
Aorta
Superior vena cava
Pulmonary veins
Pulmonary arteries
Heart:
Right atrium
Right ventricle
Inferior vena cava
Heart:
Left atrium
Left ventricle
Coronary arteries
Right lung
Left lung
Femoral vein
Femoral artery

FIGURE 12.1 The cardiorespiratory system.

travels through two separate circulatory systems. The right side of the heart pumps blood to the lungs in what is called **pulmonary circulation,** and the left side pumps blood through the rest of the body in the **systemic circulation.**

Oxygen-poor blood travels through the **superior vena cava** and **inferior vena cava** into the heart's right upper chamber, the **right atrium.** After the right atrium fills, it contracts and pumps blood into the heart's right lower chamber, the **right ventricle.** When the right ventricle is full, it contracts and pumps blood through the pulmonary arteries into the lungs. There, blood picks up oxygen and discards carbon dioxide, which is expelled during exhalation. The newly oxygenated blood flows from the lungs through the pulmonary veins into the heart's **left atrium.** When the left atrium fills, it contracts and pumps blood into the **left ventricle.** When the left ventricle fills, it pumps blood through the **aorta**—the body's largest artery—for distribution to the rest of the body's blood vessels. The path of blood flow through the heart and cardiorespiratory system is illustrated in Figure 12.2.

Each heartbeat consists of two basic parts: diastole and systole. During **diastole,** the time when the heart relaxes in between beats, the atria and ventricles fill with blood. At the end of diastole, the atria contract (atrial systole), which pumps blood into the ventricles. The atria then relax. During **systole,** the ventricles contract (ventricular systole) to pump blood out of the heart.

Blood pressure, the force exerted by blood on the walls of the blood vessels, is created by the pumping action of the heart and the resistance of the blood vessels. This is an important concept because high blood pressure is treated by medicines that work on contraction as well as on the overall resistance of the blood vessels.

The heartbeat—the sequence of contractions of the heart's four chambers—is controlled by electrical and nerve impulses. These signals originate in a bundle of specialized cells in the right atrium called the *sinoatrial node* or *pacemaker.*

TERMS

pulmonary circulation The part of the circulatory system controlled by the right side of the heart: the circulation of blood between the heart and the lungs.

systemic circulation The part of the circulatory system controlled by the left side of the heart: the circulation of blood between the heart and the rest of the body.

vena cava Either of two large veins (superior vena cava and inferior vena cava) through which blood is returned to the right atrium of the heart (plural, *venae cavae*).

atrium Either of the two upper chambers of the heart (left or right) in which blood collects before passing to the ventricles (plural, *atria*).

ventricle Either of the two lower chambers of the heart (left or right) that pump blood to the lungs and other parts of the body.

aorta The largest artery in the body; receives blood from the left ventricle and distributes it to the body.

diastole The relaxation phase of the heart.

systole The contraction phase of the heart.

blood pressure The force exerted by the blood on the walls of the blood vessels; created by the pumping of the heart and the resistance of the blood vessels.

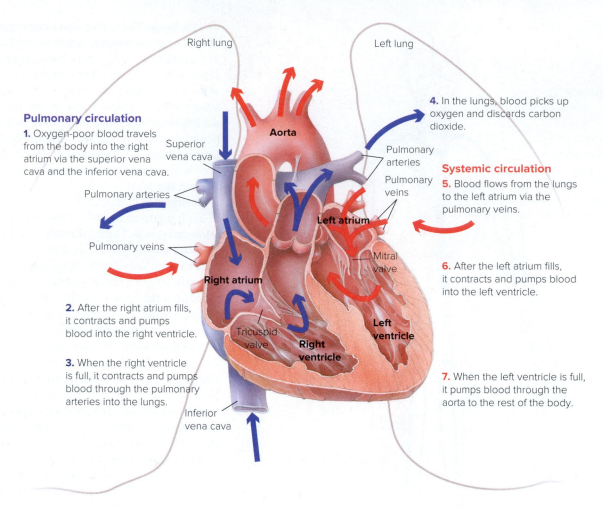

Pulmonary circulation

1. Oxygen-poor blood travels from the body into the right atrium via the superior vena cava and the inferior vena cava.

Superior vena cava

Pulmonary arteries

Pulmonary veins

Right atrium

2. After the right atrium fills, it contracts and pumps blood into the right ventricle.

3. When the right ventricle is full, it contracts and pumps blood through the pulmonary arteries into the lungs.

Tricuspid valve

Right ventricle

Inferior vena cava

Right lung

Left lung

Aorta

4. In the lungs, blood picks up oxygen and discards carbon dioxide.

Pulmonary arteries

Pulmonary veins

Left atrium

Mitral valve

Left ventricle

Systemic circulation

5. Blood flows from the lungs to the left atrium via the pulmonary veins.

6. After the left atrium fills, it contracts and pumps blood into the left ventricle.

7. When the left ventricle is full, it pumps blood through the aorta to the rest of the body.

FIGURE 12.2   Circulation in the heart. Blue arrows indicate oxygen-poor blood; red arrows indicate oxygen-rich blood.

Blood vessels are classified by size and function. **Veins** carry blood to the heart, whereas **arteries** carry blood away from the heart. Veins have thin walls, but arteries have thick elastic walls that enable them to expand and relax with the volume of blood being pumped through them.

After leaving the heart, the aorta branches into smaller and smaller vessels. The smallest arteries branch still further into **capillaries**—tiny vessels with walls only one cell thick. The capillaries deliver oxygen- and nutrient-rich blood to the tissues and pick up oxygen-poor,

carbon-dioxide-laden blood. From the capillaries, this blood empties into small veins (*venules*) and then into larger veins that return it to the heart to repeat the cycle.

Blood pumped through the chambers of the heart does not reach the cells of the heart, so the organ has its own network of arteries, veins, and capillaries. Two large vessels, the right and left **coronary arteries,** branch off the aorta and supply the heart muscle with oxygenated blood (Figure 12.3). Blockage of a coronary artery is the leading cause of heart attacks.

> **QUICK STATS**
>
> More than **1 in 3** American adults has at least one form of cardiovascular disease.
>
> —American Heart Association, 2016

> **TERMS**
>
> **vein** A vessel that carries blood to the heart.
>
> **artery** A vessel that carries blood away from the heart.
>
> **capillary** A small blood vessel that exchanges oxygen and nutrients between the blood and the tissues.
>
> **coronary artery** A blood vessel branching from the aorta that provides blood to the heart muscle.

RISK FACTORS FOR CARDIOVASCULAR DISEASE

Researchers have identified a variety of factors associated with an increased risk of developing cardiovascular disease. They are grouped into two categories: major risk factors and contributing risk factors. Some risk factors are linked to

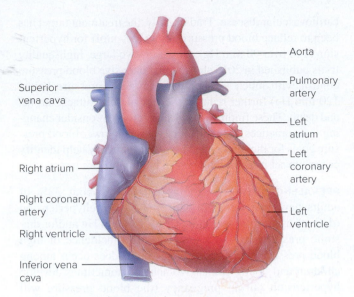

FIGURE 12.3 **Blood supply to the heart.**

(Labels on figure:)
Superior vena cava
Right atrium
Right coronary artery
Right ventricle
Inferior vena cava
Aorta
Pulmonary artery
Left atrium
Left coronary artery
Left ventricle

controllable aspects of lifestyle and can therefore be changed, referred to as modifiable risk factors. Others are beyond our control.

Major Risk Factors That Can Be Changed

The American Heart Association (AHA) identifies these major risk factors for CVD that can be changed: tobacco use, high blood pressure, unhealthy blood cholesterol levels, physical inactivity, obesity, and diabetes. Most Americans, including young adults, have at least one major risk factor for CVD.

Tobacco Use Annually, nearly one in five deaths is attributable to smoking. People who smoke a pack of cigarettes a day have twice the risk of heart attack as nonsmokers; smoking two or more packs a day triples the risk. When smokers have heart attacks, they are two to three times more likely than nonsmokers to die from them. Cigarette smoking also doubles the risk of stroke.

Smoking harms the cardiovascular system in the following ways: It damages the lining of arteries. It reduces the level of high-density lipoproteins (HDL), or "good" cholesterol. It raises the levels of triglycerides and low-density lipoproteins (LDL), or "bad" cholesterol. Nicotine increases blood pressure and heart rate. The carbon monoxide in cigarette smoke displaces oxygen in the blood, reducing the amount of oxygen available to the body. Smoking causes **platelets** to stick

together in the bloodstream, leading to clotting, and it speeds the development of fatty deposits in the arteries.

You don't have to smoke to be affected. The risk of developing heart disease increases up to 30% among those exposed to environmental tobacco smoke, also known as second-hand smoke, at home or at work. As of 2014, researchers estimate that nearly 34,000 nonsmokers die from heart disease each year as a result of exposure to environmental tobacco smoke.

Recently, electronic cigarettes (or e-cigarettes) have become popular, especially among teenagers and young adults. As of 2014, approximately 2.4 million middle and high school students were current (past 30-day) users of electronic cigarettes. Notably, e-cigarettes contain nicotine, which causes addiction, may harm brain development, and could lead to continued tobacco product use among youth. The Centers for Disease Control and Prevention (CDC) has identified electronic cigarettes as an area of concern due to the potential harm to public health in the United States.

High Blood Pressure High blood pressure, or **hypertension,** is a risk factor for many forms of cardiovascular disease, including heart attacks and stroke.

Blood pressure, the force exerted by the blood on the vessel walls, is created by the pumping action of the heart and the resistance of the arteries. High blood pressure occurs when too much force is exerted against the walls of the arteries. Many factors affect blood pressure, such as exercise or excitement. Short periods of high blood pressure are normal, but chronic high blood pressure is a health risk.

Health care professionals measure blood pressure with a stethoscope and an instrument called a *sphygmomanometer.* At home you can track your own blood pressure by using an electronic blood pressure monitor, and some new technologies measure blood pressure with wearable devices. A normal blood pressure reading for a healthy adult is below 120 systolic and below 80 diastolic. Blood pressure readings at this level are classified as prehypertension because they begin to carry risk. High blood pressure (hypertension) in adults is defined as equal to or greater than 140 over 90 mm Hg (Table 12.1); it is diagnosed based on the average of several readings taken at different times.

In about 90% of people with high blood pressure, the underlying cause is unknown. This type of high blood pressure is called *primary* (or *essential*) *hypertension* and is probably due to a combination of genetic and environmental factors, including obesity, stress, excessive alcohol intake, inactivity, and a diet high in sodium and solid fats. In the remaining 10% of people, the condition is caused by an identifiable underlying illness and is referred to as *secondary hypertension.* Although hypertension often cannot be cured, it can be managed with lifestyle changes and medications.

platelets Cells in the blood that are necessary for the formation of blood clots.   **TERMS**

hypertension Sustained abnormally high blood pressure.

Table 12.1	Blood Pressure Classification for Healthy Adults			
CATEGORY[a]	SYSTOLIC (mm Hg)		DIASTOLIC (mm Hg)	
Normal[b]	below 120	and	below 80	
Prehypertension	120–139	or	80–89	
Hypertension[c]				
Stage 1	140–159	or	90–99	
Stage 2	160 and above	or	100 and above	

[a]When systolic and diastolic pressures fall into different categories, the higher category should be used to classify blood pressure status.

[b]The risk of death from heart attack and stroke begins to rise when blood pressure is above 115/75.

[c]Based on the average of two or more readings taken at different physician visits. In people older than 50, systolic blood pressure greater than 140 mm Hg is a much more significant CVD risk factor than diastolic blood pressure.

SOURCE: National Heart, Lung, and Blood Institute. 2011. *The Seventh Report of the Joint National Committee on Prevention, Detection, Evaluation, and Treatment of High Blood Pressure* (NIH Publication No. 03-5233). Bethesda, MD: National Heart, Lung, and Blood Institute. These guidelines are under development, according to the National Heart, Lung, and Blood Institute (http://www.nhlbi.nih.gov/health-pro/guidelines/current/hypertension-jnc-7).

CAUSES High blood pressure results from an increased output of blood by the heart or from increased resistance to blood flow in the arteries. The latter condition can be caused by constriction of smooth muscle surrounding the arteries or by **atherosclerosis,** a disease process that causes arteries to become clogged and narrowed. (Atherosclerosis is discussed in detail later in this chapter.) Atherosclerosis also scars and hardens arteries, making them less elastic and further increasing blood pressure. When a person has high blood pressure, the heart must work harder than normal to force blood through the narrowed and stiffened arteries, straining both the heart and the arteries.

HEALTH RISKS High blood pressure is often called a silent killer because it usually has no symptoms. A person may have high blood pressure for years without realizing it. But during that time, it slowly damages vital organs and increases the risk of heart attack, congestive heart failure, stroke, kidney failure, and blindness. The risk of death from heart attack or stroke begins to rise even within the "normal" range, when blood pressure is above 115 over 75 mm Hg, well below the traditional 140 over 90 mm Hg cutoff for a diagnosis of hypertension. People with blood pressure in the range referred to as prehypertension are at increased risk of heart attack and stroke.

An appropriate blood pressure target for risk reduction may depend on a person's age and other risk factors for cardiovascular disease. Traditionally, the treatment target has been to reduce blood pressure below the cutoff for hypertension (140 over 90 mm Hg). However, two large, high-quality trials published in 2015 showed that intensive blood pressure control with much lower targets (systolic pressure below 120 mm Hg) further reduced the risk of heart attack, stroke, and death. These findings may lead doctors to consider changing their practices so that they target much lower blood pressure goals for their patients. Future research may help identify criteria to set more individualized blood pressure targets.

PREVALENCE Hypertension is common. About 33% of adults have hypertension, and 30% have prehypertension (defined as systolic pressure of 120–139 mm Hg and/or diastolic pressure of 80–89 mm Hg). The incidence of high blood pressure increases with age, but it does occur among children and young adults. Women can sometimes develop hypertension during pregnancy (the blood pressure will usually return to normal following pregnancy). High blood pressure is two to three times more common in women taking oral contraceptives, especially in obese and older women; this risk increases with the duration of use. The rate of hypertension is highest in African Americans (42–44%). Among African Americans, compared with other groups, the disorder is often more severe, more resistant to treatment, and more likely to be fatal at an early age.

TREATMENT Primary hypertension cannot be cured, but it can be controlled. Because hypertension has no early warning signs, it is crucial to have your blood pressure tested at least once every two years (and more often if you have other CVD risk factors). In fact, experts now advise that anyone with hypertension or prehypertension monitor their own blood pressure several times each week.

Lifestyle changes are recommended for everyone with prehypertension and hypertension. These changes include weight reduction, regular exercise, a healthy diet, and moderation of alcohol use. The DASH diet (see Chapter 9) is recommended specifically for people with high blood pressure. Sodium restriction is also helpful for most people with hypertension. The 2015–2020 Dietary Guidelines for Americans recommend restricting sodium consumption to less than 2300 mg (~1 teaspoon of table salt) per day for all adults and children age 14 and over. Adults with prehypertension and hypertension would particularly benefit from lowered blood pressure. For these individuals, further reduction to 1500 mg per day can result in even greater blood pressure reduction.

QUICK STATS

1 out of every 3 U.S. adults has high blood pressure; only half have it under control.

—National Center for Health Statistics, 2016

atherosclerosis A form of cardiovascular disease in which the inner layers of artery walls are made thick and irregular by plaque deposits; arteries become narrow and blood supply can be reduced. **TERMS**

Nearly 80% of dietary salt in the typical American diet is found in processed food and drinks. It follows, then, that the easiest way to achieve population-wide reduction is for the food industry to lower the amount of salt added to food products. Reductions in supplemental salt in restaurant food have also been suggested; some cities now require warnings listed next to dishes with high amounts of sodium. Obviously, self-prepared meals offer the greatest control over dietary salt intake. For people whose blood pressure is not adequately controlled with lifestyle changes, medication can be prescribed.

High Cholesterol   *Cholesterol* is a fatty, waxlike substance that circulates through the bloodstream. It is an important component of cell membranes, sex hormones, vitamin D, the fluid that coats the lungs, and the protective sheaths around nerves. Adequate cholesterol is essential for the proper functioning of the body. Excess cholesterol, however, can clog arteries and increase the risk of CVD. There are two primary sources of cholesterol: the liver, which manufactures it, and dietary sources.

GOOD VERSUS BAD CHOLESTEROL   Cholesterol is carried in the blood in protein-and-lipid packages called **lipoproteins**. **Low-density lipoproteins (LDLs)** (18–27 nm) shuttle cholesterol from the liver to the organs and tissues that require it. LDLs are known as "bad" cholesterol because, if the body has more than it can use, the excess is deposited in the blood vessels. LDLs can then accumulate and be deposited in artery walls. They can then be oxidized by free radicals, which speeds inflammation and damage to artery walls and increases the likelihood of a blockage. If coronary arteries are blocked, the result may be a heart attack; if an artery carrying blood to the brain is blocked, a stroke may occur. **High-density lipoproteins (HDLs),** or "good" cholesterol, are the smallest of the lipoproteins (6–12.5 nm). They shuttle unused cholesterol back to the liver for recycling. By removing cholesterol from blood vessels, HDLs help protect against atherosclerosis.

BLOOD CHOLESTEROL GUIDELINES   The risk for CVD increases with higher blood cholesterol levels, especially LDL. The National Cholesterol Education Program recommends lipoprotein testing at least once every five years for all adults, beginning at age 20. The recommended test measures total cholesterol, LDL cholesterol, HDL cholesterol, and triglycerides (another blood fat). In general, high LDL, total cholesterol, and triglyceride levels, combined with low HDL levels, are associated with a higher risk for CVD. You can reduce this risk by lowering LDL, total cholesterol, and triglycerides. Raising HDL is important because a high HDL level seems to offer protection from CVD even in cases where total cholesterol is high. This appears to be especially true for women.

In 2013, the American College of Cardiology (ACC) and the American Heart Association released updated guidelines on the treatment of high blood cholesterol. These recommendations differ drastically from previous recommendations, and are still under review by multiple medical groups. Notably, the new guidelines no longer recommend treating to a target cholesterol level (the idea that "lower is better" is no longer included). Rather, these new guidelines suggest assessing a person's risk of developing cardiovascular disease over the next 10 years, and treating this level. The ACC and AHA identified four groups of people, based on observations made during multiple published clinical trials, who would benefit from treatment of high blood cholesterol levels (see Table 12.2).

The 2013 ACC/AHA guidelines also offer recommendations for people to modify their lifestyles either prior to developing or while already suffering from high cholesterol. These lifestyle guidelines include maintaining a healthy diet, engaging in regular aerobic exercise, avoiding tobacco products, and maintaining a healthy weight. These recommendations are vitally important in managing the risk of CVD and are often the first step in managing high cholesterol—before any medications are prescribed.

Table 12.2

People Who Benefit from Treatment of High Cholesterol

1. People age 75 and under with known cardiovascular disease, including previous heart attacks, chest pain due to partially clogged arteries, history of invasive treatment for clogged arteries, previous stroke, or previous clogged arteries in the limbs.
2. People age 21 and over with high LDL levels, 190 mg/dl or greater.
3. People ages 40–75 with a history of diabetes, an LDL level 70–189 mg/dl, and no known history of cardiovascular disease.
4. People ages 40–75 without diabetes or known cardiovascular disease but with a high risk of developing it over the next 10 years and an LDL level over 70 mg/dl.*

*10-year cardiovascular risk is calculated using a new tool available on the AHA website (https://professional.heart.org/professional/GuidelinesStatements/PreventionGuidelines/UCM_457698_Prevention-Guidelines.jsp).

SOURCE: Stone, N. J., et al. 2013. ACC/AHA guideline on the treatment of blood cholesterol to reduce atherosclerotic cardiovascular risk in adults. A report of the American College of Cardiology/American Heart Association Task Force on Practice Guidelines. *Journal of the American College of Cardiology.*

The updated cholesterol guidelines have been controversial because they eliminated the previous guidelines for targeting specific levels of LDL and HDL based on people's individual risk. Rather than target specific LDL and HDL levels, the new guidelines suggest statin therapy administered at different intensity doses if lifestyle modifications have not adequately lowered cholesterol levels. *Statins* are the primary cholesterol-lowering medications used today. *High-intensity* therapy is defined as a statin dosage that reduces the LDL level by greater than or equal to 50%, whereas *moderate-intensity* therapy reduces LDL level by 30–50%. Statins dramatically reduce the risk of CVD in individuals with high cholesterol levels. These medications may also decrease CVD risk even in those without high cholesterol levels. Of course, with any medication, side effects must be weighed against the potential benefits. The primary side effect seen with statins is muscle cramping, or myositis, which is usually mild and can be avoided by switching to a different kind of statin.

BENEFITS OF CONTROLLING CHOLESTEROL People can cut their heart attack risk by about 2% for every 1% that they reduce their total blood cholesterol levels. Previous studies have suggested that people who treat their high total cholesterol can reduce their risk of heart attack by 40%. Studies indicate that treating elevated LDL and raising HDL levels not only reduces the likelihood that arteries will become clogged but also may reverse deposits on artery walls.

Physical Inactivity

An estimated 40–60 million Americans are so sedentary that they are at high risk for developing CVD. Exercise is a key component in the fight against heart disease. It lowers CVD risk by helping to decrease blood pressure and resting heart rate, increase HDL levels, maintain desirable weight, improve the condition of blood vessels, and prevent or control diabetes. One study found that women who accumulated at least three hours of brisk walking each week cut their risk of heart attack and stroke by more than 50%.

Obesity

Death from CVD is two to three times more likely in obese people (**body mass index, or BMI** ≥ 30) than it is in lean people (BMI = 18.5–24.9), and for every 5-unit increase in BMI, a person's risk of death from coronary heart disease increases by 30%.

Excess body fat is strongly associate with hypertension, inactivity, and increasing age. With excess weight, there is also more blood to pump and the heart has to work harder. This causes chronically elevated pressures within the heart chambers that can lead to ventricular **hypertrophy** (enlargement). Eventually the heart muscle can start to fail, known as congestive heart failure.

> **body mass index (BMI)**   A calculated measure of human body shape; the ratio of mass (in kilograms) divided by height (in meters) squared: weight/height^2
>
> **hypertrophy**   Abnormal enlargement of an organ.
>
> **TERMS**

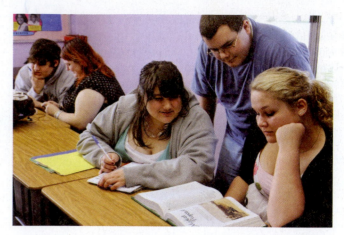

Being overweight or obese is a major risk factor for cardiovascular disease, but physical activity, including walking, can lower that risk. Modest weight loss can also reduce CVD risk.

© Stephan Gladieu/Getty Images

Diabetes

As described in Chapter 11, *diabetes mellitus* is a disorder characterized by elevated blood glucose levels due to an insufficient supply or inadequate action of insulin. Diabetes doubles the risk of CVD for men and triples the risk for women. The most common cause of death in adults with diabetes is CVD.

People with diabetes have higher rates of other CVD risk factors, including hypertension, obesity, and unhealthy blood

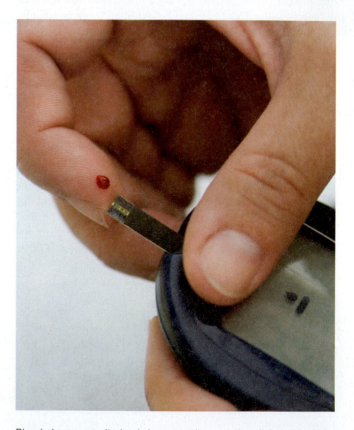

Blood glucose monitoring is important in managing diabetes and its associated risks.

© Michael Krasowitz/Photographer's Choice/Getty Images

lipid levels (typically, high triglyceride levels and low HDL levels). The elevated blood glucose and insulin levels that occur in diabetes can damage the endothelial cells that line the arteries, making them more vulnerable to atherosclerosis. Diabetics also often have platelet and blood coagulation abnormalities that increase the risk of heart attack and stroke. People with prediabetes (when the blood sugar levels are elevated but not high enough to diagnose diabetes) also face an increased risk of CVD.

In people with prediabetes, a healthy diet and exercise are the most effective tools in preventing diabetes. For people with diabetes, a healthy diet, exercise, and careful control of glucose levels are recommended to reduce the chances of developing complications. Even people whose diabetes is under control face a high risk of CVD, so control of other risk factors is critical.

Contributing Risk Factors That Can Be Changed

Other CVD risk factors that can be changed include triglyceride levels, metabolic syndrome, inflammation, psychological and social factors, and alcohol and drug use.

High Triglyceride Levels   Like cholesterol, **triglycerides** are blood fats that are obtained from food and manufactured by the body. High triglyceride levels are a reliable predictor of heart disease, especially if associated with other risk factors, such as low HDL levels, obesity, and diabetes. Factors contributing to elevated triglyceride levels include excess body fat, physical inactivity, cigarette smoking, type 2 diabetes, excessive alcohol intake, very high-carbohydrate diets, and certain diseases and medications.

A full lipid profile should include testing and evaluation of triglyceride levels. For people with borderline high triglyceride levels, increased physical activity, reduced intake of added sugars, and weight reduction can help bring levels down into the healthy range. For people with high triglyceride levels, drug therapy may be recommended if initial strategies are ineffective. Moderating alcohol intake and avoiding use of tobacco products are also important.

Insulin Resistance and Metabolic Syndrome   As people gain weight and become less active, their muscles, fat, and liver become less sensitive to the effect of insulin—a condition known as *insulin resistance*. As the body becomes increasingly insulin resistant, the pancreas must secrete more and more insulin (hyperinsulinemia) to keep glucose levels

QUICK STATS

85% of people with type 2 diabetes also have metabolic syndrome.

—National Heart, Lung, and Blood Institute, 2015

Table 12.3	Characteristics of Metabolic Syndrome*
FACTOR	**CRITERIA**
Large waistline (abdominal obesity)	35 or more inches (88 cm) for women 40 or more inches (102 cm) for men
High triglyceride level	150 mg/dl or higher Or taking medication to treat high triglycerides
Low HDL level	Less than 50 mg/dl for women Less than 40 mg/dl for men Or taking medication to treat low HDL
High blood pressure	130/85 mm Hg or higher (one or both numbers) Or taking medication to treat high blood pressure
High fasting blood sugar	100 mg/dl or higher Or taking medication to treat high blood sugar

*A person having three or more factors listed here is diagnosed with metabolic syndrome.

SOURCE: Adapted from National Heart, Lung, and Blood Institute. 2015. *How Is Metabolic Syndrome Diagnosed?* (http://www.nhlbi.nih.gov /health/health-topics/topics/ms/diagnosis).

within a normal range. Eventually even high levels of insulin may become insufficient, and blood glucose levels start to rise (hyperglycemia), setting the stage for prediabetes and, if not addressed, eventually for type 2 diabetes.

Those who have insulin resistance tend to have several other related risk factors. This cluster of abnormalities is called *metabolic syndrome* or *insulin resistance syndrome* (Table 12.3). Metabolic syndrome significantly increases the risk of CVD—more so in women than in men. It is estimated that about 23% of the adult U.S. population has metabolic syndrome.

To reduce your risk of developing metabolic syndrome, choose a healthy diet and get plenty of aerobic exercise. Reducing calorie intake to prevent weight gain or losing weight if needed also reduces insulin resistance. The amount and type of carbohydrate intake is also important. Diets high in simple carbohydrates, such as white sugar and white flour (high-glycemic-index foods), can raise levels of glucose and triglycerides while lowering HDL, thus contributing to metabolic syndrome and CVD. This is particularly true for people who are already sedentary and overweight. For people prone to insulin resistance, eating more protein, vegetables, and fiber while limiting fat, added sugars, and starches may be beneficial.

Inflammation   Inflammation plays a key role in the development of CVD. When an artery is injured by hypertension, smoking, cholesterol, or other factors, the body's response is to produce inflammation. A substance called *C-reactive protein (CRP)* is released into the bloodstream during the inflammatory response, and high levels of CRP indicate a

triglyceride   A type of blood fat that can be a predictor of heart disease.

TERMS

substantially elevated risk of heart attack and stroke. It has also been proposed that CRP by itself may harm the coronary arteries. Gum disease involves another type of inflammation that may moderately influence the progress of heart disease. Lifestyle changes and certain drugs can reduce CRP levels.

Psychological and Social Factors   Many of the psychological and social factors that influence other areas of wellness are also important risk factors for CVD.

STRESS   Excessive stress can strain the heart and blood vessels over time and contribute to CVD. When you experience stress, stress hormones activate the sympathetic nervous system. As described in Chapter 2, the sympathetic nervous system causes the fight-or-flight response. This response increases heart rate and blood pressure so that more blood is distributed to the heart and other muscles in anticipation of physical activity; these changes place increased stress on the arteries. Blood glucose concentrations and cholesterol also increase to provide a source of energy, and the platelets become activated so that they will be more likely to clot in case of injury. If you are healthy, you can tolerate the cardiovascular responses that take place during stress. But if you already have CVD, stress can lead to adverse outcomes such as abnormal heart rhythms (arrhythmias) and heart attacks.

CHRONIC HOSTILITY AND ANGER   Certain traits in the hard-driving "Type A" personality—hostility, cynicism, and anger—are associated with increased risk of heart disease.

SUPPRESSING PSYCHOLOGICAL DISTRESS   Consistently suppressing anger and other negative emotions may also be hazardous to a healthy heart. People who hide psychological distress appear to have higher rates of heart disease than people who experience similar distress but share it with others.

DEPRESSION   Depression appears to increase the risk of CVD in healthy people, and it definitely increases the risk of adverse cardiac events in those who already have heart disease.

The relationship between depression and CHD is complex and not fully understood. Depressed people may be more likely to smoke or be sedentary. They may not consistently take prescribed medications, and they may not cope well with having an illness or undergoing a medical procedure. Depression also causes physiological changes; for example, it elevates basal levels of stress hormones, which induce a variety of stress-related responses.

ANXIETY   Evidence suggests that chronic anxiety and anxiety disorders (such as phobias and panic disorder) are associated with up to a threefold increased risk of CHD, heart attack, and sudden cardiac death. People with anxiety are more likely to have a subsequent adverse cardiac event after having a heart attack.

SOCIAL ISOLATION   Social isolation and low social support (living alone, or having few friends or family members) are associated with an increased incidence of CHD and poorer

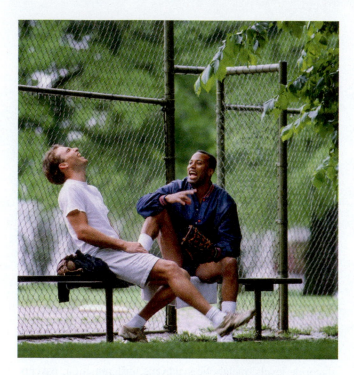

A strong social support network is a major antidote to stress and can help promote and support a healthy lifestyle that includes opportunities for exercise and relaxation.
© Corbis RF/Alamy

outcomes after the first diagnosis of CHD. Elderly men and women who report less emotional support from others before they have a heart attack are almost three times more likely to die in the first six months after the heart attack. A strong social support network is a major antidote to stress. Friends and family members can also promote and support a healthy lifestyle.

LOW SOCIOECONOMIC STATUS   Low socioeconomic status and low educational attainment are social factors associated with an increased risk of CVD. These associations are complex and likely due to a variety of factors, including lifestyle, diet, and access to health care, among others.

Alcohol and Drugs   Although moderate drinking (defined as no more than one or two drinks per day for men and no more than one drink per day for women) may have health benefits for some people, drinking alcohol in excess raises blood pressure and can increase the risk of stroke and heart failure. Stimulant drugs, particularly cocaine and methamphetamines—and associated stimulants, such as designer drugs including ecstasy (MDMA)—can also cause serious cardiac problems, including heart attack, stroke, and sudden cardiac death.

Major Risk Factors That Can't Be Changed

A number of major risk factors for cardiovascular disease cannot be changed. These include family history of CVD (genetics), aging, male gender, and ethnicity.

Genetics   Multiple genes contribute to the development of CVD—the umbrella term for diseases of the heart and blood vessels—and its associated risk factors, such as high cholesterol, hypertension, diabetes, and obesity. Having a favorable set of genes decreases your risk of developing CVD; having an unfavorable set of genes increases your risk. Risk, however, may be modified by lifestyle factors such as whether you smoke, exercise, or eat a healthy diet.

Age   About 70% of all heart attack victims are age 65 and over, and about 75% who suffer fatal heart attacks are over 65. For people over 55, the incidence of stroke more than doubles in each successive decade. However, even people in their thirties and forties, especially men, can have heart attacks.

Gender   Although CVD is the leading killer of both men and women in the United States, men face a greater risk of heart attack than women, especially earlier in life. Until age 55, men also have a greater risk of hypertension. The incidence of stroke is also higher for males than females, until age 65. By age 75, however, this gender gap nearly disappears.

Race and Ethnicity   Rates of heart disease vary among racial and ethnic groups in the United States, with African Americans having much higher rates of hypertension, heart disease, and stroke than other groups (see the box "Gender, Race/Ethnicity, and Cardiovascular Disease"). Mexican Americans were also found to have a higher rate of stroke than non-Hispanic whites, and Hispanic women have higher rates of angina (a warning sign of blocked coronary arteries) than non-Hispanic white women. Asian Americans historically have had far lower rates of CVD than white Americans.

Possible Risk Factors Currently Being Studied

In recent years, other possible risk factors for cardiovascular disease have been identified. Elevated levels of homocysteine, an amino acid circulating in the blood, are associated with an increased risk of CVD. Homocysteine appears to damage the lining of blood vessels, resulting in inflammation and the development of fatty deposits in artery walls. These changes can lead to the formation of clots and blockages in arteries, which in turn can cause heart attacks and strokes.

Several infectious agents have been identified as possible culprits in the development of CVD. *Chlamydia pneumoniae,* a common cause of flulike respiratory infections, has been found in sections of clogged, damaged arteries but not in sections of healthy arteries.

Other factors currently under investigation include a specific type of LDL called lipoprotein(a) or Lp(a), LDL particle size, blood levels of iron, and blood levels of uric acid.

MAJOR FORMS OF CARDIOVASCULAR DISEASE

Although deaths from cardiovascular disease have declined dramatically over the past 60 years, it remains the leading cause of death in the United States. According to the CDC, heart disease killed approximately 614,000 Americans in 2014. Figure 12.4 shows the death rates among population groups due to heart disease in 2014, the most recent year for which data are available.

The main forms of CVD are atherosclerosis, coronary heart disease and heart attack, stroke, peripheral arterial disease, congestive heart failure, congenital heart disease, rheumatic heart disease, and heart valve problems. Many forms are interrelated and have elements in common; we treat them separately here for the sake of clarity. Hypertension, which is both a major risk factor and a form of CVD, was described earlier in the chapter.

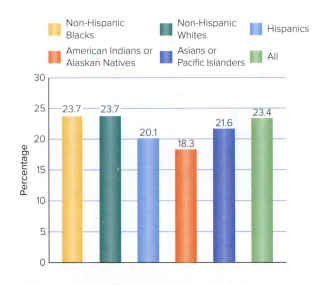

VITAL STATISTICS

FIGURE 12.4   Percentage of U.S. deaths due to heart disease, by race and ethnicity.

SOURCE: National Center for Health Statistics. 2015. LCWK1: Deaths, percent of total deaths, and death rates for the 15 leading causes of death in 5-year age groups, by race and sex: United States, 1999–2014 and LCWK2: Deaths, percent of total deaths, and death rates for the 15 leading causes of death in 10-year age groups, by race and sex: United States, 1999–2014 (http://www.cdc.gov/nchs/nvss/mortality_tables.htm).

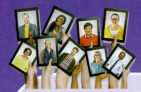

Cardiovascular disease is the leading cause of death for all Americans, but significant differences exist between men and women and among racial/ethnic groups in the incidence, diagnosis, and treatment of this deadly disease.

CVD in Women

CVD has been thought of as a "man's disease," but it actually kills more women than men. Polls indicate that women vastly underestimate their risk of dying of a heart attack and overestimate their risk of dying of breast cancer. In reality, nearly 1 in 3 women dies of CVD, whereas 1 in 31 dies of breast cancer. And although CVD typically does not develop in women younger than age 50, recent research suggests that the number of CVD deaths in women aged 35–45 may be increasing.

The hormone estrogen, produced naturally by a woman's ovaries until menopause, improves blood lipid concentrations and reduces other CVD risk factors. For several decades, many physicians encouraged menopausal women to take hormone replacement therapy (HRT), which includes estrogen, to relieve menopause symptoms and presumably to reduce their risk of CVD. However, some studies found that HRT may actually *increase* a woman's risk for heart disease and other health problems, including breast cancer.

When women have heart attacks, they are more likely than men to die within a year and are less likely than men to report the usual symptoms of a heart attack, such as chest pain. Additionally, women are likely to report less specific symptoms, which may obscure the diagnosis. These symptoms include fatigue; weakness; shortness of breath; nausea; vomiting; and pain in the abdomen, neck, jaw, and back. Women are also more likely to have pain at rest, during sleep, or with mental stress. A woman who experiences these symptoms should be persistent in seeking accurate diagnosis and appropriate treatment.

Women should be aware of their CVD risk factors and consult with a physician to assess their risk and determine the best way to prevent CVD.

CVD in African Americans and Other Racial/Ethnic Groups

African Americans are at substantially higher risk of death from CVD than other groups. The rate of hypertension among African Americans is among the highest in the world. African Americans tend to develop hypertension at an earlier age than non-Hispanic whites, and their average blood pressures are much higher. African Americans have a higher risk of stroke; have strokes at younger ages; and, if they survive, have more significant stroke-related disabilities. Some experts recommend that African Americans be given antihypertensive drugs when blood pressure reaches 130/80 rather than the typical 140/90 cutoff for hypertension.

A number of genetic and biological factors may contribute to CVD in African Americans. For instance, a higher sensitivity to dietary sodium may lead to greater blood pressure elevation in response to a given amount of sodium. African Americans may also experience less dilation of blood vessels in response to stress, an attribute that also raises blood pressure for all racial/ethnic groups.

Heredity also plays a large role in the tendency to develop diabetes, another important CVD risk factor that is more common in blacks than whites. However, Latinos are even more likely to develop diabetes and insulin resistance, and at a younger age, than African Americans. There is variation within the Latino population, however; a higher prevalence of diabetes occurs among Mexican Americans and Puerto Ricans and a relatively lower prevalence among Cuban Americans.

Racial and ethnic minorities are more likely than non-Hispanic whites to be poor, and low income is associated with reduced access to health care and healthy dietary options for CVD prevention.

Discrimination may also play a role in CVD. Physicians and hospitals may treat the medical problems of non-whites differently from those of whites. Discrimination, low income, and other forms of deprivation may also increase stress, which is linked with hypertension and CVD. Lack of insurance coverage and less-advanced medical technologies in hospitals that serve minority and low-income neighborhoods may also play a role.

All Americans, regardless of background, are advised to have their blood pressure checked regularly, exercise on a regular basis, eat a healthy diet, manage stress, and avoid tobacco products. Tailoring your lifestyle to any risk factors that may be especially relevant for you can also be helpful in some cases. Discuss your particular risk profile with your physician to help identify the lifestyle changes most appropriate for you.

Atherosclerosis

Atherosclerosis is a form of arteriosclerosis, or thickening and hardening of the arteries. In atherosclerosis, arteries become narrowed by deposits of fat, cholesterol, and other substances (Figure 12.5). The process begins when the endothelial cells (cells that line the arteries) become damaged, most likely through a combination of factors such as smoking, high blood pressure, high insulin or glucose levels, and deposits of oxidized LDL particles. The body's response to this damage results in inflammation and changes in the artery lining that create a magnet for LDL, platelets, and other cells. These cells build up and cause a bulge in the wall of the artery. As these deposits, called **plaques,** accumulate in artery walls, the arteries lose their elasticity and their ability to expand and

> **plaque** A deposit of fatty (and other) substances on the inner wall of an artery. **TERMS**

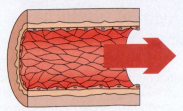

1. A healthy artery allows blood to flow through freely.

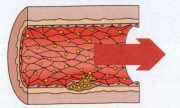
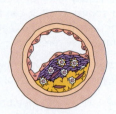

2. Plaque buildup begins when endothelial cells lining the arteries are damaged by smoking, high blood pressure, oxidized LDL cholesterol, and other causes. Excess cholesterol particles collect beneath these cells.

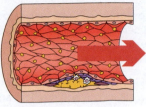
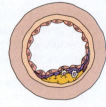

3. In response to the damage, platelets and other types of cells collect at the site. A fibrous cap forms, isolating the plaque within the artery wall. An early-stage plaque is called a fatty streak.

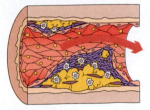
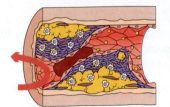
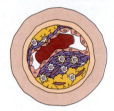

4. Chemicals released by cells in and around the plaque cause further inflammation and buildup. An advanced plaque contains LDL cholesterol, white blood cells, connective tissue, smooth muscle cells, platelets, and other compounds.

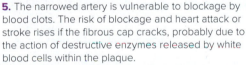

5. The narrowed artery is vulnerable to blockage by blood clots. The risk of blockage and heart attack or stroke rises if the fibrous cap cracks, probably due to the action of destructive enzymes released by white blood cells within the plaque.

6. If a clot is traveling through the bloodstream, it may become trapped in the narrowed artery at the site of the plaque buildup, cutting off blood supply and oxygen to tissue.

FIGURE 12.5 **Atherosclerosis: The process of cardiovascular disease.**

contract, restricting blood flow. Once narrowed by a plaque, an artery is vulnerable to blockage by blood clots. The risk of life-threatening clots and heart attacks increases if the fibrous cap covering a plaque ruptures.

If the heart, brain, or other organs are deprived of blood and the oxygen it carries, the effects of atherosclerosis can be deadly. Coronary arteries, which supply the heart with blood, are particularly susceptible to plaque buildup, a condition called **coronary heart disease (CHD)** or *coronary artery disease (CAD)*. The blockage of a coronary artery causes a heart attack, and blockage of a cerebral artery (leading to the brain) causes a stroke. Blockage of an artery in a limb causes *peripheral arterial disease,* a condition that causes pain and may require amputation of the affected limb.

The main risk factors for atherosclerosis are tobacco use, physical inactivity, high blood cholesterol levels, high blood pressure, and diabetes. Atherosclerosis often begins in childhood: Autopsy studies of young trauma victims have revealed atherosclerosis of the coronary arteries in adolescents.

Coronary Artery Disease and Heart Attack

The most common form of heart disease is CHD caused by atherosclerosis. When one of the coronary arteries becomes blocked, the result is a **heart attack,** or *myocardial infarction (MI)*. During a heart attack, the heart muscle (the myocardium) is damaged, and part of it may die from lack of oxygenated blood. Although a heart attack may come without warning, it usually results from a chronic disease process.

coronary heart disease (CHD)   Heart disease caused by atherosclerosis in the arteries that supply blood to the heart muscle; also called *coronary artery disease (CAD)*.   **TERMS**

heart attack   Damage to, or death of, heart muscle, resulting from a failure of the coronary arteries to deliver enough blood to the heart; also known as *myocardial infarction (MI)*.

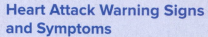

Heart Attack Warning Signs and Symptoms

The most common symptoms of a heart attack for both men and women are the following:

• *Chest pain or discomfort* in the center or left side of the chest that usually lasts for more than a few minutes or goes away and comes back. It can feel like pressure, squeezing, fullness, or pain. It also can feel like heartburn or indigestion. It can be mild or severe.

• *Upper body discomfort* in one or both arms, the back, shoulders, neck, jaw, or upper part of the stomach (above the navel).

• *Shortness of breath* may be the only symptom, or it may occur before or along with chest pain or discomfort. It can occur when you are resting or doing mild physical activity.

But remember these additional facts:

• Heart attacks can start slowly and cause only mild pain or discomfort. Symptoms can be mild or more intense and sudden. Symptoms also may come and go over several hours.

• People who have high blood sugar (diabetes) may have no symptoms or very mild ones. Heart attacks without symptoms or with very mild symptoms are called silent heart attacks.

• The most common symptom, in both men and women, is chest pain or discomfort.

• Women are somewhat more likely than men to experience shortness of breath; nausea and vomiting; unusual tiredness (sometimes for days); and pain in the back, shoulders, and jaw.

• Other possible symptoms include breaking out in a cold sweat, light-headedness or sudden dizziness, or a change in the pattern of usual symptoms.

The signs and symptoms of a heart attack can develop suddenly or slowly—within hours, days, or weeks of a heart attack. If you think you or someone you know might be having heart attack symptoms or a heart attack, don't ignore it or feel embarrassed to call for help. **Call 9-1-1 right away.** Here's why:

• Acting fast can save a life. Every minute matters. Never delay calling 9-1-1 to do anything you think might help.

• An ambulance is the best and safest way to get to the hospital. Emergency medical services (EMS) personnel start lifesaving treatments right away. People who arrive at the hospital by ambulance often receive faster treatment.

• The 9-1-1 operator or EMS technician can give you advice. You might be told to chew (or crush) and swallow an aspirin, unless there is a medical reason for you not to take one.

Stroke Warning Signs and Symptoms

The symptoms of stroke are distinctive because they happen quickly:

• Sudden numbness or weakness of the face, arm, or leg (especially on one side of the body)

• Sudden confusion, trouble speaking, or understanding speech

• Sudden trouble seeing in one or both eyes

• Sudden trouble walking, dizziness, loss of balance or coordination

• Sudden severe headache with no known cause.

An acronym to help you remember the most common symptoms of a stroke is FAST (facial drooping, arm weakness, speech difficulty, and time to call 9-1-1). If you believe someone

---

Heart attack symptoms may include chest pain or pressure; arm, neck, or jaw pain; difficulty breathing; excessive sweating; nausea and vomiting; and loss of consciousness. Most people having a heart attack suffer chest pain, but about one-third of heart attack victims do not. Women, older adults, and people with diabetes and certain forms of CVD are the most likely groups to experience heart attacks without chest pain.

Angina   Arteries narrowed by disease may still be open enough to deliver sufficient amounts of oxygenated blood to the heart. At times, however—during stress or exertion, for example—the heart needs more oxygen than can flow through narrowed arteries. When the need for oxygen exceeds the supply, chest pain, called **angina pectoris,** may occur.

Angina pain is usually felt as an extreme tightness in the chest and heavy pressure behind the breastbone or in the shoulder, neck, arm, hand, or back. Angina may be controlled in a number of ways (with drugs and surgical or nonsurgical

procedures), but its course is unpredictable. Over a period ranging from hours to years, the narrowing may go on to full blockage and a heart attack.

Arrhythmias and Sudden Cardiac Death   The pumping of the heart is controlled by electrical impulses from the sinus node that maintain a regular heartbeat of 60–100 beats per minute. If this electrical conduction system is disrupted, the heart may beat too quickly, too slowly, or in an irregular fashion—a condition known as an **arrhythmia.**

> **angina pectoris**   Pain in the chest, and often in the left arm and shoulder, caused by the heart muscle not receiving enough oxygenated blood. The pain is usually brought on by exercise or stress.
>
> **arrhythmia**   A change in the heartbeat's normal, regular pattern.
>
> **TERMS**

is having a stroke, call 9-1-1 immediately. Ischemic strokes, the most common type, can be treated with a drug called t-PA, which dissolves blood clots. The drug must be administered within three hours, but to be evaluated and receive treatment in time, patients must get to the hospital within 60 minutes.

A transient ischemic attack (TIA) has the same signs and symptoms as a stroke. However, TIA symptoms usually last less than 1–2 hours (although they may last up to 24 hours). A TIA may occur only once in a person's lifetime or more often and can be a warning sign for future strokes. At first, it may not be possible to tell whether someone is having a TIA or stroke. All stroke-like symptoms require medical care.

Sudden Cardiac Arrest Signs

In sudden cardiac arrest (SCA), the heart stops beating suddenly and unexpectedly. As a result, blood stops flowing to the brain and other vital organs. The patient suddenly becomes unresponsive and stops breathing, and if he or she does not receive treatment within minutes, death occurs. Usually, the first sign of SCA is loss of consciousness (fainting). At the same time, no heartbeat (or pulse) can be felt. Some people may have a racing heartbeat or feel dizzy or light-headed just before they faint. Within an hour before SCA, some people experience chest pain, shortness of breath, nausea, or vomiting.

If you are with someone who experiences these symptoms, begin CPR and call 9-1-1 immediately. Rapid treatment of SCA with a defibrillator can be lifesaving. A defibrillator is a device that sends an electric shock to the heart to restore its normal rhythm. Automated external defibrillators (AEDs) can be used by bystanders to save the lives of people who are having SCA. These portable devices often are found in public places, such as shopping malls, golf courses, businesses,

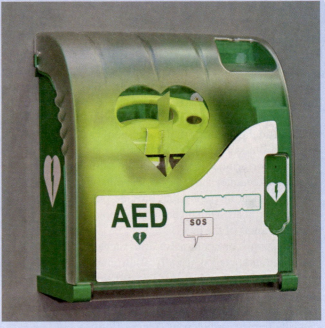

© Baloncici/123RF

airports, airplanes, convention centers, hotels, sports venues, and schools.

SOURCES: National Heart, Lung, and Blood Institute. 2013. *What Are the Symptoms of a Heart Attack?* (http://www.nhlbi.nih.gov/health/health-topics/topics/heartattack/signs); National Institute of Neurological Disorders and Stroke. 2013. *Know Stroke. Know the Signs. Act in Time.* (http://www.ninds.nih.gov/disorders/stroke/knowstroke.htm); National Heart, Lung, and Blood Institute. 2011. *What Is Sudden Cardiac Arrest?* (http://www.nhlbi.nih.gov/health/health-topics/topics/scda).

Arrhythmias can cause symptoms ranging from imperceptible to severe and even fatal.

Sudden cardiac death, also called *cardiac arrest,* is most often caused by an arrhythmia called *ventricular fibrillation,* a kind of quivering of the ventricle that makes it ineffective in pumping blood. If ventricular fibrillation continues for more than a few minutes, it is generally fatal. Cardiac defibrillation, in which an electrical shock is delivered to the heart, can be effective in jolting the heart into a more

efficient rhythm. Training in the use of AEDs is available from organizations such as the American Red Cross and the American Heart Association.

Helping a Heart Attack Victim

Most deaths from heart attacks occur within two hours of the first onset of symptoms. Unfortunately, many heart attack victims wait more than two hours before getting help. If you or someone you are with shows any of the signs of heart attack listed in the box "Warning Signs and Symptoms of Heart Attack, Stroke, or Cardiac Arrest," take immediate action. Call for help—even if the person denies something is wrong. Many experts also suggest that the heart attack victim *chew* and swallow one adult aspirin tablet (325 mg) as soon as possible after symptoms begin. Aspirin has an immediate anticlotting effect.

If the victim loses consciousness, a qualified person should immediately check for a pulse and start administering emergency **cardiopulmonary resuscitation (CPR)** if no

> **TERMS**
>
> **sudden cardiac death** A nontraumatic, unexpected death from sudden cardiac arrest, most often due to arrhythmia; in most instances, victims have underlying heart disease.
>
> **cardiopulmonary resuscitation (CPR)** A technique involving mouth-to-mouth breathing and/or chest compressions to keep oxygen flowing to the brain.

pulse is found. Damage to the heart muscle increases with time. If the person receives emergency care quickly enough, a clot-dissolving agent or emergency invasive procedure can be used to break up the clot in the coronary artery.

Detecting and Treating Heart Disease   Currently the most common initial screening tool for CHD is the stress, or exercise, test. During an exercise stress test, a patient runs or walks on a treadmill or pedals a stationary cycle while being monitored for abnormalities with an **electrocardiogram (ECG or EKG).** Certain characteristic changes in the heart's electrical activity while under stress can reveal particular heart problems, such as restricted blood flow. Exercise testing can also be performed in conjunction with imaging techniques such as nuclear medicine or echocardiography that provide pictures of the heart, which can help pinpoint abnormal areas of the heart.

If symptoms or noninvasive tests suggest CHD, the next step is usually a coronary **angiogram,** performed in a cardiac catheterization lab. If a problem is found, it is commonly treated with a metal stent or **balloon angioplasty,** which is performed by specially trained cardiologists (Figure 12.6).

Other treatments, ranging from medication to major surgery, are also available. Along with a low-fat diet, regular exercise, and smoking cessation, one frequent recommendation for people at intermediate to high risk for CVD is to take a low-dose (81 mg) aspirin tablet every day. Aspirin helps prevent platelets in the blood from sticking to arterial plaques and forming clots, and it also reduces inflammation.

Prescription drugs can help control heart rate, dilate arteries, lower blood pressure, and reduce the strain on the heart—improving both the quality and length of life in heart patients. In patients with CHD, cholesterol-lowering statins are effective in preventing heart attacks; statins also have beneficial anti-inflammatory effects. In **coronary bypass surgery,** surgeons remove a healthy blood vessel—usually a vein from the patient's leg—and graft it from the aorta to one or more coronary arteries to bypass a blockage.

Stroke

A **stroke,** also called a *cerebrovascular accident (CVA),* occurs when the blood supply to the brain is cut off and brain tissue subsequently dies.

Types of Strokes   There are two major types of strokes (Figure 12.7).

ISCHEMIC STROKE   An **ischemic stroke** is caused by a blockage in a blood vessel. There are two types of ischemic strokes: A *thrombotic stroke* is caused by a **thrombus,** which is a blood clot that forms in a cerebral or carotid artery that has been narrowed or damaged by atherosclerosis. An *embolic stroke* is caused by an **embolus,** which is a wandering

blood clot that is carried in the bloodstream and may become wedged in a cerebral artery. Ischemic strokes, account for 87% of all strokes.

HEMORRHAGIC STROKE   A **hemorrhagic stroke** occurs when a blood vessel in the brain bursts, spilling blood into the surrounding tissue. Cells normally nourished by the vessel are deprived of blood and cannot function. In addition, accumulated blood from the burst vessel may put pressure on surrounding brain tissue, causing damage and even death. There are two types of hemorrhagic strokes: In an *intracerebral hemorrhage,* a blood vessel ruptures within the brain. About 10% of strokes are caused by intracerebral hemorrhages. In a *subarachnoid hemorrhage,* a blood vessel on the brain's surface ruptures and bleeds into the space between the brain and the skull. About 3% of strokes are of this type.

Hemorrhages can be caused by head injuries or the bursting of a malformed blood vessel, or **aneurysm,** which is a blood-filled pocket that bulges out from a weak spot in the artery wall. Aneurysms in the brain may remain stable and never break. But when they do, the result is a hemorrhagic stroke. Aneurysms may be caused or worsened by hypertension.

The Effects of a Stroke   The interruption of the blood supply to any area of the brain prevents the nerve cells there

TERMS

electrocardiogram (ECG or EKG)   A test to detect cardiac abnormalities by evaluating the electrical activity in the heart.

angiogram   A picture of the arterial system taken after injecting a dye that is opaque to X-rays.

balloon angioplasty   A technique in which a catheter with a deflated balloon on the tip is inserted into an artery; the balloon is then inflated at the point of obstruction in the artery, pressing the plaque against the artery wall to improve blood supply.

coronary bypass surgery   Surgery in which a blood vessel is grafted from the aorta to a point below an obstruction in a coronary artery, improving the blood supply to the heart.

stroke   Impeded blood supply to some part of the brain, resulting in the destruction of brain cells; also called a *cerebrovascular accident (CVA).*

ischemic stroke   Impeded blood supply to the brain caused by a clot obstructing a blood vessel.

thrombus   A blood clot that forms in a blood vessel that has already been damaged by plaque buildup; the clot may lead to stroke.

embolus   A blood clot that breaks off from its place of origin in a blood vessel and travels through the bloodstream.

hemorrhagic stroke   Impeded blood supply to the brain caused by the rupture of a blood vessel.

aneurysm   A sac or outpouching formed by a distention or dilation of the artery wall.

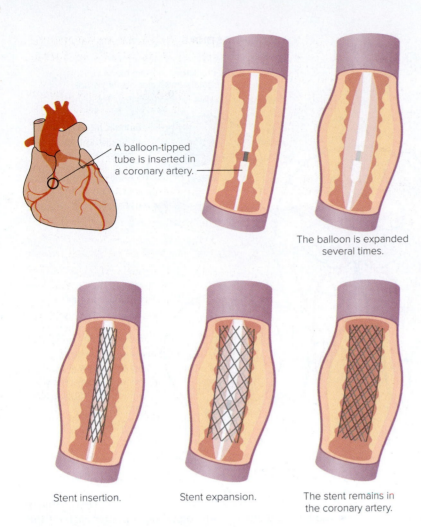

A balloon-tipped tube is inserted in a coronary artery.

The balloon is expanded several times.

Stent insertion.

Stent expansion.

The stent remains in the coronary artery.

FIGURE 12.6 **Balloon angioplasty and stenting.**

from functioning—in some cases causing death. Stroke survivors usually have some lasting disability. A stroke may cause paralysis, walking disability, speech impairment, memory loss, or changes in behavior. The severity of the stroke and how long the effects last depend on which brain cells have been injured, how widespread the damage is, how effectively the body can restore the blood supply, and how rapidly other areas of the brain can take over the functions of the damaged areas.

Detecting and Treating Stroke Effective treatment requires the prompt recognition of symptoms and correct diagnosis of the type of stroke.

A quick way to recognize a stroke is to ask the person to do four simple things:

1. Ask the person to smile. If her smile droops on one side, or if she is unable to move or open one side of her mouth, she may be having a stroke.

2. Ask the person to hold his arms or legs out. If the person cannot move one arm/leg or hold one arm/leg still, it may be a sign of a stroke.

3. Ask the person to repeat a simple, short sentence, such as "Take me out to the ball game." If she has trouble speaking or cannot speak, a stroke is possible.

4. Ask the person whether he has any decreased sensation, numbness, or abnormal tingling in his legs, arms, or other body parts.

If someone has difficulty performing any of these tests, follow the steps described in the box "Warning Signs and Symptoms of Heart Attack, Stroke, or Cardiac Arrest." Remember the acronym FAST, and call 9-1-1 for help if needed. Many people have strokes without knowing it. These "silent strokes" do not cause any noticeable symptoms while they are occurring. Although they may be mild, silent strokes leave their victims at a higher risk for subsequent and more serious strokes. They also contribute to loss of mental and cognitive skills.

Some stroke victims have a **transient ischemic attack (TIA),** or "ministroke," days, weeks, or months before they have a full-blown stroke. A TIA produces temporary stroke-like symptoms, such as weakness or numbness in an arm or a leg, speech difficulty, or dizziness. These symptoms are brief, often lasting just a few minutes, and do not cause permanent damage. TIAs should be taken as warning signs of a stroke, however, and anyone with a suspected TIA should get immediate medical attention.

A person with stroke symptoms should be rushed to the hospital. A **computed tomography (CT)** scan, which uses a computer to construct an image of the brain from X-rays, can assess brain damage and determine the type of stroke. Newer techniques using MRI and ultrasound are becoming increasingly available and should improve the speed and accuracy of stroke diagnosis.

If tests reveal that a stroke is caused by a blood clot—and if help is sought within a few hours of the onset of symptoms—the blockage can be treated with the same kind of clot-dissolving drugs that are used to treat coronary artery blockages. If the clot is dissolved quickly enough, brain damage is minimized and symptoms may disappear.

If detection and treatment of stroke come too late, rehabilitation and prevention of further events is the only treatment. Although damaged or destroyed brain tissue does not normally regenerate, nerve cells in the brain can make new pathways, and some functions can be taken over by other parts of the brain. Some spontaneous recovery starts immediately after a stroke and continues for a few months.

transient ischemic attack (TIA) A small stroke; **TERMS** usually a temporary interruption of blood supply to the brain, causing numbness or difficulty with speech.

computed tomography (CT) The use of computerized X-ray images to create a cross-sectional depiction (scan) of tissue density.

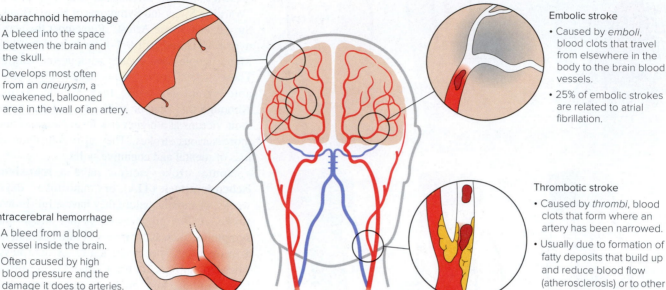

HEMORRHAGIC STROKE
- 13% of strokes.
- Caused by ruptured blood vessels followed by blood leaking into tissue.
- Usually more serious than ischemic stroke.

Subarachnoid hemorrhage
- A bleed into the space between the brain and the skull.
- Develops most often from an *aneurysm,* a weakened, ballooned area in the wall of an artery.

Intracerebral hemorrhage
- A bleed from a blood vessel inside the brain.
- Often caused by high blood pressure and the damage it does to arteries.

ISCHEMIC STROKE
- 87% of strokes.
- Caused by blockages in brain blood vessels; potentially treatable with clot-busting drugs.
- Brain tissue dies when blood flow is blocked.

Embolic stroke
- Caused by *emboli,* blood clots that travel from elsewhere in the body to the brain blood vessels.
- 25% of embolic strokes are related to atrial fibrillation.

Thrombotic stroke
- Caused by *thrombi,* blood clots that form where an artery has been narrowed.
- Usually due to formation of fatty deposits that build up and reduce blood flow (atherosclerosis) or to other artery conditions.

FIGURE 12.7 Types of stroke.

SOURCE: Adapted from *Harvard Health Letter,* April 2000. Harvard University. Artwork by Harriet Greenfield, reprinted with permission.

Some people recover completely in a matter of days or weeks, but most stroke victims who survive must adapt to some disability.

Peripheral Arterial Disease

Peripheral arterial disease (PAD) refers to atherosclerosis in the leg or arm arteries, which can eventually limit or completely obstruct blood flow. The same process that occurs in the heart arteries can occur in any artery of the body.

The risk of PAD is significantly increased in people with diabetes and people who use tobacco products. The likelihood of needing an amputation is increased in those who continue to use tobacco products, and PAD in people with diabetes tends to be extensive and severe.

Symptoms of PAD include claudication and rest pain. *Claudication* is aching or fatigue in the affected leg with exertion, particularly walking, which resolves with rest. Claudication occurs when leg muscles do not get adequate blood and oxygen supply. *Rest pain* occurs when the limb artery is unable to supply adequate blood and oxygen even when the body is not physically active. This occurs when the artery is significantly narrowed or completely blocked. PAD is the leading cause of amputation in people over 50.

Congestive Heart Failure

When the heart cannot maintain its regular pumping rate and force, fluid begins to back up. When extra fluid seeps through capillary walls, edema (swelling) results, usually in the legs and ankles, but sometimes in other parts of the body as well. Fluid can collect in the lungs and interfere with breathing, particularly when a person is lying down. This condition is called **pulmonary edema,** and the entire process is known as **congestive heart failure.** About 5.1 million Americans suffer from heart failure. Treatment includes reducing the workload on the heart, modifying salt intake, and using drugs that help the body eliminate excess fluid. The risk of heart failure increases with age, and being overweight is a significant independent risk factor.

Other Forms of Heart Disease

Other, less common, forms of heart disease include congenital heart defects, rheumatic heart disease, and heart valve disorders.

TERMS

peripheral arterial disease (PAD)
Atherosclerosis in the arteries in the legs (or less commonly, the arms) that can impede blood flow and lead to pain, infection, and loss of the affected limb.

pulmonary edema   The accumulation of fluid in the lungs.

congestive heart failure   A condition resulting from the heart's inability to pump enough blood to keep up with the body's metabolic needs; blood backs up in the veins leading to the heart, causing an accumulation of fluid in various parts of the body.

Congenital Heart Defects   About 40,000 children born each year in the United States have a defect or malformation of the heart or major blood vessels. These conditions are collectively referred to as **congenital heart defects,** and they cause about 3600 deaths a year. Most of the common congenital defects can now be accurately diagnosed and treated with medication or surgery. The most common congenital defects are holes in the wall that divides the chambers of the heart. Such defects cause the heart to produce a distinctive sound, making diagnosis relatively simple. Another common defect is *coarctation of the aorta*—a narrowing, or constriction, of the aorta. Heart failure may result unless the constricted area is repaired by surgery.

Hypertrophic cardiomyopathy occurs in approximately 1 out of every 500 people in the United States and is the most common cause of sudden death among athletes younger than age 35. It causes the heart muscle to become hypertrophic (enlarged), primarily in the septum, which is the area between the two ventricles. People with hypertrophic cardiomyopathy are at high risk for sudden death, mainly due to serious arrhythmias. Hypertrophic cardiomyopathy may be identified by a **murmur** and diagnosed using echocardiography. Possible treatments include medication and a pacemaker or an internal defibrillator. If the hypertrophy is mainly in the septum, some of the septum can be surgically removed or a nonsurgical procedure can be done to kill off the extra muscle.

Rheumatic Heart Disease   **Rheumatic fever,** a consequence of certain types of untreated streptococcal throat infections, is a leading cause of heart failure worldwide. Rheumatic fever can permanently damage the heart muscle and heart valves, a condition called *rheumatic heart disease (RHD)*. Symptoms of strep throat include the sudden onset of a sore throat, painful swallowing, fever, swollen glands, headache, nausea, and vomiting. If left untreated, up to 3% of strep infections progress into rheumatic fever. Rheumatic fever affects primarily children between the ages of 5 and 15 years.

---

congenital heart defect   A defect or malformation of the heart or its major blood vessels, present at birth.

hypertrophic cardiomyopathy   An inherited condition in which there is an enlargement of the heart muscle, especially the muscle between the two ventricles.

murmur   An abnormal heart sound indicating turbulent blood flow through a valve or hole in the heart.

rheumatic fever   A disease, mainly of children, characterized by fever, inflammation, and pain in the joints. It often damages the heart valves and muscle, a condition called rheumatic heart disease.

mitral valve prolapse (MVP)   A condition in which the mitral valve billows out during ventricular contraction, allowing leakage of blood from the left ventricle into the left atrium.

TERMS

Heart Valve Disorders   Age, previous heart attacks, congenital defects, and certain types of infections can cause abnormalities in the valves between the chambers of the heart. Heart valve problems generally fall into two categories—the valve fails to open fully, or it fails to close completely. In either case, blood flow through the heart is impaired.

The most common heart valve disorder is **mitral valve prolapse (MVP),** which occurs in about 3% of the population. MVP is characterized by a billowing of the mitral valve, which separates the left ventricle and left atrium, during ventricular contraction. In some cases, blood leaks from the ventricle into the atrium. Most people with MVP have no symptoms and need no treatment.

PROTECTING YOURSELF AGAINST CARDIOVASCULAR DISEASE

You can take several important steps now to lower your risk of developing cardiovascular disease (Figure 12.8). CVD can begin very early in life. Reducing CVD risk factors when you are young can pay off with many extra years of life and health.

Eat Heart-Healthy

For most Americans, eating a heart-healthy diet involves decreasing saturated and trans fat intake, eating a high-fiber diet, reducing sodium intake and increasing potassium intake, avoiding excessive alcohol consumption, and eating foods rich in omega-3 fatty acids.

In addition to these familiar guidelines, a few specifics pertain to heart health: (1) Plant stanols and sterols, found in some types of trans-fat-free margarines and other products, reduce the absorption of cholesterol in the body and help lower LDL levels. (2) Folic acid, vitamin B-6, and vitamin B-12 lower homocysteine levels, and folic acid has also been found to reduce the risk of hypertension. (3) Diets rich in calcium may help prevent hypertension and possibly stroke by reducing insulin resistance and platelet aggregation. (4) There appears to be a close association between vitamin D deficiency and cardiovascular disease. However, studies have failed to show benefits to replacement of low vitamin D levels with supplemental dietary vitamin D. (5) Replacing some animal proteins with soy protein (such as tofu) may help lower LDL cholesterol. Healthy carbohydrates are important for people with insulin resistance, prediabetes, or diabetes. Finally, (6) reduced calorie intake also helps control body weight—an extremely important risk factor for CVD.

A diet plan that reflects many of the recommendations described here was released as part of a study called Dietary Approaches to Stop Hypertension, or DASH. The DASH study found that a diet low in fat and high in fruits, vegetables, and low-fat dairy products reduces blood pressure. See Chapter 9 and visit https://www.nhlbi.nih.gov/health/health-topics/topics/dash for details about the DASH diet plan.

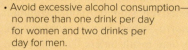

Do More

- Eat a diet rich in fruits, vegetables, whole grains, and low-fat or fat-free dairy products. Eat five to nine servings of fruits and vegetables each day.

- Eat several servings of high-fiber foods each day.

- Eat two or more servings of fish per week; try a few servings of nuts and soy foods each week.

- Choose unsaturated fats rather than saturated and trans fats.

  - Be physically active; do both aerobic exercise and strength training on a regular basis.

  - Achieve and maintain a healthy weight.

- Develop effective strategies for handling stress and anger. Nurture old friendships and family ties, and make new friends; pay attention to your spiritual side.

- Obtain recommended screening tests and follow your physician's recommendations.

Do Less

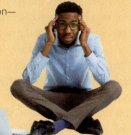

- Don't use tobacco in any form: cigarettes, spit tobacco, cigars and pipes, bidis and clove cigarettes.

- Limit consumption of trans fats and saturated fats.

- Limit consumption of salt to no more than 2300 mg of sodium per day (1500 mg if you have or are at high risk for hypertension).

- Avoid exposure to environmental tobacco smoke.

- Avoid excessive alcohol consumption— no more than one drink per day for women and two drinks per day for men.

- Limit consumption of added sugars and refined carbohydrates.

- Avoid excess stress, anger, and hostility.

FIGURE 12.8 **Strategies for reducing your risk of cardiovascular disease.**
© Rubberball/Getty Images; © Vladyslav Starozhylov/Alamy

Exercise Regularly

You can significantly reduce your risk of CVD with a moderate amount of physical activity. In addition to aerobic exercise for building and maintaining cardiovascular health, strength training helps reduce body fat and improves lipid levels and glucose metabolism. The more exercise you get, the less likely you are to develop or die from CVD.

Avoid Tobacco Products

The number-one risk factor for CVD that you can control is smoking. If you smoke, quit. If you don't smoke, don't start. If you live or work with people who smoke, take steps to prevent or stop your exposure.

Manage Your Blood Pressure, Cholesterol Levels, and Stress/Anger

If you have no CVD risk factors, have your blood pressure measured by a trained professional at least once every two years. Yearly tests are recommended if you have risk factors. If your blood pressure is high, follow your physician's advice on how to lower it. All people age 20 and over should have their cholesterol checked at least once every five years.

BASIC FACTS ABOUT CANCER

Cancer is the abnormal, uncontrolled multiplication of cells, which can ultimately cause death if left untreated.

Tumors

Most cancers take the form of tumors, although not all tumors are cancerous. A **tumor** (or *neoplasm*) is a mass of tissue that serves no physiological purpose. It can be benign, like a wart, or malignant, like most lung cancers.

Benign (noncancerous) **tumors** are made up of cells similar to the surrounding normal cells and are enclosed in a membrane that prevents them from penetrating neighboring tissues. They are dangerous only if their physical presence interferes with body functions. A benign brain tumor, for example, can cause death if it blocks the blood supply to the brain.

Ask Yourself

QUESTIONS FOR CRITICAL THINKING AND REFLECTION

Do you know what your blood pressure and cholesterol levels are? If not, is there a reason you don't know? Is something preventing you from getting this information about yourself? How can you motivate yourself to have these easy but important health checks?

TERMS

cancer   The abnormal, uncontrolled multiplication of cells.

tumor   A mass of tissue that serves no physiological purpose; also called a *neoplasm*.

benign tumor   A tumor that is not cancerous.

The term **malignant tumor** is synonymous with cancer. A malignant tumor can invade surrounding structures, including blood vessels, the **lymphatic system,** and nerves. It can also spread to distant sites via the blood and lymphatic circulation, producing invasive tumors in almost any part of the body. A few cancers, like leukemia (cancer of the blood), do not produce a mass but still have the fundamental property of rapid, uncontrolled cell proliferation. For this reason, such diseases are malignant and are considered to be a form of cancer.

Cancer begins when a change (or mutation) in a cell occurs that allows the cell to grow and divide when it should not. In adults, cells normally multiply at a rate just sufficient to replace dying cells. In contrast, a malignant cell divides into new cells without regard for normal control mechanisms and gradually produces a mass of abnormal cells, or a tumor. A pea-sized mass is made up of about a billion cells, so a single tumor cell must go through many divisions, often taking years, before the tumor grows to a noticeable size.

Eventually a tumor becomes large enough to cause symptoms or to be detected directly. In the breast, for example, a tumor may be felt as a lump or diagnosed as cancer by an X-ray or **biopsy.** In less accessible locations, like the lung, a tumor may be noticed only after it has grown considerably and may then be detected only by an indirect symptom, such as a persistent cough or unexplained bleeding. In the case of leukemia, changes in the blood are eventually noticed as increasing fatigue, infection, or abnormal bleeding.

Metastasis

Metastasis is the spread of cancer cells from one part of the body to another. Metastasis occurs because cancer cells do not stick to each other as strongly as normal cells do and therefore may move away from the site of the *primary tumor* (the cancer's original location). After cancer cells break away, they can pass through the lining of lymph or blood vessels to invade nearby tissue. They can also travel to different parts of the body where they establish new cancer cells. This traveling and seeding process is called *metastasizing,* and the new tumors are called *secondary tumors* or *metastases.* The ability of cancer cells to metastasize makes early cancer detection critical. To cure cancer, every cancerous cell must be removed or destroyed. Once cancer cells enter either the lymphatic system or the bloodstream, it is extremely difficult to stop their spread to other organs of the body.

Remission

A significant number of cancer cases go into **remission,** which in some cases lasts for years. In remission, signs and symptoms of cancer disappear, and the disease is considered to be under control. Remission typically results from treatment, but, rarely, some cancer patients enter remission spontaneously.

The Incidence of Cancer

Each year more than 1.6 million people in the United States are diagnosed with cancer. Most will be cured, or live many years past their initial cancer diagnosis. In fact, the American Cancer Society (ACS) estimates that the **five-year survival rate** for all cancers diagnosed between 2005 and 2011 is 69%. Figure 12.9 shows the number of new cases of cancer each year, and the number of deaths. Overall, men are more likely than women to die.

Until 1991, the number of cancer deaths increased fairly steadily in the United States, largely due to a wave of lethal lung cancers among men caused by smoking. In 1991, the cancer death rate in men began to fall. The cancer death rate in women began to fall in 2003. However, death rates from cancer are not declining as fast as those from heart disease, in large part because of the differing effects that quitting smoking has on disease risk. Heart-related damage from smoking reverses more quickly and more significantly than does cancer-related damage from smoking.

Still, many more people could be saved from cancer. The overwhelming majority of skin cancers could be prevented by protecting the skin from excessive sun exposure, and the majority of lung cancers could be prevented by avoiding exposure to tobacco smoke. Thousands of cases of colon, breast, and uterine cancers could be prevented by improving diet and controlling body weight. Regular screenings and self-examinations have the potential to save an additional 100,000 lives per year.

THE CAUSES OF CANCER

Although scientists do not know everything about what causes cancer, they have identified genetic, environmental, and lifestyle factors that increase the risk of developing cancer.

TERMS

malignant tumor   A tumor that is capable of spreading and thus is cancerous.

lymphatic system   A system of vessels that returns proteins, lipids, and other substances from fluid in the tissues to the circulatory system.

biopsy   The removal of a small piece of body tissue to allow for microscopic examination; a needle biopsy uses a needle to remove a small sample of tissue, but some biopsies require surgery.

metastasis   The spread of cancer cells from one part of the body to another.

remission   A period during the course of cancer in which there are no symptoms or other evidence of disease.

five-year survival rate   The percentage of patients diagnosed with a certain disease who will be alive five years after the date of diagnosis; used to estimate the prognosis of a particular disease.

New cases	Deaths	Male	Female	New cases	Deaths
34,780 (4%)	6,910 (2%)	Oral cavity and pharynx	Brain and other nervous system	10,420 (1%)	6,610 (2%)
46,870 (6%)	6,750 (2%)	Melanoma of the skin	Melanoma of the skin	29,510 (4%)	3,380 (1%)
117,920 (14%)	85,920 (13%)	Lung and bronchus	Thyroid	49,350 (6%)	1,070 (.4%)
13,460 (2%)	12,720 (4%)	Esophagus	Lung and bronchus	106,470 (13%)	72,160 (26%)
28,410 (3%)	18,280 (6%)	Liver and intrahepatic bile duct	Breast	246,660 (29%)	40,450 (14%)
27,670 (3%)	21,450 (7%)	Pancreas	Liver and intrahepatic bile duct	10,820 (1%)	8,890 (3%)
39,650 (5%)	9,240 (3%)	Kidney and renal pelvis	Pancreas	25,400 (3%)	23,330 (7%)
70,820 (8%)	26,020 (8%)	Colon and rectum	Kidney and renal pelvis	23,050 (3%)	5,000 (2%)
58,950 (7%)	11,820 (4%)	Urinary bladder	Colon and rectum	63,670 (8%)	23,170 (8%)
180,890 (21%)	26,120 (8%)	Prostate	Ovary	22,280 (3%)	14,240 (5%)
34,090 (4%)	14,130 (4%)	Leukemia	Uterine corpus	60,050 (7%)	10,470 (4%)
40,170 (5%)	11,520 (4%)	Non-Hodgkin lymphoma	Leukemia	26,050 (3%)	10,270 (4%)
			Non-Hodgkin lymphoma	32,410 (4%)	8,630 (3%)
841,390 (100%)	314,290 (100%)	All sites	All sites	843,820 (100%)	281,400 (100%)

VITAL STATISTICS

FIGURE 12.9 **Estimated number of new cancer cases and deaths by sex and by site, United States, 2016.** Estimated new cases are based on 1998–2012 incidence rates reported by the North American Association of Central Cancer Registries, representing 89% of the U.S. population. Estimated deaths are based on 1998–2012 U.S. mortality data, National Center for Health Statistics, Centers for Disease Control and Prevention.

SOURCE: American Cancer Society. 2016. *Cancer Facts and Figures, 2016.* Atlanta, GA: American Cancer Society.

© amanaimages/Getty RF.

The Role of DNA

Heredity and genetics are important factors in a person's risk of cancer. Certain genes may predispose some people to cancer, and specific genetic mutations have been associated with cancer.

Some mutations are inherited and others are caused by environmental agents including radiation, environmental substances, and chemical substances in air pollution.

The most prominent example of an inherited genetic mutation associated with increased cancer risk involves the *BRCA* gene. Women who inherited an altered copy of this gene face a significantly increased risk of breast and ovarian cancer. Testing and identification of hereditary cancer risks can be helpful for some people, especially if it leads to increased attention to controllable risk factors and better medical screening.

Tobacco Use

Smoking is responsible for an estimated 32% of all cancer deaths, including 83% of lung cancer deaths for men and 76% of such deaths for women. Overall, tobacco use is responsible for nearly one in five American deaths—approximately 480,000 premature deaths each year. The U.S. Surgeon General has reported that tobacco use is a direct cause of several types of cancer. In addition to lung and bronchial cancer, tobacco use is linked to cancer of the larynx, mouth, pharynx, esophagus, stomach, pancreas, kidneys, bladder, and cervix.

Dietary Factors

How important is diet in cancer prevention? The relationship between food and cancer risk is complex and controversial. The foods you eat contain many biologically active compounds, and your food choices may either increase your cancer risk by exposing you to potentially dangerous compounds or reduce your risk through consumption of potentially protective ones.

The following dietary factors may affect cancer risk:

- *Dietary fat and meat.* Diets high in fat and meat may contribute to certain cancers, including colon, stomach, and prostate cancers. Certain types of fats may be riskier than others. Omega-6 polyunsaturated fats are associated with a higher risk of certain cancers; omega-3 fats are not.

- *Alcohol.* Alcohol is associated with an increased incidence of several cancers. Women who have two to five drinks daily have about 1.5 times the cancer risk of women who drink no alcohol. Alcohol and tobacco interact as risk factors for oral cancer.

- *Fried foods.* High levels of the chemical acrylamide (a probable human carcinogen) are found in starch-based foods that have been fried or baked at high temperatures, especially french fries and certain types of snack chips and crackers.

- *Fiber.* Further study is needed to clarify the relationship between fiber intake and cancer risk, but experts still recommend a high-fiber diet for its overall positive effect on health.

- *Fruits and vegetables.* Researchers have identified many mechanisms by which food components may act against cancer. Some may prevent carcinogens from forming in the first place or block them from reaching or acting on target cells. Others boost enzymes that detoxify carcinogens and render them harmless. Some essential nutrients help reduce the harmful effects of carcinogens; for example, vitamin C, vitamin E, selenium, and the **carotenoids** (vitamin A precursors) may help block cancer by acting as antioxidants.

Many other anticancer agents in the diet fall under the broader heading of **phytochemicals,** which are substances in plants that help protect against chronic diseases. One of the first to be identified was sulforaphane, a potent anticarcinogen found in broccoli. Sulforaphane induces the cells of the liver and kidney to produce higher levels of protective enzymes, which then neutralize dietary carcinogens. Most fruits and vegetables contain beneficial phytochemicals, and researchers are just beginning to identify them. Figure 12.10 summarizes dietary and other strategies for reducing cancer risk.

Inactivity and Obesity

The American Cancer Society recommends maintaining a healthy weight throughout life with a balanced diet and physical activity, and by achieving and maintaining a healthy weight if you are currently overweight or obese. Obesity in middle and later age has been shown to increase risk for many cancers, and now evidence suggests that weight gain in early adulthood also puts us at risk—in women, particularly for endometrial and post-menopausal breast cancers, and in men, for colorectal cancer.

Carcinogens in the Environment

Some carcinogens occur naturally in the environment, like viruses and the sun's UV rays. Others are manufactured or synthetic substances that show up occasionally in the general environment but more often in the work environments of specific industries.

Microbes   It is estimated that 15–20% of the world's cancers are caused by microbes, including viruses, bacteria, and parasites, although the percentage is much lower in

> **TERMS**
>
> **carotenoid**   Any of a group of yellow-to-red plant pigments that can be converted to vitamin A by the liver; many act as antioxidants or have other anticancer effects. The carotenoids include beta-carotene, lutein, lycopene, and zeaxanthin.
>
> **phytochemical**   A naturally occurring substance found in plant foods that may help prevent chronic diseases such as cancer and heart disease; *phyto* means "plant."

Do More

- Eat a varied, plant-based diet that is high in fiber-rich foods such as legumes and whole grains.

- Eat 7–13 servings of fruits and vegetables every day, favoring foods from the following categories:
    - Cruciferous vegetables
    - Citrus fruits
    - Berries
    - Dark green leafy vegetables
    - Dark yellow, orange, or red fruits and vegetables

- Be physically active.

- Maintain a healthy weight.

- Practice safer sex (to avoid HPV infection).

- Protect your skin from the sun with appropriate clothing and sunscreen.

- Perform regular self-exams (skin self-exam for all, testicular self-exam for men, breast self-awareness for women).

- Obtain recommended screening tests and discuss with your physician any family history of cancer.

Do Less

- Don't use tobacco in any form:
    - Cigarettes
    - Spit tobacco
    - Cigars and pipes
    - Bidis and clove cigarettes

- Avoid exposure to environmental tobacco smoke.

- Limit consumption of fatty meats and other sources of saturated fat.

- Avoid excessive alcohol consumption.

- Limit consumption of salt.

- Don't eat charred foods, and limit consumption of cured and smoked meats and meat and fish grilled in a direct flame.

- Avoid occupational exposure to carcinogens.

- Limit exposure to UV radiation from sunlight.

- Avoid tanning lamps or beds.

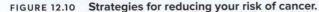

FIGURE 12.10   **Strategies for reducing your risk of cancer.**

© C Squared Studios/Getty Images RF; © Stockdisc/PunchStock RF; © Stockdisc/PunchStock RF; © Robyn Mackenzie/123RF

industrialized countries like the United States. Certain types of human papillomavirus are known to cause oropharyngeal cancer, cervical cancer, and other cancers, and the *Helicobacter pylori* bacterium has been linked to stomach cancer. Hepatitis viruses B and C together cause as many as 80% of the world's liver cancers.

Ingested Chemicals   Some compounds added to food, such as the nitrates and nitrites found in processed meat, are potentially dangerous. Although nitrates and nitrites are not themselves carcinogenic, they can combine with substances in the stomach and be converted to nitrosamines, which are highly potent carcinogens. Foods cured with nitrites, as well as those cured by salt or smoke, have been linked to esophageal and stomach cancer, and they should be eaten only in modest amounts.

Environmental and Industrial Pollution   Pollutants in the air have long been suspected of contributing to the incidence of lung cancer. Although fewer than 2% of cancer deaths are caused by general environmental pollution, such as substances in our air and water, exposure to carcinogenic materials in the workplace is a more serious problem. Occupational exposure to specific carcinogens may account for about 4% of cancer deaths. With increasing industry and government regulation, we can anticipate that the industrial sources of cancer risk will continue to diminish, at least in the United States.

Radiation   All sources of radiation are potentially carcinogenic, including medical X-rays, radioactive substances (radioisotopes), and UV rays from the sun. Successful efforts have been made to reduce the amount of radiation needed for mammograms, dental X-rays, and medical X-rays. Sunlight is an important source of radiation, and care should be taken to avoid excessive exposure.

> **QUICK STATS**
>
> Worldwide, **8.2 million** people died of cancer in 2012.
> —World Health Organization, 2015

Ask Yourself

QUESTIONS FOR CRITICAL THINKING AND REFLECTION

What do you think your risks for cancer are? Do you have a family history of cancer, or have you been exposed to carcinogens? How about your diet and exercise habits? What can you do to reduce your risks?

DETECTING, DIAGNOSING, AND TREATING CANCER

Early cancer detection often depends on our willingness to be aware of changes in our own body and to make sure we keep up with recommended screening tests. Although treatment success varies with individual cancers, cure rates have increased—sometimes dramatically—in this century, especially for cancers that are diagnosed at their early stages.

Detecting Cancer

Self-monitoring is the first line of defense. By being aware of the risk factors in your own life, your immediate family's cancer history, and your own history, you may bring a problem to the attention of a physician long before it would have been detected at a routine physical. In addition to self-monitoring, the ACS recommends routine cancer checkups, as well as specific screening tests for certain cancers (Table 12.4).

Diagnosing Cancer

Methods for determining the exact location, type, and extent of a cancer continue to improve. A biopsy may be performed to confirm the type of tumor. Several diagnostic imaging techniques have replaced exploratory surgery for some patients. They include MRIs, CT scanning, and ultrasonography.

Treating Cancer

The ideal cancer therapy would kill or remove all cancerous cells while leaving normal tissue untouched. Sometimes this is almost possible, as when a surgeon removes a small superficial tumor of the skin. Usually the tumor is less accessible, and some combination of surgery, radiation therapy, and chemotherapy must be applied instead. Some patients choose to combine conventional therapies with alternative treatments.

For most cancers, surgery is a definitive treatment. Surgically removing all the cancerous cells from the body can result in a long-lasting cure. This is particularly true for early cancers of the breast, prostate, lung, and colon. When the cancer is more advanced or involves nearby lymph nodes, patients may require chemotherapy or radiation therapy in addition to surgery.

Chemotherapy, or the use of medications to kill cancer cells, has been in use since the 1940s. Many of these drugs work by interfering with DNA synthesis and replication in rapidly dividing cells. Normal cells, which usually grow slowly, are not significantly destroyed by these drugs. However, some normal tissues such as intestinal, hair, and blood-forming cells are always growing, and damage to these tissues produces the unpleasant side effects of chemotherapy, including nausea, vomiting, diarrhea, and hair loss.

Chemotherapy can be used in a variety of settings, depending on the type of cancer and the timing in which the drugs are given. When the goal of treatment is cure (that is, completely eradicating all cancer cells), chemotherapy is often given either before or after surgery. Patients with cancers that are not thought to be curable (that is, not

> **chemotherapy**   The treatment of cancer with chemicals that selectively destroy cancerous cells. **TERMS**

SITE/TESTS AND PROCEDURES	DESCRIPTION	LINKS FOR MORE INFORMATION
BREAST		
Mammography	Mammograms are the best way to find breast cancer early, when it is easier to treat. These imaging tests, which involve low-dose X-rays, are recommended every 1 to 2 years for women starting at age 45 and especially between 50 and 74, or as long as they are in good health.	CDC: www.cdc.gov/cancer/breast/basic_info/screening.htm NCI: www.cancer.gov/types/breast/mammograms-fact-sheet www.cancer.gov/types/breast/patient/breast-screening-pdq
Breast awareness	Routine examination of the breasts by health care providers or by women themselves starting in their 20s has not been shown to reduce deaths from breast cancer. However, any lump or other unusual change in the breast needs to be promptly reported to a doctor.	ACS: www.cancer.org/treatment/understandingyourdiagnosis /examsandtestdescriptions/ mammogramsandotherbreastimagingprocedures/index
CERVIX		
Pap and HPV cytology tests	Pap tests can find abnormal cells in the cervix that may turn into cancer, and they can find cervical cancer early, when the chance of a cure is high. Testing every 3 to 5 years should begin at age 21 and end at age 65, if results have been normal. Women who have been vaccinated against HPV still need HPV tests.	CDC: www.cdc.gov/cancer/cervical/basic_info/screening.htm NCI: www.cancer.gov/types/cervical/pap-hpv-testing-fact-sheet www.cancer.gov/types/cervical/patient/cervical-screening-pdq
COLON		
Colonoscopy and sigmoidoscopy	A sigmoidoscopy every 5 years or a colonoscopy every 10 years between the ages of 50 and 75 can reduce the likelihood of death from colorectal cancer and can detect abnormal polyps that can be removed before they turn into cancer. The virtual colonoscopy has not been shown to reduce deaths from colorectal cancer.	CDC: www.cdc.gov/cancer/colorectal/basic_info/screening.htm NCI: www.cancer.gov/types/colorectal/screening-fact-sheet www.cancer.gov/types/colorectal/patient/colorectal -screening-pdq
High-sensitivity fecal occult blood test (FOBT)	This yearly multiple-stool, take-home test reduces death from colorectal cancer and is recommended for people between ages 50 and 75. If a positive result is found, the test is followed by a colonoscopy or sigmoidoscopy.	ACS: www.cancer.org/healthy/findcancerearly /examandtestdescriptions/faq-colonoscopy-and -sigmoidoscopy
LUNG		
Low-dose computed tomography (LDCT)	This imaging test has been shown to reduce lung cancer deaths among heavy smokers (30 pack-years*) between ages 55 and 74 or 80 who still smoke or have quit within the last 15 years.	CDC: www.cdc.gov/cancer/lung/basic_info/screening.htm NCI: www.cancer.gov/types/lung/patient/lung-screening-pdq
OVARY AND UTERUS		
CA-125 blood test, transvaginal ultrasound	There is no evidence that any screening test reduces deaths from ovarian cancer. However, these tests can help in diagnosing ovarian cancer. Women should report any unexpected bleeding or spotting to a doctor.	CDC: www.cdc.gov/cancer/ovarian/basic_info/screening.htm NCI: www.cancer.gov/types/ovarian/patient/ovarian-screening-pdq www.cancer.gov/types/uterine/patient/endometrial -screening-pdq
PROSTATE		
Prostate-specific antigen (PSA)	Although this blood test, which is often done with a digital rectal exam, can detect prostate cancer at an early stage, it is more likely to lead to overdiagnosis and overtreatment than to reduce deaths from prostate cancer. Starting at age 50, men should talk to a doctor about the pros and cons of this test. African American men and men whose father or brother had prostate cancer before age 65 should talk to a doctor about this test starting at age 45.	CDC: www.cdc.gov/cancer/prostate/basic_info/screening.htm NCI: www.cancer.gov/types/prostate/psa-fact-sheet

*A pack-year is calculated by multiplying the number of packs of cigarettes smoked per day by the number of years the person has smoked. For example, smoking 2 packs per day for 10 years is equal to 20 pack-years; smoking one-half pack per day for 10 years is equal to 5 pack-years.

SOURCES: American Cancer Society (ACS). 2015. *Exams and Tests to Find and Diagnose Cancer* (http://www.cancer.org/healthy/findcancerearly /examandtestdescriptions/index); Centers for Disease Control and Prevention (CDC). 2015. *Cancer Prevention and Control: Cancer Screening Tests* (http://www.cdc .gov/cancer/dcpc/prevention/screening.htm); National Cancer Institute (NCI). 2015. *Screening Tests* (http://www.cancer.gov/about-cancer/screening/screening-tests).

all of the cancer cells can be destroyed) can still benefit from chemotherapy. This is often referred to as *palliative chemotherapy*.

Radiation therapy uses a beam of X-rays or gamma rays directed at the tumor to kill tumor cells. With sophisticated techniques, the harmful rays are directed precisely at the cancerous cells, in order to minimize damage to surrounding normal cells. Radiation therapy is usually less toxic for the patient than either surgery or chemotherapy, and it can be performed on an outpatient basis.

COMMON TYPES OF CANCER

Cancers are classified according to the types of cells that give rise to them:

• **Carcinomas** arise from *epithelia*—tissues that cover external body surfaces, line internal tubes and cavities, and form the secreting portion of glands. This type of cancer is the most common. Major sites include the skin, breast, uterus, prostate, lungs, and gastrointestinal tract.

• **Sarcomas** arise from connective and fibrous tissues such as muscle, bone, cartilage, and the membranes covering muscles and fat.

• **Lymphomas** are cancers of the lymph nodes, part of the body's infection-fighting system.

• **Leukemias** are cancers of the blood-forming cells, which reside chiefly in the bone marrow.

Cancers vary greatly in how easily they can be detected and how well they respond to treatment. In general, it is difficult for an **oncologist** or **hematologist** to predict how a specific cancer will behave because each one arises from a unique set of changes in a single cell. In the sections that follow, we look more closely at the most common cancers and their causes, as well as how they are detected and treated.

Lung Cancer

Lung cancer accounts for about 14% of all new cancer diagnoses and is the most common cause of cancer death in the United States: It is responsible for about 160,000 deaths each year. Since 1987, lung cancer has surpassed breast cancer as the leading cause of cancer death in women.

Risk Factors The chief risk factor for lung cancer is tobacco smoke, which currently accounts for 30% of all cancer deaths and 90% of lung cancer deaths. When smoking is combined with exposure to other carcinogens, such as asbestos particles or certain pollutants, the risk of cancer can be multiplied by a factor of 10 or more.

The smoker is not the only one at risk. Environmental tobacco smoke (ETS) is a human carcinogen—even brief exposure can cause serious harm. Long-term exposure to ETS increases the risk of lung cancer.

Detection and Treatment Lung cancer is difficult to detect at an early stage and hard to cure even when detected early. Symptoms of lung cancer do not usually appear until the disease has advanced to the invasive stage. Signs and symptoms such as a persistent cough, chest pain, or recurring bronchitis may be the first indication of a tumor's presence. Spiral CT scans, a computer-assisted body imaging technique, can detect lung cancer in high-risk patients significantly earlier than chest X-rays. Besides CT scanning, a diagnosis can usually be made by chest X-ray or by studying the cells in sputum.

If caught early, localized cancers can be treated with surgery alone. The majority of patients are diagnosed with advanced disease, however, and radiation and chemotherapy are often used in addition to surgery. The five-year survival rate for all stages combined is only 17%. Phototherapy, gene therapy, and immunotherapy (vaccines) are being studied in hopes of improving these statistics.

Ask Yourself

QUESTIONS FOR CRITICAL THINKING AND REFLECTION
Most people think of cancer as a death sentence, but is that necessarily true? Have you or has anyone you know had an experience with cancer? If so, what was the outcome? Have you ever considered whether you might be at increased risk for some types of cancer? Have you taken any steps to reduce your risk?

Colon and Rectal Cancer

Another common cancer in the United States is colon and rectal cancer (also called *colorectal cancer*). Although there are effective screening methods for colorectal cancer, it is the third most common type of cancer.

Risk Factors Age is a key risk factor for colon and rectal cancer; the vast majority of cases are diagnosed in people aged 50 and over. Heredity also plays a role. Many cancers arise from preexisting **polyps**, which are small growths on the wall of the colon that may gradually develop into

---

TERMS

carcinoma   Cancer that originates in epithelial tissue (skin, glands, and lining of internal organs).

sarcoma   Cancer arising from bone, cartilage, or striated muscle.

lymphoma   A tumor originating from lymphatic tissue.

leukemia   Cancer of the blood or the blood-forming cells.

oncologist   A specialist in the diagnosis and treatment of cancer.

hematologist   A specialist in the diagnosis and treatment of blood disorders, including cancers such as leukemia and lymphoma.

polyp   A small, usually harmless mass of tissue that projects from the inner surface of the colon or rectum.

malignancies. The tendency to form colon polyps appears to be determined by specific genes, so many colon cancers may be due to inherited gene mutations.

Excessive alcohol use and smoking may increase the risk of colorectal cancer. Regular physical activity appears to reduce a person's risk, whereas obesity increases risk. A diet rich in fruits, vegetables, and whole grains is associated with lower risk. However, research findings on whether dietary fiber prevents colon cancer have been mixed. Studies have suggested a protective role for folic acid, magnesium, vitamin D, and calcium; in contrast, high intake of refined carbohydrates, simple sugars, red meat, processed meats, and smoked meats and fish may increase risk.

Regular use of nonsteroidal anti-inflammatory drugs such as aspirin and ibuprofen may decrease the risk of colon cancer and other cancers of the digestive tract. These agents are not currently recommended for colorectal cancer prevention, although several studies are under way to determine if the protective benefit of these drugs is greater than the risk of other negative health effects.

Detection and Treatment

If identified early, precancerous polyps and early-stage cancers can be removed before they become malignant or spread. Because polyps may bleed as they progress, common warning signs of colon cancer are bleeding from the rectum and a change in bowel habits.

Regular screening tests are recommended beginning at age 50 (earlier for people with a family history of the disease or who are otherwise at high risk). A yearly stool blood test can detect small amounts of blood in the stool long before obvious bleeding would be noticed. More involved screening tests are recommended at 5- or 10-year intervals. These tests include a sigmoidoscopy or colonoscopy, during which a flexible fiber-optic device is inserted through the rectum and the colon is examined and polyps biopsied or removed. Screening is effective, and studies demonstrate that it can prevent up to 76–90% of colon cancers. Still, only about half of U.S. adults have undergone any of these tests.

Surgery is the primary treatment for colon and rectal cancer. Radiation and chemotherapy may be used before surgery to shrink a tumor or after surgery to destroy any remaining cancerous cells. The five-year survival rate is 90% for colon and rectal cancers detected early and 65% overall.

Breast Cancer

Breast cancer is the most common cancer in women. In men, breast cancer occurs rarely. In the United States, about one woman in eight will develop breast cancer during her lifetime. Each year, about 247,000 American women are diagnosed with breast cancer and about 41,000 die from it.

QUICK STATS

14.5 million Americans with a history of cancer were alive in January 2014.
—American Cancer Society, 2016

Fewer than 2% of breast cancer cases occur in women under age 35, but incidence rates increase quickly with age. About 50% of cases are diagnosed in women aged 45–65.

Risk Factors

Genetics play a very important role in breast cancer. A woman who has two close relatives with breast cancer is more than four times more likely to develop the disease than a woman who has no close relatives with it. Even though genetic factors are important, inherited mutations in breast cancer susceptibility genes account for only approximately 5–10% of all breast cancer cases.

Other risk factors include early onset of menstruation, late onset of menopause, having no children or having a first child after age 30, current use of hormone replacement therapy, obesity, and alcohol use. Estrogen may be a unifying element for many of these risk factors. Estrogen circulates in a woman's body in high concentrations between puberty and menopause. Fat cells also produce estrogen, and estrogen levels are higher in obese women. Alcohol can interfere with estrogen metabolism in the liver and increase estrogen levels in the blood. Estrogen promotes the growth of cells in responsive sites, including the breast and the uterus, so any factor that increases estrogen exposure may raise breast cancer risk. A dramatic drop in rates of breast cancer from 2001 to 2004 was attributed in part to reduced use of hormone replacement therapy by women over age 50 beginning in July 2002. Millions of women stopped taking the hormones after research from the Women's Health Initiative linked hormone replacement therapy with an increased risk of breast cancer and heart disease.

Eating a low-fat, vegetable-rich diet, exercising regularly, limiting alcohol intake, and maintaining a healthy body weight can minimize the chance of developing breast cancer, even for women at risk from family history or other factors. Despite some popular myths, studies have shown that breast cancer incidence is not increased by underwire bras, antiperspirants, breast implants, or abortions.

Early Detection

A cure is most likely if breast cancer is detected early, so regular screening is a good investment, even for younger women. The ACS recommends the following for the early detection of breast cancer:

- *Mammography.* A **mammogram** is a low-dose breast X-ray that can identify about 80–90% of breast cancers at an early stage, before physical symptoms develop. The ACS recommends that women at average risk for breast cancer begin annual mammograms at age 45; at age 55, women should have

mammogram A low-dose X-ray of the breasts used to check for early signs of breast cancer. **TERMS**

mammograms every other year. However, the ACS also states that women aged 40–44 and women over the age of 55 may choose to have annual mammograms. Some controversy surrounds the best age to start mammographic screening. Some groups have argued that the rates of false-positive mammograms are higher between ages 40 and 50; thus, the U.S. Preventive Services Task Force, for example, advises that women should wait until age 50 to begin routine screening.

- **Breast awareness.** The ACS no longer recommends breast self-exams (BSE) or clinical breast exams, but many doctors still do, and a woman should be familiar with her breasts and alert her health care provider to any changes right away. The following are warning signs of breast cancer but can also be caused by other conditions: A new lump in the breast or underarm; Thickening or swelling of part of the breast; irritation or dimpling of breast skin; redness or flaky skin in the nipple area or the breast; pulling in of the nipple or pain in the nipple area; nipple discharge other than breast milk, including blood; any change in the size or the shape of the breast; and pain in any area of the breast. Women who do choose to perform BSE should review the recommended technique with their health care provider. Most breast lumps and changes are benign but should be checked by a health care provider.

Additional screenings may be recommended for women at increased risk for breast cancer. Studies show that MRI may be better than mammography at detecting breast abnormalities in some women. The ACS recommends both an annual mammogram and an annual MRI for women who are at high risk for breast cancer, such as those who carry a *BRCA* mutation. **Ultrasonography** (use of sound waves to create images of soft tissue) is not a standard screening tool for breast cancer, but it is often used as a follow-up test if a mammogram reveals an abnormality in breast tissue.

Treatment   If a lump is detected, it may be scanned by ultrasonography and biopsied to see if it is cancerous. In most cases, the lump is found to be a cyst or other harmless growth, and no further treatment is needed. If the lump contains cancer cells, a variety of surgeries may be indicated, ranging from a lumpectomy (removal of the lump and surrounding tissue) to a mastectomy (removal of the breast).

Analyzing the tumor specimen with special stains can help predict the risk of breast cancer recurrence and help identify women who will benefit most from additional therapy; women can then make more informed treatment decisions. Treatment with **monoclonal antibodies,** such as trastuzumab, is an option for about 15–20% of patients diagnosed with breast cancer.

If the tumor is discovered before it has spread to the adjacent lymph nodes or outside the breast, the patient has a 99% chance of surviving more than five years. The relative survival rate for all stages is 89% at five years.

Strategies for Prevention   A number of drugs have been proposed for the prevention of breast cancer, especially in high-risk patients. A family of drugs called *selective estrogen receptor modulators* (*SERMs*) acts like estrogen in some tissues of the body but blocks estrogen's effects in others. One SERM, tamoxifen, has long been used in breast cancer treatment because it blocks the action of estrogen in breast tissue. In 1998, the U.S. Food and Drug Administration (FDA) approved the use of tamoxifen to reduce the risk of breast cancer in healthy women who are at high risk for the disease. However, the drug has serious potential side effects, including increased risk of blood clots and uterine cancer. Another SERM, raloxifene, was approved in 2007 for the reduction of invasive breast cancer risk in postmenopausal women at high risk for breast cancer. Compared to tamoxifen, raloxifene has been shown to pose a slightly lower risk of blood clots and uterine cancer, but the risk is still higher than that of a placebo. Raloxifene has also been shown to improve bone mineral density.

Prostate Cancer

The prostate gland is located at the base of the bladder in men and completely surrounds the male's urethra; if enlarged, it can block the flow of urine. Prostate cancer is the most common cancer in men and the second leading cause of cancer death in men. In the United States, nearly 181,000 new cases are diagnosed and more than 26,000 men die from the disease each year.

Risk Factors   Age is the strongest predictor of risk, with approximately 60% of cases of prostate cancer diagnosed in men over age 65. Inherited genetic predisposition may be responsible for 5–10% of cases, and men with a family history of the disease should be particularly vigilant about screening. African American men and Jamaican men of African descent have the highest rates of prostate cancer of any groups in the world. Both genetic and lifestyle factors may be involved.

Diets that are high in calories, dairy products, and animal fats and also low in plant foods have been implicated as possible culprits, as have obesity, inactivity, and a history of sexually transmitted diseases. Type 2 diabetes and insulin resistance are also associated with prostate cancer. Soy foods, tomatoes, and cruciferous vegetables are being investigated for their possible protective effects.

Detection   Warning signs of prostate cancer can include changes in urinary frequency, weak or interrupted urine flow, painful urination, and blood in the urine.

---

ultrasonography   An imaging method in which sound waves are bounced off body structures to create an image on a TV monitor; also called *ultrasound*.

TERMS

monoclonal antibody   An antibody designed to bind to a specific cancer-related target.

Techniques for early detection include a digital rectal examination and the **prostate-specific antigen (PSA) test.** Currently there is insufficient data in support of or against routine screening with the PSA test. The ACS recommends that men be provided information about the benefits and limitations of the tests and that both the exam and the PSA test be offered annually, beginning at age 50, for men who are at average risk of prostate cancer, do not have any major medical problems, and have a life expectancy of at least 10 years. Men at high risk, including African Americans and those with a family history of the disease, should consider beginning screening at age 45. Men with multiple family members who have been diagnosed with the disease should begin screening at age 40.

PSA testing has been a subject of controversy among experts for several years because of its tendency to yield misleading results, leading to further testing, including biopsies, that can potentially cause harm. This potential harm is especially a concern for older men (over age 75), who are more likely to die of other causes even if they have slow-growing prostate cancer. In older men, most prostate cancers are not deadly, making treatment pointless and potentially harmful.

Treatment   Treatments vary based on the stage of the cancer and the patient's age. A small, slow-growing tumor in an older man may be treated with watchful waiting and no initial therapy because he is more likely to die from another cause before his cancer becomes life-threatening. More aggressive treatment would be indicated for younger men or those with more advanced cancers. Treatment may involve *radical prostatectomy* (surgical removal of the prostate). Although radical surgery has an excellent cure rate, it is major surgery and often results in **incontinence** or erectile dysfunction. Minimally invasive surgery, which utilizes a laparoscopic or robotic approach, can sometimes be performed with fewer complications and quicker recovery.

A less invasive alternative involves surgical implantation of radioactive seeds. Radiation from the seeds destroys the tumor and much of the normal prostate tissue but leaves surrounding tissue relatively untouched. Alternative or additional treatments include external radiation, hormonal therapy, cryotherapy, and chemotherapy. Several new treatments for advanced prostate cancer have recently been approved by the FDA, including a cancer vaccine known as sipuleucel-T.

Survival rates for all stages of this cancer have improved steadily since 1940; the five-year survival rate is now nearly 100%.

Cancers of the Female Reproductive Tract

Several types of cancer can affect the female reproductive tract, and a few of these cancers are relatively common.

Cervical Cancer   Cancer of the cervix occurs in women in their twenties and thirties. In the United States, approximately 13,000 women are diagnosed with cervical cancer each year, and the disease kills more than 4000 women annually.

Cervical cancer is largely a sexually transmitted disease. Virtually all cases of cervical cancer stem from infection by the human papillomavirus (HPV), a group of about 100 related viruses that also cause common warts and genital warts. When certain types of HPV are introduced into the cervix, usually by an infected sex partner, the virus infects cervical cells, causing them to divide and grow. If unchecked, this growth can develop into cervical cancer. Cervical cancer is associated with multiple sex partners and is extremely rare in women who have not had heterosexual intercourse. Smoking, immunosuppression, and prolonged use of oral contraceptives also have been associated with increased risk.

Screening for the changes in cervical cells that precede cancer is done chiefly by means of the **Pap test.** During a pelvic exam, loose cells are scraped from the cervix and examined under a microscope to see whether they are normal. If cells are abnormal but not yet cancerous, the patient has a condition commonly referred to as *cervical dysplasia.* Sometimes such abnormal cells spontaneously return to normal, but in about one-third of cases the cellular changes progress toward malignancy. If this happens, the abnormal cells must be removed, either surgically or with a cryoscopic (ultra-cold) probe or localized laser treatment. When abnormal cells are in a precancerous state, the small patch of dangerous cells can be removed completely.

Without timely surgery, the malignant cells invade the cervical wall and spread to the uterus and adjacent lymph nodes. At this stage, chemotherapy and radiation may be used to kill the cancer cells, but chances for a complete cure are reduced. Even when a cure can be achieved, it often requires surgical removal of the uterus.

Because the Pap test is highly effective, all women between ages 21 and 65 should be tested. The recommended schedule for testing depends on risk factors, the type of Pap test performed, and whether the Pap test is combined with HPV testing. Two HPV vaccines have been approved by the FDA for the prevention of cervical cancer. Women who receive one of the vaccines should continue to receive routine Pap tests because the vaccines do not protect against all types of the virus.

---

prostate-specific antigen (PSA) test   A screening test for prostate cancer that measures blood levels of prostate-specific antigen (PSA).

incontinence   The inability to control the flow of urine.

Pap test   A scraping of cells from the cervix for examination under a microscope to detect cancer.

TERMS

Uterine, or Endometrial, Cancer Cancer of the lining of the uterus (the *endometrium*) most often occurs after the age of 55. The risk factors are similar to those for breast cancer, including prolonged exposure to estrogen, early onset of menstruation, late menopause, never having been pregnant, and obesity. Type 2 diabetes is also associated with increased risk. The use of oral contraceptives or hormone therapies that contain estrogen plus progestin does not appear to increase risk.

Endometrial cancer often presents with abnormal vaginal bleeding in a postmenopausal woman. It is treated surgically, commonly by *hysterectomy,* or removal of the uterus. Radiation treatment, hormones, and chemotherapy may be used in addition to surgery. When the tumor is detected at an early stage, about 95% of patients are alive and disease-free five years later. When the disease has spread beyond the uterus, the five-year survival rate is less than 67%.

Ovarian Cancer Although ovarian cancer is rare compared with cervical or uterine cancer, it causes more deaths than the other two combined. About 22,000 women were diagnosed with ovarian cancer in 2016, and an estimated 14,000 deaths resulted from this cancer in the same year. There are often no warning signs of ovarian cancer. Early symptoms may include increased abdominal size and bloating, urinary urgency, and pelvic pain. It cannot be detected by Pap tests or any other simple screening method and is often diagnosed late in its development, when surgery and other therapies are unlikely to be successful.

The risk factors are similar to those for breast and endometrial cancers: increasing age (most ovarian cancer occurs after age 60), never having been pregnant, a family history of breast or ovarian cancer, obesity, and specific genetic mutations including *BRCA1* and *BRCA2*. A high number of ovulations appears to increase the chance that a cancer-causing genetic mutation will occur, so anything that lowers the number of lifetime ovulation cycles—pregnancy, breastfeeding, or use of oral contraceptives—reduces a woman's risk of ovarian cancer.

Women with symptoms or who are at high risk because of family history or because they harbor a mutant gene may be offered screening with a pelvic exam, ultrasound, and blood test. Ovarian cancer is treated by surgical removal of both ovaries, the fallopian tubes, and the uterus. Radiation and chemotherapy are sometimes used in addition to surgery. When the tumor is localized to the ovary, the five-year survival rate is 92%. However, it is diagnosed this early only 15% of the time. For all stages, the five-year survival rate is only 46%.

Skin Cancer

Skin cancer is the most common type of cancer, but it is often not included in cancer incidence and mortality statistics because many types of skin cancer are easily curable. Of the approximate 3.5 million cases of skin cancer diagnosed each year, about 76,000 are of the most serious type, **melanoma.**

Risk Factors Almost all cases of skin cancer can be traced to excessive exposure to **ultraviolet (UV) radiation** from the sun, including longer-wavelength ultraviolet A (UVA) and shorter-wavelength ultraviolet B (UVB) radiation. UVB radiation causes sunburns and can damage the eyes and the immune system. UVA is less likely to cause an immediate sunburn, but it damages connective tissue and leads to premature aging of the skin, giving it a wrinkled, leathery appearance. (Tanning lamps and tanning salon beds emit mostly UVA radiation.) Both UVA and UVB radiation have been linked to the development of skin cancer, and the National Toxicology Program has declared both solar and artificial sources of UV radiation, including sunlamps and tanning beds, to be known human carcinogens.

Both severe, acute sun reactions (sunburns) and chronic low-level sun reactions (suntans) can lead to skin cancer. People with fair skin have less natural protection against skin damage from the sun and a higher risk of developing skin cancer, whereas people with naturally dark skin have a considerable degree of protection. Lighter-skinned people are about 10 times more likely to develop melanoma, but darker-skinned people are still at risk.

Severe sunburns in childhood have been linked to a significantly increased risk of skin cancer in later life, so children in particular should be protected. According to the Skin Cancer Foundation, the risk of skin cancer doubles in people who have had five or more sunburns in their lifetime. Because of damage to the ozone layer of the atmosphere, there is a chance that we may all be exposed to increasing amounts of UV radiation in the future. Other risk factors for skin cancer include having many moles (particularly large ones), spending time at high altitudes, and a family history of the disease.

Types of Skin Cancer There are three main types of skin cancer, named for the types of skin cells from which they develop. **Basal cell carcinoma** (usually benign) and **squamous cell carcinoma** (malignant) together account for about 95% of the skin cancers diagnosed each year.

TERMS

melanoma A malignant tumor of the skin that arises from pigmented cells, usually a mole.

ultraviolet (UV) radiation Light rays of a specific wavelength emitted by the sun; most UV rays are blocked by the ozone layer in the upper atmosphere.

basal cell carcinoma Benign skin cancer of the base of the outermost layer of the skin.

squamous cell carcinoma Malignant cancer of the surface of the outermost layer of the skin.

If you consistently use sun-protective clothing, sunscreen, and common sense, you can lead an active outdoor life *and* protect your skin against most sun-induced damage.

Clothing

• **Wear long-sleeved shirts and long pants.** Consider clothing made from special sun-protective fabrics; these garments have an ultraviolet protection factor (UPF) rating, similar to the SPF for sunscreens.

• **Wear a hat.** A good choice is a broad-brimmed hat or a legionnaire-style cap that covers the ears and neck. Wear sunscreen on your face even if you are wearing a hat.

• **Wear sunglasses.** Exposure to UV rays can damage the eyes and cause cataracts.

Sunscreen

• **Use a sunscreen and lip balm with a sun protection factor (SPF) of 15 or higher.** An SPF rating refers to the amount of time you can stay out in the sun before you burn, compared with not using sunscreen. For example, a product with an SPF of 15 would allow you to remain in the sun without burning 15 times longer, on average, than if you didn't apply sunscreen.

• **Apply sunscreen correctly and often.** Shake sunscreen before applying. Apply it 30 minutes before exposure to

allow it time to bond to the skin. Reapply sunscreen frequently and generously to all sun-exposed areas. A higher SPF does not mean you can use less. Reapply sunscreen 15–30 minutes after sun exposure begins and then every two hours after that and following activities, such as swimming, that could remove sunscreen.

Time of Day and Location

• **Avoid sun exposure between 10 a.m. and 4 p.m.,** when the sun's rays are most intense.

• **Consult the day's UV index, which predicts UV levels on a 0–11+ scale, to get a sense of the amount of sun protection you'll need.** You can download a free UV index app from the U.S. Environmental Protection Agency or find index ratings from the National Weather Service.

Tanning Salons

• **Avoid tanning salons.** Tanning beds and lamps emit mostly UVA radiation, increasing your risk of premature skin aging (such as wrinkles) and skin cancer.

• **If you really want a tan, consider using a sunless tanning product.** Lotions, creams, and sprays containing the color additive dihydroxyacetone (DHA) are approved by the FDA for tanning.

They are usually found in chronically sun-exposed areas, such as the face, neck, hands, and arms. They usually appear as pale, waxlike, pearly nodules or red, scaly, sharply outlined patches. These cancers are often painless, although they may bleed, crust, and form an open sore on the skin.

Melanoma is by far the most dangerous skin cancer because it spreads so rapidly. It can occur anywhere on the body, but the most common sites are the back, chest, abdomen, and lower legs. A melanoma usually appears at the site of a preexisting mole. The mole may begin to enlarge, become mottled or varied in color (colors can include blue, pink, and white), or develop an irregular surface or irregular borders. Tissue invaded by melanoma may also itch, burn, or bleed easily.

Prevention   One of the major steps you can take to protect yourself against all forms of skin cancer is to avoid lifelong overexposure to sunlight. Blistering, peeling sunburns from unprotected sun exposure are particularly dangerous, but suntans—whether from sunlight or from tanning lamps—also increase your risk of developing skin cancer later in life. People of every age, especially babies and children, need to be protected from the sun with **sunscreens** and protective clothing. For a closer look at sunlight and skin cancer, see the box "Sunscreens and Sun-Protective Clothing."

Detection and Treatment   Make it a habit to examine your skin regularly. Most of the spots, freckles, moles, and blemishes on your body are normal; you were born with some of them, and others appear and disappear throughout your life. But if you notice an unusual growth, discoloration, sore that does not heal, or mole that undergoes a sudden or progressive change, see your physician or dermatologist immediately.

> **sunscreen**   A substance used to protect the skin from UV rays; usually applied as a lotion, cream, or spray.
>
> **TERMS**

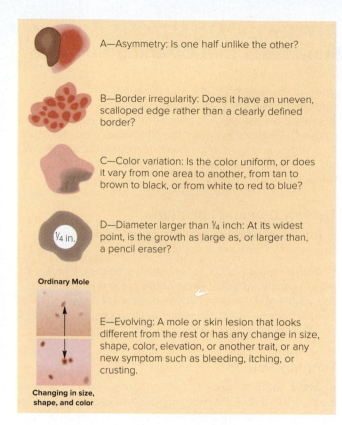

A—Asymmetry: Is one half unlike the other?

B—Border irregularity: Does it have an uneven, scalloped edge rather than a clearly defined border?

C—Color variation: Is the color uniform, or does it vary from one area to another, from tan to brown to black, or from white to red to blue?

¼ in.

D—Diameter larger than ¼ inch: At its widest point, is the growth as large as, or larger than, a pencil eraser?

Ordinary Mole

E—Evolving: A mole or skin lesion that looks different from the rest or has any change in size, shape, color, elevation, or another trait, or any new symptom such as bleeding, itching, or crusting.

Changing in size, shape, and color

FIGURE 12.11 **The ABCDE test for melanoma.** To see a variety of photos of melanoma and benign moles, visit the National Cancer Institute's Visuals Online site (http://visualsonline.cancer.gov).

Figure 12.11 illustrates the characteristics of a possible melanoma—asymmetry; border irregularity; color variations; a diameter greater than ¼ inch; and changes in the size, shape, or color of the mole. If someone in your family has had multiple skin cancers or melanomas, consult a dermatologist for a complete skin examination and discussion of your particular risk.

Since 2011, the FDA has approved several new therapies for metastatic melanoma. For example, ipilimumab is a monoclonal antibody that activates the body's anticancer immune response and was approved for patients with previously untreated metastatic melanoma. For melanoma, the five-year survival rate is 98% if the tumor is localized but only 63% if the cancer has spread to adjacent lymph nodes. Improvements in survival are anticipated with the use of these new immune-based treatments.

Testicular Cancer

Testicular cancer is relatively rare, accounting for only 1% of cancer in men (about 8000 cases per year), but it is the most common cancer in men aged 20–35. It is much more common among European Americans than among Latinos, Asian Americans, or African Americans. It is also relatively common among men whose fathers had testicular cancer. Men with undescended testicles are at increased risk for testicular cancer, and for this reason that condition should be corrected in early childhood. Self-examination may help in the early detection of testicular cancer (see the box "Testicle Self-Examination"). Tumors are treated by surgical removal of the testicle and, if the tumor has spread, by chemotherapy; radiation treatment is used only rarely. The five-year survival rate for testicular cancer is 95%.

Ask Yourself

QUESTIONS FOR CRITICAL THINKING AND REFLECTION

Has anyone you know had cancer? If so, what type of cancer was it? What were its symptoms? Based on the information presented so far in this chapter, did the person have any of the known risk factors for the disease?

TIPS FOR TODAY AND THE FUTURE

A growing body of research suggests that you can take an active role in preventing CVD and many cancers by adopting a wellness-focused lifestyle.

RIGHT NOW YOU CAN:

- Make an appointment to have your blood pressure and cholesterol levels checked.
- Plan to replace one high-fat and one high-sugar item in your diet with one that is high in fiber. For example, replace a doughnut with a bowl of whole-grain cereal.
- Buy multiple bottles of sunscreen and put them in places where you will most likely need them, such as your backpack, gym bag, or car.
- Check the cancer screening guidelines in this chapter and make sure you are up-to-date on yours.
- If you are a woman, develop breast self-awareness. If you are a man, do a testicular self-exam.

IN THE FUTURE YOU CAN:

- Track your eating habits for one week and then compare them to the DASH eating plan. Make adjustments to bring your diet closer to the DASH recommendations.
- Learn where to find information about daily UV radiation levels in your area, and learn how to interpret the information. Many local newspapers and television stations (and their websites) report current UV levels every day.
- Gradually add foods with abundant phytochemicals to your diet.

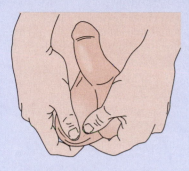

The best time to perform a testicular self-exam is after a warm shower or bath, when the scrotum is relaxed.

First, stand in front of a mirror and look for any swelling of the scrotum. Then examine each testicle with both hands. Place the index and middle fingers under the testicle and the thumbs on top. Roll the testicle gently between the fingers and thumbs. Don't worry if one testicle seems slightly larger than the other; that's common. Also, expect to feel the epididymis, which is the soft, sperm-carrying tube at the rear of the testicle.

Perform a self-exam each month. If you find a lump, swelling, or nodule, see a physician right away. The abnormality may not be cancer, but only a physician can make a diagnosis.

Other possible signs of testicular cancer include a change in the way a testicle feels, a sudden collection of fluid in the scrotum, a dull ache in the lower abdomen or groin, a feeling of heaviness in the scrotum, or pain in a testicle or the scrotum.

SOURCES: Testicular Cancer Resource Center. 2012. *How to Do a Testicular Self Examination* (http://tcrc.acor.org/tcexam.html); National Cancer Institute. 2013. *General Information about Testicular Cancer* (http://www.cancer.gov/cancertopics/pdq/treatment/testicular/Patient).

SUMMARY

- The cardiovascular system circulates blood throughout the body. The heart pumps blood to the lungs via the pulmonary artery and to the body via the aorta.

- The six major risk factors for CVD that can be changed or controlled are tobacco use, high blood pressure, unhealthy cholesterol levels, inactivity, overweight or obesity, and diabetes.

- Effects of smoking include lower HDL levels, increased blood pressure and heart rate, and increased risk of blood clots.

- Hypertension occurs when blood pressure exceeds normal levels most of the time. It weakens the heart, scars and hardens arteries, and can damage the eyes and kidneys.

- High LDL and low HDL cholesterol levels contribute to clogged arteries and increase the risk of developing CVD.

- Physical inactivity, obesity, and diabetes are interrelated and are associated with high blood pressure and unhealthy cholesterol levels.

- Contributing risk factors that can be changed include high triglyceride levels, metabolic syndrome, inflammation, and psychological and social factors.

- Risk factors for CVD that can't be changed include being over 65, being male, being African American, and having a family history of CVD.

- Atherosclerosis is a progressive hardening and narrowing of arteries that can lead to restricted blood flow and even complete blockage.

- Heart attacks are usually the result of a long-term disease process. Warning signs of a heart attack include chest discomfort, shortness of breath, nausea, and sweating.

- A stroke occurs when the blood supply to the brain is cut off by a blood clot or hemorrhage. A transient ischemic attack (TIA) may be a warning sign of an impending stroke.

- Congestive heart failure occurs when the heart's pumping action becomes less efficient and fluid collects in the lungs or in other parts of the body.

- Dietary changes that can protect against CVD include decreasing your intake of fat and cholesterol, and increasing your intake of fiber by eating more fruits, vegetables, and whole grains.

- CVD risk can also be reduced by exercising regularly, avoiding tobacco and environmental tobacco smoke, knowing and managing your blood pressure and cholesterol levels, and developing effective ways of handling stress and anger.

- Cancer is the abnormal, uncontrolled multiplication of cells; it can cause death if untreated.

- A malignant tumor can invade surrounding structures and spread to distant sites via the blood and lymphatic system, producing additional tumors.

- A malignant cell divides without regard for normal growth. As tumors grow, they produce signs or symptoms that are determined by their location in the body.

- Mutagens include radiation, viral infection, and chemical substances in food and air.

- Cancer-promoting dietary factors include meat, especially red and processed meat; certain types of fats; and alcohol. Diets high in fruits and vegetables are linked to a lower risk of cancer.

- Other possible causes of cancer include inactivity and obesity, certain viruses and chemicals, and radiation.

- Self-monitoring and regular screening tests are essential to early cancer detection. Methods of cancer diagnosis include MRI scanning, CT scanning, and ultrasound. Treatment methods usually consist of some combination of surgery, chemotherapy, and radiation.

- Lung cancer kills more people than any other type of cancer. Tobacco smoke is the primary cause.

- Colon and rectal cancers are linked to age, heredity, obesity, and a diet rich in processed meat and low in fruits and vegetables. Most colon cancers arise from preexisting polyps.

- Breast cancer affects about one in eight women in the United States. Although there is a genetic component to breast cancer, diet and hormones are also risk factors.

- Prostate cancer is chiefly a disease of aging; diet and lifestyle probably are factors in its occurrence. Early detection is possible through rectal examinations and PSA blood tests.

- Cancers of the female reproductive tract include cervical, uterine, and ovarian cancers. The Pap test is an effective screening test for cervical cancer.

- Abnormal cellular changes in the skin, often a result of exposure to the sun, cause skin cancer, as does chronic exposure to certain chemicals. Skin cancers include basal cell carcinoma, squamous cell carcinoma, and melanoma.

- Testicular cancer can be detected early through self-examination.

FOR MORE INFORMATION

American Academy of Dermatology. Provides information about skin cancer prevention.

http://www.aad.org

American Cancer Society. Provides a wide range of free materials on the prevention, diagnosis, and treatment of cancer.

http://www.cancer.org

American Heart Association (AHA). Provides information about hundreds of topics relating to cardiovascular disease; the AHA's website links to several sites focusing on specific heart-related topics.

http://www.heart.org

American Institute for Cancer Research. Provides information about lifestyle and cancer prevention, especially nutrition.

http://www.aicr.org

Cancer Guide: Steve Dunn's Cancer Information Page. Provides links to many good cancer resources on the Internet and advice about how to make the best use of the information.

http://www.cancerguide.org

Clinical Trials. Information about clinical trials for new cancer treatments can be accessed at the following sites:

http://www.cancer.gov/clinicaltrials

http://www.centerwatch.com

Dietary Approaches to Stop Hypertension (DASH). Provides information about the design, diets, and results of the DASH study, including tips on how to follow the DASH diet at home.

http://www.nhlbi.nih.gov/health/resources/heart/hbp-dash-index

EPA/Sunwise. Provides information about the UV index and the effects of sun exposure, with links to sites with daily UV index ratings for cities in the United States and other countries.

http://www.epa.gov/sunwise/uvindex.html

The Heart: The Engine of Life. An online museum exhibit containing information about the structure and function of the heart, how to monitor your heart's health, and how to maintain a healthy heart.

https://www.fi.edu/heart-engine-of-life

MedlinePlus: Blood, Heart, and Circulation Topics. Provides links to reliable sources of information on many topics relating to cardiovascular health.

https://www.nlm.nih.gov/medlineplus/bloodheartandcirculation.html

MedlinePlus Cancer Information. Provides news and links to reliable information on a variety of cancers and cancer treatment.

http://www.nlm.nih.gov/medlineplus/cancers.html

National Cancer Institute. Provides information about treatment options, screening, and clinical trials.

http://www.cancer.gov

National Comprehensive Cancer Network (NCCN). Presents treatment guidelines for physicians and patients related to the treatment of various cancers; these guidelines were developed by a group of leading cancer centers.

http://www.nccn.org

National Heart, Lung, and Blood Institute. Provides information about and interactive applications for a variety of topics relating to cardiovascular health and disease, including cholesterol, smoking, obesity, hypertension, and the DASH diet.

http://www.nhlbi.nih.gov/

National Stroke Association. Provides information and referrals for stroke victims and their families as well as a stroke risk assessment.

http://www.stroke.org

National Toxicology Program. The federal program that creates regular reports listing the substances known or reasonably assumed to cause cancer in humans.

http://ntp.niehs.nih.gov/

Oncolink/The University of Pennsylvania Cancer Center Resources. Contains information about different types of cancer and answers to frequently asked questions.

http://www.oncolink.org

Your Disease Risk Index. Includes interactive risk assessments as well as tips for preventing common cancers.

http://www.yourdiseaserisk.wustl.edu/

SELECTED BIBLIOGRAPHY

American Cancer Society. 2015. *Breast Cancer Facts and Figures 2015–2016.* Atlanta, GA: American Cancer Society.

American Cancer Society. 2016. *Cancer Facts and Figures 2016.* Atlanta, GA: American Cancer Society.

Adly, G., and R. Plakogiannis. 2013. Reinitiating aspirin therapy for primary prevention of cardiovascular events in a patient post–aspirin–induced upper gastrointestinal bleed: A case report and review of literature. *Annals of Pharmacotherapy* 47(2): e8.

Bibbins-Doming, K., et al. 2010. Projected effect of dietary salt reductions on future cardiovascular disease. *New England Journal of Medicine* 362(7): 590–599.

Bouvard, V., et al. 2015. Carcinogenicity of consumption of red and processed meat. *Lancet Oncology* 16 (16): 1599–1600

Bucholz, E. M., et al. 2016. Life expectancy after myocardial infarction, according to hospital performance. *New England Journal of Medicine* 375(14): 1332–1342.

Cao, S., et al. 2015. The health effects of passive smoking: An overview of systematic reviews based on observational epidemiological evidence. *PLoS One* 10(10): e0139907.

Castellsaqué, X., et al. 2016. HPV involvement in head and neck cancers. Comprehensive assessment of biomarkers in 3680 patients. *Journal of the National Cancer Institute* 108(6).

Centers for Disease Control and Prevention. 2015. Current cigarette smoking among adults—United States, 2005–2014. *MMWR* 64(44): 1233–1240.

Centers for Disease Control and Prevention. 2015. *Heart Disease Statistics and Maps* (http://www.cdc.gov/heartdisease/facts.htm).

Centers for Disease Control and Prevention. 2015. *Vital Signs: E-Cigarette Ads and Youth* (http://www.cdc.gov/vitalsigns/ecigarette-ads/index.html).

Demeyer, D., et al. 2015. Mechanisms linking colorectal cancer to the consumption of (processed) red meat: A review. *Critical Reviews in Food Science and Nutrition*, May 15.

Farvid, M. S., et al. 2016. Fruit and vegetable consumption in adolescence and early adulthood and risk of breast cancer: Population based cohort study. *British Medical Journal* 353: i2343.

Guan, W., et al. 2015. Race is a key variable in assigning lipoprotein(a) cutoff values for coronary heart disease risk assessment: The Multi-Ethnic Study of Atherosclerosis. *Arteriosclerosis, Thrombosis, and Vascular Biology* 35(4): 996–1001.

Han, X., et al. 2015. Body mass index at early adulthood, subsequent weight change and cancer incidence and mortality. *International Journal of Cancer* 135(12): 2900–2909.

Heinl, R. E., et al. 2016. Comprehensive cardiovascular risk reduction and cardiac rehabilitation in diabetes and the metabolic syndrome. *Canadian Journal of Cardiology* 32(10S2): S349–S357.

James, P. A., et al. 2014. 2014 Evidence-based guideline for the management of high blood pressure in adults: report from the panel members appointed to the Eighth Joint National Committee (JNC 8). *Journal of the American Medical Association* 311(5): 507–520.

Jemal, A., et al. 2015. Prostate cancer incidence and PSA testing patterns in relation to USPSTF screening recommendations. *Journal of the American Medical Association* 314(19): 2054–2061.

Kaiser, J. 2016. Tests of blood-borne DNA pinpoint tissue damage: Assays spot cell death from diabetes, cancer, and more. *Science* 351(6279): 1253

Kassianos, A. P., et al. 2015. Smartphone applications for melanoma detection by community, patient and generalist clinician users: A review. *British Journal of Dermatology* 172(6): 1507–1518.

Li, X., et al. 2016. Effectiveness of prophylactic surgeries in BRCA1 or BRCA2 mutation carriers: A meta-analysis and systematic review. *Clinical Cancer Research*, March 15 (epub ahead of print).

Mendis, S., et al., eds. 2011. *Global Atlas on Cardiovascular Disease Prevention and Control.* Geneva, Switzerland: World Health Organization (in collaboration with the World Heart Federation and World Stroke Organization).

Moore S. C., et al. 2016. Leisure-time physical activity and risk of 26 types of cancer in 1.44 million adults. *JAMA Internal Medicine.* DOI: 10.1001/jamainternmed.2016.1548.

Mozaffarian, D., et al. 2016. *Heart disease and stroke statistics—2016 Update: A report from the American Heart Association. Circulation* 133: e38-e360.

Myers, E. R., et al. 2015. Benefits and harms of breast cancer screening: A systematic review. *Journal of the American Medical Association* 314(15): 1615–1634.

National Center for Health Statistics. 2016. *Health, United States, 2015: With Special Feature on Racial and Ethnic Health Disparities.* Hyattsville, MD: National Center for Health Statistics.

National Heart, Lung, and Blood Institute. 2015. *How Is Metabolic Syndrome Diagnosed?* (http://www.nhlbi.nih.gov/health/health-topics/topics/ms/diagnosis).

National Toxicology Program. 2014. *Report on Carcinogens,* 13th ed. Research Triangle Park, NC: USDHHS Public Health Service.

Pham, T., et al. 2016. The effect of serum 25-hydroxyvitamin D on elevated homocysteine concentrations in participants of a preventive health program. *PLos One* 11(8): e061368.

Razdan, S. N., et al. 2016. Quality of life among patients after bilateral prophylactic mastectomy: A systematic review of patient-reported outcomes. *Quality of Life Research* 25(6):1409–1421.

Rothwell, P. M., et al. 2016. Effects of aspirin on risk and severity of early recurrent stroke after transient ischaemic attack and ischaemic stroke: time-course analysis of randomised trials. *Lancet* 388(10042): 365–375.

Semsarian, C., et al. 2015. New perspectives on the prevalence of hypertrophic cardiomyopathy. *Journal of the American College of Cardiology.* 65(12): 1249–1254.

Shi, S., et al. 2016. Depression and risk of sudden cardiac death and arrhythmias: a meta-analysis. *Psychosomatic Medicine,* 13 Sep [epub ahead of print].

Sonnenburg, J. L., and F. Bäckhed. 2016. Diet–microbiota interactions as moderators of human metabolism. *Nature* 535: 56–64.

SPRINT Research Group. 2015. A randomized trial of intensive versus standard blood-pressure control. *New England Journal of Medicine* 373(22): 2103–2116.

Stone, N. J., et al. 2013. ACC/AHA guideline on the treatment of blood cholesterol to reduce atherosclerotic cardiovascular risk in adults: A report of the American College of Cardiology/American Heart Association Task Force on Practice Guidelines. *Journal of the American College of Cardiology.*

Torre, L. A., et al. 2016. Cancer statistics for Asian Americans, Native Hawaiians, and Pacific Islanders, 2016: Converging incidence in males and females. *CA: A Cancer Journal for Clinicians* 66(3): 182–202.

U.S. Department of Health and Human Services. 2014. *The Health Consequences of Smoking—50 Years of Progress: A Report of the Surgeon General.* Atlanta, GA: U.S. Department of Health and Human Services, Centers for Disease Control and Prevention, National Center for Chronic Disease Prevention and Health Promotion, Office on Smoking and Health.

U.S. Departments of Health and Human Services and Agriculture. 2015. *2015–2020 Dietary Guidelines for Americans* (http://health.gov/dietaryguidelines/2015/guidelines/).

Widmer, R. J., et al. 2015. The Mediterranean diet, its components, and cardiovascular disease. *American Journal of Medicine* 128(3): 229–238.

Wilson, K. M., et al. 2015. Calcium and phosphorus intake and prostate cancer risk: A 24-y follow-up study. *American Journal of Clinical Nutrition* 101(1): 173–183.

World Health Organization. 2015. Fact Sheet No. 297: Cancer (http://www.who.int/mediacentre/factsheets/fs297/en).

Xie, X., et al. 2015. Effects of intensive blood pressure lowering on cardiovascular and renal outcomes: Updated systematic review and meta-analysis. *Lancet* S0140-6736(15)00805-3.

Zhang, Z. M., et al. 2016. Race and sex differences in the incidence and prognostic significant of silent myocardial infarction in the Atherosclerosis Risk in Communities (ARIC) study. *Circulation* 133(22): 2141–2148.

BEHAVIOR CHANGE STRATEGY
Modifying Your Diet for Heart Health and Cancer Prevention

When we think about the health benefits of fruits and vegetables, we usually focus on the fact that they are rich in carbohydrates, dietary fiber, and vitamins and low in fat. A benefit that we may overlook is that they contain specific cancer-fighting compounds (phytochemicals) that help slow, stop, or even reverse the process of cancer. The National Cancer Institute (NCI) reports that people who eat five or more servings a day of fruits and vegetables have half the risk of cancer of those who eat fewer than two. According to the NCI, seven to nine servings or more per day are optimal.

Most Americans need to double the amount of fruits and vegetables they eat every day. Begin by monitoring your diet for one or two weeks to assess your current intake; then look for ways to incorporate these foods into your diet in easy and tasty ways. Here are some tips to get you started.

Breakfast

- Drink pure fruit juice every morning.
- Add raisins, berries, or sliced fruit to cereal, pancakes, or waffles. Top bagels with tomato slices.
- Try a fruit smoothie made from fresh or frozen fruit and orange juice or low-fat yogurt.

Lunch

- Choose vegetable soup or salad with your meal.

- Replace potato chips or french fries with cut-up vegetables.
- Add extra chunks of fruits or vegetables to salads.
- Add vegetables such as roasted peppers, cucumber slices, shredded carrots, avocado, or salsa to sandwiches.
- Drink tomato or vegetable juice instead of soda (watch for excess sodium).

Dinner

- Choose a vegetarian main course, such as stir-fry or vegetable stew. Have at least two servings of vegetables with every dinner.
- Microwave vegetables and sprinkle them with a little Parmesan cheese.
- Substitute vegetables for meat in casseroles and pasta and chili recipes.
- At the salad bar, pile your plate with healthful vegetables and use low-fat or nonfat dressing.

Snacks and On the Go

- Keep ready-to-eat fruits and vegetables on hand (apples, plums, pears, and carrots).
- Keep small packages of dried fruit in the car (try dried apples, apricots, peaches, pears, and raisins).

- Make ice cubes from pure fruit juice and drop them into regular or sparkling water.
- Freeze grapes for a cool summer treat.

The All-Stars

Different fruits and vegetables contribute different vitamins, phytochemicals, and other nutrients, so be sure to get a variety. The following types of produce are particularly rich in nutrients and phytochemicals:

- Cruciferous vegetables (e.g., broccoli, cauliflower, cabbage, bok choy, brussels sprouts, kohlrabi, turnips)
- Citrus fruits (e.g., oranges, lemons, limes, grapefruit, tangerines)
- Berries (e.g., strawberries, raspberries, blueberries)
- Dark green leafy vegetables (e.g., spinach, chard, collards, beet greens, kale, mustard greens, romaine and other dark lettuces)
- Deep yellow, orange, and red fruits and vegetables (e.g., carrots, pumpkin, sweet potatoes, winter squash, red and yellow bell peppers, apricots, cantaloupe, mangoes, papayas)

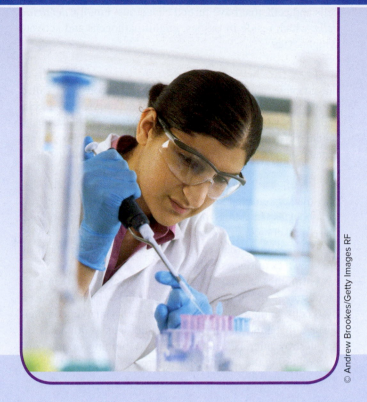

© Andrew Brookes/Getty Images RF

CHAPTER OBJECTIVES

- Explain the body's physical and chemical defenses against infection

- Describe the step-by-step process by which infectious diseases are transmitted

- Identify the major types of pathogens, the diseases they cause, and possible treatments for them

- Discuss steps you can take to support your immune system

- Discuss the symptoms, risks, and treatments for the major sexually transmitted infections

- List strategies for protecting yourself from sexually transmitted infections

CHAPTER **13**

Immunity and Infection

Countless microscopic organisms live around, on, and in us. Although most microbes are beneficial, many of them can cause **infections** and infectious diseases including sexually transmitted infections. But the constant vigilance of our immune system keeps them at bay and our bodies healthy. The immune system protects us not just from **pathogens** but also from cancer. This chapter introduces you to the mechanisms of immunity and infection, as well as strategies for keeping yourself well in a world of disease-causing microorganisms.

THE BODY'S DEFENSE SYSTEM

Our bodies have very effective ways of protecting themselves against invasion by foreign organisms. The immune system is the body's collective set of defenses that includes surface barriers as well as the specialized cells, tissues, and organs that carry out the immune response. The first line of defense is a formidable array of physical and chemical barriers. When these barriers are breached, cellular processes of the immune system come into play. Together these defenses provide an effective response to nearly all the invasions that our bodies experience.

Physical and Chemical Barriers

The skin, the body's largest organ, prevents many microorganisms from entering the body. Although many bacterial and fungal organisms live on the surface of the skin, few can penetrate it except through a cut or break.

All body cavities and passages that are exposed to the external environment are lined with mucous membranes, which secrete mucus and contain cells designed to prevent the passage of unwanted organisms and particles. These areas include the mouth, nostrils, eyelids, bronchioles, vagina, and other organs of the respiratory, digestive, and urogenital tracts. Skin and mucous membranes are made of epithelial tissue, which consists of one or more layers of closely packed cells with almost no space between cells. The fluids that cover epithelial tissue, such as tears, saliva, and vaginal secretions, are rich in enzymes and other proteins that break down and destroy many microorganisms.

> **TERMS**
>
> **infection**   Invasion of the body by a microorganism.
>
> **pathogen**   A microorganism that causes disease.

The respiratory tract is lined not only with mucous membranes but also with cells having hairlike protrusions called *cilia*. The cilia sweep foreign matter up and out of the respiratory tract. Particles that are not caught by this mechanism may be expelled from the system by a cough.

The Immune System: Cells, Tissues, and Organs

Beyond surface barriers, the **immune system** operates through a remarkable information network involving billions of white blood cells that protect the body when a threat arises. These white blood cells are produced continuously throughout life.

The immune system can be thought of as two systems. The *innate immune system* consists of cells that can recognize pathogenic microorganisms and are the first responders to those pathogens. The *adaptive immune system* consists of cells (called T cells and B cells) that can recognize pathogenic microorganisms and that have the remarkable ability to improve and accelerate their responses after exposure to those pathogens. The complete elimination of a pathogen involves the coordinated activities of both systems. An important cell type that is at the nexus of the innate and adaptive immune systems is the dendritic cell.

Cells of the Innate Immune System
The cells of the innate immune system recognize pathogens as "foreign" and kill them, but they cannot develop a memory of these pathogens. Thus, they respond the same way no matter how many times a pathogen invades. *Neutrophils,* one type of white blood cell, travel in the bloodstream to areas of invasion, attacking and ingesting pathogens. *Eosinophils,* white blood cells that occur in mucosal tissues such as those in the gastrointestinal tract and the mammary glands, provide innate immunity to certain microbes. *Macrophages,* or "big eaters," act as scavengers, devouring pathogens and worn-out cells. *Natural killer cells* directly destroy virus-infected

cells and cells that have turned cancerous. Finally, *dendritic cells,* which reside in tissues, engulf pathogens and activate lymphocytes.

Cells of the Adaptive Immune System
The cells of the adaptive immune system are white blood cells called **lymphocytes.** The two main types of lymphocytes are T cells and B cells, which differ in function. Whereas cells of the innate immune system can recognize a cell as foreign, lymphocytes are capable of exquisite specificity and of immunological memory.

Antigens and Antibodies
All of your body cells display markers on their surfaces that identify them as "self" to lymphocytes. Invading microbes also display markers, and these markers identify them as foreign, or "nonself," to lymphocytes. Nonself markers that trigger an immune response are known as **antigens.**

Antibodies are specialized proteins that circulate in your bloodstream and are present in most body fluids. Produced by B cells, antibodies have complementary markers on their surface that bind to antigens on microbes. Antibodies do not destroy microbes directly, but by binding to antigens, antibodies tag the microbe for destruction by other types of immune cells.

T Cells and B Cells
Each T and B cell has receptors that allow it to recognize one specific antigen. The immune system produces T and B cells with many receptor types, each capable of recognizing a different antigen, meaning the immune system can recognize nearly all disease-causing microbes. When a B cell lymphocyte or T cell lymphocyte encounters the antigen for which it is specific, it proliferates, producing many more lymphocytes that are specific to the same antigen. These daughter cells then differentiate into cells with specific immune functions and attack the invading organisms. **B cells** become plasma cells that secrete antibodies. **T cells** differentiate into helper T cells, killer T cells, or suppressor T cells (also called regulatory T cells). Some B and T cells become memory B and T cells, which can mount a rapid and powerful response should they encounter the same invader months or even years in the future.

The Inflammatory Response
When injured or infected, the body reacts by producing an inflammatory response. Macrophages engulf the invading microbe and produce substances that convey danger to other cells of the immune system. The resulting inflammatory response triggered by **histamine** (a chemical that also contributes to the allergic response) causes blood vessels to dilate and fluid to flow out of capillaries into the injured tissue. This activity produces increased heat, swelling, and redness in the affected area. White blood cells are drawn to the area and attack the invaders, in many cases destroying them. This entire reaction is the immune response, as described in the next section. At the site of infection there may be *pus*—a collection of dead white blood cells and debris resulting from the encounter.

TERMS

immune system   The body's collective system of defenses that includes surface barriers as well as the specialized cells, tissues, and organs that carry out the immune response.

lymphocyte   A type of white blood cell that carries out important functions in the immune system.

antigen   A substance that triggers the immune response.

antibody   A specialized protein, produced by white blood cells, that can recognize specific antigens.

B cell   A type of lymphocyte that produces antibodies.

T cells   Cells that are responsible for cell-mediated adaptive immune reactions. Helper T cells activate macrophages and promote activation of B cells and killer T cells. Killer T cells kill cells infected with viruses and other intracellular pathogens.

histamine   A chemical responsible for the dilation and increased permeability of blood vessels in the inflammatory response.

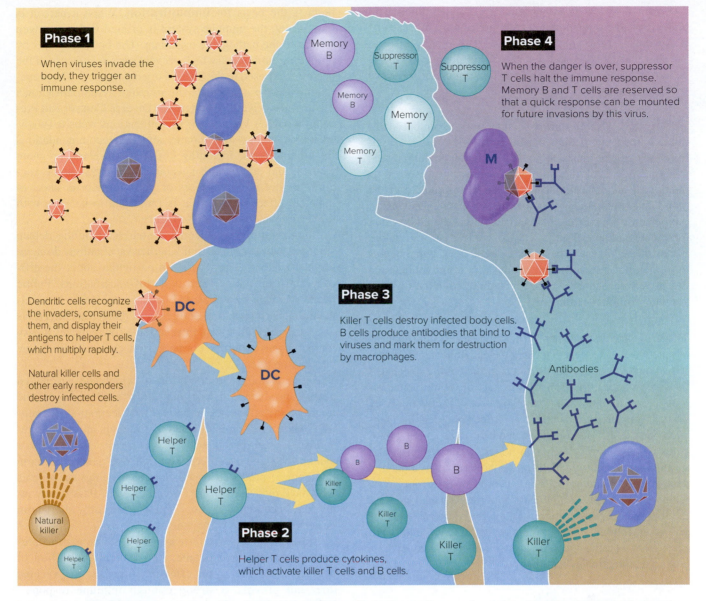

Phase 1

When viruses invade the body, they trigger an immune response.

Dendritic cells recognize the invaders, consume them, and display their antigens to helper T cells, which multiply rapidly.

Natural killer cells and other early responders destroy infected cells.

DC

DC

Natural killer

Helper T

Helper T

Helper T

Helper T

Helper T

Phase 2

Helper T cells produce cytokines, which activate killer T cells and B cells.

Killer T

Killer T

Killer T

Killer T

Killer T

B

B

B

Phase 3

Killer T cells destroy infected body cells. B cells produce antibodies that bind to viruses and mark them for destruction by macrophages.

Antibodies

Memory B

Memory B

Memory T

Memory T

Suppressor T

Memory T

Phase 4

When the danger is over, suppressor T cells halt the immune response. Memory B and T cells are reserved so that a quick response can be mounted for future invasions by this virus.

Suppressor T

M

FIGURE 13.1 The immune response. Once invaded by a pathogen, the body mounts a complex series of reactions to destroy the invader. Pictured here are the phases of the immune response as the body works to destroy a virus.

The Immune Response   The activities of the innate and adaptive immune systems are integrated to generate a coordinated and usually highly effective immune response. Figure 13.1 illustrates how this happens:

• *Phase 1: Recognition.* If a pathogen breaches the body's physical and chemical barriers, it initiates the first phase of the immune response by arousing dendritic cells at the site of pathogen entry. They engulf the pathogen and migrate to nearby lymphoid tissue. There the dendritic cells activate helper and killer T cells by presenting fragments of pathogen proteins to T cells. Antigen carried into lymphoid tissue also activates B cells.

• *Phase 2: Proliferation.* The activated helper and killer T cells multiply, thereby amplifying the immune response

to the pathogen. Helper T cells produce special growth stimulants called cytokines, which then further stimulate the activation and proliferation of killer T cells and B cells.

• *Phase 3: Elimination.* The activated T and B cells then undergo a transformation to become either memory cells or effector cells. The effector cells mediate elimination of the pathogen. If the infecting pathogen is a virus or an intracellular bacterium, then killer T cells destroy body cells that are infected with that pathogen. Activated B cells become memory B cells or plasma cells, which are antibody-producing factories. The antibodies bind to extracellular pathogens (those outside body cells) and mark them for destruction by macrophages and natural killer cells.

- *Phase 4: Slowdown.* Regulatory T cells inhibit lymphocyte proliferation and induce lymphocyte death, causing a slowdown of the immune response. This process restores "resting" levels of B and T cells. Some memory T and B cells remain and can initiate a rapid response if the same pathogen reappears in the future.

Immunity   Usually, after an infection, a person is immune to the same pathogen. This **immunity,** or insusceptibility, occurs because some of the lymphocytes created during phase 2 of the immune response are reserved as memory T and B cells. They continue to circulate in the blood and lymphatic system for years or even for the rest of the person's life. If the same antigen enters the body again, the memory T and B cells recognize and destroy it before it can cause illness. The ability of memory lymphocytes to remember previous infections and improve immune defenses if the same microbe is encountered in the future is known as **adaptive immunity.**

The Lymphatic System   The lymphatic system consists of a network of vessels that carry a clear fluid called lymph. It also includes organs and structures, such as the spleen and the lymph nodes, that function as part of the immune system. The lymphatic vessels pick up excess fluid from body tissues; this fluid may contain microbes and dead or damaged body cells. Macrophages, dendritic cells, and lymphocytes congregate in the lymph nodes; when lymph passes through a node, foreign cells and debris are filtered out and destroyed. If immune cells in a lymph node recognize an antigen, the adaptive immune response will be triggered. As the immune response progresses, a lymph node actively involved in fighting an infection may fill with cells and swell. Physicians use the location of swollen lymph nodes as a clue to an infection's location.

Immunization

The ability of the immune system to remember previously encountered organisms and retain its strength against them is the basis for **immunization.** When a person is immunized, the immune system is primed with an antigen similar to the pathogenic organism. The body responds by producing antibodies, which prevent serious infection if the person is exposed to the disease organism itself. The preparations used to manipulate the immune system are known as **vaccines.** Visit the Centers for Disease Control and Prevention (CDC) Vaccines & Immunizations website (www.cdc.gov/vaccines) for updates and the recommendations for other groups, including children, travelers, pregnant women, and adults with special health risks. Some vaccines require multiple doses or periodic booster shots to maintain effectiveness, so it is important to keep up with the recommended vaccine schedule.

Immunization has become a source of public debate among people who question whether vaccinations do more harm than good. They worry in particular about the efficacy and safety of certain types of vaccinations. Public health officials are concerned because decreases in vaccination rates can result in outbreaks of dangerous infectious diseases, especially since international travel makes it easy for pathogens to cross borders from countries with low vaccination rates.

Active immunity, a condition in which the vaccinated person produces his or her own antibodies to the microorganism, can be acquired by vaccination or naturally when a person is infected and mounts an immune response to the pathogen. This contrasts with *passive immunity,* which is conferred by injecting gamma globulin (antibodies) produced by other human beings or animals who have recovered from a given disease. Passive immunity does not confer memory and provides only short-term protection against a pathogen.

Most childhood vaccines are effective enough to prevent disease in most people. For a small proportion of people, a vaccine is not effective—that is, the vaccine does not provoke a strong enough immune response. Protection from infection is provided by those around them, as long as they live, work, and travel around people who have been vaccinated and are themselves protected. The same is true for people who cannot be vaccinated due to young age or underlying medical conditions (such as cancer treatment).

Keeping vaccination rates consistently high over time is necessary to maintain protection. Before the development of the measles vaccine in 1963, nearly everyone in the United States got measles, and hundreds died from measles every year. In the five years before the vaccine was introduced, about 400–500 deaths and 48,000 hospitalizations from measles occurred annually. Following widespread vaccination, the United States was declared measles-free in 2000, meaning measles is not constantly present. However, outbreaks have continued to occur, with infection brought into the United States by unvaccinated travelers (Americans or foreign visitors) who get measles while they are in other countries. People with measles can

immunity   Resistance to infection.

TERMS

adaptive immunity   Immunity to infection acquired by the activation of antigen-specific lymphocytes in response to infection or immunization. Adaptive immunity results in immunological memory.

immunization   The process of conferring a person with immunity to a pathogen by administering a vaccine.

vaccines   A preparation of killed or weakened microorganisms, inactivated toxins, or components of microorganisms that is administered to stimulate an immune response; a vaccine protects against future infection by the pathogen.

easily spread it to others who are not vaccinated or otherwise protected (e.g., from past infection).

Vaccines are approved by the Advisory Committee on Immunization Practices—the advisors for the CDC—and the Committee on Infectious Diseases—the advisors for the American Academy of Pediatrics (AAP). Both the AAP and the CDC advisory committees have expert knowledge in virology, microbiology, statistics, epidemiology, and pathogenesis—knowledge necessary for reviewing and evaluating studies on vaccine efficacy and safety.

To further ensure their safety, vaccines are tested in larger numbers of people for longer periods of time than drugs are before being licensed. For example, the human papillomavirus (HPV) vaccine was tested in 30,000 women, the conjugate pneumococcal vaccine was tested in 40,000 children, and each of the current rotavirus vaccines was tested in 70,000 children before being licensed. No other type of medication receives this degree of scrutiny.

Additionally, safety mechanisms such as the Vaccine Adverse Event Reporting System (VAERS) and the Vaccine Safety Datalink Project monitor adverse events reported after licensure. Side effects from immunization are usually mild, such as soreness at the injection site. Any risk from a vaccine must be balanced against the risk posed by the diseases it prevents. For example, the last major U.S. epidemic of rubella in 1964–1965 infected 12.5 million Americans, caused 11,000 miscarriages, killed 2000 infants, and resulted in 20,000 infants being born with rubella-caused birth defects. Since the introduction of the vaccine and the maintenance of high vaccination rates, U.S. rubella cases have dropped to an average of about 10 per year. Worldwide, however, an estimated 100,000 babies are born each year with birth defects due to rubella infection in pregnant women.

Allergy: A Case of Mistaken Identity

An estimated 50 million Americans are affected by **allergies.** In a person with an allergy, the immune system reacts to a harmless substance as if it were a harmful pathogen.

> **QUICK STATS**
>
> **Within 6 years of the HPV vaccine's introduction, the prevalence of HPV infection in vaccinated sexually active 14- to 24-year-old females in the United States dropped from 19% to 2%.**
>
> —Markowitz, et al., *Pediatrics*, 2016

For the most part, allergy symptoms—stuffy nose, sneezing, wheezing, skin rashes, and so on—are the result of the immune response.

Substances that provoke allergies are known as **allergens;** they may cause a response if they are inhaled or swallowed or if they come in contact with the skin. Common allergens include pollen, animal dander, dust mites and cockroaches, molds and mildew, foods, and insect stings.

The Allergic Response Although allergies are an adverse response to environmental antigens that are not pathogenic, this type of immune response in fact evolved as a protective response to certain types of pathogens, particularly parasitic worms. Most allergic reactions are due to the production of a special type of antibody known as *immunoglobulin E (IgE)*. Initial exposure to a particular allergen sensitizes the immune system by causing the production of allergen-specific IgE, which binds to special IgE receptors on mast cells. When the body is subsequently exposed to the allergen, the allergen binds to IgE antibodies that are bound by IgE receptors on certain white blood cells called mast cells, thereby causing the mast cells to release large amounts of histamine and other compounds that cause allergic symptoms.

Histamine has many effects, including increasing the inflammatory response and stimulating mucus production. In the nose, histamine may cause congestion and sneezing; in the eyes, itchiness and tearing; in the skin, redness, swelling, and itching; in the intestines, bloating and cramping; and in the lungs, coughing, wheezing, and shortness of breath. In some people, an allergen can trigger an **asthma** attack. Symptoms—wheezing, tightness in the chest, shortness of breath, and coughing—often occur immediately, within minutes of exposure.

Asthma is caused by both chronic inflammation of the airways and spasm of the muscles surrounding the airways. The spasm causes constriction, and the inflammation causes the airway linings to swell and secrete extra mucus, which further obstructs the passages.

> **TERMS**
>
> **allergy** An immune response to normally innocuous foreign chemicals and proteins that is characterized by specific symptoms usually caused by mast cell activity; also called *hypersensitivity*.
>
> **allergen** A substance that triggers an allergic reaction.
>
> **asthma** A disease in which chronic inflammation and periodic constriction of the airways cause wheezing, shortness of breath, and coughing.

An asthma attack is initiated by an irritating stimulus in the bronchial tubes. The stimulus may be an inhaled allergen, such as pollen, dust mites, mold, animal dander, or cockroach droppings, or it can be a nonallergen stimulus, such as exercise, cold air, pollutants, tobacco smoke, infection, or stress. In women with asthma, hormonal changes that occur as menstruation starts may increase vulnerability to attacks. Both environmental and genetic factors contribute to the development of asthma.

The most serious, but rare, kind of allergic reaction is **anaphylaxis,** which results from a release of histamine throughout the body. Anaphylactic reactions can be life threatening because symptoms may include swelling of the throat, extremely low blood pressure, fainting, heart arrhythmia, and seizures. Anaphylaxis is a medical emergency, and treatment requires immediate injection of epinephrine. People at risk for anaphylaxis should wear medical alert identification and keep self-administrable epinephrine readily available.

Climate Change and Allergies The predicted global changes in climate are likely to exacerbate allergies, including allergic rhinitis and asthma. Global warming is influencing plant and fungal reproduction and thus is influencing both spatial and temporal production of allergens. If warm weather periods lengthen, then the period of pollen release also will be prolonged and the amount of pollen released may increase. Thus, politicians and policymakers must become involved in reducing the impact of climate change on human health.

Dealing with Allergies If you suspect you might have an allergy, visit your physician or an allergy specialist. You may be able to avoid or minimize exposure to allergens by changing your environment or behavior. For example, removing carpets from the bedroom and using special bedding can reduce dust mite contact. Also, medications are available for allergy sufferers. Many over-the-counter antihistamines are effective at controlling symptoms, and prescription coritcosteroids delivered by aerosol markedly reduce allergy symptoms. A third approach is immunotherapy, in which a person is desensetized to a particular allergen through the administration of gradually increasing doses of the allergen over a period of months or years.

QUICK STATS

About **8.6%** of children and **7.4%** of adults currently have asthma in the United States.

—Centers for Disease Control and Prevention, 2016f

---

anaphylaxis A severe systemic hypersensitive reaction to an allergen characterized by difficulty breathing, low blood pressure, heart arrhythmia, seizure, and sometimes death.

incubation period The period when bacteria or viruses are actively multiplying inside the body's cells; usually a period without symptoms of illness.

TERMS

THE SPREAD OF DISEASE

The immune system is operating at all times, maintaining its vigilance when you're well and fighting invaders when you're sick.

Symptoms and Contagion

The symptoms you experience during an illness are related to the phase of infection and the actions of your immune system. During the first phase of infection, or **incubation period,** when viruses or bacteria are actively multiplying before the immune system has gathered momentum, you may not have any symptoms of the illness, but you may be contagious. During the second and third phases of the immune response, you may still be unaware of the infection, or you may "feel a cold coming on." Symptoms first appear during the *prodromal period,* which follows incubation. If you have acquired immunity, the infection may be eradicated during the incubation period or the prodromal period. In this case it does not develop into a full-blown illness.

Many symptoms of an illness are actually due to the body's immune response rather than to the actions or products of the invading organism. For example, fever is caused by the release of certain cytokines by macrophages and other cells during the immune response. These cytokines travel in the bloodstream to the brain and cause the body's thermostat to be reset to a higher level. The resulting elevated temperature helps the body fight against pathogens by enhancing immune responses.

You may be contagious before you experience any symptoms, and you are contagious as long as your body is releasing infectious microbes. This means that you can transmit an illness without knowing you're infected or catch an illness from someone who doesn't appear to be sick. Similarly, your symptoms may continue after the pathogens have been mostly destroyed, when you are no longer infectious.

The Chain of Infection

Infectious diseases are transmitted from one person to another through a series of steps—a chain of infection. New infections can be prevented by interfering with any step in this process. The chain of infection has six major links:

1. *Pathogen.* The infectious disease cycle begins with a pathogen that enters the body.

2. *Reservoir.* The pathogen has a natural environment—called a **reservoir**—in which it typically lives. This reservoir can be a person or an animal. A person who is the reservoir for a pathogen may be ill or may be an asymptomatic carrier who, although having no symptoms, can spread infection.

3. *Portal of exit.* To transmit infection, the pathogen must leave the reservoir through some portal of exit. In the case of a human reservoir, portals of exit include saliva, the mucous membranes, blood, feces, and nose and throat discharges.

4. *Means of transmission.* Transmission can occur directly or indirectly. In *direct transmission,* the pathogen is passed from one person to another without an intermediary. In *indirect transmission,* animals or insects such as rats, ticks, and mosquitoes serve as **vectors,** carrying the pathogen from one host to another. Pathogens can also be transmitted via contaminated soil, food, or water or from inanimate objects, such as eating utensils, doorknobs, and handkerchiefs.

5. *Portal of entry.* To infect a new host, a pathogen must have a portal of entry into the body. Pathogens can enter through direct contact with or penetration of the skin or mucous membranes, inhalation, or ingestion. Pathogens that enter the skin or mucous membranes can cause a local infection of the tissue, or they may penetrate into the bloodstream or lymphatic system, thereby causing a **systemic infection.**

6. *The new host.* Once in the new host, a variety of factors determine whether the pathogen will be able to establish itself and cause infection. People with a strong immune system or resistance to a particular pathogen are less likely to become ill than are people with poor immunity. If conditions are right, the pathogen will multiply and produce disease in the new host. In such a case, the new host may become a reservoir from which a new chain of infection can be started.

Interrupting the chain of infection at any point can prevent disease. Strategies for breaking the chain include both public health measures and individual action. For example, a pathogen's reservoir can be isolated or destroyed, as when a sick individual is placed under quarantine or when insects or animals carrying pathogens are killed. Public sanitation practices, such as sewage treatment and the chlorination of drinking water, can also kill pathogens. Transmission can be disrupted through strategies like hand washing and the use of face masks. Immunization and the treatment of infected hosts can stop the pathogen from multiplying, producing a serious disease, and being passed on to a new host.

Epidemics and Pandemics

The rapid spread of a disease or health condition is called an **epidemic.** Although the word is usually used in reference to infectious diseases, it is also used for health conditions that are not caused by an infectious organism. For example, it is often said that obesity and diabetes have reached epidemic proportions in the United States.

An important underlying premise of the concept of "epidemic" is that the occurrence of the disease is greater than what is expected normally. Thus, the common cold, which occurs with great frequency, is never classified as an epidemic. Conversely, the term *epidemic* is used to refer to outbreaks of diseases that are not widespread. For example, when 10 infants died in California in 2010 from whooping cough, the incident was referred to as an epidemic.

When an epidemic is widespread, it is called a **pandemic.** In contrast to the term *epidemic,* the term *pandemic* refers exclusively to infectious disease. Human history has been punctuated by numerous pandemics of various diseases, including bubonic plague, smallpox, and influenza. One of the most severe influenza pandemics occurred in 1918–1919, following World War I, when 20–40% of the world's population became ill and as many as 40 million people died.

Not all widespread infectious diseases are pandemics. An infectious disease is said to be endemic when it habitually exists in a certain region. Endemic diseases generally occur at low frequency in particular populations or regions. For example, malaria is endemic to low-altitude areas of northern and eastern South Africa.

H1N1 Influenza   In 2009, an outbreak of influenza caused by a virus never before identified as a cause of human illness sparked fears of a worldwide influenza pandemic. The influenza A virus mutates frequently during replication, and it can also exchange genes with other influenza A viruses, including strains that infect domestic and wild animals. The H1N1 strain resulted from a combination of genes from four viruses: two from swine flu viruses, one from an avian (bird) flu virus, and one from a human flu virus. The addition of the gene from a human virus meant that humans could be infected with it, and, because it was new, they had no prior immunity.

TERMS

reservoir   A long-term host in which a pathogen typically lives.

vector   An insect, rodent, or other organism that carries and transmits a pathogen from one host to another.

systemic infection   An infection spread by the blood or lymphatic system to large portions of the body.

epidemic   A rapidly spreading disease or health-related condition.

pandemic   A widespread epidemic.

In June 2009, with cases reported in 74 countries, the World Health Organization declared that a flu pandemic was under way. By February 2010, the WHO reported up to 86 million cases and up to nearly 18,000 deaths. By May of that year, flu activity had tapered off and declined to normal levels, but the same influenza A (H1N1) virus was the predominant strain during the 2013–2014 influenza season. The WHO continues to track trends globally, and the CDC continues to recommend H1N1 vaccination for persons aged 6 months to 24 years and people aged 25–64 years who are at high risk.

H5N1 Influenza Since 1998, scientists have been monitoring the progress of another influenza A virus known as H5N1, or avian (bird) influenza. This strain infects chickens, ducks, and geese as well as wild birds; it doesn't pass easily to humans or among humans, but when it does, it is deadly. According to the WHO, more than 700 humans have been infected with Asian H5N1 virus since November 2003. The infections have occurred primarily in Indonesia, Vietnam, and Egypt, although European countries also reported infections. The first case of Asian H5N1 in the Americas was in a traveler who went from China to Canada in January 2014. Although H5N1 infections of humans have been rare, approximately 60% of the infected people died.

PATHOGENS, DISEASES, AND TREATMENTS

The pathogens that cause infectious diseases include bacteria, viruses, fungi, protozoa, and parasitic worms (Figure 13.2). Infections can occur almost anywhere in or on the body. Examples of common infections are bronchitis, which is an infection of the airways (bronchi); meningitis, infection of the tissue surrounding the brain and spinal cord; and conjunctivitis, infection of the layer of cells surrounding the eyes.

Bacteria

The most abundant living things on earth are **bacteria,** which are single-celled organisms that usually reproduce by splitting in two to create a pair of identical cells. Bacteria are often classified by their shape: bacilli (rod-shaped), cocci (spherical), spirochete (spiral-shaped), or vibrios (comma-shaped).

Many species of bacteria are beneficial, but some are pathogenic, causing disease in their hosts. About 100 species of bacteria can cause disease in humans. We harbor both helpful and harmful bacteria on our skin and in our gastrointestinal and reproductive tracts. The human colon contains helpful bacteria that produce certain vitamins and help digest nutrients. Helpful bacteria also keep harmful bacteria in check by competing for food and resources and secreting substances toxic to pathogenic bacteria.

Pneumonia Inflammation of the lungs, called **pneumonia,** may be caused by infection with bacteria, viruses, or fungi, or by contact with chemical toxins or irritants. Pneumonia can be serious if the alveoli (air sacs) become clogged with fluid, thus preventing oxygen from reaching the bloodstream. Pneumonia often follows another illness, such as a cold or the flu, but the symptoms are typically more severe—fever, chills, shortness of breath, increased mucus production, and cough. Pneumonia is one of the 10 leading causes of death for Americans; people most at risk for severe infection include those under age 2 or over age 75 and those with chronic health problems such as heart disease, asthma, or HIV. Worldwide, pneumonia is the leading cause of death for children under 5 years of age.

The most common cause of bacterial pneumonia is *Streptococcus pneumoniae*, or pneumococcus. A vaccine is available for pneumococcal pneumonia and is recommended for all adults age 65 and over and others at risk. Mycoplasma is a very small bacterium; *M. pneumoniae* causes a mild form of pneumonia often called "walking pneumonia." Outbreaks of infection with mycoplasmas are relatively common among young adults, especially in crowded settings such as dormitories. Bacterial pneumonia can be treated with antibiotics, which we will discuss shortly.

Meningitis Inflammation of the *meninges,* the protective membranes covering the brain and spinal cord, is called **meningitis.** Inflammation is usually caused by infection of the fluid surrounding the brain. The infection can be caused by a bacterium, virus, fungus, or parasite. Most cases of meningitis are viral; they are usually mild and resolve without medical intervention. Bacterial meningitis, however, can be life threatening and requires immediate treatment with

TERMS

bacterium A microscopic single-celled organism with a cell wall (plural, *bacteria)*. Bacteria may be helpful or harmful to humans.

pneumonia Inflammation of the lungs, typically caused by infection or exposure to chemical toxins or irritants.

meningitis Infection of the meninges (membranes covering the brain and spinal cord).

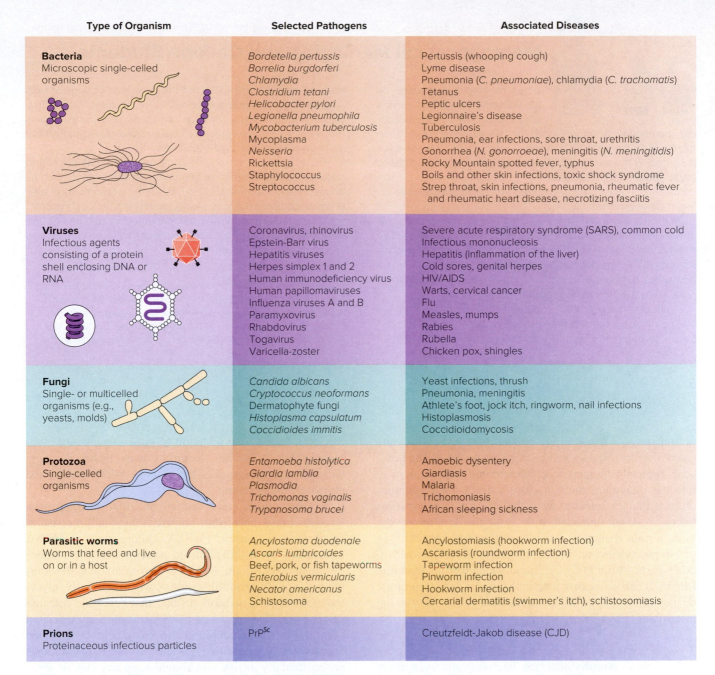

Type of Organism	Selected Pathogens	Associated Diseases
Bacteria Microscopic single-celled organisms	*Bordetella pertussis* *Borrelia burgdorferi* *Chlamydia* *Clostridium tetani* *Helicobacter pylori* *Legionella pneumophila* *Mycobacterium tuberculosis* Mycoplasma *Neisseria* Rickettsia Staphylococcus Streptococcus	Pertussis (whooping cough) Lyme disease Pneumonia (*C. pneumoniae*), chlamydia (*C. trachomatis*) Tetanus Peptic ulcers Legionnaire's disease Tuberculosis Pneumonia, ear infections, sore throat, urethritis Gonorrhea (*N. gonorroeae*), meningitis (*N. meningitidis*) Rocky Mountain spotted fever, typhus Boils and other skin infections, toxic shock syndrome Strep throat, skin infections, pneumonia, rheumatic fever and rheumatic heart disease, necrotizing fasciitis
Viruses Infectious agents consisting of a protein shell enclosing DNA or RNA	Coronavirus, rhinovirus Epstein-Barr virus Hepatitis viruses Herpes simplex 1 and 2 Human immunodeficiency virus Human papillomaviruses Influenza viruses A and B Paramyxovirus Rhabdovirus Togavirus Varicella-zoster	Severe acute respiratory syndrome (SARS), common cold Infectious mononucleosis Hepatitis (inflammation of the liver) Cold sores, genital herpes HIV/AIDS Warts, cervical cancer Flu Measles, mumps Rabies Rubella Chicken pox, shingles
Fungi Single- or multicelled organisms (e.g., yeasts, molds)	*Candida albicans* *Cryptococcus neoformans* Dermatophyte fungi *Histoplasma capsulatum* *Coccidioides immitis*	Yeast infections, thrush Pneumonia, meningitis Athlete's foot, jock itch, ringworm, nail infections Histoplasmosis Coccidioidomycosis
Protozoa Single-celled organisms	*Entamoeba histolytica* *Giardia lamblia* *Plasmodia* *Trichomonas vaginalis* *Trypanosoma brucei*	Amoebic dysentery Giardiasis Malaria Trichomoniasis African sleeping sickness
Parasitic worms Worms that feed and live on or in a host	*Ancylostoma duodenale* *Ascaris lumbricoides* Beef, pork, or fish tapeworms *Enterobius vermicularis* *Necator americanus* Schistosoma	Ancylostomiasis (hookworm infection) Ascariasis (roundworm infection) Tapeworm infection Pinworm infection Hookworm infection Cercarial dermatitis (swimmer's itch), schistosomiasis
Prions Proteinaceous infectious particles	PrP^{Sc}	Creutzfeldt-Jakob disease (CJD)

FIGURE 13.2   Pathogens and associated infectious diseases.

antibiotics. Symptoms of meningitis include fever, a severe headache, stiff neck, sensitivity to light, and confusion. Symptoms can appear quickly or over a few days. Immediate treatment is needed because death can occur within hours. Today *Neisseria meningitidis* (meningococcus) and *Streptococcus pneumoniae* (pneumococcus) are the leading

causes of bacterial meningitis, particularly in adolescents and young adults (see the box "Meningococcal Meningitis and College Students").

The disease is fatal in about 10% of cases, and about 10–20% of people who recover have permanent disabilities, including brain damage, seizures, and hearing loss. Worldwide, meningitis kills about 170,000 people each year, particularly in the so-called meningitis belt in sub-Saharan Africa.

Strep Throat and Other Streptococcal Infections
Streptococcus is the genus name of a group of bacteria that cause several diseases in humans. Streptococcal pharyngitis,

streptococcus   Any of a genus (*Streptococcus*) of spherical bacteria; streptococcal species can cause skin infections, strep throat, rheumatic fever, pneumonia, scarlet fever, and other diseases.

TERMS

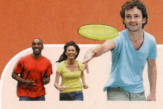

WELLNESS ON CAMPUS
Meningococcal Meningitis and College Students

When meningitis is caused by the bacterium *Neisseria meningitidis,* it is called meningococcal meningitis. Although rates of this disease have been declining since the 1990s, it still causes deaths. The disease is spread by the exchange of respiratory and throat secretions (as in coughing and sneezing) and through person-to-person contact (as in kissing); it can readily spread among people living in close quarters.

In the United States, nearly 30% of meningitis cases occur in adolescents and young adults, and there is an increased risk in college students. Lifestyle factors, such as crowded living situations, irregular sleep patterns, sharing of personal items, bar patronage, and smoking (active or passive) all increase the risk for meningococcal meningitis.

A vaccine is available that protects against four of the five most common strains of meningitis. Because rates of the disease rise beginning in early adolescence and peak between ages 15 and 20, the CDC and the American College Health Association recommend vaccination for all unvaccinated first-year college students living in dormitories, and some schools require it. Visit www.immunize.org/laws/menin.asp to find out more about specific state mandates.

Meningococcal meningitis is treated with antibiotics, and often those who have direct contact with the patient, such as housemates, roommates, and romantic partners, are also given antibiotics. Besides being vaccinated, you can protect yourself against meningococcal meningitis by getting enough sleep, not smoking and not being around tobacco smoke, and avoiding people who are sick.

SOURCES: Centers for Disease Control and Prevention. 2016. *Meningitis* (http://www.cdc.gov/meningitis); Vaccines.gov. n.d. *College & Young Adults* (http://www.vaccines.gov/who_and_when/college/); American College Health Association. 2015. *Meningitis on Campus*: Know Your Risk (http://www.acha.org/ACHA/Resources/Topics/Meningitis.aspx).

---

or strep throat, is characterized by a red, sore throat with white patches on the tonsils, swollen lymph nodes, fever, and headache. Typically the streptococcus bacterium is spread from an infected individual through close contact via respiratory droplets that are released when the infected person sneezes or coughs. If left untreated, strep throat can develop into the more serious rheumatic fever. A particularly virulent type of streptococcus can invade the bloodstream, spread to other parts of the body, and produce dangerous systemic illness. It can also cause a serious but rare infection of the deeper layers of the skin, a condition called necrotizing fasciitis or "flesh-eating strep."

Toxic Shock Syndrome and Other Staphylococcal Infections **Staphylococcus** bacteria are commonly found on the skin and in the nasal passages of healthy people. For example, *Staphylococcus aureus* occurs on 15–40% of people who show no signs of disease. Occasionally, however, staphylococci enter the body and cause an infection, ranging from minor skin infections such as boils to very serious conditions such as blood infections and pneumonia. The risk of a serious staph infection is higher in persons with certain medical conditions, including people suffering from malnutrition, alcoholism, intravenous drug use, diabetes, or kidney failure.

Staphylococcus aureus is responsible for many cases of toxic shock syndrome (TSS). The bacteria produce a toxin that causes a massive proliferation of T cells that can bind to it. The staphylococcus toxins are referred to as "super antigens" because the massive proliferation of T cells results in excessive production of pro-inflammatory cytokines. This "cytokine storm" causes tissue damage, widespread coagulation of blood in the blood vessels, and ultimately organ failure.

A serious antibiotic-resistant infection is caused by a staphylococcus bacterium known as methicillin-resistant *Staphylococcus aureus* (MRSA). Many cases of MRSA infection occur in hospitalized patients, and these infections tend to be severe. MRSA is also common in the community (outside hospital settings), where it usually infects the skin, causing painful lesions that resemble infected spider bites. The spread of MRSA infection is associated with places where people are in close contact with one another, such as locker rooms and playing fields; athletes are particularly at risk and should keep any cuts or abrasions covered.

Tuberculosis Caused by the bacterium *Mycobacterium tuberculosis,* **tuberculosis (TB)** is a chronic bacterial infection that usually affects the lungs, though it can

> **TERMS**
>
> **staphylococcus** Any of a genus (*Staphylococcus*) of spherical, clustered bacteria commonly found on the skin or in the nasal passages; staphylococcal species may enter the body and cause conditions such as boils, pneumonia, toxic shock syndrome, and severe skin infections.
>
> **tuberculosis (TB)** A chronic bacterial infection that usually affects the lungs.

affect other organs as well. TB is spread via the respiratory route. Symptoms include coughing, fatigue, night sweats, weight loss, and fever. Between 10 and 15 million Americans have been infected with *M. tuberculosis* and continue to carry it. Only about 10% of people with latent TB infections actually develop an active case of the disease; the immune system usually prevents the disease from becoming active. In the United States, active TB is most common among people infected with HIV, recent immigrants from countries where TB is endemic, and those who live in inner cities.

Many strains of tuberculosis respond to antibiotics, but only over a course of treatment lasting 6–12 months. Failure to complete treatment can lead to relapse and the development of strains of antibiotic-resistant bacteria. Multidrug-resistant TB (MDR TB) is resistant to at least two of the best anti-TB drugs. Extensively drug-resistant TB (XDR TB) is resistant to those drugs as well as some second-line drugs. XDR TB is relatively rare, but patients with this form of TB have fewer and less effective treatment options. TB is a leading cause of death in people with HIV infection.

Tick-borne Infections   Lyme disease is one such infection, and it accounts for more than 25,000 cases per year. It is spread by the bite of a tick that is infected with the spiral-shaped bacterium *Borrelia burgdorferi*. Ticks acquire the bacterium by ingesting the blood of an infected animal; they can then transmit the microbe to their next host. The deer tick is responsible for transmitting Lyme disease bacteria to humans in the northeastern and north-central United States; on the Pacific Coast, the culprit is the western black-legged tick.

Symptoms of Lyme disease vary but typically occur in three stages. In the first stage, about 80% of victims develop a bull's-eye-shaped red rash expanding from the area of the bite, usually about two weeks after the bite occurs. The second stage occurs weeks to months later in 10–20% of untreated patients; symptoms may involve the nervous and cardiovascular systems and can include impaired coordination, partial facial paralysis, and heart rhythm abnormalities. These symptoms usually disappear on their own within a few weeks. The third stage, which occurs in about half of untreated people, can develop months or years after the tick bite and usually consists of chronic or recurring arthritis. Lyme disease can also cause fetal damage or death at any stage of pregnancy. Lyme disease is treatable at all stages, although arthritis symptoms may not resolve completely. Lyme disease is preventable by avoiding contact with ticks or by removing a tick before it has had the chance to transmit the infection.

Rocky Mountain spotted fever and typhus are caused by the *rickettsia* bacterium and are also transmitted via tick bites. Rocky Mountain spotted fever is characterized by sudden onset of fever, headache, and muscle pain, followed by development of a spotted rash.

Other Bacterial Infections   The following are a few of the many other infections caused by bacteria:

- *Ulcers.* Up to 90% of ulcers are caused by infection with the bacterium *Helicobacter pylori*. If tests show the presence of *H. pylori,* antibiotics often cure the infection and the ulcers.

- *Tetanus.* Also known as lockjaw, tetanus is caused by the bacterium *Clostridium tetani,* which thrives in deep puncture wounds and produces a deadly toxin. Worldwide more than 200,000 people die from tetanus each year.

- *Clostridium difficile.* Another type of *Clostridium* bacteria, called *Clostridium difficile* (*C. diff*), has joined MRSA as a major emerging threat in American health care settings, particularly hospitals. It causes inflammation of the colon, resulting in diarrhea, fever, and nausea. Most cases of *C. diff* infection respond to a new class of antibiotics that selectively kills *C. diff* without affecting the many bacterial species that populate the normal, healthy intestine. The CDC recommends that doctors, nurses, and other health care providers wash their hands frequently to reduce the spread of the bacterium.

- *Pertussis.* Also known as whooping cough, pertussis is a highly contagious respiratory illness caused by the bacterium *Bordetella pertussis*. Those at high risk include infants and children who are too young to be fully vaccinated and those who have not completed the primary vaccination series. Adolescents and adults become susceptible when immunity from vaccination wanes, so a booster shot is recommended at 11–12 years or during adolescence and thereafter every 10 years.

- *Urinary tract infections (UTIs).* Infection of the bladder and urethra is most common among sexually active women, but UTIs can occur in anyone. The bacterium *Escherichia coli* (*E. coli*) is the most common infectious agent, responsible for about 80% of all UTIs.

Antibiotic Treatments   **Antibiotics** are both naturally occurring and synthetic substances that can kill bacteria or inhibit their growth. Antibacterial antibiotics are categorized based on their mechanism of action. The majority of antibiotics inhibit the synthesis of the bacterial cell wall. The second largest group interferes with the production of bacterial proteins. A third class prevents the replication of the bacterial DNA.

Antibiotics have saved millions of lives. However, their overuse and misuse have led to the emergence of antibiotic-resistant bacteria. A bacterium can become

> **antibiotic**   A synthetic or naturally occurring substance that kills or inhibits the growth of bacteria, fungi, or protozoa.   **TERMS**

resistant from a chance genetic mutation or through the transfer of genetic material from one bacterium to another. When exposed to antibiotics, resistant bacteria can grow and flourish while the antibiotic-sensitive bacteria die off. Eventually an entire colony of bacteria can develop resistance to one or more antibiotics and become very difficult to treat. Antibiotic-resistant strains of many common bacteria have developed, including strains of gonorrhea, salmonella, and tuberculosis. Antibiotic resistance is a major factor contributing to the rise in problematic infectious diseases.

Resistance is promoted when people fail to take the full course of an antibiotic or when they inappropriately take antibiotics for viral infections. Another possible source of resistance is the use of antibiotics in agriculture, which is estimated to account for 50–80% of the 25,000 tons of antibiotics used annually in the United States.

You can help prevent the development of antibiotic-resistant strains of bacteria by using antibiotics properly:

• Don't ask your doctor for an antibiotic every time you get sick. Antibiotics are helpful for bacterial infections but are ineffective against viruses.

• Use antibiotics as directed, and finish the full course of medication even if you begin to feel better.

• Never take an antibiotic without a prescription. If you take an antibiotic for a viral infection, your illness will not improve.

Viruses

A **virus** is a microscopic organism consisting of genetic material covered by a protein coat. Viruses lack the enzymes essential to energy production and protein synthesis in normal animal cells, and they can replicate only inside the cells of another organism. Once a virus is inside the host cell, it sheds its protein covering and exploits the host's cellular machinery to produce more viruses like itself. Most contagious diseases are caused by viruses.

The Common Cold A cold may be caused by any of more than 200 viruses that attack the lining of the nasal passages. Cold viruses are almost always transmitted by hand-to-hand contact. To lessen your risk of contracting a cold, wash your hands frequently; if you touch someone else, avoid touching your face until after you've washed your hands.

If you catch a cold, over-the-counter cold remedies may relieve your symptoms, but they do not eliminate the virus. The jury is still out on whether other remedies, including zinc gluconate lozenges, echinacea, and vitamin C, relieve symptoms or shorten the duration of a cold. Researchers are also studying antiviral drugs that target the most common types of

cold viruses. Antibiotics will not affect a viral infection but will help treat a bacterial sinus infection.

Influenza Commonly called the flu, **influenza** is an infection of the respiratory tract caused by the influenza virus. Compared to the common cold, influenza is a more serious illness, usually including a fever and extreme fatigue. Most people who get the flu recover within one to two weeks, but some develop potentially life-threatening complications, such as pneumonia. The highest rates of infection occur in children. Influenza is highly contagious and is spread via respiratory droplets. The most effective way to prevent the flu is through annual vaccination. The CDC recommends vaccination for all people age 6 months and over.

Measles, Mumps, and Rubella Worldwide, more than 600,000 people die each year from measles. Measles is a highly contagious disease, and before the introduction of vaccines, more than 90% of Americans contracted measles by age 15. Rubella, if it infects a pregnant woman, can be transmitted to a fetus, causing miscarriage, stillbirth, and severe birth defects, including deafness, eye and heart defects, and mental impairment. Mumps generally causes swelling of the parotid (salivary) glands, located just below and in front of the ears. This virus can also cause meningitis and, in males, inflammation of the testes.

Chickenpox, Cold Sores, and Other Herpesvirus Infections The **herpesviruses** are a large group of viruses. Once infected, the host is never free of the virus. The virus lies latent within certain cells and becomes active periodically, producing symptoms. Herpesviruses are particularly dangerous for people with a depressed immune system, as in the case of HIV infection. The family of herpesviruses includes the Varicella-zoster virus, which causes chickenpox and shingles; Herpes simplex virus (HSV) types 1 and 2, which cause cold sores and the sexually transmitted infection herpes; and Epstein-Barr virus (EBV), which causes infectious mononucleosis.

TERMS

virus A very small infectious agent composed of nucleic acid (DNA or RNA) surrounded by a protein coat; lacks an independent metabolism and reproduces only within a host cell.

influenza Infection of the respiratory tract by the influenza virus, which is highly infectious and prone to variation; the form changes rapidly; commonly known as the flu.

herpesvirus A large family of viruses responsible for cold sores, mononucleosis, chickenpox, shingles, and the sexually transmitted infection herpes; causes latent infections.

Two herpesviruses that can cause severe infections in people with AIDS or who have a suppressed immune system are cytomegalovirus (CMV), which infects the lungs, brain, colon, and eyes, and human herpesvirus 8 (HHV-8), which has been linked to Kaposi's sarcoma, a cancer of the connective tissue.

Viral Hepatitis   Viral **hepatitis** is a term used to describe several different infections that cause inflammation of the liver. Hepatitis is usually caused by one of the three most common hepatitis viruses. Hepatitis A virus (HAV) causes the mildest form of the disease and is usually transmitted by food or water contaminated by sewage or an infected person. Hepatitis B virus (HBV) is usually transmitted sexually. Hepatitis C virus (HCV) can also be transmitted sexually, but it is much more commonly passed through direct contact with infected blood via injection drug use or—prior to the development of screening tests—blood transfusions. HBV and, to a lesser extent, HCV can also be passed from a pregnant woman to her child.

Symptoms of acute hepatitis infection can include fatigue, **jaundice,** abdominal pain, loss of appetite, nausea, and diarrhea. Most people recover from hepatitis A within a month or so. However, 5–10% of people infected with HBV and 85–90% of people infected with HCV become chronic carriers of the virus, capable of infecting others for the rest of their lives. Some chronic carriers remain asymptomatic, while others slowly develop chronic liver disease, cirrhosis, or liver cancer.

The extent of HCV infection has been recognized only recently, and most infected people are unaware of their condition. To ensure proper treatment and prevention, testing for HCV may be recommended for people at risk, including people who have injected drugs (even once); who received a blood transfusion or a donated organ prior to July 1992; who have engaged in high-risk sexual behavior; or who have had body piercing, tattoos, or acupuncture involving unsterile equipment.

Human Papillomavirus (HPV)   The more than 200 types of HPV cause a variety of warts (noncancerous skin tumors), including common warts on the hands, plantar warts on the soles of the feet, and genital warts around the genitalia. Depending on their location, warts may be removed using over-the-counter preparations or professional methods such as laser surgery or cryosurgery. Because HPV infection is chronic, warts can reappear despite treatment. HPV causes the majority of cases of cervical cancer. Three vaccines are available, targeting the types of HPV linked to the majority of HPV-caused cancers. Vaccination is recommended for all girls and boys aged 11 or 12; women can get the HPV vaccine through age 26 and men, through age 21.

Treating Viral Illnesses   Antiviral drugs typically work by interfering with some part of the viral life cycle; for example, they may prevent a virus from entering body cells or from successfully reproducing within cells. Antivirals are currently available to fight infections caused by HIV, influenza, herpes simplex, varicella-zoster, HBV, and HCV. Most other viral diseases must simply run their course.

Fungi

A **fungus** is an organism that reproduces by spores and feeds on organic matter. Only about 50 of the many thousands of species of fungi cause disease in humans, and these diseases are usually restricted to the skin, mucous membranes, and lungs. Some fungal diseases are extremely difficult to treat because spores are an especially resistant dormant stage of the organism.

Candida albicans is a common fungus found naturally in the vagina of most women. When excessive growth occurs, the result is itching and discomfort, commonly known as a yeast infection.

Other common fungal conditions, including athlete's foot, jock itch, and ringworm, affect the skin. These three conditions are usually mild and easy to cure. Fungi can also cause systemic diseases that are severe, life threatening, and extremely difficult to treat. Fungal infections can be especially deadly in people with impaired immune systems.

Protozoa

Protozoa are single-celled organisms that can cause a range of diseases in humans. Millions of people in developing countries suffer from protozoal infections.

Malaria, caused by a parasitic protozoan of the genus *Plasmodium,* is a major killer worldwide; each year there are 350–500 million new cases of malaria globally and more than 1 million deaths, mostly among infants and children. Drug-resistant strains of malaria have emerged, requiring new medicines.

Giardiasis is caused by *Giardia lamblia,* a single-celled parasite that lives in the intestines of humans and animals. Giardiasis is characterized by nausea, diarrhea, bloating, and

---

TERMS

hepatitis   Inflammation of the liver, which can be caused by infection, drugs, or toxins.

jaundice   Increased bile pigment levels in the blood, characterized by yellowing of the skin and the whites of the eyes.

fungus   A single-celled or multicelled organism that reproduces by spores and feeds on organic matter; examples include molds, mushrooms, and yeasts. Fungal diseases include yeast infections, athlete's foot, and ringworm.

protozoan   A microscopic single-celled organism that often produces recurrent, cyclical attacks of disease; plural, *protozoa.*

malaria   A severe, recurrent, mosquito-borne infection caused by the parasitic protozoan *Plasmodium.*

giardiasis   An intestinal disease caused by the parasitic protozoan *Giardia lamblia.*

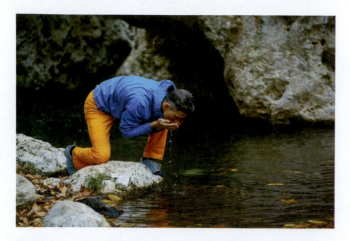

Even seemingly pristine mountain streams can be contaminated with the protozoan *Giardia lamblia,* as many unwary hikers and campers have discovered. Symptoms of giardiasis include abdominal pain, bloating, and diarrhea.

© Vitaliy Mateha/123RF

abdominal cramps, and it is among the most common water-borne diseases in the United States. People may become infected with *Giardia* if they consume contaminated food or water or pick up the parasite from the contaminated surface of an object such as a bathroom fixture, diaper pail, or toy.

Parasitic Worms

The **parasitic worms** are the largest organisms that can enter the body to cause infection. Worms, including intestinal parasites such as the tapeworm and hookworm, cause a variety of relatively mild infections. Pinworm, the most common worm infection in the United States, primarily affects young children. Smaller worms known as flukes infect organs such as the liver and lungs and, in large numbers, can be deadly. Worm infections generally originate from contaminated food or drink and can be prevented by careful attention to hygiene.

Emerging Infectious Diseases

Emerging infectious diseases are infections whose incidence in humans has increased or threatens to increase in the near future. They include both known diseases that have experienced a resurgence, such as tuberculosis and cholera, and diseases that were previously unknown or confined to specific areas, such as the Zika and Ebola viruses.

Selected Infections of Concern Although the chances of the average American contracting an exotic infection are very low, emerging infections are a concern to public health officials and represent a challenge to all nations in the future.

ZIKA DISEASE Zika virus is transmitted by several species of *Aedes* mosquitoes; it can also spread through sex with a man infected with Zika, and it can pass from a pregnant

woman to her fetus. The virus was discovered in Uganda in 1947 and arrived in Southeast Asia shortly thereafter. By 2014, it had spread across the Pacific Islands and into the Americas; as of mid-2016, active virus transmission has been reported throughout most of South and Central America, the Caribbean (including Puerto Rico), Mexico, and parts of Florida.

In most people, Zika symptoms are very mild, lasting a week or less, and may include fever, rash, and joint pain. However, a small proportion of people infected with Zika develop a neurological condition called Guillain-Barré syndrome, usually characterized by muscle weakness; this condition typically resolves within a few weeks or several months. Of greater concern are the effects of Zika during pregnancy. Following reports in Brazil of an increase in the number of babies born with microcephaly (small head size) and other serious brain anomalies to mothers infected with Zika, researchers examined the virus as a possible cause. In 2016, the CDC confirmed that, on the basis of the available evidence, Zika can cause birth defects including microcephaly, impaired growth, eye defects, hearing loss, and possibly other problems.

The specific geographic areas where Zika virus is spreading are likely to change over time, and research is ongoing into its effects and the best strategies for testing and prevention. The mosquitoes that carry Zika are found in many parts of the world, including much of the United States, and not only are they aggressive daytime biters but they are also active at night. For up-to-date information, visit the CDC Zika website (www.cdc.gov/zika).

EBOLA Ebola virus disease (EVD) is caused by Ebola virus, which is transmitted to people from wild animals. Infected people can then transmit the virus to others through direct contact with blood or body fluids or objects that have been contaminated. EVD is a severe infection with an average fatality rate of about 50%. Ebola is rare, but outbreaks have occurred periodically since it was first identified in 1976. There is no vaccine; it is treated with supportive care, and spread of the infection is controlled by identifying and isolating the sick and their close contacts. As of June 2016, about 28,600 cases had been reported worldwide, with about 12,000 deaths. The outbreak in West Africa that began in March 2014 was the largest in history. The most severely affected countries were Guinea, Liberia, and Sierra Leone. Four cases were treated in the United States: one a traveler from West Africa (the only death in the United States), two health care workers who treated him, and a medical aid worker who had worked in Guinea. On January 14, 2016, the WHO declared that the outbreak was at its end, although occasional flare-ups may still occur.

> **parasitic worm** A pathogen that causes intestinal and other infections; includes tapeworms, hookworms, pinworms, and flukes.
>
> **TERMS**

WEST NILE VIRUS West Nile virus is carried by birds and then passed to humans when mosquitoes bite first an infected bird and then a person. In the United States, West Nile virus has caused infections in humans in 46 states and the District of Columbia. About 20% of infected people develop fever and other moderate symptoms, such as muscle aches and nausea; less than 1% develop a serious neurological illness such as meningitis or encephalitis. Since 1999, when West Nile virus disease was first identified in the United States, more than 40,000 cases and 1,700 deaths have been reported.

PATHOGENIC ESCHERICIA COLI *E. coli* bacteria live in the intestines of humans and animals and are an essential component of gut immunity. However, some strains of *E. coli* cause diarrhea; six types cause disease. Since 2006, there have been 24 multistate outbreaks of *E. coli*-caused disease. These outbreaks have been caused by contaminated foods including lettuce, spinach, sprouts, hazelnuts, processed meats, frozen foods, poultry, and beef sold both in grocery store chains and in restaurants. However, people also can become infected in other ways, such as by swallowing contaminated swimming pool water and through contact with an infected animal—for example, by petting an animal and then not washing hands before eating. Pets and animals at exhibits such as petting zoos can be healthy but carry pathogens on their bodies that can be passed to humans. The CDC website has guidelines for preventing infection.

HANTAVIRUS Hantavirus infection can cause a deadly disease called hantavirus pulmonary syndrome (HPS). In North America, the deer mouse, the white-footed mouse, the rice rat, and the cotton rat are carriers of hantaviruses. People can become infected when rodent urine and droppings that contain the virus get into the air, for example, after they dry out. Since 1993, 606 cases of HPS have been counted in the lower 48 states, with an average fatality rate of 36%.

Factors Contributing to Emerging Infections

What's behind this rising tide of infectious diseases? Contributing factors are complex and interrelated. New or increasing drug resistance has been found in organisms that cause malaria, tuberculosis, gonorrhea, influenza, AIDS, and pneumococcal and staphylococcal infections. Some bacterial strains now appear to be resistant to all available antibiotics. Another factor is poverty. More than 1 billion people live in extreme poverty, and half the world's population has no regular access to essential drugs. Population growth, urbanization, overcrowding, and migration (including the movement of refugees) also spread infectious diseases. A poor public health infrastructure is often associated with poverty and social upheaval, but problems such as contaminated water supplies can occur even in industrial countries. Inadequate vaccination has led to the reemergence of diseases such as diphtheria and pertussis. Natural disasters such as hurricanes also disrupt the public health infrastructure, leaving survivors with contaminated water and food supplies and no shelter from disease-carrying insects.

International tourism and trade are also factors, as they open the world to infectious agents. For example, the ongoing outbreak of Zika virus in Brazil is believed to be due to a combination of increased numbers of foreign travelers attending the 2014 FIFA World Cup and a large population of *Aedes* mosquitoes in the region. And food now travels long distances to our table, and microbes are transmitted along with it. Mass production of food increases the likelihood that a chance contamination can lead to mass illness.

Other causes can be traced to human behaviors–for example, the widespread use of injectable drugs, which rapidly transmits HIV infection and hepatitis. Changes in sexual behavior also, over the past 40 years have led to a proliferation of old and new sexually transmitted infections. And the use of day care facilities for children has led to increases in the incidence of several infections that cause diarrhea. Finally, the lengthening of warm periods and a change to shorter or milder winters may enable pathogenic species and, for some pathogens, their insect vectors to expand their range into countries or states where they once had not existed or had been rare.

Immune Disorders

Considering the complexity of the immune system, it is not surprising that the system sometimes fails to operate properly, resulting in disease. When the immune system breaks down, "self" may be misread and attacked as "nonself," and the result is an autoimmune disease. In most autoimmune diseases, the immune system targets or destroys specific tissues. For example, in type 1 diabetes, the insulin-producing cells of the pancreas are destroyed. In multiple sclerosis, the protective coating around nerves is destroyed. In Hashimoto's thyroiditis, the thyroid gland is destroyed. In rheumatoid arthritis, the membranes lining the joints are destroyed. In systemic lupus erythematosus, destructive inflammation affects the joints, blood vessels, heart, lungs, brain, and kidneys.

The causes of autoimmune diseases are not well understood. The rates of many autoimmune diseases are much higher in women than in men. About 2 million Americans have lupus, and 80% of them are women. Among the estimated 1% of Americans with rheumatoid arthritis, women outnumber men three to one. A number of studies in animal models and humans indicate that gut microbes have a role in susceptibility or resistance to the development of autoimmune disease. Because diet can affect the composition of gut microbiota, there is increasing interest in the role of diet in the occurrence of specific autoimmune diseases.

As explained in Chapter 12, cancer cells are cells that have mutated in ways that allow them to multiply uncontrollably. The immune system detects cells that have recently become abnormal and destroys them just as it would a foreign cell. However, some types of cancer cells actually suppress immune responses.

In recent years, conventional cancer treatments have been augmented with a treatment known as immunotherapy. The goal of immunotherapy is to stimulate the patient's immune

Ask Yourself

QUESTIONS FOR CRITICAL THINKING AND REFLECTION

Have you ever had any of the illnesses described in the preceding sections? How were you exposed to the disease? Could you have taken any precautions to avoid it?

system to attack tumor cells. One immunotherapeutic strategy involves administering tumor-specific antibodies to the patient to stimulate the immune system to recruit macrophages to destroy the tumor cells. Another strategy is to infuse the patient with immune cells, such as dendritic cells. This is the basis of the vaccine for prostate cancer, the first FDA-approved cancer vaccine. This vaccine does not cure cancer but can extend patients' lives by several months.

SUPPORTING YOUR IMMUNE SYSTEM

The immune system does an amazing job of protecting you from illness, but you can help ensure its optimal functioning by choosing healthy behaviors. Here are some general guidelines for supporting your immune system:

- Eat a balanced diet and maintain a healthy weight.

- Get enough sleep. Experimental studies have shown that people who sleep fewer than six hours per night have compromised immune function. Quality sleep is as important as sufficient sleep. *Sleep quality* refers to a collection of measurable components, including the length of time it takes to fall asleep, duration of sleep, the amount of time spent asleep as a proportion of the total time spent in bed, frequency of awakenings, and feeling refreshed or tired upon awakening.

- Exercise, but not when you're sick. Exercise helps you stay healthy. It also staves off stress, which can weaken your immune system.

- Don't smoke. Smoking decreases the levels of some immune cells.

- If you drink alcohol, do so only in moderation. Excessive drinking can interfere with normal immune system functioning.

- Make sure you get enough Vitamin D. Vitamin D is made in the skin upon exposure to sunlight. It is not always possible to get sufficient sunlight exposure.

- Wash your hands frequently. When soap and water are not available, use hand sanitizer. Make sure the product is at least 60% alcohol, but avoid sanitizers that contain *triclosan*. Triclosan has been detected in the breast milk, urine, and plasma of people who use products containing it.

- Avoid contact with people who are contagious with an infectious disease.

- Make sure you drink water only from clean sources. Unpurified water from lakes and streams can carry pathogens, even if it seems pristine.

- Avoid contact with disease carriers such as rodents, mosquitoes, and ticks. Never touch or feed wild animals or rodents.

- Practice safer sex.

- Do not use injectable drugs of any kind.

- Make sure you have received all your recommended vaccinations, and keep them up-to-date. Your physician can tell you exactly what immunizations you need and when you should have them.

THE MAJOR STIs

Sexually transmitted infections (STIs)—also still called **sexually transmitted diseases (STDs)**—spread from person to person mainly through sexual activity. STIs are a particularly insidious group of illnesses because a person can be infected and be able to transmit the disease, yet not look or feel sick. The Centers for Disease Control and Prevention (CDC) estimates that the cost of STIs to the health care system in the United States exceeds $16 billion per year.

The following seven STIs pose major health threats:

- HIV/AIDS
- Chlamydia
- Gonorrhea
- Human papillomavirus (HPV)
- Herpes
- Hepatitis
- Syphilis

STIs can cause serious complications if left untreated and pose risks to a fetus or newborn. STIs can result in long-term consequences, including chronic pain, infertility, stillbirths, genital cancers, and death. The CDC estimates that at least 24,000 American women become infertile each year as a result of undiagnosed and untreated STIs. In fact, the rate of STIs is among the highest in the United States of any industrialized nation. The Centers for Disease Control and Prevention (CDC) estimates that 110 million Americans are infected with an STI and that over 20 million Americans become newly infected with an STI each year. The total number of people infected is higher than the number of new cases because some infections, such as HIV and genital herpes, are not curable and so persist. Young people aged 15–24 account for half of STI cases in the United States.

> **sexually transmitted infection (STI) or sexually transmitted disease (STD)** An infection that is transmitted mainly by sexual contact; some can also be transmitted by other means. **TERMS**

HIV Infection and AIDS

HIV causes AIDS. With recent advances in the treatment of **human immunodeficiency virus (HIV),** people infected with the virus are now living almost as long as people not infected with it. Adequate treatment is not accessible, however, for most people worldwide. Untreated HIV infection may advance to **acquired immunodeficiency syndrome (AIDS)** within 8–10 years of diagnosis. This stage of HIV infection is defined by a severely compromised immune system and the presence of opportunistic infections.

Many experts believe that the global HIV epidemic peaked in the late 1990s, at about 3.5 million new infections per year, compared with an estimated 2.1 million new infections in 2015. Despite a slowing of the epidemic, AIDS remains a primary cause of death in Africa and continues to be a major cause of mortality around the world (see the box "HIV/AIDS around the World").

In the United States, about 1.2 million people are living with HIV. The incidence of HIV has leveled off at about 45,000 new infections annually. More than 670,000 Americans with an AIDS diagnosis have died since the start of the epidemic in 1981. Today, 1 in 8 Americans infected with HIV are unaware of their HIV status.

What Is HIV Infection?

HIV infection is a chronic disease that progressively damages the body's immune system, making an otherwise healthy person less able to resist a variety of infections and disorders. Normally, when a virus or other pathogen enters the body, it is targeted and destroyed by the immune system. But HIV attacks the immune system itself, invading and taking over **CD4 T cells** (white blood cells that fight infection), macrophages, and other essential elements of the immune system. HIV enters a human cell and converts its own genetic material, RNA, into DNA. It then inserts this DNA into the chromosomes of the host cell. The viral DNA is not only instrumental in producing new copies of HIV, but it also seriously reduces immune functions.

Immediately following infection with HIV, billions of infectious particles are produced every day. For a time, the immune system keeps pace, also producing billions of new cells. Unlike the virus, however, the immune system cannot make new cells indefinitely; as long as the virus keeps replicating, it wins in the end. The destruction of the immune system is signaled by the loss of CD4 T cells. As the number of CD4 cells declines, an infected person may begin to experience mild to moderately severe symptoms. A person is diagnosed with AIDS when the number of CD4 cells in the blood drops below a certain level (200/µl). People with AIDS are vulnerable to several serious **opportunistic (secondary) infections**.

The first weeks after being infected with HIV are called the *primary infection* phase. Most, but not all, infected people develop flulike symptoms about two to four weeks after being exposed to the virus. During primary HIV infection, people have large amounts of HIV in the bloodstream and genital fluids, making it easier to transmit the virus. Several months later, infected people develop antibodies to the virus, so commonly available tests will show a positive result. The next phase of HIV infection is the chronic **asymptomatic** (symptom-free) stage, also called the *latency* phase. This period can last from 2 to 20 years, averaging 11 years in untreated adults. During this time, the virus progressively infects and destroys the cells of the immune system. Even if they are symptom-free, people infected with HIV can transmit the disease to others.

Transmitting the Virus

HIV lives only within cells and body fluids, not outside the body. It is transmitted by blood and blood products, semen, vaginal and cervical secretions, and breast milk. It cannot live in air, in water, or on objects or surfaces such as toilet seats, eating utensils, or telephones. A person is not at risk of HIV infection by being in the same classroom, dining room, or even household with someone who is infected.

The three main routes of HIV transmission are specific kinds of sexual contact; direct exposure to infected blood; and contact between an HIV-infected woman and her child during pregnancy, childbirth, or breastfeeding.

HIV is more likely to be transmitted by unprotected anal or vaginal intercourse than by other sexual activities. During vaginal intercourse, male-to-female transmission is more likely to occur than female-to-male transmission. HIV has been found in preejaculatory fluid, which means that transmission can occur before ejaculation. Being the receptive partner during unprotected anal intercourse is the riskiest of all sexual activities. Oral–genital contact carries some risk of transmission, although less than anal or vaginal intercourse.

> **QUICK STATS**
>
> HIV/AIDS is ranked as the **eighth leading cause** of death among Americans aged 25–34 years.
>
> —National Center for Health Statistics, 2016

TERMS

human immunodeficiency virus (HIV) The virus that causes HIV infection and AIDS.

acquired immunodeficiency syndrome (AIDS) An advanced stage of HIV infection.

HIV infection A chronic, progressive viral infection that damages the immune system.

CD4 T cell A type of white blood cell that helps coordinate the activity of the immune system; the primary target of HIV infection. A decrease in the number of these cells correlates with the severity of HIV-related illness.

opportunistic (secondary) infection An infection caused when organisms take the opportunity presented by a primary (initial) infection to multiply and cause a new, different infection.

asymptomatic Showing no signs or symptoms of a disease.

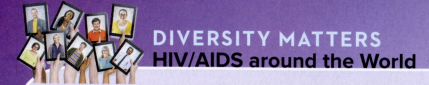

DIVERSITY MATTERS
HIV/AIDS around the World

In 2016, the world marked the 35th year since cases of what we now know as AIDS were reported in gay men in California and New York. A year later, similar cases were being described in hemophiliacs, individuals who had received blood transfusions, injection drug users, infected women, and their newborn infants. With this change in demographics came the knowledge and awareness that AIDS was not just a disease of gay men. Cases in women were becoming increasingly more commonplace in central Africa, announcing the epidemic in the heterosexual community on the global level. Since the year of the first report of HIV/AIDS, more than 70 million people have been infected and more than 34 million have died.

Global Disparities in HIV/AIDS

The vast majority of cases have occurred in economically emerging countries, where heterosexual contact is the primary means of transmission. Sadly, HIV continues to disproportionately affect nonwhite racial and ethnic populations and the poor. Adolescent girls and young women are at particularly high risk; they make up 11% of the global population but accounted for 20% of new adult HIV infections in 2015. The gender imbalance is even more pronounced in sub-Saharan Africa, the hardest-hit region, where women accounted for 56% of new infections in 2015. Factors at the root of this disparity include harmful gender norms and inequalities, violence,

poverty, and lack of access to sexual and reproductive health services.

Other key populations at risk worldwide include gay men and other men who have sex with men, people who inject drugs, sex workers, transgender people, prisoners, clients of sex workers, and other sex partners of at-risk populations. These groups are often marginalized and stigmatized, reducing their access to services, which in turn increases rates of infection. The distribution of new HIV infections among key populations varies by region: People who inject drugs account for about half of HIV infections in eastern Europe and central Asia, whereas men who have sex with men account for half of new infections in western and central Europe and North America. In some cities in Africa, HIV prevalence among sex workers is over 70%.

HIV/AIDS Prevention and Treatment Gains and Challenges

Despite the ongoing tragedy of the epidemic, strides have been made in treatment and prevention measures. By 2015, an estimated 17 million people were accessing updated treatment, more than double the number receiving treatment in 2010. Due to these scaled-up efforts, the rate of new infections and deaths has declined in some regions. For example, since 2010 in eastern and southern Africa, the number of people receiving treatment increased by over 50% and AIDS-related deaths dropped

by 36%. Treating HIV with effective drugs not only prolongs life and decreases suffering, but it also reduces the spread of the virus because individuals who have received treatment are generally much less infectious than those who have not.

Efforts to combat AIDS are complicated by political, economic, and cultural barriers. Education and prevention programs are often hampered by resistance from social and religious institutions and by the taboo on openly discussing sexual issues. Condoms are not commonly used in many countries, and women in many societies do not have control over sexual situations to insist that men use condoms. Empowering women is a crucial priority in reducing the spread of HIV. In particular, reducing sexual violence against women, promoting financial independence, and increasing women's education and employment opportunities are essential.

Successful prevention approaches include STI treatment and education, public education campaigns about safer sex, and syringe exchange programs for injection drug users. Efforts are ongoing to improve access to barrier protective devices such as condoms. Male circumcision has been shown to reduce the risk of heterosexually acquired HIV infection in men by about 60%; voluntary adult male circumcision is recommended by the World Health Organization (WHO) as part of HIV prevention programs in regions with HIV epidemics among heterosexuals and with high HIV and low male circumcision prevalence. The partial

The presence of lesions, blisters, or inflammation from other STIs in the genital, anal, or oral areas makes it two to nine times easier for the virus to be passed. Spermicides may also cause irritation and increase the risk of HIV transmission. Studies of the widely used spermicide non-oxynol-9 (N-9) have found that frequent use may cause vaginal and rectal irritation, increasing the risk of transmission of HIV and other STIs. The WHO recommends that spermicides containing N-9 not be used for protection against HIV and STIs. Condoms or lubricants with N-9 should never be used during anal intercourse because

N-9 damages the lining of the rectum, providing an entry point for HIV and other STIs.

The risk of HIV transmission during oral sex is generally considered to be low but may be increased if a person has oral sores or other damage to the gums or tissues in the mouth.

Studies in economically emerging nations with high rates of HIV infection have found that circumcised males have a lower risk of HIV infection than uncircumcised males.

Direct contact with the blood of an infected person is another major route of HIV transmission. Needles and

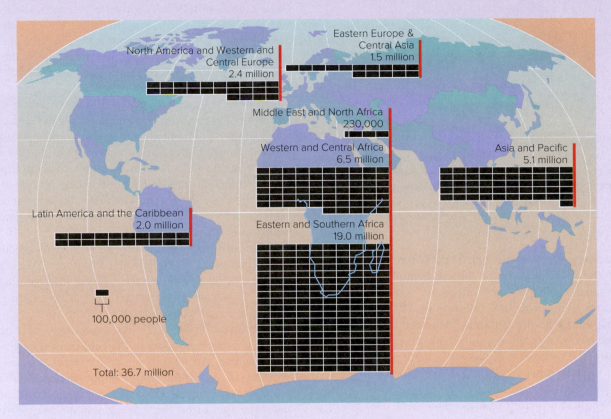

North America and Western and Central Europe
2.4 million

Eastern Europe & Central Asia
1.5 million

Middle East and North Africa
230,000

Western and Central Africa
6.5 million

Asia and Pacific
5.1 million

Latin America and the Caribbean
2.0 million

Eastern and Southern Africa
19.0 million

100,000 people

Total: 36.7 million

Approximate number of people living with HIV/AIDS in 2015.

protection provided by circumcision does not eliminate the need for condom use. The effectiveness for HIV prevention of consistent condom use is estimated to be about 70-80%.

Despite progress, according to the Joint United Nations Programme on HIV/AIDS (UNAIDS), without a scale-up in prevention and treatment efforts, the epidemic will continue to outrun the response. UNAIDS launched a fast-track strategy in 2014 that aims to greatly step up the response in low- and middle-income countries, with the goal of ending the epidemic by 2030. For 2020, UNAIDS set a 90-90-90 treatment target:

• 90% of people living with HIV know their status.

• 90% of people living with HIV who know their status are receiving treatment.

• 90% of people on treatment have suppressed viral loads.

SOURCE: Joint United Nations Programme on HIV/AIDS. 2016. *Global AIDS Update 2016.* Geneva: UNAIDS; Joint United Nations Programme on HIV/AIDS. 2016. *On the Fast-Track to End AIDS: 2016–2021 Strategy.* Geneva: UNAIDS.

syringes used to inject drugs (including heroin, cocaine, and anabolic steroids) are usually contaminated with the user's blood.

In the past, before effective screening was available, some people were infected with HIV through blood transfusions and other medical procedures involving blood products. All blood in licensed U.S. blood banks and plasma centers is now screened thoroughly for HIV.

The final major route of HIV transmission is mother-to-child, also called *vertical* or *perinatal transmission,* which can occur during pregnancy, childbirth, or breastfeeding.

Without intervention, the likelihood of HIV transmission from mother to child is 20–45%; however, transmission may be prevented by providing antiretroviral medications to both mother and child during those stages in which transmission is known to occur.

Populations of Special Concern for HIV Infection

In 2015, the CDC estimated that 75% of HIV-positive Americans were men. Among Americans newly diagnosed with HIV infection, the most common means of HIV exposure is sexual activity between men (Figure 13.3).

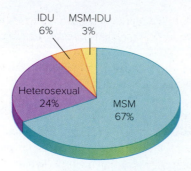

IDU
6%

MSM-IDU
3%

Heterosexual
24%

MSM
67%

* MSM = Men who have sex with men
IDU = Injection drug users

FIGURE 13.3 **Routes of HIV transmission among Americans newly diagnosed with HIV infection in 2014.**

SOURCE: Centers for Disease Control and Prevention. 2015. *HIV Surveillance Report, 2014*, Vol. 26 (http://www.cdc.gov/hiv/library/reports/surveillance).

Men who have sex with men (MSM) represent about 4% of the male population in the United States but accounted for 67% of new infections and 52% of all Americans living with HIV infection in 2014. In 2011, a third of MSM who did not know they were HIV infected reported having a recent unprotected anal sexual encounter with an HIV-negative or unknown-status partner. Only 67% of sexually active MSM reported getting an HIV test in the past year. An additional 3% of new infections were MSM who had a history of intravenous drug use. Young men in particular are at risk, in part because they tend to engage in unsafe sexual practices such as unprotected anal intercourse.

Drug and alcohol use has also been associated with risky sexual behavior and is directly or indirectly associated with HIV acquisition in this population. Use of meth-amphetamine and club drugs, as well as the recreational use of erectile dysfunction drugs, has been associated with risky sexual behavior and HIV infection in MSM.

Disproportionately high rates of HIV infection also occur in certain racial and ethnic groups, as well as among the poor. In 2014, blacks represented 44% of new HIV cases even though they make up only 12% of the U.S. population. Black women accounted for 62% of new HIV infec-

QUICK STATS

54% of Americans aged 18–64 have been tested for HIV at least once.

—Kaiser Family Foundation, 2016

tions among women; 91% were infected through heterosexual contact. Hispanics accounted for 24% of all new HIV infections in 2014; they represent 17% of the population. These patterns of HIV infection reflect complex social, economic, and behavioral factors. Reducing the rates of HIV transmission and AIDS death in nonwhite racial and ethnic groups, women, and high-risk groups requires addressing problems of poverty, discrimination, and drug abuse.

Symptoms   As described earlier, in the days or weeks following infection with HIV, most people develop symptoms, which can include fever, fatigue, rashes, headache, swollen lymph nodes, body aches, night sweats, sore throat, nausea, and ulcers in the mouth. Symptoms of primary infection can last from a few days to more than a month. Because these symptoms are similar to those of many common viral illnesses, the condition often goes undiagnosed.

Diagnosis of HIV at this very early stage of infection is extremely beneficial. People with early-stage HIV can make lifestyle changes to improve their overall health during this period. They can also protect their partners during this phase, when viral levels are high.

Other than the initial flulike symptoms, most people have few if any symptoms in the first months or years of HIV infection. As the immune system weakens, however, a variety of symptoms can develop—persistent swollen lymph nodes; lumps, rashes, sores, or other growths on or under the skin or on the mucous membranes; persistent yeast infections; unexplained weight loss; fever and drenching night sweats; dry cough and shortness of breath; persistent diarrhea; easy bruising and unexplained bleeding; profound fatigue; memory loss; difficulty with balance; tremors or seizures; changes in vision, hearing, taste, or smell; changes in mood and other psychological symptoms; and persistent or recurrent pain. Many of these symptoms can also occur with a variety of other illnesses.

People with HIV infection are highly susceptible to opportunistic infections, as noted earlier. The infection most often seen in the United States among people with HIV is *Pneumocystis* **pneumonia,** a fungal infection. **Kaposi's sarcoma,** a previously rare form of cancer, is common in HIV-infected men. Women with HIV infection often have frequent and difficult-to-treat vaginal yeast infections. Cases of tuberculosis (TB) are increasingly being reported in people with HIV.

Diagnosis   Three general types of HIV diagnostic tests are currently available:

- **HIV antibody tests,** performed on blood or oral fluids, check whether the body is producing antibodies against the HIV virus; these tests usually detect infection within 3–12 weeks after exposure.

TERMS

***Pneumocystis* pneumonia**   A fungal infection common in people infected with HIV.

Kaposi's sarcoma   A form of cancer characterized by purple or brownish lesions that are generally painless and occur anywhere on the skin; usually appears in persons infected with HIV.

HIV antibody test   A blood test to determine whether a person has been infected with HIV; becomes positive within weeks or months of exposure.

- **Combination HIV antigen/antibody tests** look both for antibodies and for an HIV antigen known as p24 (part of the virus itself). Because the antigen is produced before antibodies develop, combination blood tests can detect HIV earlier in the course of infection (usually two to six weeks after exposure), compared to antibody-only tests.
- **Nucleic acid tests (NATs)** test directly for HIV RNA in the blood and can usually detect HIV within one to four weeks after infection; the test is expensive and not routinely used for initial screening.

The different settings in which HIV testing can be done affect which types of tests are offered and how soon the results are available. A positive result is always confirmed with follow-up tests. Because it takes time for HIV RNA, p24 antigens, and HIV antibodies to become detectible, it is important to consider the timing of testing. The window period—the time between infection with HIV and when a test can accurately detect it—varies with the type of test and with the individual. If you get an HIV test within three months after a potential HIV exposure and the result is negative, get tested again in three months. Testing for HIV is recommended for everyone (see the box "Getting an HIV Test").

If a person is diagnosed as **HIV positive,** the next step is to determine the disease's severity to plan appropriate treatment. The status of the immune system can be gauged by taking CD4 T cell measurements every few months. The infection itself can be monitored by tracking the viral load (the amount of virus in the body) with blood tests that measure HIV RNA (NAT tests).

A diagnosis of AIDS, the most severe form of HIV infection, is given if a person is HIV positive and either has developed an infection defined as an AIDS indicator or has a severely damaged immune system (as measured by CD4 T cell counts).

In the United States, every state has laws that require doctors, clinics, and laboratories to report all diagnosed cases of HIV and AIDS to public health authorities, who use this information to track the spread of the disease. Despite efforts to safeguard confidentiality and prohibit discrimination, mandatory reporting of HIV infection remains controversial. If people believe they are risking their jobs, friends, or social acceptability, they may be less likely to get tested. The CDC recommends that states continue to provide opportunities for people to be tested anonymously, including via home tests.

> **combination HIV antigen/antibody test** A blood test that detects the presence of HIV p24 antigen, an early marker for HIV infection, as well as HIV antibodies.
>
> **HIV nucleic acid test (NAT)** A test used to detect the presence of HIV RNA and to determine the viral load (the amount of HIV in the blood).
>
> **HIV positive** A diagnosis resulting from the presence of HIV in the bloodstream; also referred to as *seropositive*.
>
> **TERMS**

Treatment Although there is no known cure for HIV infection, medications can significantly alter the course of the disease and extend life. The drop in the number of U.S. AIDS deaths since 1996 is in large part due to the increasing use of combinations of new drugs.

The main types of antiviral drugs used against HIV/AIDS are reverse transcriptase inhibitors, protease inhibitors, integrase inhibitors, and entry inhibitors. These drugs either block HIV from replicating itself or prevent it from infecting other cells. Research has shown that using combinations of antiviral drugs can sometimes reduce HIV in the blood to undetectable levels. More than 30 drugs are now available to treat HIV, including three once-a-day tablets (containing a combination of HIV medications). However, people on antiviral drugs can still transmit the infection, and concerns are growing that even these very aggressive treatments are starting to fail and that drug-resistant strains of HIV are developing rapidly. In addition to antiviral drugs, most patients with low CD4 T cell counts take a variety of antibiotics to help prevent opportunistic infections such as pneumonia, tuberculosis, and other bacterial and fungal infections.

In some cases, medications are used to prevent infection in people who have been exposed to HIV, such as victims of sexual assault and health care workers with potential exposure to HIV-infected blood or body fluids. This type of treatment, called postexposure prophylaxis (PEP), should begin as soon as possible after exposure, but always within 72 hours. PEP treatment usually lasts 28 days.

The cost of treatment for HIV continues to be an area of major concern. Costs are tremendous even for relatively wealthy countries, but 95% of people with HIV infection live in poor countries, where treatments are unlikely to be available to anyone except the wealthiest few. Pharmaceutical companies, the World Bank, and the international community are working to lower drug costs and provide aid for developing regions.

HIV treatment is also challenging because taking the combination drugs is complicated, and the drugs have short-term side effects that may cause people to stop taking them. Drug resistance develops quickly if the medicines are taken inconsistently. The drugs can also have long-term side effects, including serious health problems in some individuals. The National Institutes of Health (NIH) has issued guidelines for HIV treatment that help patients and their doctors with decisions about treatment.

Prevention Research on the development of a safe, effective, and inexpensive vaccine to stop the spread of HIV worldwide has been ongoing. Approaches to prevention include abstinence, consistent condom use with all sexual acts, and needle exchange programs for persons who use intravenous drugs. The FDA has approved a drug to be taken by people who do not have HIV but are at high risk for it. It is called a pre-exposure prophylaxis (PrEP), meaning that it is a prevention method intended to be used with other methods for reducing HIV risk.

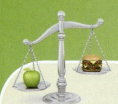

CRITICAL CONSUMER
Getting an HIV Test

Who and How Often?

The CDC recommends that everyone between the ages of 13 and 64 be tested for HIV at least once as part of routine health care. The CDC hopes that routine HIV testing will increase the likelihood that people with HIV will be diagnosed earlier. People with certain risk factors should be tested more often. The CDC recommends testing at least once a year for anyone who answers yes to any of the following:

- Are you a man who has had sex with another man?

- Have you had sex—anal or vaginal—with an HIV-positive partner?

- Have you had more than one sex partner since your last HIV test?

- Have you injected drugs and shared needles or "works" (e.g., water or cotton) with others?

- Have you exchanged sex for drugs or money?

- Have you been diagnosed with or sought treatment for another STI?

- Have you been diagnosed with or received treatment for hepatitis or TB?

- Have you had sex with someone who could answer yes to any of the above questions or someone whose sexual history you don't know?

In addition, CDC guidelines state that sexually active gay and bisexual men may benefit from more frequent testing (e.g., every three to six months).

Physician or Clinic Testing

Your physician, student health clinic, Planned Parenthood, public health department, or local AIDS association can arrange your HIV test. Testing usually costs $50–$100, but public clinics often charge little or nothing. The standard test involves drawing a sample of blood that is sent to a lab, where it is checked using one or more of the available test types. For accuracy and early diagnosis, the CDC recommends laboratory tests done in the following sequence:

1. Combination test; if it is positive for antibodies and/or p24 antigen, this is followed by

2. Specialized antibody test, which confirms which type of HIV is present

3. If findings from the second test are indeterminate or contradictory, a NAT test is done to confirm if HIV RNA is present

It may take a week or more for the results of these tests to become available, and you'll be asked to call or come in personally to obtain your results, which should also include appropriate counseling.

Alternative tests are available at some clinics. The Orasure test uses oral fluid, which is collected by swabbing the inside of the mouth. Rapid tests are available at some locations. These tests involve the use of blood or oral fluid and can provide results in as little as 20 minutes. If a rapid test is positive for HIV infection, a confirming test will be performed. Most rapid tests are antibody tests, which may be less likely than combination tests to detect HIV infection in the first few weeks following exposure. Similarly, blood tests may detect infection earlier than oral fluid tests, because the level of antibodies in oral fluid is lower than in blood.

Before you get an HIV test, be sure you understand what will be done with the results. Results from confidential tests may still become part of your medical record and be reported to state and

---

How Can You Protect Yourself?   Although AIDS cannot be cured, infection can be prevented. You can protect yourself by avoiding behaviors that may bring you into contact with HIV. This means making careful choices about sexual activity and not sharing needles if you inject drugs.

In a sexual relationship, the current and past behaviors of you and your partner determine the amount of risk involved. If you are uninfected and in a mutually monogamous relationship with another uninfected person, you are not at risk for HIV. For anyone not involved in a long-term, mutually monogamous relationship, abstinence from any sexual activity that involves the exchange of body fluids is the only sure way to prevent HIV infection (Figure 13.4).

People who inject drugs should avoid sharing needles, syringes, filters, or anything that might have blood on it. Needles can be decontaminated with a solution of bleach and water, but this is not a foolproof procedure, and HIV can survive in a syringe for a month or longer. HIV can also survive boiling.

For more guidelines and tips, see the box "Preventing STIs."

Chlamydia

Chlamydia trachomatis causes **chlamydia,** the most prevalent bacterial STI in the United States. Both men and women are susceptible to chlamydia, but, as with most STIs, women bear the greater burden because of possible complications and consequences of the disease. Rates of chlamydia in women were about two times those in men in 2015. For women, the highest rates of infection occur among 15- to 24-year-olds. For men, the highest rates occur among 20- to 24-year-olds.

> **chlamydia**   An STI transmitted by the bacterium *Chlamydia trachomatis*.   **TERMS**

federal public health agencies. If you decide you want to be tested anonymously, ask your physician about an anonymous test, or use a home test.

Home Testing

Home test kits for HIV cost $40–$70. Avoid test kits sold on the Internet that are not approved by the U.S. Food and Drug Administration (FDA). As of this printing, two HIV home-testing devices were approved by the FDA: Home Access and OraQuick. Positive results with either test kit need to be confirmed with follow-up testing. To use the Home Access test, you prick a finger with a supplied lancet, blot a few drops of blood onto blotting paper, and mail it to the company's laboratory. In about a week (or within three business days for more expensive "express" tests), you call a toll-free number to find out your results. Anyone testing positive is routed to a trained counselor, who can provide emotional and medical support. The OraQuick HIV test, manufactured by Ora-sure, was approved by the FDA in July 2012. This home test is the first rapid HIV test approved for home use. Like the Orasure test available to clinics, the OraQuick home test uses a sample taken from the mouth and returns results in 20 minutes. The results of home test kits are completely anonymous. Anyone testing positive should call a medical doctor or the OraQuick Consumer Support Center for counseling and routes to care.

Understanding the Results

A negative test result means that no evidence of infection was found—no antibodies or, if you had a combination test, p24 antigens. However, as noted earlier, it may take three weeks or even longer for the infection to be detectible. Therefore, an infected person may get a false-negative result. If you test negative but your risk of infection is high, ask about obtaining a NAT test, which allows for very early diagnosis. If you engage in any risky behaviors, get retested frequently.

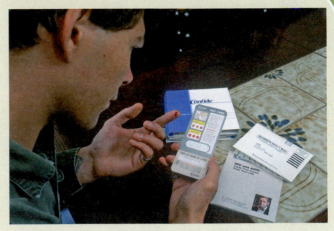
© Yvonne Hemsey/Getty Images

A positive result means that you are infected. Seek medical care and counseling immediately. Rapid progress is being made in treating HIV, and treatments are potentially much more successful when started early. For more information about testing, visit the CDC National HIV, STD, and Hepatitis Testing website (www.hivtest.org).

SOURCES: Centers for Disease Control and Prevention. 2016. *HIV Basics: Testing* (http://www.cdc.gov/hiv/basics/testing.html); AIDS.gov. 2015. *HIV Test Types* (https://www.aids.gov/hiv-aids-basics/prevention /hiv-testing/hiv-test-types/index.html); Centers for Disease Control and Prevention and Association of Public Health Laboratories. 2014. *Laboratory Testing for the Diagnosis of HIV Infection: Updated Recommendations* (http://dx.doi.org/10.15620/cdc.23447); U.S. Food and Drug Administration. 2013. *Testing for HIV* (http://www.fda.gov /BiologicsBloodVaccines/SafetyAvailability/HIVHomeTestKits /ucm126460.htm).

If left untreated, it can lead to pelvic inflammatory disease (PID). Chlamydia also greatly increases a woman's risk for infertility and ectopic (tubal) pregnancy. The CDC currently recommends annual chlamydia testing for all sexually active women aged 25 and under and for older women who are at increased risk (such as those who have multiple sex partners).

Chlamydia can also lead to infertility in men, although not as often as in women. In men under age 35, chlamydia is the most common cause of epididymitis, which is inflammation of the sperm-carrying ducts. In men, up to half of all cases of **urethritis,** inflammation of the urethra, are caused by chlamydia.

Infants of infected mothers can acquire the infection through contact with the pathogen in the birth canal during delivery.

Symptoms   Most people experience few or no symptoms from chlamydia infection, increasing the likelihood that they will inadvertently spread the infection to their partners.

In men, chlamydia symptoms can include painful urination, a slight watery discharge from the penis, and sometimes pain around the testicles. Women may notice increased vaginal discharge, burning with urination, pain or bleeding with intercourse, and lower abdominal pain. The exact time from chlamydia infection to symptomatic disease is unknown, though it may range up to 12 weeks.

Diagnosis and Treatment   Chlamydia is diagnosed through laboratory tests on a urine sample or a small amount of fluid from the urethra, cervix, rectum, or vagina. Once chlamydia has been diagnosed, the infected person and his or her partner(s) are given antibiotics—usually doxycycline for a week or azithromycin, which can cure infection in one dose.

> **urethritis**   Inflammation of the tube that carries urine from the bladder to the outside opening.   **TERMS**

High Risk

Unprotected anal sex is the riskiest sexual behavior, especially for the receptive partner.

Unprotected vaginal intercourse is the next riskiest, especially for women, who are much more likely to be infected by an infected male partner than vice versa.

Oral sex is probably considerably less risky than anal and vaginal intercourse but can still result in HIV transmission.

Sharing of sex toys is considered low risk but carries a theoretical risk of transmission because they can carry blood, semen, or vaginal fluid.

Use of a condom reduces risk considerably but not completely for any type of intercourse. Anal sex with a condom is riskier than vaginal sex with a condom; oral sex with a condom is less risky, especially if the man does not ejaculate.

Hand-genital contact and deep kissing are less risky but could still theoretically transmit HIV; the presence of cuts or sores increases risk.

Sex with only one uninfected and totally faithful partner is without risk, but effective only if both partners are uninfected and completely monogamous.

Activities that don't involve the exchange of body fluids carry no risk: hugging, massage, closed-mouth kissing, masturbation, phone sex, and fantasy.

Abstinence is completely without risk. For many people, it can be an effective and reasonable method of avoiding HIV infection and other STIs during certain periods of life.

No Risk

FIGURE 13.4 **What's risky and what's not: The approximate relative risk of HIV transmission in various sexual activities.** (For additional information about the risk of acquiring HIV from certain types of exposures, visit http://www.cdc.gov/hiv/risk/estimates/riskbehaviors.html.)

Testing and treatment of partners is important. When it is unlikely that a partner will seek medical treatment, the CDC recommends that an extra prescription for antibiotics be provided to the patient or medications provided to give to his or her partner. This strategy, called *expedited partner therapy,* is legal and encouraged in some states under certain circumstances.

Gonorrhea

Gonorrhea is caused by the bacterium *Neisseria gonorrhoeae.* Nearly 400,000 new cases of gonorrhea were reported to the CDC in 2015, a significant increase from the previous year. Because the infection often causes no symptoms, only about 50% of actual infections are reported, and the number of new infections may be much higher. The incidence rates peak among 15- to 24-year-olds. Like chlamydia, untreated gonorrhea can cause PID in women and urethritis and epididymitis in men. An infant passing through the birth canal of an infected

mother may contract *gonococcal conjunctivitis,* an eye infection that can cause blindness if not treated.

Symptoms In males, the incubation period for gonorrhea is brief, generally two to seven days. The first symptoms are due to urethritis, which causes urinary discomfort and a thick, yellowish white or yellowish green discharge from the penis. Up to half of infected males have very minor symptoms or none at all.

Most females with gonorrhea are asymptomatic. Those who have symptoms often experience pain with urination, increased vaginal discharge, and severe menstrual cramps.

Rectal gonorrhea infections in men and women may be associated with pus or blood in the feces or rectal pain and itching. Pharyngeal infections in men and women often do not cause symptoms; however, they may be associated with sore throat or pus on the tonsils.

Diagnosis and Treatment Gonorrhea is detectable by several tests. Depending on the test, samples of urine, vaginal, cervical, urethral, throat, or rectal fluids may be collected. Antibiotics are used to treat gonorrhea, but increasing drug resistance is a major concern. As such, the recommended treatment is a combination of ceftriaxone (an injectable cephalosporin) along with a single dose of azithromycin regardless of chlamydia testing results.

Pelvic Inflammatory Disease

Pelvic inflammatory disease (PID) is a major complication in 10–40% of women who have been infected with either gonorrhea or chlamydia and have not received treatment. PID occurs when the initial infection travels upward beyond the cervix into the uterus, oviducts, ovaries, and pelvic cavity. PID may be serious enough to require hospitalization and sometimes surgery. Even if the disease is treated successfully, about 25% of affected women will have long-term problems, such as a continuing susceptibility to infection, ectopic pregnancy, infertility, and chronic pelvic pain.

PID is the leading cause of infertility in young women, often going undetected until the inability to become pregnant leads to further evaluation. Risk factors include have a new or multiple sex partners, having a sex partner who has other sex partners at the same time, and inconsistent use of condoms. Smokers have twice the risk of PID compared to nonsmokers. Using an intrauterine device for contraception increases the risk of PID, though this is primarily confined to the first three weeks after insertion, and risk of an STI-related cause is greatly reduced for women with only one uninfected sexual partner.

gonorrhea A sexually transmitted bacterial infection caused by the bacterium *Neisseria gonorrhoeae* that usually affects mucous membranes.

pelvic inflammatory disease (PID) An ascending infection that progresses from the vagina and cervix to the uterus, oviducts, and pelvic cavity.

TERMS

Before you begin a sexual relationship with someone, talk with your potential partner about HIV, safer sex, and condom use. (For tips on how to talk to your partners about STIs, visit www.gytnow.org/talking-to-your-partner/). The following guidelines may help you avoid infection:

- Don't drink alcohol or use drugs in sexual situations. Mood-altering drugs can affect your judgment and make you more likely to take risks. Having sex when intoxicated significantly increases the risk of exposure to STIs.

- Limit the number of partners. Avoid sexual contact with people who have HIV or an STI or who have engaged in risky behaviors in the past, including unprotected sex and injection drug use.

- Use condoms during every act of intercourse including oral sex. Condoms do not provide perfect protection, but they greatly reduce your risk of contracting an infection. Multiple studies show that regular condom use can reduce the risk of several diseases, including HIV, chlamydia, gonorrhea, HPV, and genital herpes.

- Use condoms properly for maximum protection.

- Avoid sexual contact that could cause cuts or tears in the skin or tissue.

- Get periodic screening tests for STIs and HIV. Sexually active women age 25 and under should be screened for gonorrhea and chlamydia at least annually, and older women at risk for STIs should be offered screening. MSM should be tested for STIs at least annually or more frequently depending on risk behaviors. As described in Chapter 12, a Pap test is recommended at age 21 and every three to five years thereafter, depending a woman's age and on whether a Pap test is combined with HPV screening. More frequent screening may be recommended for women who have compromised immune systems or abnormal screening results. All adults aged 13–64 should be tested at least once for HIV.

- Get vaccinated. All sexually active men and women should be vaccinated against hepatitis B. All MSM should be vaccinated against hepatitis A. Young men and women age 26 years and under should consider getting vaccinated against HPV; the vaccine protects against the strains that cause most (but not all) cases of cervical cancer and genital warts.

- Get prompt treatment for any STIs you contract. Make sure your partner gets tested and receives treatment, too. In some parts of the country, expedited partner therapy may allow your health care provider to give you a prescription or medications for your partner (consult your health care provider to see if this is available in your area). Don't have sex until both of you have completed your treatment.

- If you inject drugs of any kind, don't share needles, syringes, or anything that might have blood on it. If your community has a syringe exchange program, use it. Seek treatment.

- If you are at risk for HIV infection, don't donate blood, sperm, or body organs. Don't have unprotected sex or share needles or syringes. Consider talking to your provider to see if PrEP is right for you. Get tested for HIV soon, and get treatment. HIV-infected people who receive early treatment generally feel better and live longer than those who delay.

Symptoms   Symptoms of PID vary greatly. Some women may be asymptomatic; others may have abdominal pain, fever, chills, nausea, and vomiting. Early symptoms are essentially the same as those described for chlamydia and gonorrhea. Symptoms often begin or worsen during or soon after a woman's menstrual period. Many women have abnormal vaginal bleeding—either bleeding between periods or heavy and painful menstrual bleeding.

Diagnosis and Treatment   Diagnosis of PID is made on the basis of symptoms, physical examination, ultrasound, and laboratory tests. **Laparoscopy** may be used to confirm the diagnosis and obtain material for cultures.

Antibiotics are usually started immediately; in severe cases, the woman may be hospitalized and given intravenous antibiotics. It is especially important that an infected woman's partners receive treatment. As many as 60% of the male contacts of women with PID are infected but asymptomatic.

Human Papillomavirus

Human papillomavirus (HPV) infection can cause several diseases, including common warts, **genital warts**, and genital cancers. HPV causes virtually all cervical cancers, as well as anal, penile, vulvar, vaginal, and some forms of

> **laparoscopy**   A method of examining the internal organs by inserting a tube containing a small light through an abdominal incision. **TERMS**
>
> **human papillomavirus (HPV)**   The pathogen that causes human warts, including genital warts, as well as anal and genital cancers.
>
> **genital warts**   A sexually transmitted viral infection characterized by growths on the genitals; also called genital HPV infection or condyloma. Persistence of HPV infection predisposes the infected person to some forms of genital cancers.

Why Do College Students Have High Rates of STIs?

• Risky sexual behavior is common. One study of college students found that fewer than half used condoms consistently and one-third had had 10 or more sex partners. Another study found that 19% of male students and 33% of female students had consented to sexual intercourse simply because they felt awkward refusing.

• College students underestimate their risk of STIs. Although students may have considerable knowledge about STIs, they often feel the risks do not apply to them—a dangerous assumption. One study of students with a history of STIs showed that more than half had unprotected sex while they were infected, and 25% of them continued to have sex without ever informing their partner(s).

• Many students are infected but don't know it. A 2006 study of asymptomatic college women revealed that nearly 10% were infected with chlamydia.

What Effect Does Alcohol or Drug Use Have on My Likelihood of Getting an STI?

• Between one-third and one-half of college students report participating in sexual activity as a direct result of being intoxicated. All too often, sexual activity while intoxicated leads to unprotected intercourse.

• Students who binge-drink are more likely to have multiple partners, use condoms inconsistently, and delay seeking treatment for STIs than are students who drink little or no alcohol. Sexual assaults occur more frequently when either the perpetrator or the victim has been drinking.

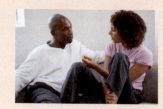

What Can Students Do to Protect Themselves against STIs?

• Limit the number of sex partners. Even people who are always in a monogamous relationship can end up with extensive potential exposure to STIs if, over the years, they have numerous relationships.

• Use condoms consistently, and don't assume it's safe to stop after you've been with a partner for several months. HIV infection, HPV infection, herpes, and chlamydia can be asymptomatic for months or years and can be transmitted at any time. If you haven't been using condoms with your current partner, start now.

• Enjoy sexuality on your own terms. Don't let the expectations of friends and partners cause you to ignore your own feelings. Let your own wellness be your first priority. If you choose to be sexually active, learn about safer sex practices.

• Get to know your partner, and talk to him or her before becoming intimate. Be honest about yourself, and encourage your partner to do the same. But practice safer sex no matter what.

---

oropharyngeal cancers (the oropharynx includes the back of the mouth and the throat). Genital HPV is usually spread through sexual activity, including oral sex.

HPV is the most common STI in the United States. About 14 million Americans become infected with HPV each year. In all, more than 80% of sexually active people will have been infected with HPV by age 50. HPV is especially common in young people, with some of the highest infection rates among college students (see the box "College Students and STIs"). Many young women contract HPV infection within three months of becoming sexually active.

There are more than 100 different strains of HPV, and different strains cause different types of infection. More than 40 types are likely to cause genital infection. Types 6 and 11 cause 90% of visible genital warts. There are at least 13 other HPV strains, including 16 and 18, that are considered high-risk strains for cancer and most often implicated in anogenital cancers (anal, cervical, penile, vaginal, and vulvar cancers).

As of June 2016, three HPV vaccines were licensed in the United States. All three vaccines protect against HPV 16 and 18, the strains that cause the most HPV-linked cancers.

Two of the vaccines protect against additional strains of the virus (two and seven strains, respectively), including those that cause other cancer cases and genital warts. All three vaccines are licensed for use in females, and two are licensed for use in males. The CDC recommends vaccination for all girls and boys aged 11–12, although the vaccine can be given as early as age 9. The vaccine is most effective when given prior to exposure to genital HPV, and this virus is so common that many young people will be exposed to it shortly after becoming sexually active. Each of the vaccines requires three injections over a period of six months. For people not vaccinated as children, vaccination is recommended for women through age 26 and for men through age 21. HPV vaccination is recommended for men who have sex with men through age 26 years who did not get any or all doses when they were younger. Immunized women should continue to receive cervical cancer screening according to current guidelines.

Symptoms   Most people infected with HPV have no visible warts or other symptoms and are not aware that they are infected and contagious to others. The good news is that the immune system usually clears the virus on its own, and infection disappears without any treatment. But in some cases, the infection persists and causes genital warts or cancers.

The types of HPV that cause cervical cancer do not produce any visible changes on the external genitals. The types that cause genital warts can produce anything from a small bump to a large, warty growth. Untreated warts can grow together to form a cauliflower-like mass. In males, they appear on the penis and often involve the urethra, appearing first at the opening and then spreading inside. The growths may cause irritation and bleeding, leading to painful urination and a urethral discharge. Warts may also appear around the anus or within the rectum. In women, warts may appear on the labia or vulva and may spread to the *perineum*, the area between the vagina and the rectum. They may also appear on the cervix.

Diagnosis and Treatment Genital warts are usually diagnosed based on the appearance of the lesions. HPV infection of the cervix is often detected on routine Pap tests. Special tests are now available to detect the presence of HPV infection and to distinguish among the more common strains of HPV, including those that cause most cases of cervical cancer.

Treatment of genital warts focuses on reducing the number and size of warts, through cryosurgery (freezing), electrocautery (burning), or laser surgery. Even after treatment and the disappearance of visible warts, the individual may continue to carry HPV in healthy-looking tissue and can probably still infect others. Cervical abnormalities that are cancerous or precancerous are treated surgically or with other techniques such as electrical excision, freezing, and laser.

Anyone who has ever had HPV infection should inform all partners and use condoms, even though they do not provide total protection. Whether or not they have had the vaccine, all women should have regular pelvic exams and Pap tests.

Genital Herpes

Up to one in six adults aged 14–49 in the United States has **genital herpes.** Worldwide, genital herpes is extremely common, and it is a major factor in HIV transmission.

Two types of herpes simplex viruses, HSV 1 and HSV 2, cause genital herpes and oral–labial herpes (cold sores). After infection, the virus lies dormant in nerve cells and can reactivate at any time. The type of virus may determine how frequently genital outbreaks occur. Compared to individuals with HSV 1 genital infections, those with HSV 2 infections tend to have more frequent outbreaks of genital lesions and shed more virus without having symptoms.

HSV 1 infection is so common that 50–80% of U.S. adults have antibodies to it (indicating previous exposure to the virus); most were exposed to HSV 1 during childhood.

HSV 2 infection usually occurs during adolescence and early adulthood, often between ages 18 and 25.

HSV 2 is almost always sexually transmitted. However, changes in sexual behaviors, specifically oral-genital contact, have contributed to increased incidence of anogenital HSV 1 infections in young adults. HSV infections spread readily whether people have active sores or are completely asymptomatic. Because HSV is asymptomatic in 80–90% of people, the infection is often acquired from a person who does not know that he or she is infected.

If you have ever had an outbreak of genital herpes, you should consider yourself always contagious and inform your partners. Avoid intimate contact when any sores are present, and use condoms during all sexual contact. One study showed that using condoms for every act of intercourse results in a 30% decrease in the transmission of herpes, compared with no condom use. Condoms are more effective in preventing the transmission of other STIs than herpes, but the same study showed that they can make a significant difference in preventing the spread of genital herpes.

Newborns can occasionally be infected with HSV, usually during passage through the birth canal of an infected mother. Such transmission is more likely to occur when HSV infection was acquired by the mother during the third trimester of pregnancy. Without treatment, 65% of newborns with HSV will die, and most who survive will have some degree of brain damage. Pregnant women who have been exposed to genital herpes should inform their physicians so that appropriate precautions can be taken to protect their babies from infection.

Symptoms Up to 90% of people who are infected with HSV have no symptoms. Those who develop symptoms often first notice them within 2–20 days of having sex with an infected partner. (However, it is not unusual for the first outbreak to occur months or even years after initial exposure.) The first episode of genital herpes frequently causes flulike symptoms in addition to genital lesions. The lesions tend to be painful or itchy and can occur anywhere on the genitals, inner thighs, or anal area. Depending on their location, they can cause considerable pain with urination. Lymph nodes in the groin may become swollen and tender. The sores usually heal within three weeks.

On average, people with a new diagnosis will experience five to eight outbreaks per year, with a decrease in the frequency of outbreaks over time. Recurrent episodes are usually less severe than the initial one, with fewer and less painful sores that heal more quickly. Outbreaks can be triggered by a

genital herpes A sexually transmitted infection caused by the herpes simplex virus. **TERMS**

number of events, including stress, illness, fatigue, sun exposure, sexual intercourse, and menstruation.

Diagnosis and Treatment Genital herpes can be diagnosed on the basis of symptoms, but laboratory testing is helpful if there is any question about the diagnosis. Several blood tests can detect the presence of HSV antibodies in the blood.

There is no cure for herpes. Once infected, a person carries the virus for life. Antiviral drugs such as acyclovir can be taken at the beginning of an outbreak to shorten the severity and duration of symptoms. Support groups are available to help people learn to cope with herpes. There is no vaccine to prevent herpes, but research is ongoing.

Hepatitis B

Hepatitis (inflammation of the liver) can cause serious and sometimes permanent damage to the liver, which can result in death in severe cases. One of the many types of hepatitis is caused by hepatitis B virus (HBV). Like HIV, HBV is found in most body fluids, including blood and blood products, semen, saliva, urine, and vaginal secretions. Hepatitis B is much more contagious than HIV infection; it is easily spread among people who live in close contact with one another. It is easily transmitted through any sexual activity that involves the exchange of body fluids. HBV is not usually spread by hugging, coughing, food or water, sharing eating utensils or drinking glasses, or casual contact. The primary risk factors for HBV infection are sexual exposure and injection drug use; having multiple sex partners greatly increases risk. HBV can also be transmitted through nonsexual close contact that could involve blood exposure, including the use of contaminated needles, razor blades, and toothbrushes. Vaccination against HBV is recommended for incoming college students.

Other forms of viral hepatitis can also be sexually transmitted. Hepatitis A is of particular concern for people who engage in anal sex; a vaccine is available and is recommended for all people at risk. Large population-based studies have demonstrated an association between hepatitis C virus (HCV) and individuals who engage in high-risk sexual encounters (multiple sex partners, unprotected sex, or sex with an HCV-infected person or injection drug user). Over the past few years, there has been a surge in safe and effective treatments to cure HCV; thus, testing and managing the care of infected individuals may help to curb this problem.

Symptoms Many people infected with HBV never develop symptoms; they have what are known as silent infections. The normal incubation period is 30–180 days. Mild cases of hepatitis cause flulike symptoms such as fever, body aches, chills, and loss of appetite. As the illness progresses, there may be nausea, vomiting, dark-colored urine, abdominal pain, and jaundice.

Most adults who have acute HBV infection recover completely within a few weeks or months. But about 5% of adults who are infected with HBV become chronic carriers of the virus, capable of infecting others for the rest of their lives. Some chronic carriers remain asymptomatic, whereas others develop chronic liver disease. Chronic hepatitis can cause cirrhosis, liver failure, and a deadly form of liver cancer.

Diagnosis and Treatment Hepatitis is diagnosed by blood tests used to analyze liver function, detect the infecting organism, and detect antibodies to the virus. There is no cure for HBV infection and no specific treatment for acute infections; antiviral drugs and immune system modulators may be used for chronic HBV infection. Vaccination against HBV is recommended for all infants and children as well as previously unvaccinated adults.

Syphilis

Syphilis, a disease that once caused death and disability for millions, can now be treated effectively with antibiotics. Syphilis rates in 2015 were higher than they had been in the previous 20 years. Specifically, rates in young men who have sex with men were high; rates of co-infection with HIV were also high in this group. In 2015, 60% of reported early cases of syphilis were among MSM. Studies have found an association between syphilis infection and the use of the Internet as a means to meet sex partners among MSM. Another trend is an increase in the proportion of cases of syphilis transmitted through oral sex.

Syphilis is caused by a spirochete called *Treponema pallidum,* a thin, corkscrew-shaped bacterium. It requires warmth and moisture to survive and dies quickly outside the human body. The disease is usually acquired through sexual contact, although infected pregnant women can transmit it to their fetuses. The pathogen passes through any break or opening in the skin or mucous membranes and can be transmitted by kissing, vaginal or anal intercourse, or oral–genital contact.

Symptoms Syphilis progresses through several stages. *Primary syphilis* is characterized by an ulcer called a **chancre** that appears within 10–90 days after exposure. The chancre is usually found at the site where the organism entered the body,

TERMS

hepatitis Inflammation of the liver, which can be caused by infection, drugs, or toxins; some forms of infectious hepatitis can be transmitted sexually.

syphilis A sexually transmitted bacterial infection caused by the spirochete *Treponema pallidum.*

chancre The sore produced by syphilis in its earliest stage.

such as the genital area, but it may also appear in other sites such as the mouth, breasts, or fingers. Chancres contain large numbers of bacteria and make the disease highly contagious when present; they are often painless and typically heal on their own within a few weeks. If the disease is not treated during the primary stage, about a third of infected individuals progress to chronic stages of infections.

Secondary syphilis is usually characterized by a skin rash that appears three to six weeks after the chancre. The rash may cover the entire body or only a few areas, but the palms of the hands and soles of the feet are usually involved. The rash is highly contagious but usually heals within several weeks or months.

If the disease remains untreated, the symptoms of secondary syphilis may recur over a period of several years; affected individuals may then lapse into an asymptomatic latent stage in which they experience no further consequences of infection. However, in about 15% of untreated syphilis cases, the individual develops *late,* or *tertiary, syphilis,* with symptoms that can appear 10–20 years after infection. Late syphilis can damage many organs of the body (brain, nerves, eyes, heart, blood vessels, liver, bones, and joints), possibly causing severe dementia, cardiovascular damage, blindness, and death.

Neurosyphilis, syphilis that invades the nervous system, can occur at any stage of the infection. Symptoms vary but may include headaches, vision or hearing loss, alterations in behavior, and disorders of movement. It is also possible that the patient has no overt symptoms at the time of diagnosis. *Ocular syphilis* is a clinical manifestation of neurosyphilis that can affect nearly any part of the eye structure. Symptoms may include decreased vision and the potential for permanent blindness. More than 200 cases of ocular syphilis were reported in 20 states in 2014–2016. Most of these cases were found in HIV-infected men who have sex with men, and few were found among heterosexual men and women not infected with HIV.

In infected pregnant women, syphilis can cross the placenta. If the mother does not receive treatment, the probable result is stillbirth, prematurity, or congenital deformity. In many cases, the infant is also born infected *(congenital syphilis)* and requires treatment.

Diagnosis and Treatment   Syphilis is diagnosed by examination of infected tissues and with blood tests. All stages can be treated with antibiotics, but damage from late syphilis can be permanent.

Other STIs

Trichomoniasis (often called *trich*) is the most prevalent nonviral STI in the United States; it is estimated to affect some 3.7 million individuals. The actual number of new infections is unknown; however, there were 225,000 office-related visits for trich in 2013. The single-celled organism that causes trich, *Trichomonas vaginalis,* is highly transmissible during penile-vaginal sex. Nonsexual transmission is rare. Up to 85% of those infected may have no or minimal symptoms. Untreated infections might last for years. Women who become symptomatic with trich develop a yellow-greenish, diffuse, or foul-smelling vaginal discharge and severe itching and vulvar irritation. Men may develop inflammation of the urethra, epididymis, or prostate. *T. vaginalis* is not visible to the naked eye; however, a physician can check urine or urethral specimens and vaginal secretions for the presence of this organism. Prompt treatment with oral metronidazole is important because studies suggest that trich may increase the risk of HIV transmission and, in pregnant women, premature delivery. If you or your partner has trich, you should both receive treatment.

Bacterial vaginosis (BV) is the most common cause of abnormal vaginal discharge in women of reproductive age. BV occurs when healthful bacteria that normally inhabit the vagina become displaced by unhealthful species. BV is generally not considered an STI but may be associated with sexual activity—for example, change in partners, multiple partners, and female same-sex relationships. Symptoms of BV include vaginal discharge with a fishy odor, and sometimes vaginal irritation. BV can place women at risk for other STIs, complications after some gynecological surgical procedures, and complications during pregnancy. BV is treated with topical and oral antibiotics.

Lymphogranuloma venereum (LGV) is an infection of the lymphatic system caused by three strains of the bacteria *Chlamydia trachomatis* (not the same strain that causes the genital STI chlamydia). The incidence of LGV in the United States is unknown; however, outbreaks have occurred in the Netherlands and other European countries among men who have sex with men. LGV is more common in men than in women; the main risk factor is being HIV positive. The first symptom is an ulcer at the site of sexual penetration that

TERMS

trichomoniasis   A protozoal infection caused by *Trichomonas vaginalis,* most commonly transmitted sexually.

bacterial vaginosis (BV)   A condition that may be linked to sexual activity; caused by an overgrowth of certain bacteria inhabiting the vagina.

lymphogranuloma venereum (LGV)   An infection of the lymphatic system caused by three strains of the bacterium *Chlamydia trachomatis*, transmitted sexually.

appears 3–30 days after exposure; there may also be swollen glands in the genital area. Among those who practice anal receptive intercourse, symptoms may include rectal ulcers, bleeding, and pain. If the infection is untreated, chronic symptoms may develop, so individuals with symptoms should see a physician. If you have this infection, your partner should be referred for testing and treatment.

Pubic lice (commonly known as *crabs*) and **scabies** are highly contagious parasitic infections. They are usually treated with topical medicines, but oral medications are sometimes needed as well. Lice infestation can require repeated treatment.

WHAT YOU CAN DO ABOUT STIs

You can take responsibility for your health and contribute to a general reduction in the incidence of STIs in three major areas: education, diagnosis and treatment, and prevention.

Education

Educational campaigns about HIV/AIDS and other STIs have paid off in changing attitudes and sexual behaviors. Levels of awareness about HIV infection among the general population are quite high, although some segments of the population are harder to reach and continue to engage in high-risk behaviors. Learning about STIs is still up to every person individually, as is applying that knowledge to personal situations.

Diagnosis and Treatment

Early diagnosis and treatment of STIs can help you avoid complications and help prevent the spread of infection.

• *Be alert for symptoms.* If you are sexually active, be alert for any sign or symptom of disease, such as a rash, a discharge, sores, or pain. Although only a physician can make a proper diagnosis of an STI, you can perform a genital self-examination between check-ups to look for early warning signs of disease, such as bumps, sores, blisters, or warts.

• *Get vaccinated.* Every young, sexually active person should be vaccinated against hepatitis B; vaccines are available for all age groups. The CDC also recommends that men who have sex with men be vaccinated against hepatitis A, and males and females aged 9–26 be vaccinated against HPV.

• *Get tested.* The CDC recommends that everyone aged 13–64 be tested for HIV at least once during routine medical care. If you are sexually active, be sure to get periodic STI checks, even if you have no symptoms. If you have a risky sexual encounter, see a physician as soon as possible.

• *Inform your partners.* Telling a partner that you have exposed him or her to an STI isn't easy. Despite the awkwardness and difficulty, it is crucial that your sex partner or partners be informed and urged to seek testing and/or treatment as quickly as possible.

• *Get treatment.* With the exception of AIDS treatments, treatments for STIs are safe and generally inexpensive. If you are receiving treatment, follow instructions carefully and complete all the medication as prescribed. Don't stop taking the medication just because you feel better or your symptoms have disappeared.

Prevention

If you choose to be sexually active, the key is to think about prevention *before* you have a sexual encounter or find yourself in the heat of the moment. Find out what your partner thinks before you become sexually involved. By thinking and talking about responsible sexual behavior, you are expressing a sense of caring for yourself, your potential partner, and your future children.

TIPS FOR TODAY AND THE FUTURE

Your immune system is a remarkable germ-fighting network, but it needs your help to work at its best.

RIGHT NOW YOU CAN:

- Make sure that you have plenty of soap on hand in your bathroom and kitchen. It does not have to be antibacterial soap.
- Start getting at least 15 more minutes of sleep each night.
- Make an appointment with your health care provider if you are worried about possible STI infection.
- Resolve to discuss condom use with your partner if you are sexually active and are not already using condoms.

IN THE FUTURE YOU CAN:

- Stock up on hand sanitizer and tissues. Put them in your backpack, car, locker, and other places where you might need to wash your hands when soap and water won't be available.
- Make an appointment with your physician to ensure your immunizations are up-to-date.
- Learn how to communicate effectively with a partner who resists safer sex practices or is reluctant to discuss his or her sexual history. Support groups and educational classes can help.

SUMMARY

- The immune system includes both surface barriers and the cells that mount the immune response.

- Physical and chemical barriers to microorganisms include skin, mucous membranes, and the cilia lining the respiratory tract.

- The immune response is carried out by white blood cells that are continuously produced in the bone marrow. Cells of the innate immune system include neutrophils, eosinophils, macrophages, dendritic cells, and natural killer cells. Cells of the adaptive immune system are lymphocytes—in particular, T cells and B cells.

- The immune response has four stages: recognition of the invading pathogen; rapid replication of killer T cells and B cells; attack by killer T cells and macrophages; and suppression of the immune response.

- Immunization is based on the body's ability to remember previously encountered organisms.

- Allergic reactions occur when the immune system responds to harmless substances as if they were dangerous pathogens.

- The step-by-step process by which infections are transmitted from one person to another involves a pathogen, its reservoir, a portal of exit, a means of transmission, a portal of entry, and a new host. Infection can be prevented by breaking the chain at any point.

- The spread of disease may result in epidemics or pandemics.

- Bacteria are single-celled organisms; some cause disease in humans. Significant bacterial infections include pneumonia, meningitis, strep throat, toxic shock syndrome, MRSA, tuberculosis, Lyme disease, and ulcers.

- Most antibiotics work by interrupting the production of new bacteria; they do not work against viruses. Bacteria can become resistant to antibiotics.

- Viruses cannot grow or reproduce themselves; viruses cause the common cold, influenza, measles, mumps, rubella, chickenpox, cold sores, mononucleosis, encephalitis, hepatitis, polio, and warts.

- Other infectious diseases are caused by certain types of fungi, protozoa, and parasitic worms.

- Autoimmune diseases occur when the body identifies its own cells as foreign.

- A healthy immune system can destroy mutant cells that may become cancerous.

- The immune system needs little help other than adequate nutrition and rest, moderate exercise, and protection from excessive stress. Vaccinations also help protect against disease.

- *Sexually transmitted infection (STI)* is used interchangeably with the term *sexually transmitted disease (STD)* and is gradually replacing it.

- Human immunodeficiency virus (HIV) affects the immune system, making an otherwise healthy person less able to resist a variety of infections.

- HIV is carried in blood and blood products, semen, vaginal and cervical secretions, and breast milk. HIV is transmitted through the exchange of these fluids.

- There is currently no cure or vaccine for HIV infection. Drugs have been developed to slow the course of the disease and to prevent or treat certain secondary infections.

- HIV infection can be prevented by making careful choices about sexual activity and not sharing drug needles.

- Chlamydia causes epididymitis and urethritis in men; in women, it can lead to pelvic inflammatory disease (PID) and infertility if untreated.

- Untreated gonorrhea can cause PID in women and epididymitis in men, leading to infertility. In infants, untreated gonorrhea can cause blindness.

- PID, usually a complication of untreated gonorrhea or chlamydia, is an ascending infection that progresses from the vagina and cervix to the uterus, oviducts, and pelvic cavity. It can lead to infertility, ectopic pregnancy, and chronic pelvic pain. Both the infected woman and her partners must receive treatment.

- Human papillomavirus (HPV) can cause genital warts and cervical cancer. The virus can be transmitted by asymptomatic people. Even after treatment, a person may continue to carry the virus in healthy-looking tissue. The immune system often clears HPV on its own.

- Genital herpes is a common viral infection that can cause painful blisters on the genitals. The virus remains in the body for life and causes recurrent outbreaks.

- Hepatitis B is an inflammation of the liver caused by one of the many types of hepatitis virus. It is transmitted through both sexual and nonsexual contact. Following an initial infection, most people recover, but some become carriers and may develop serious complications.

- Syphilis is a highly contagious infection caused by the spirochete *T. pallidum*. It can be treated with antibiotics. The disease progresses through three stages. Untreated, it can lead to organ damage, deterioration of the central nervous system, and death.

- Trichomoniasis is a protozoal infection that is readily transmitted by penile-vaginal sex.

- Other diseases that can be transmitted sexually or are linked to sexual activity include bacterial vaginosis, lymphogranuloma venereum, pubic lice, and scabies. Any STI that causes sores or inflammation can increase the risk of HIV transmission.

- Individuals can contribute to a reduction in the incidence of STIs by educating themselves, having any infections diagnosed and treated, and practicing preventive strategies.

FOR MORE INFORMATION

Alliance for the Prudent Use of Antibiotics. Provides information about the proper use of antibiotics and tips for avoiding infections.
http://emerald.tufts.edu/med/apua/

American Academy of Allergy, Asthma & Immunology. Provides information and publications; pollen counts are available from the website.

http://www.aaaai.org

American Autoimmune-Related Diseases Association. Provides background information, coping tips, and an online knowledge quiz about autoimmune diseases.

http://www.aarda.org

American College of Allergy, Asthma & Immunology. Provides information for patients and physicians; website includes an extensive glossary of terms related to allergies and asthma.

http://www.acaai.org

American College Health Association (ACHA). Offers free brochures on STIs, alcohol use, acquaintance rape, and other health issues.

http://www.acha.org/ACHA/Resources/Topics/Sexual
_Health.aspx

American Social Health Association (ASHA). Provides written information on STIs and referrals for those infected; sponsors support groups for people with herpes and HPV infections.

http://www.ashastd.org

Black AIDS Institute. Provides public health information about a variety of topics including testing, treatment, vaccines, and health care access; focuses on black people and the black community.

http://www.blackaids.org

The Body: The Complete HIV/AIDS Resource. Provides information about prevention, testing, and treatment and includes an online risk assessment.

http://www.thebody.com

CDC National Center for Emerging and Zoonotic Infectious Diseases. Provides extensive information on a wide variety of infectious diseases.

http://www.cdc.gov/ncezid/

CDC National Prevention Information Network. Provides extensive information and links for HIV/AIDS and other STIs.

http://www.cdcnpin.org

CDC National STD and AIDS Hotlines. Callers can obtain information, counseling, and referrals for testing and treatment. The hotlines offer information on more than 20 STIs and include Spanish and TTY services.

800-342-AIDS or 800-227-8922

800-344-SIDA (Spanish)

800-243-7889 (TTY, deaf access)

CDC: Vaccines & Immunizations. Provides information and answers to frequently asked questions about vaccines and immunizations.

http://www.cdc.gov/vaccines

HIV InSite: Gateway to AIDS Knowledge. Provides information about prevention, education, treatment, statistics, clinical trials, and new developments; from the University of California, San Francisco.

http://hivinsite.ucsf.edu

It's Your Sex Life (IYSL). Provides information on prevention, education related to STIs, and messages to support making responsible decisions related to sexual health.

http://www.itsyoursexlife.com/gyt/talk/talking-to-your-partner/

Joint United Nations Programme on HIV/AIDS (UNAIDS). Provides statistics and information on the international HIV/AIDS situation.

http://www.unaids.org

MedlinePlus: Sexually Transmitted Diseases. Provides a clearinghouse of links and information on STIs and other sexual health topics; maintained by the CDC.

http://www.nlm.nih.gov/medlineplus/sexuallytransmitteddiseases
.html

http://www.nlm.nih.gov/medlineplus/sexualhealthissues.html

The NAMES Project Foundation, AIDS Memorial Quilt. Includes the story behind the quilt, images of quilt panels, and information and links relating to HIV infection.

http://www.aidsquilt.org

National Foundation for Infectious Diseases. Provides information about a variety of diseases and disease issues.

http://www.nfid.org

National Institute of Allergy and Infectious Diseases. Includes fact sheets about many topics relating to allergies and infectious diseases, including tuberculosis and sexually transmitted infections.

http://www.niaid.nih.gov

Planned Parenthood Federation of America. Provides information about STIs, family planning, and contraception.

http://www.plannedparenthood.org

World Health Organization: Infectious Diseases. Provides fact sheets about many emerging and tropical diseases as well as information about current outbreaks.

http://www.who.int/topics/infectious_diseases/en

World Health Organization (WHO): Sexually Transmitted Infections. Provides information on international statistics and prevention efforts.

http://www.who.int/topics/sexually_transmitted_infections/en

SELECTED BIBLIOGRAPHY

AIDS.gov. 2015. CDC Supports New WHO Early Release HIV Treatment and PrEP Guidelines (https://aidsinfo.nih.gov/news/1611/cdc-supports-new-who-early-release-hiv-treatment-and-prep-guidelines).

AIDS.gov. 2015. Pre-Exposure Prophylaxis (PrEP) (http://aids.gov/hiv-aids-basics/prevention/reduce-your-risk/pre-exposure-prophylaxis/).

AIDS.gov. 2015. Sexual Risk Factors (https://www.aids.gov/hiv-aids-basics/prevention/reduce-your-risk/sexual-risk-factors/).

AIDS.gov. 2015. Statement by the HHS Panel on Antiretroviral Guidelines for Adults and Adolescents Regarding Results from the START and TEMPRANO Trials (https://aidsinfo.nih.gov/news/1592/statement-from-adult-arv-guideline-panel—start-and-temprano-trials).

American College Health Association. 2015. American College Health Association-National College Health Assessment II: Reference Group Executive Summary Spring 2015. Hanover, MD: American College Health Association.

Bradley, H., et al. 2014. Seroprevalence of herpes simplex virus types 1 and 2—United States, 1999–2010. Journal of Infectious Diseases 209(3): 325–333.

Cantor, A. G., et al. 2016. Screening for syphilis: Updated evidence report and systematic review for the U.S. Preventive Services Task Force. Journal of the American Medical Association 315(21): 2328–2337.

Centers for Disease Control and Prevention. 2012. Principles of Epidemiology in Public Health Practice. 3rd ed. Atlanta, GA: U.S. Department of Health and Human Services.

Centers for Disease Control and Prevention. 2015a. Epidemiology and Prevention of Vaccine-Preventable Diseases, 13th ed. Washington, DC: Public Health Foundation.

Centers for Disease Control and Prevention. 2015a. *Expedited Partner Therapy* (http://www.cdc.gov/std/ept/).

Centers for Disease Control and Prevention. 2015b. *HIV Surveillance Report, 2014,* Vol. 26 (http://www.cdc.gov/hiv/library/reports/surveillance).

Centers for Disease Control and Prevention. 2015c. Measles—United States, January 4-April 2, 2015. *MMWR* 64(14): 373–376.

Centers for Disease Control and Prevention. 2015d. *Reported Tuberculosis in the United States, 2014* (https://www.cdc.gov/tb/statistics /reports/2014/table1.htm).

Centers for Disease Control and Prevention. 2015e. Sexually transmitted diseases treatment guidelines, 2015. *MMWR* 64(3): 1–137.

Centers for Disease Control and Prevention. 2015f. Use of 9-valent human papillomavirus (HPV) vaccine: Updated HPV vaccination recommendations of the Advisory Committee on Immunization Practices (ACIP). *MMWR* 64(11): 300–304.

Centers for Disease Control and Prevention. 2015g. *West Nile Virus: Statistics and Maps* (https://www.cdc.gov/westnile/statsmaps/index.html)

Centers for Disease Control and Prevention. 2016a. *Antibiotic/Antimicrobial Resistance* (https://www.cdc.gov/drugresistance/index.html).

Centers for Disease Control and Prevention. 2016b. *Sexually Transmitted Disease Surveillance 2015.* Atlanta: U.S. Department of Health and Human Services.

Centers for Disease Control and Prevention. 2016c. *Frequently Asked Questions about Measles in the U.S.* (http://www.cdc.gov/measles/about /faqs.html)

Centers for Disease Control and Prevention. 2016d. *Surveillance for Viral Hepatitis-United States, 2014* (http://www.cdc.gov/hepatitis/statistics /2014surveillance/commentary.htm).

Centers for Disease Control and Prevention. 2016e. Notifiable disease and mortality tables. *MMWR* 64(52): ND923-ND940.

Centers for Disease Control and Prevention. 2016f. *National Data: Most Recent Asthma Data.* (http://www.cdc.gov/asthma/most_recent_data.htm).

Centers for Disease Control and Prevention and Association of Public Health Laboratories. 2014. *Laboratory Testing for the Diagnosis of HIV Infection: Updated Recommendations* (DOI: 10.15620/cdc.23447).

Centers for Disease Control and Prevention, National Center for HIV/AIDS, Viral Hepatitis, STD and TB prevention, Division of HIV/AIDS Prevention. 2015. *HIV in the United States: At a Glance* (http://www .cdc.gov/hiv/statistics/overview/ataglance.html).

D'Amato, G., et al. 2015. Effects on asthma and respiratory allergy of climate change and air pollution. *Multidisciplinary Respiratory Medicine* 10: 39.

Do Prado, M. F., et al. 2012. Antimicrobial efficacy of alcohol-based gels with a 30-s application. *Letters in Applied Microbiology* 54(6): 564–567.

Goulder, P. J., S. R. Lewin, and E. M. Leitman. 2016. Paediatric HIV infection: the potential for cure. *Nature Reviews Immunology* 16: 259–271.

Hay, P. E., et al. 2016. Which sexually active young female students are most at risk of pelvic inflammatory disease? A prospective study. *Sexually Transmitted Infections* 92(1): 63–66.

Henry J. Kaiser Family Foundation. 2016. *HIV Testing in the United States* (http://kff.org/hivaids/fact-sheet/hiv-testing-in-the-united-states/).

Irwin, M. R., 2012. Sleep and infectious disease risk. *Sleep* 35(8): 1025–1026.

Jemal, A., et al. 2013. Annual report to the nation on the status of cancer, 1975–2009, featuring the burden and trends in human papillomavirus (HPV)–associated cancers and HPV vaccination coverage levels. *Journal of the National Cancer Institute* 105: 175–201.

Joint United Nations Programme on HIV/AIDS (UNAIDS). 2016. *Global AIDS Update 2016.* Geneva: UNAIDS.

Lam, C. B., and E. S. Lefkowitz. 2013. Risky sexual behaviors in emerging adults: Longitudinal changes and within-person variations. *Archives of Sexual Behaviors* 42(4): 523–532.

Lamb, A. K., et al. 2011. Reducing asthma disparities by addressing environmental inequities: A case study of Regional Asthma Management and Prevention's advocacy efforts. *Family & Community Health* 34: S54–S62.

Larru, B., and P. Offit. 2014. Communicating vaccine science to the public. *Journal of Infection* 69 (Suppl. 1): S2-S4.

Lehtinen, M., et al. 2012. Overall efficacy of HPV-16/18 AS04-adjuvanted vaccine against grade 3 or greater cervical intraepithelial neoplasia: 4-year end-of-study analysis of the randomised, double-blind PATRI-CIA trial. *Lancet Oncology* 13(1): 89–99.

Markowitz, L. E., et al. 2016. Prevalence of HPV after introduction of the vaccination program in the United States. *Pediatrics,* 137(3): e20151968.

McKenzie, J. F., and R. R. Pinger. 2015. *Introduction to Community and Public Health.* 8th ed. Burlington, MA: Jones & Bartlett Learning.

Moreira, E. D., Jr., et al. 2016. Safety profile of the 9-valent HPV vaccine: a combined analysis of 7 phase III clinical trials. *Pediatrics* 138(2): e20154387.

Murray, K. A., et al. 2015. Global biogeography of human infectious diseases. *Proceedings of the National Academy of Sciences* 112(41): 12746–12751.

National Center for Health Statistics. 2016. Deaths: Final data for 2014. *National Vital Statistics Reports* 65(4);

National Institute of Allergy and Infectious Diseases. 2016. *Immune Cells* (https://www.niaid.nih.gov/topics/immunesystem/Pages/default.aspx)

National Institutes of Health. 2015. *The HIV Life Cycle* (http://aidsinfo.nih .gov/education-materials/fact-sheets/19/73/the-hiv-life-cycle).

Petrosky, E., et al. 2015. Use of 9-valent human papillomavirus (HPV) vaccine: Updated HPV vaccination recommendations of the Advisory Committee on Immunization Practices. *MMWR* 64: 300–304.

Piot, P., and T. Quinn. 2013. The AIDS pandemic—A global health paradigm. *New England Journal of Medicine* 368(23): 2210–2218.

Price, M. J., et al. 2016. Proportion of pelvic inflammatory disease cases caused by Chlamydia trachomatis: Consistent picture from different methods. *Journal of Infectious Diseases,* June 3.

Rashid, H., et al. 2012. Vaccination and herd immunity: What more do we know? *Current Opinion in Infectious Diseases* 25(3): 243–249.

Rasmussen, S. J., et al. 2016. Zika virus and birth defects—reviewing the evidence for causality. *New England Journal of Medicine* 374: 1981–1987.

Robinson, C. L. Advisory Committee on Immunization Practices recommended immunization schedules for persons aged 0 through 18 years—United States, 2016. *MMWR* 65(4): 86–87.

Satterwhite, C. L., et al. 2013. Sexually transmitted infections among U.S. women and men: Prevalence and incidence estimates, 2008. *Sexually Transmitted Diseases* 40(3).

Seehan, M. D., and W. Phipatanaul. 2015. Difficult to control asthma: Epidemiology and its link with environmental factors. *Current Opinion in Allergy and Clinical Immunology* 15(5): 397–401.

Smith, D. K., et al. 2015. Condom effectiveness for HIV prevention by consistency of use among men who have sex with men in the United States. *Journal of Acquired Immune Deficiency Syndrome* 68(3): 337–344.

Tamimi, A. H., et al. 2015. Impact of the use of an alcohol-based hand sanitizer in the home on reduction in probability of infection by respiratory and enteric viruses. *Epidemiology and Infection* 143(15): 3335–3341.

Taylor, D. J. 2016. Is insomnia a risk factor for decreased influenza vaccine response? *Behavioral Sleep Medicine* 14: 1–18.

Tobian, A., et al. 2009. Male circumcision for the prevention of HSV-2 and HPV infections and syphilis. *New England Journal of Medicine* 360: 1298–1309.

Toh, Z. Q., et al. 2015. Reduced dose human papillomavirus vaccination: An update of the current state-of-the-art. *Vaccine* 33: 5042–5050.

U.S. Food and Drug Administration. 2015. *Patient Information—Gardasil 9* (http://www.fda.gov/downloads/BiologicsBloodVaccines/Vaccines /ApprovedProducts/UCM426460.pdf).

Vásquez-Otero, O., et al. 2016. Dispelling the myth: Exploring associations between the HPV vaccine and inconsistent condom use among college students. *Preventive Medicine* http://dx.doi.org/10.1016/j.ypmed .2016.10.007.

World Health Organization. 2016. Government of Nigeria reports 2 wild polio cases, first since July 2014 (http://www.who.int/mediacentre /news/releases/2016/nigeria-polio/en).

World Health Organization. 2016. *Male Circumcision for HIV Prevention* (http://www.who.int/hiv/topics/malecircumcision/en).

World Health Organization. 2016. *Rubella: Fact Sheet* (http://www.who.int /mediacentre/factsheets/fs367/en).

BEHAVIOR CHANGE STRATEGY
Talking about Condoms and Safer Sex

The time to talk about safer sex is before you begin a sexual relationship. But even if you've been having unprotected sex with your partner, you can still start practicing safer sex now.

There are many ways to bring up the subject of safer sex and condom use with your partner. Be honest about your concerns, and stress that protection against STIs means that you care about yourself and your partner. You may find that your partner shares your concerns and also wants to use condoms. He or she may be happy and relieved that you have brought up the subject of safer sex.

However, if he or she resists the idea of using condoms, you may need to negotiate (see the dialogue suggestions). Stress that you both deserve to be protected and that sex will be more enjoyable when you aren't worrying about STIs. If you and your partner haven't used condoms before, buy some and familiarize yourselves with how to use them. Once you feel more comfortable handling condoms, you'll be able to use them correctly and incorporate them into your sexual activity. Consider trying the female condom as well.

If your partner still won't agree to use condoms, think carefully about whether you want to have a sexual relationship with this person. Maybe he or she is not the right partner for you.

IF YOUR PARTNER SAYS . . .	TRY SAYING . . .
"They're not romantic."	"Worrying about AIDS isn't romantic, and with condoms we won't have to worry." or "If we put one on together, a condom could be fun."
"I don't have any kind of disease! Don't you trust me?"	"Of course I trust you, but anyone can have an STI and not even know it. This is just a way to take care of both of us."
"I forgot to bring a condom. Let's just do it without a condom this time."	"It only takes one time to get pregnant or to get an STI. I just can't have sex unless I know I'm as safe as I can be." or "I never have sex without a condom. Let's go get some." or "I have some, right here."
"I don't like sex as much with a rubber. It doesn't feel the same."	"This is the only way I feel comfortable having sex, but believe me, it'll still be good even with protection! And it lets us both just focus on each other instead of worrying about all that other stuff." or "They might feel different, but let's try." or "Sex won't feel good if we're worrying about diseases." or "How about trying the female condom?"
"But I love you."	"Being in love can't protect us from diseases." or "I love you, too. We still need to use condoms."
"But we've been having sex without condoms."	"I want to start using condoms now so we won't be at any more risk." or "We can still prevent infection or reinfection."
"I don't know how to use them."	"I can show you—want me to put it on for you?"
"No one else makes me use a condom!"	"This is for both of us . . . and I won't have sex without protection. Let me show you how good it can be—even with a condom."
"I'm [or you're] on the pill."	"But that doesn't protect us from STIs, so I still want to be safe, for both of us."

SOURCES: Dialogue from San Francisco AIDS Foundation. 1998. Condoms for Couples (http://www.thebody.com/content/art2492.html#romantic).

CHAPTER OBJECTIVES

- Explain the concept of environmental health and how it has developed
- Explain how population growth affects the earth's environment
- Explain the impact of energy use and production on the environment
- Describe the causes and effects of air pollution
- Describe the causes and effects of water pollution
- Describe the problem of solid waste disposal and its impact on the environment and human health
- Identify environmental issues related to chemical pollution and hazardous waste
- Identify environmental issues related to radiation pollution
- Explain the concept of noise pollution and its impacts

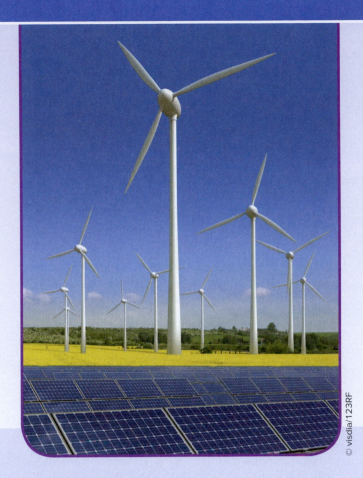

© visdia/123RF

CHAPTER **14**

Environmental Health

We are constantly reminded of our intimate relationship with everything that surrounds us—our **environment.** Although the planet provides us with food, water, air, and everything else that sustains life, it also provides us with natural occurrences—earthquakes, tsunamis, hurricanes, drought, and changes in climate—that destroy life and disrupt society. Humans have always had to struggle against the environment to survive. Today, in addition to dealing with natural disasters, we also have to find ways to protect the environment from the harmful by-products of our way of life.

This chapter introduces the concept of environmental health and explains how the environment affects us. It also discusses the ways humans affect the planet and its resources—focusing in particular on energy use and production, air and water pollution, solid waste disposal, chemical and radiation pollution, and noise pollution.

ENVIRONMENTAL HEALTH DEFINED

The field of **environmental health** grew out of efforts to control communicable diseases. These discoveries led to systematic garbage collection, sewage treatment, filtration and chlorination of drinking water, food inspection, and the establishment of public health enforcement agencies.

These efforts to control and prevent communicable diseases changed the health profile of the industrialized world. Americans rarely contract cholera, typhoid fever, plague,

> **environment**   The natural and human-made surroundings in which we spend our lives.
>
> **environmental health**   The collective interactions of humans with the environment and the short-term and long-term health consequences of those interactions.
>
> **TERMS**

diphtheria, or other diseases that once killed large numbers of people; but these diseases have not been eradicated worldwide.

In the United States, a huge, complex public health system is constantly at work behind the scenes attending to the details of these critical health concerns. Every time the system is disrupted, danger recurs. After any disaster that damages a community's public health system—whether a natural disaster such as a hurricane or a human-made disaster such as a terrorist attack—prompt restoration of basic health services becomes crucial to human survival. Every time we venture beyond the boundaries of our everyday world, whether traveling to a poorer country or camping in a wilderness area, we are reminded of the importance of these basics: clean water, sanitary waste disposal, safe food, and insect and rodent control.

Over the past few decades, the focus of environmental health has expanded and become more complex, for several reasons. We now recognize that environmental pollutants contribute not only to infectious diseases and immediate symptoms but to many chronic diseases as well. In addition, technological advances have increased our ability to affect and damage the environment. Further, rapid population growth (more than doubling in the past 50 years), which has resulted partly from past environmental improvements, means that ever more people are consuming and competing for resources, increasing human environmental impact.

Environmental health encompasses all the interactions of humans with their environment and the health consequences of these interactions. Fundamental to this definition is a recognition that we hold the world in trust for future life on earth. Our responsibility is to pass on a world no worse, and preferably better, than the one we live in today. Although many environmental problems are complex and seem beyond the control of the individual, there are ways that every person can make a difference to the future of the planet.

Ask Yourself

QUESTIONS FOR CRITICAL THINKING AND REFLECTION

How often do you think about the environment's impact on your personal health? In what ways do your immediate surroundings (your home, neighborhood, school, workplace) affect your well-being? In what ways do you influence the health of your personal environment?

POPULATION GROWTH AND CONTROL

Throughout most of history, humans have been a minor pressure on the planet. About 300 million people were alive in the year 1 CE (Common Era); by the time Europeans were settling in the Americas 1600 years later, the world population had increased gradually to a little over half a billion. But then it began rising exponentially—zooming to 1 billion by about 1800, more than doubling by 1930, and then doubling again in just 40 years (Figure 14.1).

The world's human population, currently over 7.3 billion, is increasing at a rate of about 80 million per year—approximately 150 people every minute. The United Nations projects that world population will reach 9.3 billion by 2050.

The average number of children per woman fell from 5 in 1950 to half that (2.5) in 2015. This decline in fertility has been happening in Western countries for decades and is now also happening in many of today's poor countries. Changes are also projected for the world's age distribution: For the first time in history, there are more older people than young children. By 2050, there will be 3.4 times the number

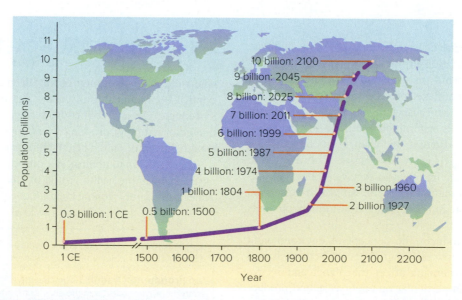

FIGURE 14.1 World population growth. The United Nations estimates that the world's population will continue to increase dramatically until it stabilizes above 10 billion people in 2100.

SOURCES: United Nations Population Division. 2015. World Population Prospects: The 2015 Revision. New York: United Nations (http://esa.un.org/unpd/wpp/); U.S. Bureau of the Census.

of people age 60 and over than of children age 4 and under.

This rapid expansion of population, particularly in the past 50 years, is generally believed to be responsible for most of the stress humans put on the environment. It is also a driving force behind many of the relatively more recent environmental health concerns, including chemical pollution, global climate change, and the thinning of the atmosphere's ozone layer.

No one knows how many people the world can support, but most scientists agree that there is a limit. A 2011 report from the United Nations' Convention on Biological Diversity states that the population's demand for resources already exceeds the earth's capacity by 20%. The primary factors that may eventually put a cap on human population are likely to be the limits of the earth's resources—food, water, land, and energy.

Although it is apparent that population growth must be controlled, population trends are difficult to influence and manage. A variety of interconnecting factors fuel the current population explosion, including high birth rates, lack of family planning, and low death rates.

To be successful, population management policies must change the condition of people's lives, especially poverty, to remove the pressures to have large families. Research indicates that the combination of improved health, better education, and increased literacy and employment opportunities for women work together with family planning to decrease birth rates.

ENVIRONMENTAL IMPACTS OF ENERGY USE AND PRODUCTION

Americans are now the second biggest energy consumers in the world; Chinese are first. We use energy to create electricity, transport us, power our industries, and run our homes. About 84% of the energy we use comes from **fossil fuels**—oil, coal, and natural gas. The remainder comes from nuclear power and renewable energy sources such as hydroelectric, wind, and solar power.

Energy consumption is at the root of many environmental problems. Automobile exhaust and the burning of oil and coal by industry and by electric power plants are primary causes of the greenhouse effect, smog, and acid precipitation (discussed in detail in later sections of the chapter). The mining of coal and the extraction and transportation of oil and natural gas cause pollution on land and in the water. The 2010 oil spill in the Gulf of Mexico was the worst environmental disaster in U.S. history and one of the largest oil spills ever to occur.

> **QUICK STATS**
>
> By 2050, the U.S. population will be nearly **400 million**; its current population is 325 million.
>
> —U.S. Census Bureau, 2016

> **fossil fuels** **TERMS** Buried deposits of decayed animals and plants that are converted into carbon-rich fuels by exposure to heat and pressure over millions of years; oil, coal, and natural gas are fossil fuels.

Environmental Threats of Extreme Energy Sources

Despite improvements in energy efficiency, the combination of global population increases and economic growth is expected to continue to drive up worldwide energy demand over time. At the same time, supplies of easily accessible oil will decline. In response, some energy companies have turned to what are often called "extreme energy sources." This term describes fossil fuels that are relatively difficult to access and extract from the environment. Accessing these energy sources requires new technologies and practices. Examples include deepwater oil rigs, tar sands oil extraction, and drilling and hydraulic fracturing ("fracking") for natural gas extraction. Critics worry that these technologies have been insufficiently studied and regulated and may pose significant new environmental risks.

Deepwater rigs extract oil that is buried deep under the ocean floor. These rigs can be difficult to manage if problems arise. A tragic example was the Deepwater Horizon rig that exploded in April 2010 in the Gulf of Mexico. As oil gushed into the water at an estimated rate of 60,000 barrels a day, it became clear that BP, the company that owned the rig, did not know how to stop it. The disaster killed thousands of birds, hundreds of endangered sea turtles, and many dolphins and other marine mammals, and the long-term health effects to the remaining wildlife are not known. The Gulf's ecosystems may need generations to recover fully, and some parts of it may never recover.

Tar sands (or oil sands) are sand deposits that are saturated with a dense form of petroleum called bitumen. The largest deposits are found in Canada, Kazakhstan, and Russia. Making liquid fuel from the oil in tar sands is an energy-intensive process. When used as fuel, the resulting molasses-like product produces two to four times the amount of greenhouse gases per barrel compared to other conventional oils. In addition, Canada's tar sands oil will need to travel through thousands of miles of leak-prone pipelines across pristine wildlife habitats in both Canada and the United States, and when it reaches shipping terminals, huge increases in oil tanker ship traffic will endanger fragile marine habitats in both countries.

Hydraulic fracturing, or "fracking," uses pressurized mixes of fluids to create cracks in rock formations deep underground, releasing natural gas. The term *fracking* is commonly used to describe both the drilling and fracturing processes in natural gas extraction. New technology and techniques have recently prompted the mining of deposits in the extensive Marcellus Shale formation, which covers large areas of the Northeast, as well as in other areas of the United States.

Critics have raised concerns about the safety of the technique, especially since many of these wells are in residential areas, near homes and schools. The specific chemicals used have not been publicly disclosed by energy companies using this technique, and reports of groundwater contamination have been verified by independent third parties. In addition, the disposal of wastewater from the fracking process (which is done by injecting the fluid deep in the ground) can induce earthquakes and has been linked to a dramatic increase in earthquakes in the central United States.

Renewable Energy

Renewable energy sources are those sources that are naturally replenished and essentially inexhaustible, such as wind and sunlight. Our best sources of renewable energy are wind power; solar power; geothermal power, which taps the heat in the earth's core; biomass, which is plant material, including trees; and biofuels, which are fuels based on natural materials such as vegetable oils and alcohol. Together with technologies that improve energy efficiency, renewable energy sources contribute to sustainability—the capacity of natural or human systems to endure and maintain well-being over time. A common definition of *sustainable development* is development that meets society's present needs without compromising the ability of future generations to meet their needs.

In 2011, President Barack Obama called for a new energy future, embracing alternative and renewable energy, ending the United States' dependence on foreign oil, and addressing the global climate crisis. The administration's "Blueprint for a Secure Energy Future" set a goal of generating 80% of the nation's electricity from "clean energy sources (including natural gas, nuclear, and clean coal)" by 2035, as well becoming the world's leader in advanced vehicle technologies. The pursuit of renewable energy sources is seen as having the potential to create new industries and generate jobs, in addition to benefiting the environment.

Alternative Fuels

The U.S. Department of Energy (DOE) is encouraging researchers and automobile manufacturers to produce vehicles that can run on alternative fuels such as ethanol. Ethanol, a form of alcohol, is a renewable and largely domestic transportation biofuel produced from fermenting plant sugars such as corn, sugarcane, and other starchy agricultural products. Ethanol use reduces the amount of imported oil required to produce gasoline, reduces overall greenhouse gas emissions from automobiles, and supports the U.S. agricultural industry.

Ethanol, however, has its critics, who say the alternative fuel may do more harm than good. Some reports show that corn-based ethanol requires more energy to produce than it yields when burned as fuel. One huge potential drawback of ethanol is the diversion of corn crops from the food supply to produce the fuel. This practice has been blamed for skyrock-

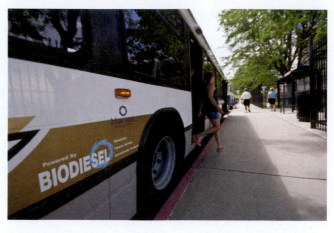

In many areas, public transit buses use alternative fuels or hybrid technology to reduce polluting emissions.
SOURCE: Pat Corkery/NREL/U.S. Department of Energy

> **QUICK STATS**
> The United States consumes **19.4 million** barrels of petroleum every day.
> —U.S. Energy Information Administration, 2016

eting food prices and food shortages around the world, which have led to food riots in several countries. The food-related concerns prompted the United Nations to call for a moratorium on food-based ethanol production until nonfood sources of alternative fuels could be developed.

Biodiesel, another alternative fuel, can be problematic depending on its material source. It is carbon neutral when the plants that are used to make it, such as soybeans and palm oil trees, absorb carbon dioxide as they grow and offset the carbon dioxide produced while making and using biodiesel. Most of the biodiesel used in the United States is made from soybean oil that is a by-product of processing soybeans for animal feed and numerous other food and nonfood products, and from waste animal fat and grease. However, in some parts of the world natural vegetation and forests have been cleared and burned to grow soybeans and palm oil trees to make biodiesel, and these negative environmental and social effects can outweigh any benefit

Hybrid and Electric Vehicles

Hybrid electric vehicles (HEVs) use two or more distinct power sources to propel the vehicle, such as an onboard energy storage system (e.g., batteries), a traditional internal combustion engine, and an electric motor. Hybrid vehicles typically have greater fuel economy than conventional cars do, and they produce fewer polluting emissions. Hybrids also tend to run with less noise than conventional vehicles. Hybrids are gaining popularity with consumers and are being used more commonly in both corporate and government vehicle fleets. A second generation of all-electric vehicles (EVs) has recently been introduced to consumer markets, taking advantage of better battery storage performance and more "quick-charging" stations, and changing consumer perceptions of the convenience of EVs.

AIR QUALITY AND POLLUTION

Air pollution is not a human invention or even a new problem. The air is polluted naturally with every forest fire, pollen bloom, and dust storm, and other natural pollutants. Humans contribute to pollution with the by-products of their activities.

Air pollution is linked to a wide range of health problems, and the very young and the elderly are among the most susceptible to its effects. For people with chronic ailments such as diabetes or heart failure, even relatively brief exposures to particulate air pollution increases the risk of death by nearly 40%, with air pollution (combustion emissions) causing about 200,000 deaths per year in the United States. Further, the children of pregnant women exposed to air pollution in urban environments have reduced birth weight, reduced intelligence (as measured by IQ), and increased incidence of obesity.

Air Quality and Smog

The U.S. Environmental Protection Agency (EPA) uses a measure called the **Air Quality Index (AQI)** to indicate whether air pollution levels pose a health concern. The AQI is used for five major air pollutants carbon monoxide (CO), sulfur dioxide (SO_2), nitrogen dioxide (NO_2), particulate matter (PM), and ground-level ozone.

The term **smog** was first used in the early 1900s in London to describe the combination of smoke and fog. What we typically call *smog* today is a mixture of pollutants, with ground-level ozone being the key ingredient. Major smog occurrences are linked to the combination of several factors: Heavy motor vehicle traffic, high temperatures, and sunny weather can increase the production of ozone. Pollutants are also more likely to build up in areas with little wind or where a topographic feature such as a mountain range or valley prevents the wind from pushing out stagnant air.

The Greenhouse Effect and Global Warming

Life on earth depends on a process known as the **greenhouse effect,** which allows for a warm atmosphere. The temperature of the earth's atmosphere depends on the balance between the amount of energy the planet absorbs from the sun (mainly as high-energy UV radiation) and the amount of energy lost back into space (as lower-energy infrared radiation). Key components of temperature regulation are carbon dioxide, water vapor, methane, and other **greenhouse gases**—so named because, like the glass panes in a greenhouse, they let through visible light from the sun but trap some of the resulting infrared radiation and reradiate it back

to the earth's surface. This process causes a buildup of heat (i.e., the greenhouse effect) that raises the temperature of the lower atmosphere (Figure 14.2).

There is scientific consensus that this natural process has been disrupted by human activity, causing **global warming** or *climate change*. The concentration of greenhouse gases is increasing because of human activity, especially the combustion of fossil fuels. Carbon dioxide levels in the atmosphere have increased rapidly in recent decades and, for the first time in recorded history, exceeded 400 parts per million in 2015. Many scientists say that 350 parts per million is the target number for the safe upper limit of carbon concentration in our atmosphere. The use of fossil fuels pumps more than 20 billion tons of carbon dioxide into the atmosphere every year. Deforestation, often by burning, also releases carbon dioxide into the atmosphere and reduces the number of trees available to convert carbon dioxide into oxygen.

The year 2015 was the warmest since record keeping began in 1880, and the 10 warmest periods have all occurred since June 1999. The average global temperature has risen more than 1.4 degrees Fahrenheit in the past century. Most scientists agree that temperatures will continue to rise, although estimates vary as to how much they will change.

If global warming persists, experts say the impact may be devastating (Figure 14.3). Possible consequences include increased rainfall and flooding in some regions, and increased drought in others; increased mortality from heat stress, urban air pollution, and tropical diseases; a poleward shift of about 50–350 miles (150–550 km) in the location of vegetation zones, affecting crop yields, irrigation demands, and forest productivity; alterations of ecosystems, resulting in possible species extinction; and increasingly rapid and drastic melting of the earth's polar ice caps.

TERMS

Air Quality Index (AQI) A measure of local air quality and what it means for health.

smog Hazy atmospheric conditions resulting from increased concentrations of ground-level ozone and other pollutants.

greenhouse effect A warming of the earth due to a buildup of greenhouse gases in the atmosphere.

greenhouse gas A gas (such as carbon dioxide) or vapor that traps infrared radiation instead of allowing it to escape through the atmosphere, resulting in a warming of the earth (the *greenhouse effect*).

global warming An increase in the earth's atmospheric temperature when averaged across seasons and geographic regions; also called *climate change*.

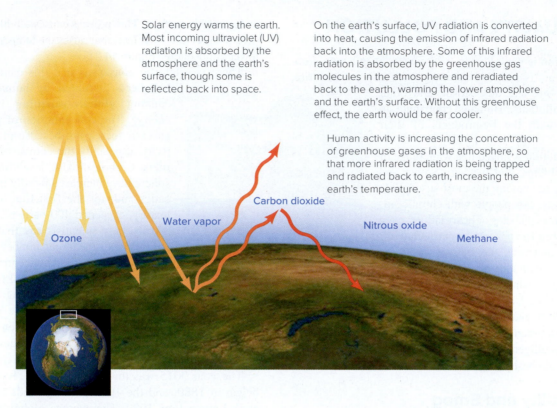

Solar energy warms the earth. Most incoming ultraviolet (UV) radiation is absorbed by the atmosphere and the earth's surface, though some is reflected back into space.

On the earth's surface, UV radiation is converted into heat, causing the emission of infrared radiation back into the atmosphere. Some of this infrared radiation is absorbed by the greenhouse gas molecules in the atmosphere and reradiated back to the earth, warming the lower atmosphere and the earth's surface. Without this greenhouse effect, the earth would be far cooler.

Human activity is increasing the concentration of greenhouse gases in the atmosphere, so that more infrared radiation is being trapped and radiated back to earth, increasing the earth's temperature.

FIGURE 14.2 **The greenhouse effect.** Key greenhouse gases that help trap heat energy in the lower atmosphere are carbon dioxide, methane, nitrous oxide, ozone, and water vapor.

© Planetary Vision Limited

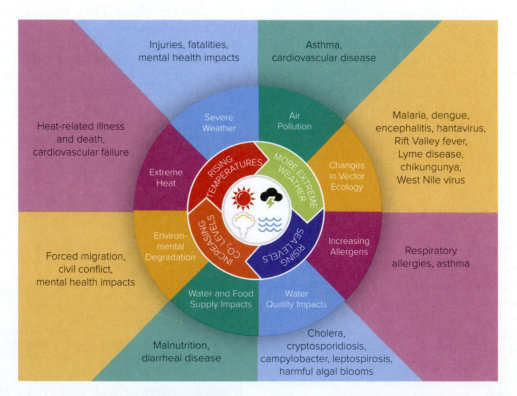

FIGURE 14.3 **Impact of climate change on human health.** Climate change can influence health and disease in many ways; the effects may vary based on location, age, socioeconomic status, and other factors.

SOURCE: Centers for Disease Control and Prevention. 2014. *Climate Effects on Health* (http://www.cdc.gov/climateandhealth/effects).

At the 2015 United Nations Climate Change Conference in Paris, France, a landmark agreement was made to limit average global warming to 2°C above preindustrial temperatures, striving for a limit of 1.5°C if possible. President Obama considered the adoption of this agreement between the 195 participating countries a "turning point for the world." According to the Paris Agreement, each country is in charge of setting its own greenhouse emissions limits, so countries must pledge sufficient reductions in order for the Agreement to be effective.

Ask Yourself

QUESTIONS FOR CRITICAL THINKING AND REFLECTION

How aware are you of the issues related to climate change, and where do you get your information? Do you think about how your lifestyle affects climate change on a day-to-day basis? Why do you think climate change is such a controversial and politically charged topic?

Thinning of the Ozone Layer

Another air pollution problem is the thinning of the atmosphere's **ozone layer,** a fragile, invisible layer about 10–30 miles above the earth's surface that shields the planet from the sun's hazardous UV rays. Since the mid-1980s, scientists have observed the seasonal appearance and growth of a hole in the ozone layer over Antarctica.

The ozone layer is being destroyed primarily by **chlorofluorocarbons (CFCs),** which are industrial chemicals that rise into the atmosphere and release chlorine atoms that destroy ozone. When the polar vortex weakens in the summer, winds richer in ozone from the north replenish the lost Antarctic ozone.

The largest and deepest ozone hole on record occurred on September 6, 2000, measured at 11.5 million square miles (29.9 million square kilometers). Although the ozone hole has been consistently smaller since then, it neared that size in 2015. At over 26 million square kilometers, it was larger than the entire continent of North America. The Antarctic ozone layer has begun to show signs of healing, but it will likely not return to its early-1980s state until about 2050, because of the long lifetimes of ozone-depleting substances in the atmosphere. Because of an international agreement that regulates the production of ozone-depleting chemicals, overall atmospheric ozone is no longer decreasing. The gradual overall recovery will include annual variations caused by weather fluctuations over Antarctica.

Without the ozone layer to absorb the sun's UV radiation, life on earth would be impossible. The potential effects of increased long-term exposure to UV light for humans include skin cancer, wrinkling and aging of the skin, cataracts and blindness, and reduced immune response. Some scientists already blame ozone loss for many cases of melanoma.

(UV radiation levels under the Antarctic hole were high enough to cause sunburn within seven minutes.)

Indoor Air Quality (IAQ)

Although most people associate air pollution with the outdoors, homes and other buildings can harbor potentially dangerous pollutants. Some of these compounds trigger allergic responses, and others have been linked to cancer and developmental problems in children. Common indoor pollutants include the following: environmental tobacco smoke (ETS); carbon monoxide and other combustion by-products from woodstoves, fireplaces, kerosene heaters and lamps, and gas ranges; volatile organic compounds (VOCs), which are gases emitted from such household items as paints, lacquers, cleaning supplies, aerosols, building materials, furnishings, and office equipment; biological pollutants, such as bacteria, dust mites, mold, and animal dander, which can cause allergic reactions and other health problems; and indoor mold, a fungus that grows in damp places, such as on shower tiles and damp basement walls.

Preventing Air Pollution

You can do a great deal to reduce air pollution. Here are a few ideas:

• Cut back on driving. Ride your bike, walk, use public transportation, or carpool in a fuel-efficient vehicle.

• Keep your car tuned up and well maintained. Keep your tires inflated at recommended pressures. To save energy when driving, avoid quick starts, stay within the speed limit, limit the use of air conditioning, and don't let your car idle unless absolutely necessary.

• Buy energy-efficient appliances and use them only when necessary. Run the washing machine, clothes dryer, and dishwasher only when you have full loads, do laundry in warm or cold water instead of hot, and don't overdry your clothes. Clean refrigerator coils and clothes dryer lint screens frequently.

• Use energy-efficient lighting: halogen, light-emitting diode (LED), or compact fluorescent bulbs (not fluorescent tubes). For more information, see the box "High-Efficiency Lighting."

• Make sure your home is well-insulated with ozone-safe agents; use insulating shades and curtains to keep heat in during winter and out during summer.

• Plant and care for trees in your yard and neighborhood. They recycle carbon dioxide, so trees work against global

ozone layer   A layer of ozone molecules in the upper atmosphere that screens out UV rays from the sun.

TERMS

chlorofluorocarbons (CFCs)   Chemicals used as spray can propellants, refrigerants, and industrial solvents, which have been implicated in the destruction of the ozone layer.

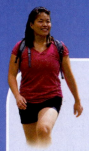

TAKE CHARGE
High-Efficiency Lighting

Lighting accounts for about 15% of all residential electricity use. Switching to energy-efficient lighting is a good way to cut your home's energy use, lower your energy bills, and reduce your environmental footprint.

The Energy Independence and Security Act (EISA) of 2007 set national performance standards for lightbulbs for the first time, requiring that basic bulbs be at least about 25% more efficient; the standards were phased in between 2012 and 2014. Traditional incandescent lightbulbs did not meet these new efficiency standards, so use of other lighting choices has grown:

• **Halogen incandescents.** More energy-efficient incandescent bulbs that also last up to three times longer than traditional bulbs.

• **Compact fluorescent lightbulbs (CFLs).** Long-lasting fluorescents that work in many types of household fixtures. These bulbs contain a very small amount of mercury and require special handling if they are broken (visit www.epa.gov/cfl for specific cleanup and recycling instructions).

• **Light-emitting diodes (LEDs).** Rapidly expanding in household use, LEDs use only about 10% of the energy and last up to 42 times longer, compared to traditional bulbs.

Although the newer styles of lightbulbs are more expensive than traditional incandescents, they save money for the user over the long term. The savings come from two differences between incandescent bulbs and high-efficiency bulbs. First, high-efficiency bulbs use much less energy by requiring less electricity to produce light. For example, a 17-watt (W) LED bulb produces as much light as a 75W incandescent lightbulb. Second, they last longer: CFLs last up to 10 times longer than conventional lightbulbs, and some LED bulbs have useful lives of more than 22 years.

To aid consumers in selecting bulbs, the Federal Trade Commission mandated Lighting Facts labels on all bulbs. Using these labels, you can compare types of bulbs and select the most appropriate one for your planned use. The brightness comparison is based on lumens rather than watts, because energy-efficient bulbs produce a brighter light with less energy—more lumens per watt than a traditional incandescent bulb.

SOURCES: U.S. Energy Information Administration. 2015. *How Much Electricity Is Used for Lighting in the United States?* (http://www.eia.gov/tools/faqs/faq.cfm?id=99&t=3); Office of Energy Efficiency & Renewable Energy. 2014. *How Energy-Efficient Light Bulbs Compare with Traditional Incandescents* (http://energy.gov/energysaver/articles/how-energy-efficient-light-bulbs-compare-traditional-incandescents); Office of Energy Efficiency & Renewable Energy. 2013. *Lighting Basics* (http://www .energy.gov/eere/energybasics/articles/lighting-basics); Federal Trade Commission. 2011. *Shopping for Lightbulbs* (http://www .consumer.ftc.gov/articles/0164-shopping-light-bulbs).

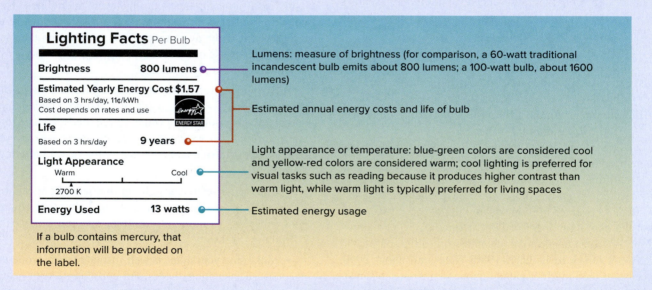

Lighting Facts Per Bulb

Brightness 800 lumens — Lumens: measure of brightness (for comparison, a 60-watt traditional incandescent bulb emits about 800 lumens; a 100-watt bulb, about 1600 lumens)

Estimated Yearly Energy Cost $1.57
Based on 3 hrs/day, 11¢/kWh
Cost depends on rates and use
ENERGY STAR

Life
Based on 3 hrs/day 9 years — Estimated annual energy costs and life of bulb

Light Appearance
Warm — Cool
2700 K — Light appearance or temperature: blue-green colors are considered cool and yellow-red colors are considered warm; cool lighting is preferred for visual tasks such as reading because it produces higher contrast than warm light, while warm light is typically preferred for living spaces

Energy Used 13 watts — Estimated energy usage

If a bulb contains mercury, that information will be provided on the label.

warming. They also provide shade and cool the air so that less air conditioning is needed.

• Before discarding a refrigerator, air conditioner, or humidifier, check with the waste hauler or your local government to ensure that ozone-depleting refrigerants will be removed prior to disposal.

• Keep paints, cleaning agents, and other chemical products tightly sealed in their original containers.

• Clean and inspect chimneys, furnaces, and other appliances regularly. Install carbon monoxide detectors.

• Always use an outside-venting hood when cooking.

WATER QUALITY AND POLLUTION

Few parts of the world have enough safe, clean drinking water, and yet few things are as important to human health.

Water Contamination and Treatment

Many cities rely at least in part on wells that tap local groundwater, but often it is necessary to tap lakes and rivers to supplement wells. Because such surface water is more likely to be contaminated with both organic matter and pathogenic microorganisms, it is purified in water treatment plants before being piped into the community. At treatment facilities, the water is subjected to various physical and chemical processes, including screening, filtration, and disinfection (often with chlorine), before it is introduced into the water supply system. **Fluoridation,** a water treatment process that reduces tooth decay by 15–40%, has been used successfully in the United States for more than 60 years.

In most areas of the United States, water systems have adequate, dependable supplies; are able to control waterborne disease; and provide water with acceptable color, odor, and taste. However, problems occur. CDC estimates that 1 million Americans become ill and 900–1000 die each year from microbial illnesses from drinking water.

Water Shortages

Water shortages are a growing concern in many regions of the world. Some parts of the United States, such as the desert West, are experiencing rapid population growth that outstrips the ability of local systems to provide adequate water to all. Groundwater pumping and the diversion of water from lakes and rivers for irrigation are further reducing the amount of water available to local communities.

Sewage

Most cities have sewage treatment systems that separate fecal matter from water in huge tanks and ponds and stabilize it so that it cannot transmit infectious diseases. After it is treated and biologically safe, the water is released back into the environment. The sludge that remains behind is often contaminated with **heavy metals** and is handled as hazardous waste. If not contaminated, sludge may be used as fertilizer, although this practice is being discouraged by scientists and some government agencies, and is not permitted in organic agriculture.

Many cities have expanded sewage treatment measures to remove heavy metals and other hazardous chemicals. This action has resulted from many studies linking exposure to chemicals such as mercury, lead, and **polychlorinated biphenyls (PCBs)** with long-term health consequences, including cancer and damage to the central nervous system.

Protecting the Water Supply

By reducing your own water use, you help preserve your community's valuable supply and lower your monthly water bill. By taking steps to keep the water supply clean, you reduce pollution overall and help protect the land, wildlife, and other people from illness. Here are some simple steps you can take to protect your water supply:

• Take showers, not baths, to minimize your water consumption. Don't let water run when you're not actively using it while brushing your teeth, shaving, or hand-washing clothes or dishes.

• Install sink faucet aerators and water-efficient showerheads, which use two to five times less water with no noticeable decrease in performance.

• Purchase a water-saving toilet, or put a displacement device in your toilet tank to reduce the amount of water used with each flush.

• Fix leaky faucets in your home. Leaks can waste thousands of gallons of water per year.

• Don't pour toxic materials such as cleaning solvents, bleach, or motor oil down the drain. Store them until you can take them to a hazardous waste collection center.

• Don't pour old medicines down the drain or flush them down the toilet. Some pharmacies will take back unused or expired medications for disposal, and many communities have drop-off days for these drugs.

Ask Yourself

QUESTIONS FOR CRITICAL THINKING AND REFLECTION

How would you describe the quality of the water where you live? Are there lakes or streams where you can safely swim or fish? What local information sources can you find about water quality in your area?

SOLID WASTE POLLUTION

Humans living in the industrialized world generate huge amounts of waste, which must be handled appropriately if the environment is to be kept safe.

TERMS

fluoridation   The addition of fluoride to the water supply to reduce tooth decay.

heavy metal   A metal with a high specific gravity, such as lead, copper, or tin.

polychlorinated biphenyl (PCB)   An industrial chemical used as an insulator in electrical transformers and linked to certain human cancers; banned worldwide since 1977 but persistent in the environment. Humans are exposed mainly through consumption of meat, fish, and dairy.

Solid Waste

The bulk of the organic food garbage produced in American kitchens is now dumped in the sewage system by way of the mechanical garbage disposal. The garbage that remains is not hazardous from the standpoint of infectious disease because there is very little food waste in it, but it does represent an enormous disposal and contamination problem.

What's in Our Garbage? The biggest single component of household trash by weight is paper products, including junk mail, glossy mail-order catalogs, and computer printouts (Figure 14.4). About 1% of the solid waste is toxic; a new source of toxic waste is the disposal of computer components in both household and commercial waste. Burning, as opposed to burial, reduces the bulk of solid waste, but it can release hazardous material into the air, depending on what is being burned. Manufacturing, mining, and other industries all produce large amounts of potentially dangerous materials that cannot simply be dumped.

Disposing of Solid Waste Since the 1960s, billions of tons of solid waste have been buried in **sanitary landfill** disposal sites. Sometimes protective liners are used around the site, and nearby monitoring wells are now required in most states. Layers of solid waste are regularly covered with thin layers of dirt until the site is filled. Some communities then plant grass and trees and convert the site into a park. Landfill is relatively stable; almost no decomposition occurs in the solidly packed waste.

Burying solid waste in landfills has several disadvantages. Burial is expensive and requires huge amounts of space. Waste can also contain chemicals such as pesticides, paints, and oils, that should not be released into the environment. Despite precautions, buried contaminants sometimes leak into the surrounding soil and groundwater.

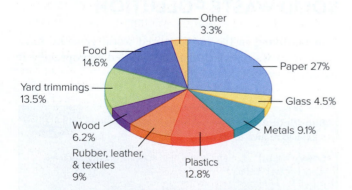

FIGURE 14.4 Components of municipal solid waste, by weight, before recycling.

SOURCE: U.S. Environmental Protection Agency. 2015. *Advancing Sustainable Materials Management: 2013 Fact Sheet* (Pub. No. EPA530-R-15-003). Washington, DC: EPA.

Table 14.1	How Long Items Take to Biodegrade

ITEM	TIME REQUIRED TO BIODEGRADE
Banana peel	2–10 days
Paper	2–5 months
Rope	3–14 months
Orange peel	6 months
Wool sock	1–5 years
Cigarette butt	1–12 years
Plastic-coated milk carton	5 years
Aluminum can	80–100 years
Plastic six-pack holder ring	450 years
Glass bottle	1 million years
Plastic bottle	Forever

Biodegradation is the process by which organic substances are broken down naturally by living organisms. Items that are **biodegradable** can break down naturally, safely, and quickly into the raw materials of nature and then disappear back into the environment. If a product is **compostable,** it may break down through *biotic* processes—those involving living organisms—as well as *abiotic* processes, which involve nonliving factors like climate and natural disasters. Table 14.1 shows the amount of time required for materials to biodegrade.

Recycling In **recycling,** many kinds of waste materials are collected and used as raw materials in the production of new products. Recycling is a good idea because it puts unwanted objects to good use, and it reduces the amount of solid waste sitting in landfills, some of which takes decades to decay naturally.

Discarded Technology: E-waste Americans scrap about 400 million consumer electronic devices each year. This "e-waste" is the fastest-growing portion of our waste stream. Junked electronic devices are toxic because they contain varying amounts of lead, mercury, and other heavy metals. Many components of electronic devices are valuable, however, and can be recycled and reused. Local and state

QUICK STATS

The average American generates **4.4 pounds** of trash per day; about 1.5 pounds of this is recycled.

—U.S. Environmental Protection Agency, 2015

TERMS

sanitary landfill A disposal site where solid wastes are buried.

biodegradable The ability of materials to break down via biotic processes—consumption by bacteria or fungi, or other biological processes.

compostable The ability of materials to break down via abiotic and biotic processes.

recycling The use of waste materials as raw materials in the production of new products.

e-waste recycling programs are becoming more common, and private companies are also getting into the e-waste recycling business. If you recycle your electronic devices, look for a "green" program or one that is certified by e-stewards, an organization that advocates for responsible e-waste recycling (www.e-stewards.org).

Reducing Solid Waste

By reducing your consumption, recycling more, and throwing away less, you can conserve landfill space and put more reusable items back into service. Here are some ideas to help you reduce solid waste:

• Buy products with the least amount of packaging you can, or buy products in bulk or packaged in recyclable containers.

• Buy recycled or recyclable products. Avoid disposables; instead use long-lasting or reusable products such as refillable pens and rechargeable batteries.

• Bring your own reusable ceramic coffee mug and metal spoon to work or wherever you drink coffee or tea. Pack your lunch in reusable containers.

• To store food, use reusable plastic or glass containers rather than foil and plastic wrap.

• Recycle your newspapers, glass, cans, paper, and other recyclables. If you receive something packaged with foam pellets, take them to a commercial mailing center that accepts them for recycling.

• Do not throw electronic items, batteries, or fluorescent lights into the trash. Take these to state-approved recycling centers; check with your local disposal service for more information.

• Start a compost pile for your organic garbage if you have a yard. If you live in an apartment, you can take your organic wastes to a community composting center, or use an indoor worm composting bin. Many communities now offer curbside collection of kitchen scraps for recycling into compost, which is sold to farms and wineries.

> ## Ask Yourself
> **?**
> ### QUESTIONS FOR CRITICAL THINKING AND REFLECTION
> What are your own waste-disposal habits? Do you recycle everything you can? Do you reuse items? Even if you are conscientious about the way you deal with waste, how could you improve your habits?

CHEMICAL POLLUTION AND HAZARDOUS WASTE

New chemical substances are continually being introduced into the environment as pesticides, herbicides, solvents, and hundreds of other products. More people and wildlife are exposed to them than ever before.

The pivotal publication of Rachel Carson's *Silent Spring* in 1962 drew attention to the problems of chemical pollution and prompted the formation of the EPA. In the 1970s, the EPA established the Superfund program to clean up the nation's uncontrolled hazardous waste sites. A national list prioritizes over 1300 sites for cleanup.

Asbestos

A mineral-based compound, asbestos was widely used for fire protection and insulation in buildings until the late 1960s. As described in Chapter 12, microscopic asbestos fibers can be released into the air when this material is applied or when it later deteriorates or is damaged. These fibers can lodge in the lungs, causing **asbestosis,** lung cancer, and other serious lung diseases. Similar conditions expose workers to risk in the coal mining industry, from coal and silica dust (black lung disease), and in the textile industry, from cotton fibers (brown lung disease).

Lead

Although lead poisoning is less of a problem than in the past, the CDC estimates that approximately half a million U.S. children aged 1–5 have blood lead levels above the cutoff at which the CDC recommends public health action. Many of these children live in poor, inner-city areas (see the box "Poverty, Gender, and Environmental Health"). No safe blood lead level has been identified for children. When lead is ingested or inhaled, it can permanently damage the central nervous system, cause mental impairment, hinder oxygen transport in the blood, and create kidney and digestive problems. Severe lead poisoning may cause coma or death. Lead exposure has been linked to attention-deficit/hyperactivity disorder (ADHD) in children. Lead can also build up in bones, where it may be released into the bloodstream during pregnancy or when bone mass is lost from osteoporosis.

Most environmental lead comes from lead-based paints. Lead paints were banned from residential use in 1978, but as many as 57 million American homes still contain them. In 2010, new guidelines were implemented requiring contractors to take special lead-containment measures when doing renovations, repairs, or painting. The use of lead in plumbing is now also banned, but some old pipes and faucets contain it; if these pipes and fixtures corrode, lead can leach into the water. The presence of lead pipes contributed to the 2014–2016 drinking water crisis in Flint, Michigan. In 2014, the city changed water suppliers to one that had higher levels of corrosive compounds but failed to add a required anticorrosive agent; lead from aging pipes leached into the drinking water. Researchers found that the incidence of elevated blood lead levels doubled in children in Flint after the water source change.

> **asbestosis** A lung condition caused by inhalation **TERMS** of microscopic asbestos fibers, which inflame the lung and can lead to lung cancer.

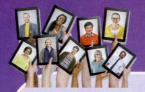
Residents of low-income and minority communities are often exposed to more environmental toxins than residents of wealthier communities are, and they are more likely to suffer from health problems caused or aggravated by pollutants.

Poor neighborhoods are often located near highways and industrial areas that have high levels of air and noise pollution; they are also common sites for hazardous waste production and disposal. Residents of substandard housing are more likely to come into contact with lead, asbestos, carbon monoxide, pesticides, and other hazardous pollutants associated with peeling paint, old plumbing, and poorly maintained insulation and heating equipment. In addition, low-income people are more likely to have jobs that expose them to asbestos, silica dust, and pesticides, and they are more likely to catch and consume fish contaminated with PCBs, mercury, and other toxins.

The most thoroughly researched and documented link among poverty, the environment, and health is lead poisoning in children. During the Flint, Michigan, water crisis, the highest blood lead levels in children were found in the most socio-economically disadvantaged neighborhood, linked to aging infrastructure. A 2013 study showed that whether they lived in a rural or urban environment, non-Hispanic blacks were more likely than non-Hispanic whites to be exposed to high soil lead concentrations. This finding was true for children age 6 and under, which is important because children may be at higher risk and more biologically vulnerable to lead exposure. The CDC and the American Academy of Pediatrics recommend annual testing of blood lead levels for all children under age 6, with more frequent testing for children at special risk.

Asthma is another health threat that appears to be linked with both environmental and socioeconomic factors. Although the number of Americans with asthma has been rising for 20 years, a recent study found a leveling and even decrease of incidence in children since 2013. Unfortunately, rates are still increasing in the poorest families. Researchers are not sure what causes asthma, but suspects include household pollutants, pesticides, air pollution, cigarette smoke, and allergens like cockroaches. These risk factors are likely to cluster in poor urban areas where inadequate health care may worsen the effects of asthma.

Gender also influences exposure to environmental hazards. In many societies, women are more often involved in day-to-day activities associated with the environment, including food preparation, agricultural work, and tasks around the home. These activities can expose women to indoor air pollution, water pollution, food-borne pathogens, agricultural chemicals, and waste contamination. Indoor pollutants, especially soot from burning wood, charcoal, and other solid fuels used for home heating and cooking, are a particular risk. Exposure to this particulate pollution increases the risk of respiratory diseases, lung cancer, and reproductive problems.

All humans are exposed to chemicals in air, food, and drinking water, and we all carry a load of chemicals in our bodies. Some of these chemicals accumulate in our bones, blood, or fatty tissues. Women are smaller than men, on average, and have a higher percentage of body fat, so chemicals that accumulate in fatty tissue may pose a relatively greater risk for women. By contrast, men may be more likely to work in industries that involve significant occupational exposures to disease-related toxins. For example, coal miners have an increased risk of lung cancer (black lung disease).

Although any chemical exposure can be a concern for health, women face the added risk of passing pollutants to a developing fetus during pregnancy or to an infant through breastfeeding. Even relatively low exposure to pollutants can result in a significant chemical body load in an infant or young child because of their small body size. And because infants and children are still developing, the effects of chemical exposure can be significant and devastating. It is not unusual for dangerous toxin exposures to be recognized first through noticeable effects on infants or children.

SOURCES: Hatta-Attisha, M., et al. 2016. Elevated blood lead levels in children associated with the Flint drinking water crisis: A spatial analysis of risk and public health response. *American Journal of Public Health* 106(2): 283-290; Akinbami, L. J., A. E. Simon, & L. M. Rosen. 2016. Changing trends in asthma prevalence among children. *Pediatrics* 137(1); Aelion, C. M., et al. 2013. Associations between soil lead concentrations and populations by race/ethnicity and income-to-poverty ratio in urban and rural areas. *Environmental Geochemistry and Health* 35(1): 1–12.

Pesticides

Pesticides are chemicals that kill unwanted pests. Herbicides (plant killers) and insecticides (insect killers) are used extensively in agriculture, and they often have toxic effects in unwanted targets, such as beneficial insects and birds. Insecticides are used primarily to prevent the spread of insect-borne diseases and to maximize food production by killing crop pests. Pesticide use has risks and benefits. For example, DDT was extremely effective in controlling mosquito-borne diseases in tropical countries and in increasing crop yields throughout the world, but it was found to harm birds, fish, and reptiles. DDT also builds up in the food chain, increasing in concentration as larger animals eat smaller ones—a process known as **biomagnification** or *bioaccumulation*. DDT was banned in the United States in 1972.

> **pesticides** Chemicals used to kill agricultural and household pests, such as weeds, insects, and rodents.
>
> **biomagnification** The accumulation of a substance in a food chain; also known as *bioaccumulation*.
>
> **TERMS**

Glyphosate (Roundup) is an herbicide that is widely used with genetically modified crops such as corn and soybeans ("Roundup-ready" crops). Toxic effects of glyphosate have been found in amphibians and humans. In 2015, California listed glyphosate as a "probable human carcinogen." Organophosphate and organochlorine pesticides have been linked to mental problems in children, such as ADHD and low IQ.

Mercury

A naturally occurring metal, mercury is a toxin that affects the brain and nervous system and may damage the kidneys and gastrointestinal tract, and increase blood pressure, heart rate, and heart attack risk. Mercury slows fetal and child development and causes irreversible deficits in brain function. Coal-fired power plants are the largest producers of mercury; other sources include mining and smelting operations and the disposal of consumer products containing mercury. Mercury persists in the environment and, like pesticides, bioaccumulates. In particular, large, long-lived fish may carry high levels of mercury.

Other Chemical Pollutants

There are tens of thousands of chemical pollutants, and the extent of their toxic effects are just beginning to be understood (see the box "Endocrine Disruption: A 'New' Toxic Threat"). They include automotive supplies (motor oil, antifreeze, transmission fluid), paint supplies (turpentine, paint thinner, mineral spirits), art and hobby supplies (oil-based paint, solvents, acids and alkalis, aerosol sprays), insecticides, batteries, computer and electronic components, and household cleaners containing sodium hydroxide (lye) or ammonia. These chemicals are dangerous when inhaled or ingested, when they contact the skin or the eyes, or when they are burned or dumped. Many cities provide guidelines about approved disposal methods and have hazardous waste collection days.

Preventing Chemical Pollution

You can take steps to reduce the chemical pollution in your community. Just as important, by reducing and eliminating the number of chemicals in your home, you may save the life of a child or animal who might encounter one of those chemicals.

• When buying products, read the labels, and buy the least toxic ones available. Choose nontoxic, nonpetrochemical cleansers, disinfectants, polishes, and other personal and household products.

• Eat and live organically. Avoid using chemical pesticides (weed, insect, and rodent killers) in the home and garden.

• Dispose of your household hazardous wastes properly. If you are not sure whether something is hazardous or don't

know how to dispose of it, contact your local environmental health office or health department.

• If you must use pesticides or toxic household products, store them in a locked place where children and pets can't get to them. Don't measure chemicals with food preparation utensils, and wear gloves whenever handling them.

• If you have your house fumigated for pest control, be sure to hire a licensed exterminator. Keep everyone, including pets, out of the house while the crew works and, if possible, for a few days after.

> ## Ask Yourself ?
>
> **QUESTIONS FOR CRITICAL THINKING AND REFLECTION**
>
> Are there any hazardous chemicals in your home, such as those found in cleaning products, solvents, paint, or batteries? Would you know what to do if one of these chemicals spilled? How would you clean it up?

RADIATION POLLUTION

Radiation comes in several forms, such as UV rays, microwaves, or X-rays, and from several sources, such as the sun, electronics, uranium, and nuclear weapons. These forms of electromagnetic radiation differ in wavelength and energy, with shorter waves having the highest energy levels.

> **QUICK STATS**
>
> There are **99 nuclear reactors** operating in the United States.
>
> —U.S. Energy Information Administration, 2016

Of most concern to health are gamma rays, which are produced by radioactive sources such as nuclear weapons, nuclear energy plants, and radon gas. These high-energy waves are powerful enough to penetrate objects and break molecular bonds. Gamma radiation cannot be seen or felt, and its effects at high doses can include **radiation sickness** and death. At lower doses, chromosome damage, sterility, tissue damage, cataracts, and cancer can occur. Other types of radiation can also affect health. For example, exposure to UV radiation from the sun or from tanning salons can increase the risk of skin cancer. The effects of some sources of radiation, such as cell phones, remain controversial.

Nuclear Weapons and Nuclear Energy

Nuclear weapons pose a health risk of the most serious kind to all species. Reducing the stockpiles of nuclear weapons is a challenge and a goal for the 21st century.

> **TERMS**
>
> **radiation** Energy transmitted in the form of rays, waves, or particles.
>
> **radiation sickness** An illness caused by excess radiation exposure, marked by low white blood cell counts and nausea; possibly fatal.

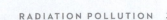

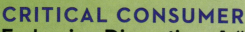

CRITICAL CONSUMER
Endocrine Disruption: A "New" Toxic Threat

In the 1970s and 1980s, scientists began to document strange occurrences in wildlife: disrupted reproduction, birth defects, tumors, and behavioral changes in birds, fish, and reptiles. The wildlife in and around the Great Lakes, an area with a history of industrial spills and contamination, was particularly affected. It was also becoming apparent that a drug given to pregnant women in the 1950s (a potent synthetic estrogen, DES) was causing infertility and rare reproductive cancers in their adult daughters.

In the mid-1990s, the influential book *Our Stolen Future* by Theo Colborn was published. Colborn suggested that toxic chemicals can cause effects other than acute toxicity (i.e., death), and that low amounts of these chemicals, over a long period of time, can cause disease. Even more concerning was the evidence that a fetus's exposure to chemicals during gestation can cause lasting changes and possible future disease in adulthood.

These chemicals, known also as **endocrine-disrupting chemicals (EDCs)** were disturbing the hormone systems of organisms. Most systems in the body rely on hormones, such as the immune, metabolic, and brain/nervous systems. A *hormone* is a chemical signal that is made in one area or organ of the body and travels to another to initiate effects. Estrogen, testosterone, and thyroid hormones are well-known examples.

Low levels of EDCs can disrupt these systems by mimicking or blocking natural hormones, causing abnormal effects. EDC exposure before and after birth may cause lifelong effects, including fertility problems, cancers, cardiovascular diseases, obesity, and mental disorders. These effects have been proven in laboratory animals and supported by observational (epidemiological) studies in humans.

Various manufactured chemicals, some in everyday products such as plastics, cosmetics, food packaging, flame retardants, pesticides, and others, are EDCs. These chemicals are known to contaminate household dust, drinking water, and food (especially meat and dairy products). Bisphenol A (BPA) is a chemical present in #7 plastic—in water bottles, the lining of canned foods, dental fillings, and cash register receipts.

The chemical has been banned in children's products in California and the European Union, and many scientists believe it should be regulated more stringently in the United States.

Traditional methods of determining chemical toxicity usually test "gross" effects: death, deformities, and tumors. These methods typically do not test low (environmental) doses of chemicals; rather, they test at high doses and extrapolate down to find "safe" exposure levels. Often, EDCs have detrimental effects at low doses but not higher ones. Therefore, a new testing paradigm must be employed that addresses physiological effects at low doses. The modern environmental movement is new, and as our scientific knowledge of these chemicals evolves and improves, so must government testing and policies surrounding the issues of EDCs, for the continued protection of human health.

What can you do?

- Educate yourself about the personal care and household products you use.

- Eat organic foods. Eat lower on the food chain.

- Avoid plastics, especially in contact with food and drinks. Do not microwave plastic containers.

- Dust, vacuum, and wipe down surfaces often.

- Avoid nonstick cookware and products.

- Avoid flame-retardant clothes and furniture.

- Avoid handling cash-register receipts. If you must, use gloves or wash your hands after handling receipts.

- Be especially cautious about exposing pregnant women, infants, and children to EDCs.

- Support legislation that will provide adequate testing and regulation of potential EDCs.

For more information and a list of EDCs visit www.endocrinedisruption.org.

Power-generating plants that use nuclear fuel also pose health problems. When **nuclear power** was first developed as an alternative to oil and coal, it was promoted as clean, efficient, inexpensive, and safe. In general, these claims have proven to be the case. Power systems in several parts of the world rely on nuclear power plants. However, despite all the built-in safeguards and regulating agencies, accidents in nuclear power plants do happen, many due to human error or following a natural disaster.

The 1986 fire and explosion at the Chernobyl nuclear power station in Ukraine caused hundreds of deaths and increased rates of genetic mutation and cancer; the long-term effects are not yet clear. The zone around Chernobyl has been sealed off to human habitation and could be unsafe for the next 24,000 years. On March 11, 2011, a 9.0 magnitude earthquake 15 miles below Japan's Honshu Island, followed by a powerful tsunami, rocked Japan's northern Fukushima Prefecture and severely damaged the Fukushima Daiichi nuclear power plant complex. Seawater was used to cool the damaged reactors, resulting in the largest release of radiation into the Pacific Ocean in history. All nuclear plants in Japan

> **endocrine-disrupting chemicals (EDCs)** **TERMS**
> Chemicals that disrupt the hormone systems of organisms.
>
> **nuclear power** The use of controlled nuclear reactions to produce steam, which in turn drives turbines to produce electricity.

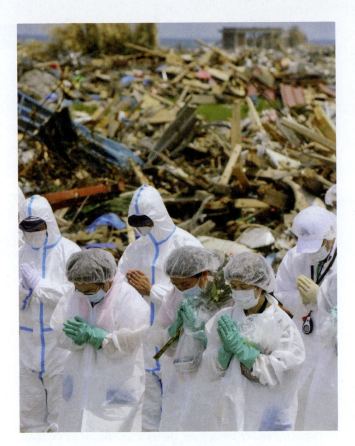

The 2011 Fukushima Daiichi nuclear disaster occurred when a tsunami, following a massive earthquake, flooded the low-lying rooms in which the plant's emergency generators were housed. The plant overheated, causing full meltdown in three of the six reactors.

© Kyodo/AP Images

were shut down until August 2015. Fisheries in the nearby area were also closed due to concern of exposure to radiation.

An additional enormous problem is disposing of the radioactive wastes these plants generate. To date, no storage method has been devised that can provide infallible, infinitely durable shielding for nuclear waste. Despite these problems, nuclear power is gaining favor again as an alternative to fossil fuels.

Medical Uses of Radiation

Another area of concern is the use of radiation in medicine, primarily in X-rays. Studies revealed that X-ray exposure is cumulative and that no level of exposure is absolutely safe. From a personal health point of view, no one should ever have a "routine" X-ray examination; each such exam should have a definite purpose, and its benefits and risks should be weighed carefully.

Radiation in the Home and Workplace

Recently there has been concern about electromagnetic radiation associated with common modern devices such as microwave ovens, computer monitors, and even high-voltage power lines. These forms of radiation do have effects on health, but research results are inconclusive.

Another controversial issue today is the effect of radiation from cell phones on health. Cell phones use electromagnetic waves (radio frequency radiation) to send and receive signals. This radiation is not directional, meaning that it travels in all directions equally, including toward the user. Factors such as the type of digital signal coding in the network, the antenna and handset design, and the position of the phone relative to the head all determine how much radiation is absorbed by a user. Studies to date have not provided conclusive evidence that cell phone use exposes users to harmful levels of radiation.

Another area of concern is **radon,** a naturally occurring radioactive gas found in certain soils, rocks, and building materials.

Avoiding Radiation

• Get only X-rays that you need, and keep a record of the date and location of every X-ray exam. Don't have a full-body CT (computed tomography) scan for routine screening; the radiation dose of one full-body CT scan is nearly 100 times that of a typical mammogram.

• Follow government recommendations for radon testing.

• Use sunscreen to protect yourself from the sun's UV radiation.

Ask Yourself

QUESTIONS FOR CRITICAL THINKING AND REFLECTION

Do you live in an area where radon is a problem? If so, has your home been checked for radon?

NOISE POLLUTION

Prolonged exposure to sounds above 80–85 **decibels** (a measure of the intensity of a sound wave) can cause permanent hearing loss. Hearing damage can occur after eight hours of exposure to sounds louder than 80 decibels. Regular exposure for longer than one minute to more than 100 decibels can cause permanent hearing loss. Children may suffer damage to their hearing at lower noise levels than those at which adults suffer damage.

Two common sources of excessive noise are the workplace and large gatherings of people at sporting events, rock concerts, and movie theaters. The Occupational Safety and Health Administration (OSHA) sets legal standards for noise in the workplace, but no laws exist regulating noise levels at concerts, which can be much louder than most workplaces.

TERMS

radon A naturally occurring radioactive gas emitted from rocks and natural building materials that can become concentrated in insulated homes, causing lung cancer.

decibel A unit for expressing the relative intensity of sounds on a scale from 0 for the average least-perceptible sound to about 120 for the average pain threshold.

Here are some ways to avoid exposing yourself to excessive noise:

• Wear ear protectors when working around noisy machinery.

• When listening to music on a headset with a volume range of 1–10, keep the volume no louder than 6. Your headset is too loud if you are unable to hear people around you speaking in a normal tone of voice. Earmuff-style headphones may be easier on the ears than earbuds, which are inserted into the ear canal. Experts warn that earbuds should not be used more than 30 minutes a day unless the volume is set below 60% of maximum; headphones can be used up to one hour.

• Avoid toys for children that make loud noise.

• Avoid loud music. Don't sit or stand near speakers or amplifiers at a concert, and don't play a car radio or stereo so high that you can't hear the traffic.

Ask Yourself

QUESTIONS FOR CRITICAL THINKING AND REFLECTION

How often do you listen to loud music? Do you ever use headphones? At what volume level do you like to listen? Do you think your listening habits pose a threat to your hearing? Would you let a child listen at the same volume level?

TIPS FOR TODAY AND THE FUTURE

Environmental health involves protecting yourself from environmental dangers and protecting the environment from the dangers created by humans.

RIGHT NOW YOU CAN:

- Turn off the lights, televisions, and stereos in any unoccupied rooms.
- Turn off power strips when not in use.
- Turn down the heat a few degrees and put on a sweater, or turn off the air conditioner and change into cooler clothes.
- Check your trash for recyclable items and take them out for recycling. If your town does not provide curbside pickup for recyclable items, find out the location of the nearest community recycling center.

IN THE FUTURE YOU CAN:

- Replace burned-out lightbulbs with halogen, LED, or compact fluorescent lightbulbs.
- Have your car checked to make sure it runs as well as it can and puts out the lowest amount of polluting emissions possible.
- Go online and find one of the many calculators available that can help you estimate your environmental footprint. After calculating your footprint, figure out ways to reduce it.

SUMMARY

• Environmental health encompasses all the interactions of humans with their environment and the health consequences of those interactions.

• The world's population is increasing rapidly, especially in the developing world. Factors that may eventually limit human population are food, availability of land and water, energy, and a minimum acceptable standard of living.

• Environmental damage from energy use and production can be limited through energy conservation and the development of nonpolluting, renewable sources of energy.

• Increased amounts of air pollutants are especially dangerous for children, older adults, and people with chronic health problems.

• Factors contributing to the development of smog include heavy motor vehicle traffic, hot weather, and stagnant air.

• Carbon dioxide and other natural gases act as a greenhouse around the earth, increasing the temperature of the atmosphere. Levels of these gases are rising through human activity; as a result, the world's climate is changing.

• The ozone layer that shields the earth's surface from the sun's UV rays has thinned and developed holes in certain regions.

• Indoor pollutants can trigger allergies and illness in the short term and chronic disease in the long term.

• Concerns with water quality focus on pathogenic organisms and hazardous chemicals from industry and households, as well as on water shortages.

• Sewage treatment prevents pathogens from contaminating drinking water; it often must also deal with heavy metals and hazardous chemicals.

• The amount of garbage is growing all the time; paper is the biggest component. Recycling can help reduce solid waste disposal problems.

• Potentially hazardous chemical pollutants include asbestos, lead, pesticides, mercury, and many household products. Proper handling and disposal are critical.

• Radiation can cause radiation sickness, chromosome damage, and cancer, among other health problems.

• Loud or persistent noise can lead to hearing loss and/or stress; two common sources of excessive noise are the workplace and rock concerts.

FOR MORE INFORMATION

Breathing Earth. Provides a simulation based on carbon dioxide emissions and birth and death rates.

http://www.breathingearth.net

CDC National Center for Environmental Health. Provides brochures and fact sheets about a variety of environmental issues.

http://www.cdc.gov/nceh/default.htm

Ecological Footprint. Calculates your personal ecological footprint based on your diet, transportation patterns, and living arrangements.

http://www.myfootprint.org

Fuel Economy. Provides information about the fuel economy of cars made since 1985 and tips on improving gas mileage.

http://www.fueleconomy.gov

Indoor Air Quality Information Hotline. Answers questions, provides publications, and makes referrals.

800-438-4318

National Lead Information Center. Provides information packets and specialist advice.

http://www.epa.gov/lead

National Oceanic and Atmospheric Administration (NOAA): Climate. Provides information about a variety of issues related to climate, including global warming, drought, and El Niño and La Niña.

http://www.noaa.gov/climate.html

National Safety Council. Provides information about lead, radon, indoor air quality, hazardous chemicals, and other environmental issues.

http://www.nsc.org/pages/home.aspx

The Post Carbon Institute: The Post Carbon Reader. A collection of diverse and provocative articles on pressing environmental problems and what can be done about them.

http://www.postcarbon.org/pcr

Student Environmental Action Coalition (SEAC). A coalition of student and youth environmental groups; the website has contact information for local groups.

http://www.seac.org

TEDX, The Endocrine Disruption Exchange. Information about endocrine-disrupting chemicals, the prenatal origins of diseases, natural gas extraction, and pesticides.

http://endocrinedisruption.org

United Nations. Several UN programs are devoted to environmental problems on a global scale; the websites provide information about current and projected trends and about international treaties developed to deal with environmental issues.

http://www.un.org/popin (Population Information Network)

http://www.unep.org (Environment Programme)

U.S. Department of Energy: Energy Efficiency and Renewable Energy (EERE). Provides information about alternative fuels and tips for saving energy at home and in your car.

http://energy.gov/eere/office-energy-efficiency-renewable-energy

U.S. Environmental Protection Agency (EPA). Provides information about EPA activities and many consumer-oriented materials. The website includes special sites devoted to global warming, ozone loss, pesticides, and other areas of concern.

http://www.epa.gov

Worldwatch Institute. A public policy research organization focusing on emerging global environmental problems and the links between the world economy and the environment.

http://www.worldwatch.org

Yale Environment 360. An online magazine offering opinion, analysis, reporting, and debate on global environmental issues.

http://e360.yale.edu

SELECTED BIBLIOGRAPHY

Aelion, C. M., et al. 2013. Associations between soil lead concentrations and populations by race/ethnicity and income-to-poverty ratio in urban and rural areas. *Environmental Geochemistry and Health* 35(1): 1–12.

American Lung Association. 2016. *State of the Air, 2016* (http://www.lung.org/our-initiatives/healthy-air/sota/).

Caiazzo, F., et al. 2013. Air pollution and early deaths in the United States. Part I: Quantifying the impact of major sectors in 2005. *Atmospheric Environment* 79: 198–208.

Centers for Disease Control and Prevention. 2015. Blood lead levels in children aged 1–5 years—United States, 2007–2012. *MMWR* 62(24): 76–80.

Centers for Disease Control and Prevention. 2015. Surveillance for waterborne disease outbreaks associated with drinking water—United States, 2011–2012. *MMWR* 64(31): 842–848.

Centers for Disease Control and Prevention. 2016. *Lead* (http://www.cdc.gov/nceh/lead).

De Coster, S., and N. vanLarebeke. 2012. Endocrine-disrupting chemicals: Associated disorders and mechanisms of action. *Journal of Environmental and Public Health,* September 6.

Grasso, M. et al. 2012. The health effects of climate change: A survey of recent quantitative research. *International Journal of Environmental Research and Public Health* 9(5): 1523–1547.

Hatta-Attisha, M., et al. 2016. Elevated blood lead levels in children associated with the Flint drinking water crisis: A spatial analysis of risk and public health response. *American Journal of Public Health* 106(2): 283–290.

Lovell, J. 2016. Q&A: What really happened to the water in Flint, Michigan? *Scientific American* (http://www.scientificamerican.com/article/q-a-what-really-happened-to-the-water-in-flint-michigan/).

Melillo, J. M., T. C. Richmond, and G. W. Yohe, Eds. 2014. *Climate Change Impacts in the United States: The Third National Climate Assessment* (http://nca2014.globalchange.gov).

Moynihan, T. 2014. *Is There Any Link between Cellphones and Cancer?* Mayo Clinic (http://www.mayoclinic.org/healthy-living/adult-health/expert-answers/cell-phones-and-cancer/faq-20057798?footprints=mine).

Petersen, M. D. et al. 2016. *One-Year Seismic Hazard Forecast for the Central and Eastern United States from Induced and Natural Earthquakes.* U.S. Geological Survey (https://pubs.er.usgs.gov/publication/ofr20161035).

Solomon, S., et al. 2016. Emergence of healing in the Antarctic ozone layer. *Science,* June 30 (epub ahead of print).

U.S. Census Bureau. 2014. *National Population Projections* (http://www.census.gov/population/projections/data/national).

U.S. Energy Information Administration. 2015. *Gasoline and Diesel Fuel Update* (http://www.eia.gov/petroleum/gasdiesel/).

U.S. Energy Information Administration. 2016. *How Many Nuclear Power Plants Are in the United States, and Where Are They Located?* (https://www.eia.gov/tools/faqs/faq.cfm?id=207&t=3).

U.S. Energy Information Administration. 2016. *How Much Oil Is Consumed in the United States?* (https://www.eia.gov/tools/faqs/faq.cfm?id=33&t=6)

U.S. Energy Information Administration. 2016. *International Energy Outlook 2016* (www.eia.gov/forecasts/ieo).

U.S. Energy Information Administration. 2016. *International Energy Statistics: Total Petroleum Consumption 2015* (http://www.eia.gov/beta/international/).

U.S. Environmental Protection Agency. 2014. *Municipal Solid Waste* (http://www.epa.gov/waste/nonhaz/municipal/index.htm).

U.S. Environmental Protection Agency. 2015. *Advancing Sustainable Materials Management: 2013 Fact Sheet* (Pub. No. EPA530-R-15-003). Washington, DC: EPA.

U.S. Environmental Protection Agency. 2016. *Superfund: National Priorities List* (https://www.epa.gov/superfund/superfund-national-priorities-list-npl).

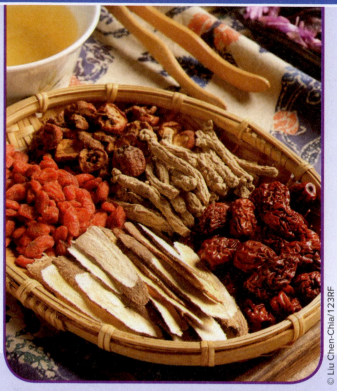
© Liu Chen-Chia/123RF

CHAPTER 15

CHAPTER OBJECTIVES

- Explain options for self-care
- Explain options for professional care
- Describe the practices of conventional medicine
- Describe integrative health practices
- Understand the costs of health care and how to pay for it

Conventional and Complementary Medicine

Today people are becoming more empowered and confident in their ability to solve personal health problems on their own. People who manage their own health care gather information and learn skills from a variety of resources. They solicit opinions and advice in order to practice safe, effective self-care, and to make decisions about seeking professional medical care—whether conventional Western medicine or complementary and alternative medicine.

This chapter will help you develop skills needed to identify and manage medical problems and to make the health care system work effectively for you.

SELF-CARE

Effectively managing medical problems involves developing several skills. First, you need to learn to be a good observer of your own body and assess your symptoms. You also must be able to decide when to seek professional advice and when you can safely deal with a problem on your own. You need to know how to safely and effectively self-treat

common medical problems. Finally, you need to know how to develop a partnership with physicians and other health care providers and how to implement treatment plans.

Self-Assessment

Symptoms are often an expression of the body's attempt to heal itself. For example, the pain and swelling that occur after an ankle injury immobilize and protect the injured joint so that healing can take place. A fever may be an attempt to inhibit the growth and reproduction of infectious agents. A cough can help clear the airways and protect the lungs.

Carefully observing symptoms also helps you identify signals that indicate you need professional help. You should begin by noting when a symptom begins, how often and when it occurs, what makes it worse, what makes it better, and whether you have any associated symptoms or illnesses. You can also monitor your body's vital signs, such as temperature and heart rate. Medical self-tests for blood pressure, blood sugar, pregnancy detection, and urinary tract infections can also help you make a more informed decision about when to seek medical help and when to self-treat.

Knowing When to See a Physician

In general, you should see a physician for symptoms that you would describe as follows:

- *Severe.* If the symptom is severe or intense, medical assistance is advised. Examples include severe pains, major injuries, and other emergencies.

- *Unusual.* If the symptom is peculiar and unfamiliar, it is wise to check it out with your physician. Examples include unexplained lumps, changes in a mole, problems with vision, difficulty swallowing, numbness, weakness, unexplained weight loss, or blood in the sputum, urine, or stool.

- *Persistent.* If the symptom lasts longer than expected, seek medical advice. Examples in adults include fever for more than five days, a cough lasting longer than two weeks, a sore that doesn't heal within a month, and hoarseness lasting longer than three weeks.

- *Recurrent.* If a symptom returns again and again, medical evaluation is advised. Examples include recurrent headaches, abdominal pain, and backache.

Sometimes a single symptom is not a cause for concern, but when the symptom is accompanied by other symptoms, the combination suggests a more serious problem. For example, a fever accompanied by neck pain can suggest meningitis.

If you evaluate your symptoms and think you need professional help, you must decide how urgent the problem is. If it is a true emergency, you should go (or ask someone to take you) to the nearest hospital emergency department. Emergencies include the following:

- Major trauma or injury especially to the head, a suspected broken bone, deep wound, severe burn, eye injury, or animal bite

- Uncontrollable bleeding or internal bleeding, as indicated by blood in the sputum, vomit, or stool

- Intolerable and uncontrollable pain or severe chest pain

- Severe shortness of breath

- Persistent abdominal pain, especially if associated with nausea and vomiting

- Poisoning or drug overdose

- Sudden numbness, weakness, or loss of function involving an arm or leg, speech difficulty, or drooping of the face

- Seizure or loss of consciousness

- Stupor, drowsiness, or disorientation that cannot be explained

- Severe or worsening reaction to an insect bite or sting, or to a medication or food, especially if accompanied by swelling of the lips, mouth, or throat, or difficulty breathing

If your problem is not an emergency but still requires medical attention, call your physician's office or contact the office's online interactive website, if available. Often you can be given medical advice over the phone or online without needing a clinical visit.

Self-Treatment

In most cases, your body can relieve your symptoms and heal the disorder. The prescriptions filled by your body's "internal pharmacy" are frequently the safest and most effective treatment, so patience and careful self-observation are often the best choices in self-treatment.

Nondrug Options Nondrug options are often easy, inexpensive, safe, and highly effective. For example, ice packs, massage, gentle yoga stretching, and neck exercises may at times be more helpful than drugs in relieving headaches and other pains. Getting adequate rest, increasing exercise, drinking more water, eating more or less of certain foods, using humidifiers, and changing ergonomics when sitting or working are some of the hundreds of nondrug options for preventing or relieving many common health problems. For a variety of disorders caused or aggravated by stress, the treatment of choice may be relaxation or other stress management strategies.

Self-Medication Self-treatment with nonprescription medications is an important part of health care. Nonprescription, or **over-the-counter (OTC), medications** are medicines that the U.S. Food and Drug Administration (FDA) has determined are safe to take without a prescription when used according to label directions.

Hundreds of products sold over-the-counter today use ingredients or dosage strengths that were available only by prescription 20 years ago. With this increased consumer choice, however, consumers have increased responsibility for using OTC drugs safely.

Although many OTC products are effective, others are unnecessary or divert attention from better ways of coping. Many ingredients in OTC drugs—an estimated 70%—have not been proven to be effective, a fact the FDA recognizes. And any drug may have risks and side effects.

Follow these simple guidelines to self-medicate safely:

- Always read labels and follow directions carefully. The information on most OTC drug labels now appears in a standard format developed by the FDA (Figure 15.1). Ingredients, directions for safe use, and warnings are clearly indicated. If you have any questions, ask a pharmacist or a qualified health care provider before using a product.

- Do not exceed the recommended dosage or length of treatment unless you discuss this with your health care provider.

> **over-the-counter (OTC) medication** A medication or product that can be purchased by a consumer without a prescription.
>
> **TERMS**

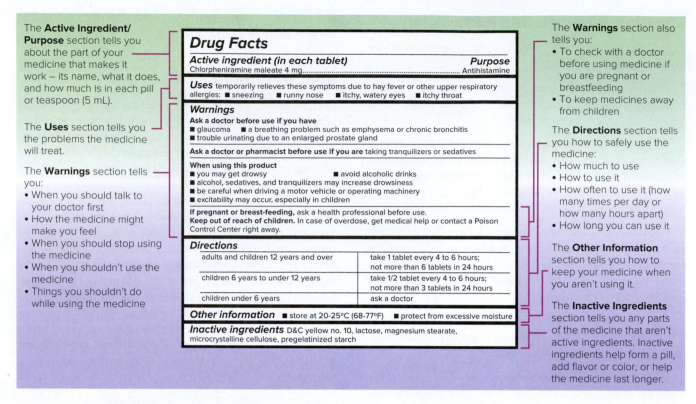

The **Active Ingredient/ Purpose** section tells you about the part of your medicine that makes it work – its name, what it does, and how much is in each pill or teaspoon (5 mL).

The **Uses** section tells you the problems the medicine will treat.

The **Warnings** section tells you:
- When you should talk to your doctor first
- How the medicine might make you feel
- When you should stop using the medicine
- When you shouldn't use the medicine
- Things you shouldn't do while using the medicine

The **Warnings** section also tells you:
- To check with a doctor before using medicine if you are pregnant or breastfeeding
- To keep medicines away from children

The **Directions** section tells you how to safely use the medicine:
- How much to use
- How to use it
- How often to use it (how many times per day or how many hours apart)
- How long you can use it

The **Other Information** section tells you how to keep your medicine when you aren't using it.

The **Inactive Ingredients** section tells you any parts of the medicine that aren't active ingredients. Inactive ingredients help form a pill, add flavor or color, or help the medicine last longer.

Drug Facts

Active ingredient (in each tablet)	Purpose
Chlorpheniramine maleate 4 mg..	Antihistamine

Uses temporarily relieves these symptoms due to hay fever or other upper respiratory allergies: ■ sneezing ■ runny nose ■ itchy, watery eyes ■ itchy throat

Warnings

Ask a doctor before use if you have
- ■ glaucoma ■ a breathing problem such as emphysema or chronic bronchitis
- ■ trouble urinating due to an enlarged prostate gland

Ask a doctor or pharmacist before use if you are taking tranquilizers or sedatives

When using this product
- ■ you may get drowsy ■ avoid alcoholic drinks
- ■ alcohol, sedatives, and tranquilizers may increase drowsiness
- ■ be careful when driving a motor vehicle or operating machinery
- ■ excitability may occur, especially in children

If pregnant or breast-feeding, ask a health professional before use.
Keep out of reach of children. In case of overdose, get medical help or contact a Poison Control Center right away.

Directions

adults and children 12 years and over	take 1 tablet every 4 to 6 hours; not more than 6 tablets in 24 hours
children 6 years to under 12 years	take 1/2 tablet every 4 to 6 hours; not more than 3 tablets in 24 hours
children under 6 years	ask a doctor

Other information ■ store at 20-25°C (68-77°F) ■ protect from excessive moisture

Inactive ingredients D&C yellow no. 10, lactose, magnesium stearate, microcrystalline cellulose, pregelatinized starch

FIGURE 15.1 **Reading and understanding OTC drug labels.**

SOURCE: U.S. Food and Drug Administration. 2015. Protecting and promoting your health.

- Use caution if you are taking other medications or supplements because OTC drugs and herbal supplements can interact with some prescription drugs. If you have questions about drug interactions, ask your health care provider or pharmacist *before* you take medicines in combination.

- Try to select medications with one active ingredient rather than a combination. A product with multiple ingredients is likely to include drugs for symptoms you don't have, which can increase side effects. Using single-ingredient products also allows you to adjust the dosage of each medication separately for optimal symptom relief with minimal side effects.

- When choosing medications, try to buy **generic drugs,** which contain the same active ingredient as brand-name products but generally at a much lower cost.

- Never take or give a drug from an unlabeled container or when you can't read the label.

- If you are pregnant or nursing or have a chronic condition such as kidney or liver disease, consult your health care provider before self-medicating.

- The expiration date marked on many medications is an estimate of how long the medication is likely to be safe and effective. However, an extensive study by the FDA found that 90% of all prescription and OTC medications are potent well after their stated expiration dates. Exceptions include tetracycline and other antibiotics, nitroglycerine, and insulin. Expiration dates are very conservative. If you have any questions about a medicine's expiration date, ask a pharmacist.

- Store your medications in a cool, dry place away from direct light and out of the reach of children.

- Use special caution with aspirin. Because of an association with a rare but serious problem known as Reye's syndrome, aspirin should not be used by children or adolescents who may have the flu, chickenpox, or any other viral illness. Outdated aspirin that has an acidic odor should be discarded.

generic drug A drug that is not registered or protected by a commercial trademark; a drug that does not have an exclusive brand name.

TERMS

Ask Yourself

QUESTIONS FOR CRITICAL THINKING AND REFLECTION

Do you often self-medicate for common medical problems, such as headaches or colds? If so, how careful are you about reading product labels and following directions? For example, would you know if you were taking two OTC medications that contained the same ingredient (such as acetaminophen or ibuprofen) at the same time?

PROFESSIONAL CARE

When self-care is not appropriate or sufficient, you need to seek professional medical care, whether by going to a hospital emergency department, or by scheduling an appointment by phone or online with your physician or another conventional health care provider. In recent years, the majority of Americans have also sought health care from practitioners of **complementary and alternative medicine (CAM)**—defined as those therapies and practices that do not form part of **conventional medicine,** which is defined as mainstream health care and medical practices taught in most U.S. medical schools and offered in most U.S. hospitals. The most frequently used CAM therapies are nonvitamin, nonmineral dietary supplements; deep breathing exercises; yoga, tai chi, and qigong; chiropractic, osteopathic manipulative treatment; meditation; massage therapy; and special diets (Table 15.1). According to the most recent Centers for Disease Control and Prevention (CDC) report, 33.2% of adults in the United States use some form of CAM. Among those who do, at least 83% use it together with conventional medicine, not in place of it.

The term *CAM* includes both the terms **complementary** and **alternative medicine:** "Complementary" means an approach that combines nonmainstream and conventional medicine. "Alternative" refers to an approach that replaces conventional medicine.

Another term, *integrative medicine,* has become widely accepted in the United States. **Integrative health** is the preferred term to use when discussing treatment options that include CAM with conventional providers or that *add* unconventional methods to conventional ones. In integrative health it is understood that conventional methods are given priority, and a CAM *modality* (technique or form), may be included if it could have additional benefits.

Consumers turn to integrative health or CAM for a variety of purposes related to health and well-being, such as boosting the immune system, lowering cholesterol levels, losing weight, quitting smoking, or enhancing memory. People with chronic conditions, including cancer, asthma, autoimmune diseases, and HIV infection, are particularly likely to try CAM therapies. Despite their popularity, many CAM practices remain controversial, and consumers need to be critically aware of safety issues. The NCCAM (now NCCIH) was established in 1992 to apply rigorous scientific methodology and standards for proving or disproving the safety and effectiveness of CAM.

The following sections examine the principles used by providers of both conventional medicine—the dominant medical system in the United States and Europe, also referred to as *standard Western medicine* or *biomedicine*—and integrative health and CAM, with particular attention to consumer issues.

Table 15.1	Use of Complementary and Alternative Therapies by Adults, 2012	
TYPE OF THERAPY		**PERCENTAGE WHO USED THERAPY IN PAST 12 MONTHS**
Nonvitamin, nonmineral dietary supplements		17.7
Deep breathing exercises		10.9
Yoga, tai chi, and qigong		10.1
Chiropractic or osteopathic manipulation		8.4
Meditation		8.0
Massage therapy		6.9
Special diets		3.0
Homeopathic treatment		2.2
Progressive relaxation		2.1
Guided imagery		1.7
Acupuncture		1.5
Energy healing therapy		0.5
Naturopathy		0.4
Hypnosis		0.1
Biofeedback		0.1
Ayurveda		0.1

SOURCE: Clarke, T.C., et al. 2015. Trends in the use of complementary health approaches among adults: United States, 2002–2012. *National Health Statistics Reports* 79: 1–16. Centers for Disease Control and Prevention, National Center for Health Statistics.

Ask Yourself

QUESTIONS FOR CRITICAL THINKING AND REFLECTION

What are your views about the use of CAM therapies? What events or information has shaped those views? Would you consider using complementary or alternative medicine?

TERMS

complementary and alternative medicine (CAM) Health care practices and products that are not considered part of conventional, mainstream medical practice as taught in most U.S. medical schools and that are not available at most U.S. health care facilities; examples of CAM practices include acupuncture and herbal remedies.

conventional medicine A system of medicine emphasizing biological and physical scientific principles; diseases are thought to be caused by identifiable physical factors and characterized by a representative set of signs and symptoms; also called *biomedicine* or *standard Western medicine.*

complementary medicine Unconventional medical practices that are used together with conventional ones.

alternative medicine Unconventional medical practices that are used instead of conventional methods.

integrative health Conventional health care practice that is sometimes augmented by adding unconventional (CAM) modalities if they could benefit the patient.

CONVENTIONAL MEDICINE

Referring to conventional medicine as "standard Western medicine" draws attention to the fact that it differs from the various medical systems that have developed in China, Japan, India, and other parts of the world. Calling it "biomedicine" reflects conventional medicine's foundation in the biological and physical sciences.

Premises and Assumptions of Conventional Medicine

One of the important characteristics of Western medicine is the belief that disease is caused by identifiable and reproducible factors. Western medicine identifies the causes of disease as pathogens (such as bacteria and viruses), physical factors (such as trauma or toxins), genetic factors, or unhealthy lifestyles that result in changes at the cellular and molecular levels. In most cases, the focus is primarily on the physical causes of illness rather than on mental or spiritual imbalance.

Another feature that distinguishes Western biomedicine from other medical systems is the concept that almost every disease is defined by a certain set of signs (*objective* physical manifestations) and symptoms (*subjective* effects perceived by an individual), and that they are similar in most patients suffering from the disease. Western medicine tends to treat diseases as biological disturbances occurring in a patient rather than as the result of mind, body, and spirit interactions.

A disease can be caused by either internal or external factors. Internal factors include anatomic or physiologic abnormalities, and defective genetic, hormonal, and immune mechanisms. External causes include infections by bacteria

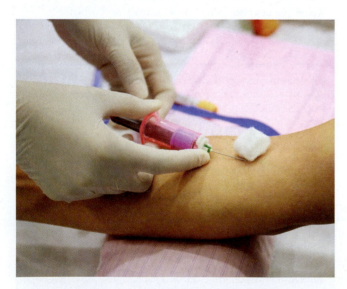

One feature that distinguishes Western biomedicine from other medical systems is the concept that almost every disease is defined by a certain set of signs and symptoms and that they are similar in most patients suffering from the disease.

© Wathanyu Sowong/123RF

and viruses, and some cases of traumatic injury. The public health measures of the 19th and 20th centuries—chlorination of drinking water, sewage disposal, food safety regulations, vaccination programs, education about hygiene, and so on—were an outgrowth of this orientation.

The implementation of public health measures is one way to control diseases; others include preventive lifestyle measures and the use of drugs and surgery. The discovery and development of sulfa drugs, antibiotics, and steroids in the 20th century, along with advances in chemistry that made it possible to identify the active ingredients in common plant-derived remedies, paved the way for the current close identification of Western medicine with **pharmaceuticals** (medical drugs, both prescription and over-the-counter). Western medicine also relies heavily on surgery and advanced medical technology to discover the physical cause of an individual's disease and to correct, remove, or destroy it.

Further, Western medicine is based on the scientific method for obtaining knowledge and explaining health-related phenomena using scientific explanations that have these characteristics:

- *Empirical.* They are based on the evidence of the senses and on objective and systematic observation, often carried out under carefully controlled conditions; they must be capable of verification by others through objective observation, which may include the use of technology (such as lab tests and physical measurement, such as blood pressure).

- *Rational.* They follow the rules of logic and are consistent with known facts.

- *Testable.* Either they are verifiable through objective observation or they lead to predictions about what should occur under defined, controlled conditions (as in randomized controlled trials).

- *Parsimonious.* They explain phenomena using the fewest causes.

- *Generality.* They can explain phenomena among other patients who have similar signs and symptoms.

- *Rigorously evaluated.* They are continuously evaluated for agreement with the evidence and known principles of parsimony and generality.

- *Tentative.* Scientists are willing to entertain the possibility that their conclusions may be faulty if new and better evidence becomes available.

Western medicine uses the scientific method in health care practice by applying the research process, a highly refined and well-established approach to exploring the causes of disease and ensuring the safety and efficacy of treatments. Research ranges from case studies—descriptions of a single

| **pharmaceuticals** Medical drugs, both prescription and over-the-counter. | **TERMS** |

patient's illness and treatment—to **randomized controlled trials (RCTs)** conducted on large populations; RCTs are considered the highest level of evidence for treatment outcomes. Conclusions made based on an RCT may be enhanced by a relatively new standard of evidence, a **meta-analysis,** which mathematically combines data from two or more methodologically similar RCTs. If several RCTs show marginal or questionable conclusions, a meta-analysis determines which way "the scale will tip" by statistically combining the data from the studies.

When results of research studies are published in medical journals, the community of scientists, physicians, researchers, and scholars has the opportunity to share the findings and enter a dialogue about the subject. Publication of research often prompts further research designed to replicate and confirm the findings, challenge the conclusions, or pursue related lines of thought or experimentation. (For guidelines on how to interpret research when it is reported in the popular media, see the box "Evaluating Health News.")

Pharmaceuticals and the Placebo Effect

In medical research, a placebo is often used when evaluating a new drug in a controlled trial (see Figure 15.2). A *placebo* is a biologically inactive substance that the subject or the experimenter cannot distinguish from the experimental drug. (For studies that don't involve drugs, such as surgery or acupuncture, a *sham* procedure is used.) Either the experimental treatment or a placebo or sham procedure is administered randomly to subjects who are unaware which they are receiving (a "blinded" trial). By comparing the effects of the experimental treatment with the effects of the placebo or sham, researchers can evaluate whether the experimental treatment is more effective than the placebo.

Researchers have consistently found that 30–40% of all patients given a placebo show some improvement. A *placebo effect* occurs when a research subject improves after receiving a placebo; the placebo effect is the difference in outcome compared to no intervention at all (no placebo and no experimental treatment). The *treatment effect* is the difference in outcome between the placebo and the experimental treatment. If the subject does not respond better to the experimental treatment compared to the placebo, then the improvement cannot be attributed to the specific actions or properties of the drug or procedure. The new science of psychoneuroimmunology (PNI) helps explain why and how the body responds to placebos, which were once considered neutral non-interventions (see Chapter 2 for more about PNI).

A placebo effect has been observed in treatment of a wide variety of conditions or symptoms, including coughing, seasickness, depression, migraines, and angina. In some cases, people given a placebo even report having the side effects associated with an actual drug.

When a skilled and compassionate medical practitioner administers a proven-effective treatment while providing the patient with a sense of confidence and hope, the positive aspects of the placebo effect can add to the benefits of the treatment—a combined treatment and placebo effect. Getting well, like getting sick, is a complex process. Anatomy, physiology, emotions, hope, beliefs, expectations, and prior experiences all contribute to the way the body reacts to medical treatments and utilizes its own healing mechanisms.

The Providers of Conventional Medicine

Conventional medicine is practiced by a wide range of health care professionals in the United States. Several kinds of professionals are permitted to practice specific fields of medicine independently, including medical doctors, osteopaths, dentists, podiatrists, and optometrists.

• **Medical doctors** are practitioners who hold a doctor of medicine (MD) degree from an accredited medical school. They are commonly called "allopathic" physicians because of their historical practice philosophy: Treatment with

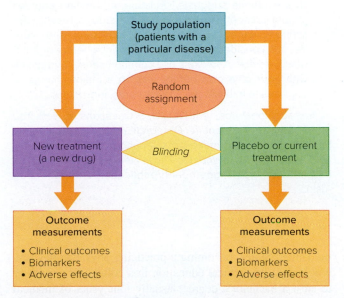

FIGURE 15.2 How a randomized control trial works.

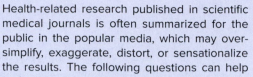

TAKE CHARGE
Evaluating Health News

Health-related research published in scientific medical journals is often summarized for the public in the popular media, which may over-simplify, exaggerate, distort, or sensationalize the results. The following questions can help you evaluate the health information about conventional medicine and CAM that you will likely encounter in popular media:

1. *Is the report based on scientific studies?* Information or advice based on carefully designed research studies has more validity than opinions, anecdotes, or casual observations.

2. *What is the source of the information?* A study published in a respected peer-reviewed scientific journal has been examined by editors and researchers who are professionally prepared to evaluate the merits of a study and its results, and its application to actual patients. Most journals include information on the funding source and the authors' affiliations that may introduce a bias or conflict of interest. Studies sponsored by drug companies or other commercial groups are suspect. Sources sponsored by universities, government agencies, professional groups (such as WebMD), and others that are rigorously peer-reviewed typically base their reports on scientific information and are considered more valid than commercial websites. Wikipedia is not considered a scientifically valid resource. When health information is critical, the consumer should review the original reference rather than rely solely on secondary interpretations.

3. *How many subjects were included in the study?* A study involving many subjects—hundreds or thousands of people—is more likely to yield reliable results than a study involving only a few subjects. Most quality studies include a "statistical power analysis" section that specifies how many subjects were necessary in order for the findings to be meaningful.

4. *Who were the subjects?* Research findings are more likely to apply to you if you share important characteristics with the study participants. For example, the results of a study on male smokers over age 60 may not be particularly meaningful for a 25-year-old female nonsmoker.

5. *What kind of study was it?* Randomized controlled trials and meta-analyses are considered the most valid. Epidemiological studies (which involve noncontrolled observations) may suggest useful information, but they cannot always establish cause-and-effect relationships. The following questions may help you to decide whether a study's results should be considered valid:

   • *Were the treatment group results compared to those of a control group or an already accepted therapy?*

   • *Were the subjects randomly assigned to the experimental groups?*

   • *Was the study blinded (to the subjects, the experimenters/evaluators, or both)?*

   • *Was it a multicenter study?* A few high-quality randomized controlled trials are multicenter studies. The results of several studies conducted in different places at different times can be mathematically combined as a meta-analysis. A well-conducted meta-analysis is considered one of the most valid types of studies.

6. *What do the statistics really say?* Are the results statistically significant? Statistical significance is usually reported as a p-value; when it is less than or equal to 0.05 or 5%, it is considered "statistically significant," meaning there is a 5% or lower probability that the findings were the result of chance. Does the study have the required number of subjects according to a statistical power analysis? Some studies report the effect size instead of or in addition to a p-value. Most of the time the effect size is more revealing than the p-value.

   If study results are given in terms of relative risk—for example, a 50% reduction in the risk of developing a disorder—you should also consider the absolute risk of the condition. For example, if the absolute risk of developing a disorder is 2%, then a medication that reduced that risk by 50% (relative risk) would lower the risk to 1%: Out of 100 people *not taking* the medication, two on average would develop the disorder; out of 100 people *taking* the medication, one would develop the disorder.

7. Is new health advice being offered? If the media report new guidelines for health behavior or medical treatment, examine the source. Be suspicious of absolutes and overstated claims that use words such as "certainty," "always," and "never." Scientifically accurate reports use words such as "results show," "for many people," and "the evidence suggests." Reliable information sources should present the limitations of a study's results, describe how the results compare with those of other studies, and consider a great deal of evidence before offering health advice. Above all, use common sense, and check with your physician before making a major change in your health habits based on news reports.

For additional tips, visit NCCIH, *9 Questions to Help You Make Sense of Scientific Research (*https://nccih.nih.gov/health/know-science/make-sense-health-research), and NIH, *Understanding Risk: What Do Those Headlines Really Mean?* (https://www.nia.nih.gov/health/publication/understanding-risk).

---

opposites (the Greek prefix *allo-* means difference, or opposition). For example, if the body is too cold, add heat; if it's too warm, cool it down; if a patient is too stimulated, administer a tranquilizer; too tranquil, give a stimulant. In the United States, becoming a practicing physician has several stages: premedical education in a college or university to earn a bachelor's degree; usually four years of medical school, which teaches basic medical skills and awards the doctor of medicine degree; and three to eight years of graduate medical study that includes a residency and possibly a specialty fellowship.

- **Doctors of osteopathic medicine** (DO) receive formal premedical education to earn a bachelor's degree; four years of osteopathic medical school leading to the DO degree; and residency and fellowship education similar to that of allopathic medical doctors over a comparable timeframe. The osteopathic philosophy emphasizes structural and functional relationships and a whole-person approach to medicine. Like allopathic physicians, osteopathic physicians practice in all of the medical and surgical specialties and subspecialties, but osteopathic physicians may also practice and specialize in osteopathic manipulative treatment.

- **Dentists** focus on the care of the teeth and mouth. They are graduates of four-year dental schools and hold the doctor of dental surgery (DDS) or doctor of medical dentistry (DMD) degree.

- **Podiatrists** are practitioners who specialize in the medical and surgical care of the feet. They hold a doctor of podiatric medicine (DPM) degree.

- **Optometrists** are practitioners trained to examine the eyes, detect eye diseases, and treat certain vision problems, most often through the use of corrective lenses. They hold a doctor of optometry (OD) degree. **Ophthalmologists** have an MD or DO degree and serve a residency or fellowship specializing in diseases of the eye. They care for all types of eye problems using drugs and surgery.

- **Nurses** or *registered nurses (RNs)* are practitioners concerned with the diagnosis and treatment of human responses to actual or potential health problems. They act to promote, maintain, or restore health. A nurse may receive advanced education to become a nurse practitioner (NP), a certified registered nurse anesthetist (CRNA), or a certified nurse midwife (CNM).

- **Physician assistants** (PAs) are nationally certified and state-licensed health care professionals who practice medicine as part of a team with physicians.

In addition to these practitioners, there are millions of other highly educated health care professionals, including physical therapists, pharmacists, medical social workers, and registered dietitians.

Choosing a Primary Care Physician

Most experts believe it is best to have a primary care physician (PCP) who gets to know you, coordinates your medical care, and refers you to specialists when you need them. Some health care insurance plans require you to identify a PCP. The primary care disciplines include family practice, internal medicine, pediatrics, and gynecology.

Many physicians coordinate your care through highly trained medical professionals such as physician assistants and nurse practitioners. These professionals perform many services that have traditionally been provided by physicians, including taking medical histories, performing physical exams, ordering laboratory and imaging studies, prescribing medications, and performing minor surgery. They work as part of a team with your doctor and are frequently able to spend more time to provide patient education and answer detailed questions about your concerns, preventive measures, and lifestyle choices.

To select a PCP, begin by making a list of possible choices. If your insurance limits the health care providers you can see, check the plan's list first. If your health plan lets you choose a physician, ask for recommendations from family, friends, coworkers, local medical societies, and the physician referral service at a local clinic or hospital. Once you have a list of possible physicians, you might want to check

TERMS

doctor of osteopathic medicine A physician who holds the doctor of osteopathy (DO) degree from an accredited osteopathic medical school; osteopathy incorporates the theories and practices of scientific medicine and includes osteopathic manual treatment.

dentist A practitioner who holds a doctor of dental surgery (DDS) or doctor of medical dentistry (DMD) degree and whose practice includes the diagnosis, treatment, and prevention of diseases and injuries of the teeth, mouth, and jaws.

podiatrist A practitioner who holds a doctor of podiatric medicine (DPM) degree and specializes in the medical and surgical care of the feet.

optometrist A practitioner who holds a doctor of optometry (OD) degree and is trained to examine the eyes, detect eye diseases, and prescribe corrective lenses.

ophthalmologist A practitioner who holds an MD or DO degree, has served a residency or fellowship specializing in diseases of the eye, and cares for all types of eye problems using drugs and surgery.

nurse A licensed health provider who is concerned with the diagnosis and treatment of human responses to actual or potential health problems and acts to promote, maintain, or restore health. Registered Nurses (RN) complete a bachelor of nursing degree. Licensed practical and vocational nurses complete a one- or two-year training program (LPN, LVN).

physician assistant A health provider who is nationally certified and licensed by his or her state to practice medicine as part of a team with physicians.

online or call the offices of those on your list to find out the following:

- Is the physician covered by your health plan and accepting new patients?
- What are the office hours, and when is the physician or office staff available?
- What do patients do if they need urgent care or have an emergency?
- Which hospitals does the physician use?
- How many other physicians are available to cover when your PCP isn't available, and who are they?
- How long does it usually take to get a routine appointment?
- Does the office send reminders about preventive services and tests such as Pap tests?
- Does the physician (or a nurse or physician assistant) give advice online or over the phone for common problems and continued care of a diagnosed problem?

A physician's practice philosophy is another important factor; most clinics provide their physicians' personal statements in brochures or online. Schedule a visit with the physician you think you would most like to use.

Choosing a Specialist

Compared to finding your PCP, your choices in finding a specialist are more limited. If you need emergency care, you may have few or no options, although you may be able to go to an accredited emergency department of a hospital you trust. If possible, go to one your PCP recommends or in which he or she has hospital privileges. For non-emergencies you may be limited to specialists covered by your insurance plan.

You should be referred to a specialist when the services you need are outside the scope of your PCP's practice. The specialist may not be a physician but rather a physical therapist, audiologist, psychologist, or another type of practitioner. In general, physician specialists are from the internal medicine subdisciplines, such as dermatology, gastroenterology, and neurology, or from the surgical subdisciplines, such as thoracic surgery, orthopedics, and neurosurgery. Some subdisciplines involve both internal medicine and surgery (gynecology, urology, and ophthalmology).

By the time of your visit, the specialist should have received a referral note from your PCP, your complete medical record, and access to all your recent lab tests and imaging studies as well as past tests that may be significant (e.g., MRIs of the spine years earlier). If your specialist refers you to another specialist, you should visit your PCP first, to keep him or her up to date on your symptoms and to discuss any questions you have about the next step in your specialized care.

Getting the Most Out of Your Medical Care

The key to making the health care system work for you lies in good communication with your physician and other members of the health care team.

The Physician–Patient Partnership The image of the all-knowing physician and the passive patient is fading. What is emerging is a physician–patient *partnership* in which the physician acts more like a consultant and the patient participates more actively (see the box "Creating Your Own Health Record"). You should expect your physician to be attentive, caring, and able to listen and clearly explain health care matters to you. You also must do your part. You need to be assertive in a firm but nonaggressive manner. You need to express your feelings and concerns, ask questions, and, if necessary, be persistent. If your physician is unable to communicate clearly with you despite your best efforts, you probably need to change physicians.

Your Physician Appointments You may be offered the opportunity to see a physician assistant or nurse practitioner who works with your physician. Physicians are often pressed for time, so prepare for office visits by writing down your key concerns and questions, along with notes about your symptoms (when they started, how long they last, what makes them better or worse, what treatments you have already tried, and so on). Bring a list of all the medications you're taking—prescription, nonprescription, and herbal. Also bring any medical records or test results your physician may not already have.

Present your concerns at the beginning of the visit to set the agenda. Be specific and concise about your symptoms, and be open and honest about your concerns. Let your physician know if you are taking any drugs, are allergic to any medications, are breastfeeding, or may be pregnant. At the end of the visit, briefly repeat the physician's diagnosis, prognosis, the purpose of any tests, and instructions you have received to make sure you understand your next steps.

The Diagnostic Process The first step in the diagnostic process is the medical history, which includes primary reason for the visit, current symptoms, past medical history, and social history (job, family life, major stressors, living conditions, and health habits). Keeping up-to-date records of your medical history can help you provide your physician with key facts about your health.

Ask Yourself

QUESTIONS FOR CRITICAL THINKING AND REFLECTION
What sort of relationship do you have with your physician? Do you think he or she understands your needs and is familiar enough with your history? Are you satisfied with this relationship?

What's your blood pressure? How about cholesterol level? What medicines are you taking? Many Americans believe that their medical records are compiled and maintained by some mysterious entity (probably called "them"). But this is not the case. We each need to be responsible for compiling our important medical records and keeping them safe and easily available to us or a caregiver in case we need the records for an emergency, or when traveling, moving, or looking for a new primary care provider. The expanding use of computerized medical records may be useful within a particular clinic or health care system, but this does not mean that every person's individual medical history has been automatically collated into a single, easy-to-find source. Computerized health records maintained by one hospital or medical care system might not be accessible by another. Ultimately each individual is responsible for keeping track of her or his own health history and records. College is a good time to start doing this for yourself, and by sharing your health knowledge and assisting family members to do the same, you are playing a more active role in your family's health care.

Personal health records should be readily accessible in case of an emergency. Some personal computerized health record systems can be purchased online, or one can be devised individually. (You can find out about various personal health records on the U.S. government's HealthIT.gov website: http://www.healthit.gov/patients-families/maintain-your-medical-record#PHR.) Whether purchased or created individually, here's what your personal health record should contain:

- Your name, emergency contact, birth date, blood type, religious preference (if any), and the date this record was compiled or updated.

- All known allergies (including medications).

- A list of all chronic conditions and the dates of their diagnosis (e.g., diabetes, high blood pressure, asthma, emphysema).

- Any hereditary diseases.

- The names and dosages of all medications you take and reasons for taking them.

- The results of tests or procedures such as blood pressure, cholesterol, vision, and others.

- The dates and reasons for all past hospitalizations and operations. If the reasons were serious or may affect future treatments (e.g., major organ involvement; devices or materials implanted surgically), a hospital discharge summary should be included.

- The dates of physical exams and any major findings.

- Vaccination schedules.

- A print-out of all laboratory test results, and a written report of any imaging studies (e.g., X-rays, CT scans, MRIs), electrocardiograms (ECGs), and special tests such as audiograms and exercise stress tests. Check to verify that dates are included.

You have the right to all of your medical records—that is, to view them or request a copy or a summary of the information. Remember, however, that you might not have access to them if your doctor's office is closed. To request copies, ask for an "authorization for the release of information form." Any fee should include only the cost of copying and postage (if you request mailing). If you see something in your medical record that you believe is incorrect or incomplete, you can request an amendment through your physician or a medical information professional, and you have the right for your amendment to be permanently included in your record.

SOURCES: MedlinePlus. Personal Health Records (www.nlm.nih.gov /medlineplus/personalhealthrecords.html); AHIMA Foundation. myPHR (www.myphr.com).

The next step is usually the physical exam, which begins with a review of vital signs: blood pressure, heart rate (pulse), breathing rate, and temperature. Depending on your primary complaint, your physician may give you a complete physical or instead focus on specific areas, such as your ears, nose, and throat.

Additionally, your physician may order medical tests. Diagnostic testing provides a wealth of information to help solve medical problems. Physicians can order imaging studies (e.g., X-rays, MRIs, or CT scans), biopsies, blood and urine tests, or **endoscopies** to view, probe, or analyze almost any part of the body.

If your physician orders a test for you, be sure you know why you need it, what the risks and benefits are for you, how you should prepare for it (e.g., by fasting or discontinuing medications or herbal remedies), and what the test will involve. Also ask what the test results mean because no test is 100% accurate—**false positives** and **false negatives** can occur—and interpretation of some tests is subjective.

Medical and Surgical Treatments Many conditions can be treated in a variety of ways; in some cases, lifestyle

TERMS

endoscopy A medical procedure in which a viewing instrument is inserted into a body cavity or opening.

false positive A test result that incorrectly detects a disorder or condition in a person who does not have the disorder or condition.

false negative A test result that fails to correctly detect a disease or condition.

changes are sufficient. When starting any treatment, make sure you know the possible risks and side effects as well as the potential benefits.

Thousands of lives are saved each year by antibiotics, insulin, and other drugs, but we pay a price for having such powerful tools. A report from the Institute of Medicine estimates that 1.5 million prescription-drug-related errors—called adverse drug events, or ADEs—occur each year in the United States. ADEs happen for several reasons:

- **Medication errors.** Physicians may overprescribe drugs, sometimes in response to pressure by patients. ADEs can occur if a physician prescribes the wrong drug or a dangerous combination of drugs. Such problems are especially prevalent among older adults, who typically take multiple medications. The risk of ADEs increases greatly with the number of medicines you take. At the pharmacy, patients may receive the wrong drug or may not be given complete information about drug risks, side effects, and interactions.

- **Off-label drug use.** Another potential problem is off-label use of drugs. Once a drug is approved by the FDA for one purpose, it can legally be prescribed (although not marketed) for purposes not listed on the label. Many off-label uses are safe and supported by some research, but both consumers and health care providers need to take special care with off-label use of medications.

- **Online pharmacies.** Although convenient, some online pharmacies may sell products or engage in practices that are illegal in the offline world, putting consumers at risk for receiving adulterated, expired, ineffective, or counterfeit drugs. The FDA recommends that consumers avoid sites that prescribe drugs for the first time without a physical exam, sell prescription drugs without a prescription, or sell medications not approved by the FDA. You should also avoid sites that do not provide access to a registered pharmacist to answer questions or that do not provide a U.S. address and phone number to contact if there's a problem. The National Association of Boards of Pharmacy sponsors a voluntary certification program for Internet pharmacies. To be certified, a pharmacy must have a state license and allow regular inspections.

- **Costs.** Spending on prescription drugs is rising faster than the rate of inflation and is now the fastest-growing portion of U.S. health care spending. Many Americans have no or limited insurance coverage for prescription drug costs. Consumers may be able to lower their drug costs by using generic versions of medications; by joining a drug discount program sponsored by a company, organization, or local pharmacy; or by investigating mail-order or Internet pharmacies.

Importing lower-cost drugs from Canada may be problematic. Canada imports U.S. drugs, and Health Canada—which provides regulation similar to the U.S. FDA—helps ensure the quality of Canadian-produced drugs, so safety should theoretically not be a concern for medicines from Canada. However, companies in Canada may make drugs for export only, thus avoiding standard regulation, and online pharmacies may claim they are operating in Canada but may be located in another country with little or no regulation. U.S. regulators have found online sites advertising Canadian drugs but shipping fake or substandard versions of medications, and shipping costs can be high. The safety of medications purchased in-person in Canada is comparable to that of the those purchased in the United States. However, a prescription from a Canadian physician may be required.

Patients share responsibility for their use of prescription drugs. Many people don't take their medications properly—skipping doses, taking incorrect doses, stopping too soon, or not taking the medication at all. An estimated 30–50% of the more than 3 billion prescriptions dispensed annually in the United States are not taken correctly and thus may not produce the desired results. Consumers can increase the safety and effectiveness of their treatment by carefully reading any prescription label and fact sheets or brochures that come with the medication. Whenever you are given a prescription, ask the following questions:

- Are there nondrug alternatives?
- What is the name of the medication, and what is it supposed to do, within what period of time?
- Can I take a generic drug rather than a brand-name one?
- Is there written information about the medication?

If written information is provided, check it for the following:

- How and when do I take the medication, how much do I take, and for how long? What should I do if I miss a dose?
- What medications, foods, drinks, or activities should I avoid when taking this drug?
- What are the side effects, and what do I do if they occur?

Surgical procedures, another staple of Western medicine, are performed more often in the United States than anywhere else in the world. Each year more than 70 million operations and related procedures are performed. About 20% are in response to an emergency such as a severe injury, and 80% are **elective surgeries,** meaning the patient can generally choose when and where to have the operation, if at all. Many elective surgeries can be done on an **outpatient** basis, so that

TERMS

elective surgery A nonemergency operation that the patient can choose to schedule.

outpatient A person receiving medical attention without being admitted to the hospital.

the patient does not have to be admitted to a hospital for the procedure.

If a health care provider suggests surgery for any reason, ask the following questions:

- Why do I need surgery at this time?
- Is a wait-and-see approach possible or advisable? If so, what are the risks?
- Are any nonsurgical options available, such as medicine or physical therapy?
- What are the risks and complications of the surgery?
- What are the anesthesia options?
- Can the operation be done on an outpatient basis?
- What can I expect before, during, and after surgery?

INTEGRATIVE HEALTH

Increasingly, more conventional Western medical providers are receptive to integrative health, and they may approve or recommend safe and effective CAM in addition to conventional treatment. Whereas conventional Western medicine tends to focus on the body, on the physical causes of disease, and on ways to eradicate pathogens in order to restore health, CAM tends to focus on the mind, body, and spirit in seeking ways to prevent diseases and restore the whole person to balance so that he or she can regain health. This is referred to as **holistic health care**—considering the whole person as a mind–body–spirit entity when diagnosing, treating, or preventing any illness or disorder. The opposite of holistic is dualistic, which refers to treating the mind and body separately.

CAM practices can be classified into several broad categories: alternative medical systems, mind–body medicine, natural products, manipulative and body-based practices, and other CAM practices. What follows is a general introduction to the five categories of CAM and a brief description of some of the more widely used therapies.

Alternative Medical Systems

Many cultures formed complete systems of medical philosophy, theory, and practice long before the current Western biomedical approach was developed. The nonconventional systems best known in the United States include traditional Chinese medicine, also known as traditional Oriental medicine, and homeopathy. Traditional medical systems have been developed in many regions of the world, including other parts of North, Central, and South America; the Middle East, India, Tibet, and Australia. In many countries, these medical approaches continue to be used today—frequently alongside Western medicine and often by physicians trained in Western medicine.

Alternative medical systems tend to have a number of concepts in common. For example, the concept of life force or energy exists in many cultures. In traditional Chinese medicine, the life force contained in all living things is called qi (sometimes spelled "chi"). Qi resembles the vis vitalis (Latin for "life force") of Greek, Roman, and European medical systems, and prana of ayurveda, a traditional medical system of India. Most traditional medical systems think of disease as a disturbance or imbalance not just of physical processes but also of forces or energies within the body, the mind, and the spirit. Treatment aims at reestablishing equilibrium, balance, and harmony.

Because the whole patient, rather than an isolated body part or disease, is treated in most comprehensive alternative medical systems, it is rare that only a single treatment approach is used. Most commonly, multiple remedies and techniques are employed together and are adjusted according to the changes in the patient's health status.

Traditional Chinese Medicine In **traditional Chinese medicine (TCM)** the free and harmonious flow of qi defines health of the body, mind, and spirit. Illness occurs when qi is deficient or the flow of qi is blocked or disturbed. TCM is believed to restore the flow of blocked qi; the goal is not only to treat illness but also to balance energy, prevent disease, and support immunity.

Two major TCM treatment methods include **herbal remedies** and **acupuncture.** Chinese herbal remedies number about 5800. In addition to herbs, plant products, fungi (mushrooms), animal parts, and minerals may be used. The use of a single medicinal substance is rare in Chinese herbal medicine; rather, several substances are combined in precise proportions, often to make a tea or soup.

An accumulating body of scientific evidence supports the medical use of acupuncture, expanding the acceptance of this CAM modality in the West and placing it on the border of conventional and nonconventional health care practice. Acupuncture is viewed in TCM as correcting disturbances in the flow of qi. Qi is believed to flow through the body along several meridians, or pathways, and there are hundreds of acupuncture points located along these meridians. The points chosen for acupuncture are highly individualized for each patient, and they change during treatment as the patient's health status changes.

TERMS

holistic health care   Practice that takes into account the whole person—body, mind, and spirit—when assessing, treating, and preventing illnesses and maintaining health.

traditional Chinese medicine (TCM)   The traditional medical system of China, which views illness as the result of a problem in the quality, quantity, balance, or flow of qi, the life force; therapies include acupuncture, herbal medicine, and massage.

herbal remedy   A medicine prepared from plants.

acupuncture   Insertion of thin needles through the skin at points along meridians—pathways through which qi is believed to flow.

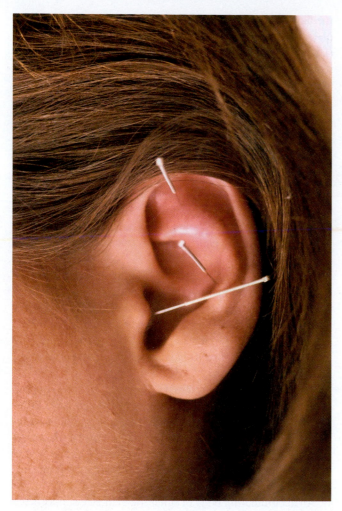

Acupuncture involves the insertion of needles at appropriate points in the skin to treat a variety of illnesses.

© Jack Star/PhotoLink/Getty Images

The World Health Organization has compiled a list of more than 40 conditions for which acupuncture may be beneficial. At a conference called by the NIH, a panel of experts cited evidence that acupuncture was effective in relieving nausea and vomiting after chemotherapy, and pain after surgery, including dental surgery. Newer studies show that acupuncture may help relieve the painful symptoms of fibromyalgia and reduce the joint pain and stiffness of osteoarthritis. There is insufficient evidence showing that acupuncture is effective for menstrual cramps, tennis elbow, carpal tunnel syndrome, asthma, and certain other conditions. Acupuncture is considered very safe, and over decades, few side effects have been reported. The FDA regulates acupuncture needles like other standard medical devices and requires that they be sterile.

Homeopathy   As a CAM system of medical practice that has unconventional origins in Germany, **homeopathy** involves treating an individual with highly diluted substances intended to trigger the body's natural system of healing. The theory is that when given in very diluted, minute quantities,

substances that produce symptoms of an illness in a healthy person will help bring about a cure in someone who is ill, and it will do this by stimulating the body's healing processes. A primary principle of homeopathy is "like cures like." Based on a patient's specific signs and symptoms, a homeopathic practitioner determines the most appropriate treatment; diluted remedies are typically administered in liquid form or applied to sweetened pellets. Although most homeopathic remedies are highly diluted, some products may be labeled as homeopathic but contain substantial amounts of active ingredients that can cause side effects or drug interactions.

Because treatments are highly individualized for each patient and difficult to explain using the conventional laws of chemistry, randomized controlled trials on homeopathy are difficult. Most clinical trials have concluded that at best there is only weak supporting evidence. Nevertheless, some states require homeopaths to be licensed and fulfill certain requirements before they are permitted to practice.

Naturopathy   **Naturopathy** is based on the premise that the body has the ability to maintain and restore optimal health. Naturopathic doctors (NDs) use both CAM and conventional approaches holistically for prevention, diagnosis, and treatment and for helping their patients minimize risks and barriers to good health. The most frequently treated conditions include allergies, chronic pain, obesity, heart disease, fertility problems, and cancer. Naturopaths can perform minor surgery such as cyst removal and skin suturing. They are also trained to use prescription medications, although their education emphasizes natural modalities for healing.

Mind–Body Medicine

Mind–body interventions make use of the integral connection between mind and body and the effect each can have on the other. They include many of the stress management techniques discussed in Chapter 2, including meditation, yoga, visualization, tai chi, and biofeedback. Psychotherapy, support groups, prayer, and music and art therapy are mind–body interventions. The placebo effect is one of the most widely known examples of mind–body interdependence. Many studies have shown evidence that mind–body interventions such as imagery, support groups, friendships, strong family relationships, meditation, prayer, and hypnotherapy can all have a positive impact on health.

homeopathy   An alternative system of practice that uses a holistic approach to diagnosis and treatment; involves administering minute doses of remedies that would, in larger quantities, produce symptoms similar to those of the illness.

naturopathy   An alternative medical system based on supporting the body's ability to heal itself and maintain optimal health by removing barriers and creating an internal and external environment that promotes health and healing.

TERMS

Clinical hypnosis is a focused state of awareness, perception, or consciousness that professionally trained practitioners use to treat a variety of physical and psychological conditions. **Hypnotherapy** is considered to be a CAM modality, although its use for certain conditions was accepted more than 40 years ago by the American Medical Association. Relatively few individuals have experienced clinical hypnotherapy or are knowledgeable about it, but many have been exposed to "stage hypnosis" and may believe that it has no legitimate clinical utility and no valid, evidence-based support. However, numerous evidence-based outcome studies have demonstrated its clinical usefulness, and brain-imaging technologies are helping to explain possible neurologic mechanisms.

Hypnotherapy involves the induction of a state of deep relaxation during which the patient is more likely to accept suggestions that can influence health and overcome conditions such as chronic pain, pain during surgery or childbirth, unhealthy habits, and anxiety and phobias. A number of NIH-sponsored reports found strong evidence for the effectiveness of hypnosis in reducing chronic pain stemming from a variety of medical conditions. Health professionals who are properly trained in hypnotherapy use this modality to augment their conventional treatments.

Natural Products

Natural products, also known as *biologically based therapies*, include substances derived from plant or animal sources. They consist primarily of herbal therapies or remedies, botanicals, and extracts from animal tissues (such as shark cartilage). Herbal remedies are a major component of all indigenous forms of medicine. Prior to the development of pharmaceuticals at the end of the 19th century, people everywhere in the world relied on materials from nature for pain relief, wound healing, and treatment of a variety of ailments. Much of the **pharmacopoeia** of present-day scientific medicine originated in the folk medicine of native people, and many prescription drugs used today have been derived from plants.

Most natural products are sold in the United States as dietary supplements and are therefore largely unregulated by the FDA. Like foods, dietary supplements must carry ingredient labels, and manufacturers are responsible for ensuring that their dietary supplements are safe and properly labeled for marketing. The FDA is responsible for monitoring the labeling and accompanying literature of dietary supplements and for overseeing their safety once they are on the market.

Well-designed clinical studies have been conducted on a number of natural products. A few commonly used herbals, their uses, and the evidence supporting their efficacy are presented in Table 15.2. Clinical trials with herbals such as St. John's wort, ginkgo biloba, and echinacea have shown only a few minor side effects. New studies are also evaluating the efficacy of varying dosages and their interactions with conventional drugs.

Although most drug–herb interactions are relatively minor compared to conventional drug–drug interactions, some can be potentially serious. Because of reports of bleeding, a popular herb, ginkgo biloba, although generally well tolerated, should be used cautiously in people suffering from clotting disorders or taking blood thinners, or prior to surgical or dental procedures involving any bleeding. St. John's wort interacts with drugs used to treat HIV infection and heart disease, and the herb may also reduce the effectiveness of oral contraceptives, antirejection drugs used in patients receiving organ transplants, and some medications used to treat infections, depression, asthma, and seizure disorders.

Another potential problem is the possibility of contaminants. In a sample of ayurvedic herbal medicine products, 20% were found to contain potentially harmful levels of lead, mercury, or arsenic. The content and potency of herbal preparations is also variable.

Studies have shown that most people do not reveal their use of CAM therapies to their conventional health care providers, a problem that can have significant health consequences. Any herbs that are used in combination with conventional drugs should be evaluated for safety by a knowledgeable health care provider such as a pharmacist.

Manipulative and Body-Based Practices

Touch and body manipulation are long-standing forms of health care. Manual healing techniques include the concept that misalignment or dysfunction in one part of the body can cause pain or dysfunction in that or another part. Correcting these misalignments can help restore optimal health.

Many manipulative and body-based practices are integral components of physical therapy and osteopathic medicine, although certain techniques fit the definition of CAM because they are not a part of conventional health care practice. The most commonly used CAM manual healing method is **chiropractic,** a method that focuses on the relationship between structure and function, primarily of the spine, joints, muscles, and the nervous system, to maintain or restore health. An important therapeutic procedure is the manipulation of joints, particularly those of the spinal column.

> **TERMS**
>
> **hypnotherapy** A mind–body technique that uses relaxation and imagery to help a patient imagine specific health outcomes and establish a belief that they can be achieved; commonly used for managing pain, phobias, and addictions.
>
> **natural products** CAM therapies that include biologically based interventions and products; examples include herbal remedies, extracts from animal tissues, and dietary supplements.
>
> **pharmacopoeia** A collection of descriptions and formulas for drugs and medicinal preparations.
>
> **chiropractic** A CAM manipulative, body-based practice that focuses on disorders of the spine, and musculoskeletal and nervous systems, and the effects of these disorders on general health; the primary treatment is manipulation of the spine and other joints.

Table 15.2   Commonly Used Herbals, Their Uses, Evidence for Their Effectiveness, and Contraindications

BOTANICAL	USE	EVIDENCE	EXAMPLES OF ADVERSE EFFECTS AND INTERACTIONS
Cranberry (*Vaccinium macrocarpon*)	Prevention or treatment of urinary tract infections	Some evidence of a modest preventive effect in some women	None known
Dandelion (*Taraxacum officinale*)	As a "tonic" against liver or kidney ailments	No conclusive evidence	May cause diarrhea in some users; people with gallbladder or bile duct problems should not take dandelion
Echinacea (*Echinacea purpurea, E. angustifolia, E. pallida*)	Stimulation of immune functions; to prevent colds and flulike diseases; to lessen symptoms of colds and flu	Some trials showed that it prevents colds and flu and helps patients recover faster from colds	Might cause liver damage if taken over long periods of time (more than 8 weeks); because it is an immune stimulant, it is not advisable to take it with immune suppressants (e.g., corticosteroids) or during chemotherapy
Evening primrose oil (*Oenothera biennis L.*)	Reduction of inflammation	Long-term supplementation effective in reducing symptoms of rheumatoid arthritis	None known
Feverfew (*Tanacetum parthenium*)	Prevention of headaches and migraines	Most trials indicate that it is more effective than placebo	Should not be used by people allergic to other members of the aster family; has the potential to increase the effects of warfarin and other anticoagulants
Garlic (*Allium sativum*)	Reduction of cholesterol	Short-term studies have found a modest effect	May interact with some medications, including anticoagulants, cyclosporine, and oral contraceptives
Ginkgo (*Ginkgo biloba*)	Improvement of circulation and memory	Improves cerebral insufficiency and slows progression of senile dementia in some patients; improves blood flow	Could increase bleeding time; should not be taken with nonsteroidal anti-inflammatory drugs (NSAIDs) like aspirin or with anticoagulants; may cause gastrointestinal disturbance
Ginseng (*Panax ginseng*)	Improvement of physical performance, memory, immune function, and glycemic control in diabetes; treatment of herpes simplex 2	No conclusive evidence exists for any of these uses	Interacts with warfarin and alcohol in mice and rats, so should probably not be used with these drugs; may cause liver damage
St. John's wort (*Hypericum perforatum*)	Treatment of depression	There is evidence that it is significantly more effective than placebo, is as effective as some standard antidepressants for mild to moderate depression, and causes fewer adverse effects	Known to interact with a variety of pharmaceuticals and should not be taken together with digoxin, theophylline, cyclosporine, indinavir, and serotonin reuptake inhibitors
Saw palmetto (*Serenoa repens*)	Improvement of benign prostatic hypertrophy	Studies show that saw palmetto may reduce mild prostate enlargement	Has no known interactions with drugs, but should probably not be taken with hormonal therapies
Valerian (*Valeriana officinalis*)	Treatment of insomnia	May help with some sleep disorders	Interacts with thiopental and pentobarbital and should not be used with these drugs

However, chiropractors also use a variety of other techniques, including exercise, patient education and lifestyle modification, nutritional supplements, and orthotics (mechanical supports and braces).

Chiropractors, or doctors of chiropractic, are trained for a minimum of four years at accredited chiropractic colleges and can go on to postgraduate training in many countries. Although specifically listed by NCCIH as one of the manipulative and body-based practices of CAM, chiropractic is accepted by many health care and health insurance providers to a far greater extent than are many other types of CAM therapies. Based on research showing the efficacy of chiropractic management in acute lower-back pain, spinal manipulation has been included in the federal guidelines for the treatment of this condition, and electrodiagnostic tests show that chiropractic is effective in controlling back pain. Promising results have also been reported with the use of chiropractic techniques in neck pain and headaches.

A word of caution is in order: Spinal manipulation must be performed only by a properly trained professional such as a chiropractor, osteopathic physician, or physical therapist who is specially trained and certified in orthopedic manual physical therapy (OMPT).

Exercise for health maintenance, promotion, and disease prevention currently fits the definition of a CAM modality. However, this is changing due to an active campaign, Exercise Is Medicine (EIM), co-launched in 2007 by the American College of Sports Medicine and the American Medical Association. A study has found that 65% of Americans would be more interested in exercising to stay healthy if advised to do so by their physicians.

The EIM initiative encourages physicians to record a patient's exercise level as a routine vital sign during clinical visits, along with pulse, respiratory rate, temperature, and blood pressure. Those who are able will be advised to exercise for 30 minutes and to stretch and engage in light muscle training for an additional 10 minutes five days each week. The EIM website (www.exerciseismedicine. org) advises physicians, other health care providers, medical educators, and the public about the benefits of exercise. Through efforts such as this, exercise is likely to transition from a CAM modality to a conventional modality and to be taught in more U.S. medical schools and to be recommended and used as a treatment in U.S. health care institutions.

Other CAM Practices

CAM practices also include traditional healing practices and energy therapies. Traditional healers may rely on touch as well as other senses, for example, sound—the shamanic clanging of a bell or the quality of a singing voice. These healers may incorporate counseling or psychological therapy in addition to prescribing herbal remedies.

Energy therapies are forms of treatment that use energy interactions between living organisms, those produced by the organism itself and those produced by outside sources such as electromagnetic energy. The recognition that the body produces electromagnetic fields has led to the development of many diagnostic procedures in Western medicine, including electroencephalography (EEG), electromyography (EMG), electrocardiography (ECG), and nuclear magnetic resonance imaging (NMRI). Energy therapies are based on the concept that energy surrounds and penetrates the body and can be influenced by movement, touch, pressure, or the placement of hands in or through the fields.

Reiki is an example of energy therapy; it is intended to correct disturbances in the flow of life energy (ki in the Japanese tradition) and enhance the body's healing powers through the use of specific hand positions on or near the patient's body. **Therapeutic touch** is derived from ancient techniques involving using the hands to detect and transmit energy (electromagnetic energy). It is based on the premise that healers can identify and correct energy imbalances by passing their hands over the patient's body.

Magnetic therapies include the application of therapeutic magnets to the body to manage pain, increase blood flow, and treat conditions such as arthritic pain. One animal study reported an increased rate of wound healing using magnets, but comprehensive literature reviews of studies on therapeutic magnets report little or no supporting evidence.

When Does CAM Become Conventional Medicine?

From a Western point of view, when ancient healers used the foxglove plant for medicinal purposes, it could be considered "alternative"—or even superstition. But when the plant's content, digitalis, was scientifically shown to be a useful pharmaceutical, it became a conventional medication for the treatment of heart disease. Because of modern research sponsored mostly by the NIH, we are seeing a number of therapeutic alternatives become mainstream medicine.

According to the NIH, in 2012, approximately 33% of adults used some form of CAM either in conjunction with or instead of standard Western health care. As new evidence emerges about the potential value of certain practices, CAM therapies are becoming commonly used in the United States, as the following examples indicate.

Tai Chi and Fibromyalgia   A once mysterious and misunderstood disorder, fibromyalgia causes chronic pain throughout the body and general fatigue. It can be partially treated with drugs, but exercise is an important component of fibromyalgia therapy because it helps maintain or improve muscle strength and function. **Tai chi,** a CAM practice with origins in ancient China, uses slow, meditative movements for maintaining and restoring health. Tai chi has long been known to offer many benefits, including gains in strength and flexibility, and it has also been shown to be helpful in pain management. A study published in 2010 in the *New England Journal of Medicine* tracked the symptoms of two groups of fibromyalgia patients: one that learned a variety of tai chi movements and another that practiced stretching exercises and received wellness counseling. Over the course

> **TERMS**
>
> **energy therapies**   Forms of CAM treatment that use varying sources of energy originating either within the body or from outside sources to promote health and healing.
>
> **Reiki**   A CAM practice intended to correct disturbances in the flow of life energy and enhance the body's healing powers through the use of various hand positions on the patient.
>
> **therapeutic touch**   A CAM practice based on the premise that healers can identify and correct energy imbalances by passing their hands over the patient's body.
>
> **magnetic therapies**   A form of alternative medicine that uses magnets to treat pain and other health problems.
>
> **tai chi**   An ancient Chinese philosophy adapted as a CAM energy modality and practiced as exercise involving slow, continuous, meditative movements accompanied by deep breathing, and used for maintaining and restoring health.

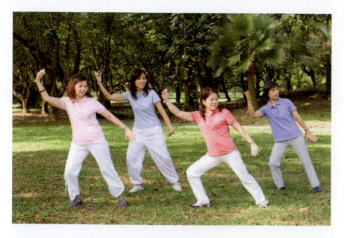

Tai chi combines gentle movements with mental focus, breathing, and relaxation. It has been shown to improve balance and stability and help people with chronic conditions cope with pain.

© Phil Date/123RF

of the study, the patients who practiced tai chi reported significantly less pain than the other group, and the benefits lasted well beyond the study's end.

CAM Therapies and Back Pain CAM therapies are used more often for back pain than for any other condition. A 2010 study showed that about 6% of adult Americans who suffer back pain have tried at least one form of alternative therapy in the hope of finding relief. The therapies most commonly used for back pain are chiropractic, massage, yoga, tai chi, and acupuncture. In this study, more than 50% of respondents said they elected to try CAM because conventional medical treatments weren't providing adequate pain relief. Nearly two-thirds said they experienced significantly reduced pain as a result of CAM therapy.

Evaluating Complementary and Alternative Therapies

CAM therapies are more difficult to investigate than conventional therapies for several reasons. One problem is that of effect size—the statistical difference in outcome between the treatment being tested and the control. Most CAM therapies have a smaller effect size than conventional treatments, making experimental outcomes difficult to detect.

Other difficulties include delayed effects (CAM therapies require longer studies and therefore more funding), variable effects (not all CAM therapies work equally well on everybody), and combination effects (several approaches used together may produce results not seen in a single approach—violating the traditional scientific tenet of parsimony). Therefore, it is important to take an active role when you are seeking medical information and advice in any modality, conventional or unconventional.

Working with Your Physician When a health issue might be serious, the NCCIH advises consumers not to seek complementary therapies without first consulting a conventional health care provider. Become informed and discuss conventional treatments that have been shown to be beneficial for your condition. If you are thinking of trying any complementary or alternative therapies, discuss these with your physician, pharmacist, or other conventional provider who is knowledgeable about your health status and is also informed about CAM or is willing to learn by consulting proper resources. If they are not informed about CAM, it may be helpful to share information from reliable, evidence-based sources with them. Areas to discuss with your physician or pharmacist include the safety of the treatment; evidence, if any, for its effectiveness; issues of timing; and the likely cost.

If appropriate, schedule a follow-up visit with your physician to assess your condition and your progress after a certain amount of time using a complementary therapy. Keep a symptom diary to track your symptoms and gauge your progress. Symptoms such as pain and fatigue are difficult to recall with accuracy, so an ongoing symptom diary is an important tool. If your physician advises against CAM and can support the advice with good evidence, you should probably not use it. If your physician is simply unreceptive or uninformed about CAM, you may need to find another physician whose health beliefs are compatible with your own. If you plan to pursue a therapy against your physician's advice, tell him or her.

For supplements, particularly botanicals, pharmacists can also be an excellent source of information; inform them about any other unconventional or conventional medications you are taking.

Questioning the CAM Practitioner You can also get information from individual practitioners, educational programs, professional organizations, and state licensing boards. Ask about education, training, licensing, and certification. If appropriate, check with local or state regulatory agencies or the consumer affairs department to determine if any complaints have been lodged against the practitioner. Some guidelines for talking with a CAM practitioner include the following:

• Ask the practitioner why he or she thinks the therapy will be beneficial for your condition. Ask for a full description of the therapy and any potential side effects. In all cases, demand an evidence-based approach.

• Describe in detail any conventional treatments you are receiving or plan to receive.

• Ask how long the therapy should continue before it can be determined if it is beneficial.

• Ask about the expected cost of the treatment. Does it seem reasonable? Will your health insurance pay some or all of the costs?

If anything an unconventional practitioner says or recommends directly conflicts with advice from your physician, discuss it with your physician before making any major changes in your current treatment regimen or lifestyle.

PAYING FOR HEALTH CARE

The U.S. health care system is one of the most advanced and comprehensive in the world, but it is also the most expensive (Figure 15.3). In 2013, Americans spent $2.7 trillion on health care, or more than $9000 per person. Many factors contribute to the high cost of health care in the United States, including the cost of advanced equipment and new technology, expensive treatments for some illnesses, aging of the population, and the demand for profits by many commercial health enterprises.

The Current System

Because of expanding health care costs and the increasing difficulty that some Americans have paying for them,

Congress passed the **Affordable Care Act** (ACA) in 2009. The bill was signed into law by President Barack Obama in 2010. The ACA's main aims are to control costs and provide more regulation of the way insurance companies cover medical expenses. Two key provisions of the ACA are that it increases preventive services and forbids insurance companies to discriminate on the basis of preexisting medical conditions (see Chapter 1).

Health care in the United States is financed by a combination of private and public insurance plans, patient out-of-pocket payments, and government assistance. Before the ACA, private insurance and individual patients paid about 55% of the total; the government paid the rest, mainly through Medicare and Medicaid. Most nonelderly Americans receive health insurance through their employers, but as medical costs increase, the number of Americans with private insurance has decreased by approximately 10% over the past two decades.

By some estimates, as many as 50 million Americans—the vast majority of them employed—had no health insurance

TERMS

Affordable Care Act A U.S. law requiring health insurance plans to include certain rights and protections (e.g., mental health and preventive services, no penalties for preexisting conditions, and the right to appeal health service charges) and requiring nearly all Americans to have health insurance coverage. The law attempts to make health care more affordable for individuals and families.

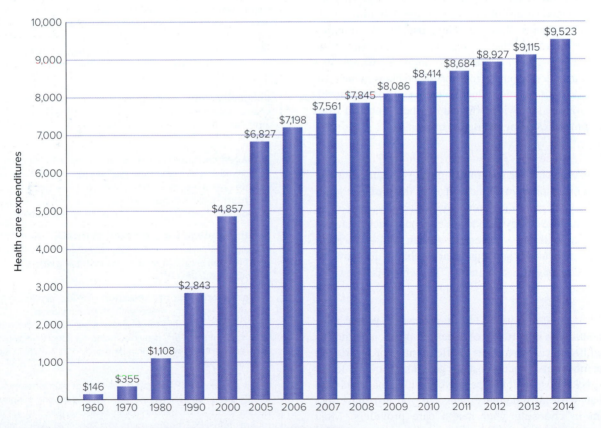

FIGURE 15.3 **Per-capita national health care expenditures, 1960–2014.**

SOURCE: National Center for Health Statistics. 2016. *Health, United States: 2015.* Hyattsville, MD: National Center for Health Statistics. Data from Health, United States, 2015.

at all prior to the ACA. Many more were underinsured, meaning they may be uninsured for periods of time, have health insurance that does not cover all needed services, and/or have high out-of-pocket costs. New and extended government health insurance programs for children reduced the number of Americans under age 18 who lack health insurance; still, 9.8 million American children were uninsured in 2010 before the ACA was available.

Health Insurance

Health insurance as required under the ACA protects you against losses incurred for medical expenses due to illness or injury. Depending on the policy, coverage may also include preventive services such as yearly exams; other physician services; medications; hospital stays; emergency department visits; physical, occupational, and speech therapy; vision care; dental coverage; and other expenses. Some insurance policies provide riders for specific CAM coverage for an additional charge. Policies differ based on the services covered, the amount of the **deductible** and **copayment,** and the limit of coverage. Of course, with many plans, the more services you add to the policy, the higher the premium. Coverage may be provided as an employment benefit or through a government-sponsored plan such as Medicaid (for certain disabled and low-income individuals) or Medicare (typically for individuals age 65 and over and those with certain illnesses). See the box "Choosing a Health Insurance Plan."

Health insurance plans are either fee-for-service (indemnity) or managed care. With both types, the individual or his or her employer pays a basic premium, usually on a monthly basis; there are often other payments as well. As part of the ACA, states now provide interactive online exchanges that supply information about various insurance plans, which can be adapted to fit an individual's needs and income level. Most insurance is provided by and can be purchased from private companies using the online exchanges.

Traditional Fee-for-Service (Indemnity) Plans
In a fee-for-service plan, or **indemnity plan,** you can go to any physician or hospital you choose. You or the provider sends the bill to your insurance company, which pays part of it. Usually you have to pay a deductible amount each year, and then the plan will pay a percentage—often 80%—of what it considers the "usual and customary" charge for covered services. You pay the remaining 20%, which is known as *coinsurance.*

Managed Care Plans
Managed care plans have agreements with a network of specified physicians, hospitals, and health care providers to offer a range of services to plan members at reduced cost. In general, you have lower out-of-pocket costs and less paperwork with a managed care plan than with an indemnity plan, but you also have less freedom in choosing your health care providers. Most Americans with job-based insurance are covered by managed care plans. These include:

- **Health maintenance organizations (HMOs)** offer members a range of services for a set monthly fee. You choose a primary care physician who manages your care and refers you to specialists if you need them. If you go outside the HMO, you have to pay for the service yourself.

- **Preferred provider organizations (PPOs)** have arrangements with physicians and other providers who have agreed to accept lower fees.

- **Point-of-service (POS) plans** are options offered by many HMOs in which you can see a specialist or a physician outside the plan, but you will have to pay most or all of the cost unless your primary care physician referred you.

Many managed care plans try to reduce costs over the long term by paying for routine preventive care, such as regular checkups and screening tests and prenatal care; they may also encourage prevention by offering health education and lifestyle modification programs for members.

Government Programs   Americans age 65 and over and younger people with certain disabilities can be covered by

> **TERMS**
>
> **deductible**   The amount you pay for services before your insurance coverage begins. For example, if your deductible is $1000, the insurance company won't pay anything for services until your expenses total $1000. The insurance company may fully cover certain services before you've reached your deductible amount.
>
> **copayment**   The amount you pay for a particular health care service; your insurance provider pays the balance. For example, for a physical exam that costs $150, you might pay your doctor's office $25 at the time of service (your copayment), and the insurance company would pay $125. The copayment amount may vary according to the type of service you received.
>
> **indemnity plan**   A health insurance plan based on a fee for each service provided; the cost is shared between you and the insurance company, and you can go to any physician or hospital you choose.
>
> **managed care plan**   A health insurance plan that contracts with providers and health care facilities (the plan's "network") to provide care at reduced costs. There are three types of managed care plans: health management organizations (HMOs), preferred provider organizations (PPOs), and point of service (POS).
>
> **health maintenance organization (HMO)**   A type of prepaid health insurance plan that covers services within a network of physicians and other professionals who are contracted with the HMO.
>
> **preferred provider organization (PPO)**   A prepaid health insurance plan that contracts with physicians, other professionals, and hospitals to provide services for discounted fees. You can go to any provider including specialists without a PCP referral. Using nonparticipating providers results in higher costs to the patient.
>
> **point-of-service (POS) plan**   A type of plan where you pay less if you use physicians, other professionals, and hospitals that belong to the plan's network, but you are required to get a referral from a PCP before going to a specialist. A POS plan combines some of the essentials of both HMO and PPO plans.

CRITICAL CONSUMER
Choosing a Health Insurance Plan

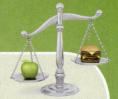

The Affordable Care Act (ACA) requires most people to obtain health insurance or pay a federal penalty. Under the ACA, a health insurance marketplace, also called health exchanges, facilitates the purchase of health insurance. But choosing a plan can be a complicated matter—confusing and intimidating. To organize your thinking about this decision, look for answers to the three questions discussed here.

1. What Does the Plan Cover?

These are the ten categories of health care services that health plans must cover to meet requirements of the ACA:

- Ambulatory patient services (care you get without being admitted to a hospital)
- Emergency services
- Hospitalization
- Maternity and newborn care
- Mental health and substance use disorder services including behavioral health treatment
- Prescription drugs
- Rehabilitative and habilitative services and devices (to help people with injuries, disabilities, or chronic conditions gain or recover mental and physical skills)
- Laboratory services
- Preventive services and chronic disease management
- Pediatric services, including oral and vision care

Insurance provided by large employers may differ slightly. You can ask for a summary of benefits and coverage to see what is covered.

2. How Much Does the Plan Cost?

You pay for health insurance in two ways—through (1) your monthly premium and (2) the out-of-pocket expenses you pay when you receive care. Out-of-pocket expenses includes deductibles, coinsurance, and copayments (see text for definitions). The higher the monthly premium you pay, the lower will be your out-of-pocket expenses.

For the ACA, the "metal categories"—bronze, silver, gold, and platinum—were created to help people choose a plan by simplifying the differences between costs and levels of coverage.

As you consider your choices, note what the total cost of care includes: your premium plus out-of-pocket costs.

Generally, your monthly insurance payment is lowest in the bronze category, but deductibles are higher and you may have more out-of-pocket costs. Platinum plans typically have the highest premiums, but deductibles and out-of-pocket costs are low. If your income qualifies you for cost-sharing reductions, you can enroll in a silver plan where you get the best of both worlds: a lower premium and a lower deductible. Out-of-pocket costs will be lower as well.

PLAN CATEGORY	THE INSURANCE COMPANY PAYS	YOU PAY
Bronze	60%	40%
Silver	70%	30%
Gold	80%	20%
Platinum	90%	10%

The "metal categories" help you determine how you and your insurance plan share total costs.

SOURCE: https://www.healthcare.gov/choose-a-plan/plans-categories/.

3. Which Doctors and Hospitals Are in Your Plan?

Every health insurance plan has a network of providers who agree to provide services to plan members for specific prices. As you've learned, plans vary in how restricted members are in relation to these networks. Some only allow members to receive services provided by doctors, specialists, or hospitals in the plan's network. Others are more flexible: They may charge less when plan members use doctors, hospitals, and other health care providers that belong to the plan's network; require members to get referrals to go outside the network; or allow members to use doctors, hospitals, and providers outside their network without a referral for an additional cost. It makes sense, then, to check the health plan and your doctor's office to make sure your desired providers are in the network of the plan you are considering.

You can get more information, browse plans, and apply for coverage at HealthCare.gov.

Medicare, a federal health insurance program that helps pay for hospitalization, physician services, and prescription drugs. As a result of limits placed on payments, however, some physicians and managed care programs have stopped accepting Medicare patients. **Medicaid** is a joint federal–state health insurance program that covers some low-income people, especially children, pregnant women, and people

TERMS

Medicare   A federal health insurance program for people age 65 and over and for younger people with certain disabilities.

Medicaid   A federally subsidized state-run plan of health care for people with low income.

with certain disabilities. The number of people and the number and cost of services covered by government programs has grown in recent years, challenging the ability of these programs to provide needed coverage. These government programs will be affected and face changes with full implementation of the ACA.

Ask Yourself

What type of health insurance coverage do you have? If you are covered by your parents' or guardians' insurance, what are the plan's benefits? If you have coverage, do you know what types of medical services are fully or partially covered? What are your copayments and deductibles? If you were faced with a medical emergency, would you know how to contact and work with your insurer to make sure your costs were covered?

TIPS FOR TODAY AND THE FUTURE

Most of the time, you can take care of yourself without consulting a health care provider. When you need professional care, you can still take responsibility for yourself by making informed decisions.

RIGHT NOW YOU CAN:

- Make sure that you have enough of your prescription medications on hand and that your prescriptions are up-to-date.
- If you take any supplements (dietary or herbal), ask your pharmacist if they can interact with any prescription drugs you are taking.
- Stock your home and car with basic first aid supplies.

IN THE FUTURE YOU CAN:

- Use professional and authoritative Internet resources to thoroughly research complementary or alternative medical treatments you are using or considering to make sure they are considered safe and effective.
- Review your medical insurance needs by checking your coverage under your parents' or guardians' policy if you are under age 26 or by checking your state's online health insurance exchange, and contact your insurance agent if you have questions about your coverage.

SUMMARY

- Informed self-care requires knowing how to evaluate symptoms. You should see a physician if symptoms are severe, unusual, persistent, or recurrent.

- Self-treatment doesn't necessarily require medication, but over-the-counter (OTC) drugs can be a helpful part of self-care.

- Conventional medicine is characterized by a focus on the physical causes of disease, the identification of signs and symptoms, the use of drugs and surgery for treatment, and the use of scientific thinking and research to understand diseases.

- Conventional practitioners include medical doctors, doctors of osteopathic medicine, podiatrists, optometrists, and dentists, as well as other highly trained professionals.

- The diagnostic process involves a medical history, a physical exam, and medical tests. Patients should ask questions about tests and treatments recommended by their providers.

- Safe use of prescription drugs requires knowledge of what the medication is supposed to do, how and when to take it, and the possible side effects.

- All surgical procedures carry risk; patients should ask many questions, including about alternatives.

- Complementary and alternative medicine (CAM) is defined as those therapies and practices that do not form part of conventional health care and medical practice as taught in most U.S. medical schools and offered in most U.S. hospitals.

- Integrative health is a term used when CAM methods are added to conventional practice—conventional methods are considered first, and CAM may be included if it could have additional benefits. The term *integrative health* or *integrative medicine* should be used in discussions with conventional providers.

- CAM is characterized by a view of health as a balance and integration of body, mind, and spirit; a focus on ways to restore the individual to optimal functioning using methods from the five fields of CAM practice as defined by the National Institutes of Health; and a body of knowledge based on the accumulated observations and experience of practitioners, often over decades or centuries, and, more recently, on the scientific evaluation of safety and efficacy.

- CAM practices can be classified into several broad categories: alternative medical systems, mind–body medicine, natural products, manipulative and body-based practices, and other CAM practices.

- Alternative medical systems such as traditional Chinese medicine and homeopathy are complete systems of medical philosophy, theory, and practice.

- Mind–body medicine includes meditation, biofeedback, group support, hypnosis, and prayer.

- Natural products include herbal remedies, botanicals, animal tissue products, and dietary supplements.

- Manipulative and body-based practices include massage and other healing techniques; the most frequently used is chiropractic.

- Other CAM practices include traditional healing practices and energy therapies.

- Because there is presently less information available about CAM and less regulation of its providers and modalities, consumers must be proactive in researching and choosing treatments, using critical thinking skills, examining the available evidence-based information available, and exercising caution.

- The Affordable Care Act and other recent government reforms of the health care system (particularly the insurance industry) aim to make affordable health insurance coverage available to more Americans.

- Health insurance plans are usually described as either fee-for-service (indemnity) or managed care plans. Indemnity plans allow consumers more choice in medical providers, but managed care plans are less expensive.

- Government programs include Medicaid for the poor and Medicare for those aged 65 and over or chronically disabled.

FOR MORE INFORMATION

Affordable Care Act. Provides information on the Affordable Care Act and the Health Insurance Marketplace.

https://www.healthcare.gov

Exercise Is Medicine. Provides information on the initiative to promote physical activity, as well as a series of factsheets with guidelines on exercise for people many different chronic conditions.

www.exerciseismedicine.org

HealthIT. Presents tips and tools related to health information technology.

https://www.healthit.gov/patients-families/

National Center for Complementary and Integrative Health (NCCIH). Provides background information and research results on many forms of CAM.

https://nccih.nih.gov

U.S. Food and Drug Administration: For Consumers. Provides materials about supplements, prescription and OTC drugs, and other FDA-regulated products.

http://www.fda.gov/ForConsumers/

SELECTED BIBLIOGRAPHY

Academic Consortium for Integrative Medicine & Health. 2016. *Member Listing* (https://www.imconsortium.org/members/members.cfm).

American Academy of Family Physicians. 2014. *Patient Protection and Affordable Care Act (ACA)* (http://www.aafp.org/advocacy/informed /coverage/aca.html).

American Association of Naturopathic Physicians. 2016. *About Naturopathic Medicine* (http://www.naturopathic.org/medicine).

American Board of Medical Specialties. 2016. *Specialty and Subspecialty Certificates* (http://www.abms.org/member-boards/specialty-subspecialty -certificates/).

American Chiropractic Association. 2015. *Facts about Chiropractic* (www .acatoday.org/News-Publications/News/Facts-About-Chiropractic).

American College of Physicians. 2009. *The ACP Evidence-Based Guide to Complementary and Alternative Medicine.* Washington, DC: American College of Physicians.

American Hospital Association. 2015. *Hospital Emergency Room Visits per 1,000 Population by Ownership Type* (http://kff.org/other/state-indicator /emergency-room-visits-by-ownership/).

Clarke, T. C., et al. 2015. Trends in the use of complementary health approaches among adults: United States, 2002-2012. *National Health Statistics Reports* 79: 1-16.

Clear Bankruptcy. 2014. *10 Leading Causes of Bankruptcy* (http://www .clearbankruptcy.com/financial-literacy/10-leading-causes-of-bankruptcy .aspx).

Commonwealth Fund. 2015. *The Problem of Underinsurance and How Rising Deductibles Will Make It Worse* (http://www.commonwealthfund .org/publications/issue-briefs/2015/may/problem-of-underinsurance).

Cowen, V. S., and V. Cyr. 2015. Complementary and alternative medicine in US medical schools. *Advances in Medical Education and Practice* 6: 113-117.

Exercise Is Medicine. 2016. *Getting Started* (http://www.exerciseismedicine .org/support_page.php?p56).

Hammer, D., et al. 2010. The intended—and unintended—consequences of healthcare reform. *Healthcare Financial Management* 64(10): 50–55.

Harris, P., et al. 2012. Prevalence of complementary and alternative medicine (CAM) use by the general population: A systematic review and update. *International Journal of Clinical Practice* 66(10): 924–939.

Health Canada. 2016. *Drugs and Health Products* (http://www.hc-sc.gc.ca /index-eng.php).

Jahnke, R., et al. 2010. A comprehensive review of health benefits of qigong and tai chi. *American Journal of Health Promotion* 24(6): e1–e25.

Kanodia, A. K., et al. 2010. Perceived benefit of complementary and alternative medicine (CAM) for back pain: A national survey. *Journal of the American Board of Family Medicine* 23(3): 354–362.

Litscher, G., et al. 2012. High-tech acupuncture and integrative laser medicine. *Evidence-Based Complementary and Alternative Medicine* (DOI: 10.1155/2012/363467).

Micozzi, M. S. 2015. *Fundamentals of Complementary and Alternative Medicine*, 5th ed. New York: Saunders..

National Center for Complementary and Integrative Health. 2016. *What Is Complementary, Alternative or Integrative Health?* (https://nccih.nih .gov/health/integrative-health).

National Center for Complementary and Alternative Medicine. 2008. *The Use of Complementary and Alternative Medicine in the United States* (http://nccam.nih.gov/news/camstats/2007/camsurvey_fs1.htm).

Sarris, J., et al. 2012. Complementary medicine, exercise, meditation, diet, and lifestyle modification for anxiety disorders: A review of current evidence. *Evidence-Based Complementary and Alternative Medicine* (DOI: 10.1155/2012/809653).

Sasson, C., et al. 2012. The changing landscape of America's health care system and the value of emergency medicine. *Academic Emergency Medicine* 19(10): 1204–1211.

Shen, P. F., et al. 2012. Acupuncture intervention in ischemic stroke: A randomized controlled prospective study. *American Journal of Chinese Medicine* 40(4): 685–693.

Society of Homeopaths. 2016. *About Homeopathy* (http://www.homeopathy -soh.org/about-homeopathy).

Spears, W., et al. 2013. Parents' perspectives on their children's health insurance: Plight of the underinsured. *Journal of Pediatrics* 162(2): 403–408.

Textbookdollars.com. 2014. *What Does Obamacare Mean for College Students?* (www.textbookdollars.com/blog/obamacare-college-students/).

U.S. Bureau of Labor Statistics. 2016. Occupational Employment and Wages Summary, 2015 (http://www.bls.gov/news.release/ocwage.nr0.htm).

U.S. Food and Drug Administration. 2015. *CFR-Code of Federal Regulations Title 21* (http://www.accessdata.fda.gov/scripts/cdrh/cfdocs/cfcfr /CFRSearch.cfm?an521:4.0.1.1.2.7.1.25.1).

U.S. Food and Drug Administration. 2016. *Information for Consumers* (http://www.fda.gov/drugs/resourcesforyou/consumers/).

Wang, C., et al. 2010. A randomized trial of tai chi for fibromyalgia. *New England Journal of Medicine* 363(8): 743–754.

Young Invincibles. 2014. *Health Care* (http://younginvincibles.org/issues /health-care/).

Zhao, X. F., et al. 2012. Mortality and recurrence of vascular disease among stroke patients treated with combined TCM therapy. *Journal of Traditional Chinese Medicine* 32(2): 173–178.

Zhuang, L. X., et al. 2012. An effectiveness study comparing acupuncture, physiotherapy, and their combination in poststroke rehabilitation: A multicentered, randomized, controlled clinical trial. *Alternative Therapies in Health and Medicine* 18(3): 8–14.

Even though you sometimes have to entrust yourself to the care of medical professionals, you are still responsible for your own behavior. Following medical instructions and advice often requires the same kind of behavioral self-management that's involved in quitting smoking, losing weight, or changing eating patterns. For example, if you have an illness or injury, you may be instructed to take medication at certain times of the day, do special exercises or movements, or change your diet.

The medical profession recognizes the importance of patient adherence and encourages different strategies to support it, such as the following:

1. Use reminders placed at home, in the car, at work, on your computer screensaver, or elsewhere that improve follow-through in taking medication and keeping scheduled appointments. To help you remember to take medications:

   - Use one of the many quality apps available for your phone or computer. (Several of the best ones are listed and reviewed at http://www.kidsmeds.org.)
   - Link taking the medication with some well-established routine, like brushing your teeth or eating breakfast.
   - Use a medication calendar, and check off each pill.
   - Use a medication organizer or pill dispenser.
   - Plan ahead; don't wait until you take the last pill to get a prescription refilled.

2. Use a journal or another form of self-monitoring to keep a detailed account of your health-related behaviors, such as taking pills on schedule, following dietary recommendations, following an exercise program, and so on.

3. Use a self-reward system so that desired behavior changes are encouraged, with a focus on short-term rewards.

4. Develop a clear image or explanation of how the medication or behavior change will improve your health, how you will look and feel, and your long-term well-being.

If these strategies don't help you stick with your treatment plan, you may need to consider other possible explanations for your lack of adherence. For example, are you confused about some aspect of the treatment? Do you find the schedule for taking your medications too complicated, or do the drugs have bothersome side effects that tempt you to avoid them? Do you feel that the recommended treatment is unnecessary or unlikely to help? Are you afraid of becoming dependent on a medication or that you'll be judged negatively if people know about your condition or treatment? A follow-up discussion with a health professional (your physician, physician assistant, nurse practitioner, dietitian, or physical therapist) and an examination of your attitudes and beliefs about your condition and treatment plan can also help improve your adherence.

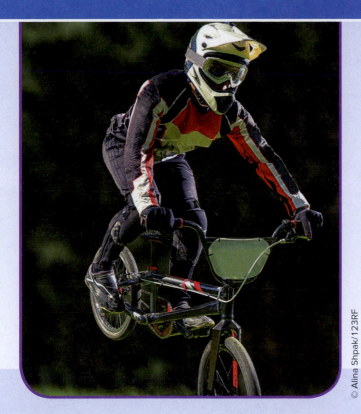

© Alina Shpak/123RF

CHAPTER 16

Personal Safety

CHAPTER OBJECTIVES

- List the most common unintentional injuries and strategies for preventing them
- Discuss violence and intentional injuries, and how to protect yourself
- List strategies for helping others in an emergency

According to the latest data from the National Center for Health Statistics, more than 190,000 Americans die each year from injuries, and many more are temporarily or permanently disabled. The economic cost of injuries is high, with over $671 billion spent each year for medical care and rehabilitation of injured people. Injuries also cause emotional suffering for injured people and their families, friends, and colleagues.

Engineering strategies such as seat belts can help lower injury rates, as can the passage and enforcement of safety-related laws, such as those requiring tamper-proof containers for over-the-counter medications. Public education can also help prevent injuries.

Ultimately, though, it is up to each person to take responsibility for his or her actions and make wise choices. Many of the same sensible attitudes, responsible behaviors, and informed decisions that optimize your wellness can improve your chances of avoiding injuries. This chapter explains how you can protect yourself and those around you from becoming the victims of unintentional and intentional injuries.

If an injury occurs when no harm is intended, it is considered an **unintentional injury.** Motor vehicle crashes, falls, and fires often result in unintentional injuries. Public health officials prefer not to use the word *accidents* to describe unintentional injuries because it suggests events beyond human control. *Injuries* are predictable outcomes that can be controlled or prevented. In contrast, an **intentional injury** is one that is purposely inflicted by yourself or by another person.

Although Americans tend to express more concern about intentional injuries, unintentional injuries are far more common. Unintentional injuries are the fifth leading cause of death among all Americans and the leading cause of death among children and young adults. Because unintentional injuries are so common, they account for more **years of potential life lost** than any other cause of death.

---

unintentional injury An injury that occurs when no harm was intended.   **TERMS**

intentional injury An injury that is purposely inflicted by yourself or by another person.

years of potential life lost The difference between an individual's life expectancy and his or her age at death.

UNINTENTIONAL INJURIES

Injury situations are generally categorized into four general classes, based on where they occur: home injuries, motor vehicle injuries, leisure injuries, and work injuries. The greatest number of disabling injuries occur in the home.

What Causes an Injury?

Most injuries are caused by a combination of human and environmental factors. Human factors are inner conditions or attitudes that lead to an unsafe state, whether physical, emotional, or psychological. A common human factor that leads to injuries is risk-taking behavior. People vary in the amount of risk they tend to take in life, but young men are especially prone to taking risks (see the box "Injuries among Young Men"). Alcohol and drug use is another common risk factor that leads to many injuries and deaths.

Psychological and emotional factors can also play a role in injuries. People sometimes act on the basis of inadequate or inaccurate beliefs about what is safe or unsafe. However, many people who have accurate information still decide to engage in risky behavior. Young people often have unsafe attitudes, such as "I won't get hurt" or "It won't happen to me." Such attitudes can lead to risk taking and ultimately to injuries.

Environmental factors leading to injury are external conditions and circumstances. They may be natural (weather conditions, the undertow of the ocean at the beach), social (a drunk driver), work-related (defective equipment, a slippery surface), or home-related (faulty wiring). Making the environment safer is an important aspect of safety. Laws are often passed to try to make our environment safer. Examples include speed limits on highways and workplace safety requirements.

Home Injuries

The most common fatal **home injuries** are the result of poisonings, falls, fires, choking, drownings, and unintentional shootings. Since 2011, the number of fatal injuries from poisonings has overtaken the number of fatal car crashes (Table 16.1).

Poisoning   More than 1 million nonfatal poisonings and 48,500 fatal poison-related incidents occur every year in the United States; 81% of poison exposures are unintentional, mainly due to prescription drug overdose. The highest number of deaths due to drug poisoning in 2014 occurred among those aged 45–54.

Prescriptions for opioid painkillers, such as codeine, hydrocodone, and morphine, are relatively easy to obtain, and these drugs can quickly become addictive, sometimes leading to overdose, sometimes to addiction. Medications are safe only when used as prescribed.

The most common type of gas poisoning is with carbon monoxide. Carbon monoxide gas is emitted by motor vehicle exhaust and some types of heating equipment. The effects of exposure to this colorless, odorless gas include headache, blurred vision, and shortness of breath, followed by dizziness, vomiting, and unconsciousness. Carbon monoxide detectors (similar to smoke detectors) are available for home use; they should be used according to the manufacturer's instructions. To prevent poisoning by gases, never operate a vehicle in an enclosed space, have your furnace inspected yearly, and use caution with any substance or device that produces potentially toxic fumes.

Keep the national poison control hotline number (800-222-1222) in a convenient location. A call to the hotline will be routed to a local poison control center, which provides expert emergency advice 24 hours a day. If a poisoning occurs, act quickly. Remove the poison from contact with the victim's eyes, skin, or mouth, or move the victim away from

> **home injuries**   Unintentional injuries and deaths **TERMS** that occur in the home and on home premises to occupants, guests, domestic servants, and trespassers; falls, burns, poisonings, suffocations, unintentional shootings, drownings, and electrical shocks are examples.

Table 16.1	Leading Causes of Deaths from Unintentional Injury, 2014			
RANK	ALL AGE GROUPS TOTAL	15–24 YEARS OLD	25–34 YEARS OLD	35–44 YEARS OLD
1	Poisoning (42,032)	Motor vehicle crash (6531)	Poisoning (9334)	Poisoning (9116)
2	Motor vehicle crash (33,736)	Poisoning (3492)	Motor vehicle crash (5856)	Motor vehicle crash (4308)
3	Fall (31,959)	Drowning (507)	Drowning (388)	Fall (504)
4	Suffocation (6580)	Non-motor vehicle transport* (205)	Fall (285)	Drowning (363)

*Includes injuries to pedestrians, cyclists, and riders of public transit not involving motor vehicles.

SOURCE: Centers for Disease Control and Prevention. 2016. *10 Leading Causes of Injury Deaths by Age Group Highlighting Unintentional Injury Deaths, United States—2014* (http://www.cdc.gov/injury/wisqars/leadingcauses.html).

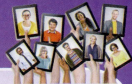

Males significantly outnumber females in early deaths, whether unintentional or intentional. Except among adults age 70 and over, the nonfatal injury rate is substantially higher in males than in females—and it peaks among young adult males (see the figure). Women are more likely to *attempt* suicide, but men are more likely to actually kill themselves. Deaths due to drug poisoning have occurred in men 1.6 times more frequently than in women. And four out of five DUI (driving under the influence) incidents involved a male driver, according to recent Centers for Disease Control and Prevention (CDC) statistics. Gender stereotypes about men and injuries do not apply in every case, but speaking generally, why do men, especially young men, have such high rates of injury?

Some researchers suggest that testosterone, a hormone that is at much higher levels in males than females, plays a role in risky and aggressive behavior. Differences in brain structure and brain activity may also influence how men and women respond to stressors and how quickly and to what degree they become verbally or physically aggressive in response to anger. Moreover, cultural ideologies that men should inhabit rigid social roles—for example, as the breadwinner, protector, or stoic warrior—can lead to emotional stress when men are faced with a reality that requires more flexibility. Ideologies that men are self-sufficient creatures may conflict with notions about love and affection; thus, if a man cannot meet a partner's expectations

for intimacy and a relationship fails, he may feel unable to ask for help and respond with a self-destructive reaction.

As gender dynamics change, the breadwinner role associated with men is now often shared with women. Both men and women work, and in some cases women are the sole breadwinners. Although ideas about men as providers haven't disappeared, fathers are now more likely to participate more fully in raising their children. Following divorce, men are more likely than women to be separated from their children, a factor cited in some suicide cases; in addition, men may be less likely than women to have sources of meaningful social support to rely on during difficult times.

Men may also have greater exposure to injury. Compared with women, men drive 60% more miles, are more likely to have access to a firearm at home, and are more likely to ride motorcycles,

operate machinery, and have jobs associated with high rates of workplace injuries. They are also more likely to engage in sports and other recreational activities that are associated with high rates of injuries. Greater access to and use of firearms plays a role in higher rates of deaths among men from assault and suicide.

SOURCES: Centers for Disease Control and Prevention: Data and Statistics (WISQARS). 2016. *Overall All Injury Causes Nonfatal Injuries and Rates per 100,000 2014, United States, All Races, Both Sexes, All Ages* (http://www.cdc.gov/injury/wisqars/nonfatal.html); Scourfield, J., and R. Evans. 2015. Why might men be more at risk of suicide after a relationship breakdown? Sociological insights. *American Journal of Men's Health* 9(5): 380–384; Stergiou-Kita, M., et al. 2016. Gender influences on return to work after mild traumatic brain injury. *Archives of Physical Medicine and Rehabilitation.* 97(2): S40–S45.

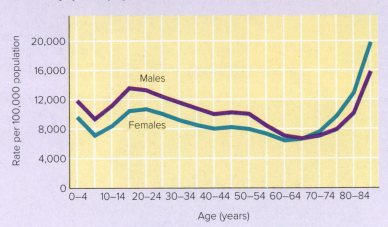

Nonfatal injury rate by age and sex.

contact with poisonous gases. Call the poison control center immediately; do not follow the emergency instructions on product labels because they may be incorrect.

Falls Most deaths from falls occur on stairs. Alcohol is a contributing factor in many falls. Strategies for preventing falls include the following:

- Install handrails and nonslip surfaces in the shower and bathtub.
- Keep floors, stairs, and outside areas clear of objects or conditions that could cause slipping or tripping, such as ice, snow, electrical cords, and toys.

- Put a light switch by the door of every room so that no one has to walk across a room to turn on a light. Use night lights in bedrooms, halls, stairs, and bathrooms.
- When climbing a ladder, use both hands. Never stand higher than the third step from the top. When using a stepladder, make sure the spreader brace is in the locked position. With straight ladders, set the base out one foot for every four feet of height.
- Don't stand on chairs to reach things.
- If there are small children in the home, place gates at the top and bottom of stairs. Never leave a baby unattended on a bed or table.

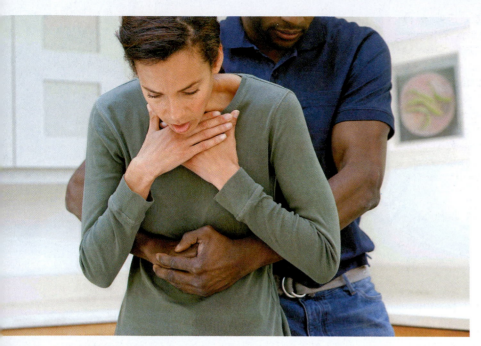

The Heimlich maneuver can save someone who is choking. Reach around the victim, making a fist and placing the thumb side of the fist just above the navel. Grasp your fist with the other hand and thrust upward and inward into the victim's abdomen. Continue with quick jerks until the object is expelled.

© Science Photo Library/Getty Images RF

- Get out as quickly as possible, and go to the designated meeting place. Don't stop for a keepsake or pet. Never hide in a closet or under a bed. Once outside, count heads to see if everyone is out. If you think someone is still inside the burning building, tell the firefighters. Never go back inside a burning building.

- If you're trapped in a room, feel the door. If it is hot or if smoke is coming in through the cracks, don't open it; use the alternative escape route. If you can't get out, go to the window and shout for help.

- Smoke inhalation is the largest cause of death and injury in fires. To avoid inhaling smoke, crawl along the floor away from the heat and smoke. Cover your mouth and nose, ideally with a wet cloth, and take short, shallow breaths.

- If your clothes catch fire, don't run. Drop to the ground, cover your face, and roll back and forth to smother the flames. Remember: stop–drop–roll.

Fires   Most fires begin in the kitchen, living room, or bedroom. Cooking is now the leading cause of home fire injuries; careless smoking is the leading cause of fire deaths, followed by problems with heating equipment and arson. A study of campus fire fatalities found that smoking materials left to smolder over time in a couch accounted for half of those fatalities in which smoking was involved.

To prevent fires, dispose of all cigarettes in ashtrays and never smoke in bed. Other strategies include proper maintenance of fireplaces, furnaces, heaters, chimneys, and electrical outlets, cords, and appliances. If you use a portable heater, keep it at least three feet away from curtains, bedding, or anything else that might catch fire. Never leave heaters on unattended.

Also, be prepared to handle fire-related situations. Plan at least two escape routes out of each room, and designate a location outside the home as a meeting place. For practice, stage a home fire drill; do this at night because that's when most deadly fires occur.

Data show that about three out of five home fire deaths occur in homes with no working smoke alarms. Install smoke detectors on every level of your home. Your risk of dying in a fire is almost twice as high if you do not use them.

These strategies can help prevent injuries in a fire:

> **QUICK STATS**
>
> About **50%** of all injuries that require medical attention occur in the home.
>
> —National Safety Council, 2016

Suffocation and Choking   Suffocation and choking represented the fourth most common cause of death in the home in 2013. Elderly people and children are especially vulnerable. Children can suffocate if they put small items in their mouths, get tangled in their crib bedding, or get trapped in airtight appliances like old refrigerators. Keep small objects out of reach of children under age 3, and don't give them raw carrots, hot dogs, popcorn, gum, or hard candy. Examine toys carefully for small parts that could come loose. Don't give plastic bags or balloons to small children.

Adults can also become choking victims, especially if they fail to chew food properly, eat hurriedly, or try to talk and eat at the same time. Many choking victims can be saved with the **Heimlich maneuver.** The American Red Cross recommends abdominal thrusts as the easiest and safest thing to do when an adult is choking. Back blows in conjunction with two-finger abdominal thrusts are an acceptable procedure for dislodging an object from the throat of an infant.

> **Heimlich maneuver**   A maneuver developed by Henry J. Heimlich, M.D., to help force an obstruction from the airway.   **TERMS**

Firearms When researchers compared rates of firearm deaths in high-income countries, they found that although the rates in most countries had declined since 2003, those in the United States, already the highest, remained unchanged. The United States has an overall firearm death rate 10 times higher than in 22 other high-income countries. The firearm homicide rate is 25 times higher, the firearm suicide rate 8 is times higher, and the unintentional gun death rate is more than 6 times higher in the United States. Over one-third of all unintended firearm deaths and nonfatal injuries involve children and young adults under 25 years of age. People who use firearms should remember the following:

- Always treat a gun as though it is loaded, even if you know it isn't.

- Never point a gun—loaded or unloaded—at anything you do not intend to shoot.

- Always unload a gun before storing it. Store unloaded firearms under lock and key, in a place separate from the ammunition.

- Always inspect firearms carefully before handling.

- If you ever plan to handle a gun, take a firearms safety course first.

- If you own a gun, buy and use a gun lock designed specifically for that weapon.

Proper storage is critical. Do not assume that young children cannot fire a gun. Even children as young as 3 have enough finger strength to pull a trigger. One study estimated that 110 children aged 0–14 die each year as a result of unintentional firearm injuries. In the overwhelming majority of child shooting cases, victims and shooters are male; and the victim has either shot himself (one-third of cases) or been shot by another child. Anyone who picks up a gun should assume it is loaded. If you plan to handle a gun, avoid alcohol and drugs, which affect judgment and coordination.

Motor Vehicle Injuries

According to the National Highway Traffic Safety Administration (NHTSA), 32,675 Americans were killed and 2.3 million injured in motor vehicle crashes in 2014. The good news is that motor vehicle deaths in this country have decreased 25% in the past decade. Worldwide, motor vehicle crashes kill 1.25 million and injure up to 50 million people each year, placing motor vehicle injuries within the top 10 leading causes of death overall. Those most involved in motor vehicle crashes are people aged 15–24. Motor vehicle injuries also result in the majority of cases of paralysis due to spinal injuries, and they are the leading cause of severe brain injury in the United States. Table 16.2 puts into context how likely Americans are to die from motor vehicle crashes versus other types of injuries.

TABLE 16.2 Lifetime Odds of Death Due to Selected Types of Injury

INJURY TYPE	LIFETIME ODDS
Suicide	1 in 97
Unintentional poisoning	1 in 103
Motor vehicle crash	1 in 113
Fall	1 in 133
Homicide (assault by firearm)	1 in 358
Pedestrian incident	1 in 672
Motorcycle rider incident	1 in 948
Drowning	1 in 1183
Exposure to fire, flames, or smoke	1 in 1454
Choking from inhalation and ingestion of food	1 in 3408
Air or space transport incident	1 in 9737
Exposure to excessive natural heat	1 in 10,784
Electric current	1 in 14,695
Contact with sharp objects	1 in 30,860
Cataclysmic storm	1 in 63,679
Hornet/bee/wasp sting	1 in 64,706
Being bitten or struck by a dog	1 in 114,622
Lightning strike	1 in 174,426

SOURCE: National Safety Council. 2016. *Lifetime Odds of Deaths for Selected Causes, U.S.* Itasca, IL: National Safety Council.

QUICK STATS

Motor vehicle injuries cost Americans more than $800 billion per year in economic and social terms.

—National Highway Traffic Safety Administration, 2015

Factors Contributing to Motor Vehicle Injuries

Common causes of motor vehicle injuries are speeding, aggressive driving, fatigue, inexperience, the use of cell phones, handheld devices and other distractions, the use of alcohol and other drugs, and the incorrect use of seat belts and other safety devices.

DISTRACTED DRIVING In 2014, motor vehicle crashes involving distracted drivers caused 3179 deaths and 431,000 injuries. Drivers in their twenties make up 27% of the distracted drivers in fatal crashes, according to the NHTSA. Distractions include visual-manual activity such as looking and using hands to type a text message (see the box "Cell Phones and Distracted Driving") and cognitive tasks such as calculating numbers or formulating a sentence. Distractions can come from outside the car as well—for example, billboards and roadside accidents—or inside the car, as in the case of a conversation with a passenger, or eating, smoking, and reaching for controls.

SPEEDING After inattentive driving, the next most common cause for car crashes is speeding and other errors in decision

WELLNESS ON CAMPUS
Cell Phones and Distracted Driving

The National Safety Council estimates that one in four motor vehicle crashes can be attributed to distractions from cell phone use. How widespread is phone use among drivers? The National Occupant Protection Use Survey reported that, at any point in the day, approximately 660,000 Americans are using cell phones or manipulating electronic devices while driving. The University of Michigan Transportation Research Institute shows that a quarter of teens respond to a text message once or more every time they drive. Similarly, 20% of teens and 10% of parents admit that they have extended, multi-message text conversations while driving.

What about college students? A survey of nearly 5000 students from 12 colleges found that 91% reported phoning and/or texting while driving. This included 87% who text at traffic lights, 60% who text on city streets or in stop-and-go traffic, and 50% who send texts while driving on the freeway. Nearly half of the respondents said they were capable or very capable of safely talking on a cell phone while driving, but only 8.5% felt that other drivers were capable of doing so. These students overestimate their ability to multitask while driving.

The visual-manual distraction of locating, dialing, text messaging, browsing, and ending a call on handheld phones increases the risk of a crash by three times. Those tasks that keep your hands and eyes from being engaged in driving the car have been shown to have a greater impact than cognitive distractions such as calculating numbers or formulating a sentence. However, research has found that, for drivers, the cognitive impairment associated with interacting with a speech-to-text system is significant and greater than that associated with activities such as listening to the radio and talking with passengers.

Drivers under age 25, who are the heaviest users of social media and cell phone technology, also generally have less skill in controlling vehicles and less efficiency in visual scanning, in addition to generally taking more risks. Their lack of experience includes less ability to handle the effects of distraction, compared to the abilities of mid-age drivers (25–64 years old).

For younger and older drivers, talking on cell phones has been found to increase the odds of severe injuries. Dialing and texting have a profound negative effect on older drivers and a somewhat negative effect on younger and mid-age drivers. Drivers over age 64 have decreased reaction times due to age-related decreased cognition and perception.

Currently, 46 states, the District of Columbia, and Guam ban all text messaging while driving; 14 states prohibit any use of a handheld phone while driving. No state bans all cell phone use in the vehicle, but 38 states and Washington, D.C., disallow all cell phone use by "novice drivers," defined as those under 18 or 19 years of age, depending on the state.

Hands-free devices are an important alternative to handheld phones (although also not entirely distraction-free). For people who live where cell phone use is legal while driving and who choose to use a phone, the following strategies may increase safety:

- Use a hands-free device so that you can keep both hands on the steering wheel.

- Be familiar with your phone and its functions, especially speed dial and redial.

- Store frequently called numbers on speed dial so that you can place calls without looking at the phone.

- If your phone has voice-activated dialing, use it.

- Let the person you are speaking with know you are driving, and be prepared to end the call at any time.

- Don't place or answer calls in heavy traffic or hazardous weather conditions.

- Don't take notes or look up phone numbers while driving.

- Time calls so that you can place them when you are at a stop.

Any kind of distraction—visual, manual, or cognitive—can contribute to an unsafe driving situation.

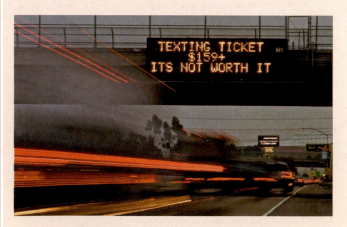
© ZUMA Press, Inc/Alamy

SOURCES: Hill, L., et al. 2015. Prevalence of and attitudes about distracted driving in college students. *Traffic Injury Prevention* 16(4): 362–367; Donmez, B., and Z. Liu. 2015. Associations of distraction involvement and age with driver injury severities. *Journal of Safety Research* 52: 23–28; Fitch, G. M., et al. 2015. Drivers' visual behavior when using handheld and hands-free cell phones. *Journal of Safety Research* 54: 105.e29–108; National Highway Traffic Safety Administration. *Facts and Statistics: What Is Distracted Driving?* (http://www.distraction.gov/stats-research-laws/facts-and-statistics.html); AAA Foundation for Traffic Safety. 2013. *Measuring Cognitive Distraction in the Automobile*. Washington, DC: AAA Foundation for Traffic Safety.

making (e.g., false assumption of others' actions, misjudgment of a gap or others' speed). As speed increases, momentum and the force of impact increase, and the time allowed for the driver to react (reaction time) decreases. Speed limits are posted to establish the safest maximum speed limit for a given area under ideal conditions; if visibility is limited or the road is wet, the safe maximum speed may be considerably lower.

AGGRESSIVE DRIVING Aggressive driving includes frequent, erratic, and abrupt lane changes; tailgating; running red lights or stop signs; passing on the shoulder; and blocking other cars trying to change lanes or pass. Aggressive drivers increase the risk of crashes for themselves and others. Injuries may also occur if aggressive drivers stop their vehicles and confront each other following an incident.

FATIGUE AND SLEEPINESS Driving requires mental alertness and attentiveness. Studies have shown that sleepiness causes slower reaction times, reduced coordination and vigilance, and delayed information processing. Research shows that even mild sleep deprivation causes deterioration in driving ability comparable to that caused by a 0.05% blood alcohol concentration—a level considered hazardous when driving.

ALCOHOL AND OTHER DRUGS Alcohol is involved in about one-third of fatal crashes. Alcohol-impaired driving is illegal in all states and the District of Columbia. The legal limit for blood alcohol concentration (BAC) is 0.08%, but people can be impaired at much lower BACs. Because alcohol affects reason and judgment as well as the ability to make fast, accurate, and coordinated movements, a person who has been drinking will be less likely to recognize that he or she is impaired. Use of many over-the-counter and all psychoactive drugs is also potentially dangerous if you plan to drive.

SEAT BELTS, AIRBAGS, AND CHILD SAFETY SEATS Although mandatory seat belt laws for adults are in effect in 49 states (not New Hampshire) and the District of Columbia, only 87% of motor vehicle occupants used seat belts in 2014, even though they are the single most effective way to reduce the risk of crash-related death. The good news is that seat belt usage was at its highest level ever.

Some people think that if they are involved in a crash they are better off being thrown free of their vehicle. In fact, the chances of being killed are 25 times greater if you are thrown from a vehicle, whether it is due to injuries caused by hitting a tree or the pavement or by being hit by another vehicle. Seat belts not only prevent you from being thrown from the car at the time of the crash but also provide protection from second collisions: If a car is traveling at 65 miles per hour (mph) and hits another vehicle, the car stops first; then the occupants stop because they, too, are traveling at 65 mph. Second collisions occur when occupants hit something inside the car, such as the dashboard or windshield. Seat belts stop these second collisions from occurring and spread the first collisions' force over the occupants' bodies.

Since 1998, all new cars and light trucks have been equipped with dual airbags—one for the driver and one for the front passenger. Many vehicles also offer side airbags, which further reduce the risk of injury. Advanced airbag systems include risk reduction technologies such as sensors to detect crash severity, seat position, passenger size, and whether a passenger is wearing a seat belt. Although airbags provide supplementary protection in the event of a collision, most are useful only in head-on collisions. They also deflate immediately after inflating and therefore do not provide protection in collisions involving multiple impacts. Airbags are not a replacement for seat belts; everyone in a vehicle should buckle up.

Airbags deploy forcefully and can injure a child or short adult who is improperly restrained or sitting too close to the dashboard, although second-generation airbags are somewhat safer for children than older devices. To ensure that airbags work safely, always follow these basic guidelines: Place infants in rear-facing infant seats in the back seat, transport children aged 12 and under in the back seat, always use seat belts and appropriate safety seats, and keep 10 inches between the airbag cover and the breastbone of the driver or passenger. If necessary, adjust the steering wheel or use seat cushions to ensure that an inflating airbag would hit you in the chest and not in the face. Children who have outgrown child safety seats but are still too small for adult seat belts alone should be secured using booster seats that ensure that the seat belt is positioned low across the hips and thighs.

Preventing Motor Vehicle Injuries
About 75% of all motor vehicle collisions occur within 25 miles of home and at speeds lower than 40 mph. Strategies for preventing motor vehicle injuries include the following:

- Obey the speed limit.
- Always wear a seat belt.
- Never drive under the influence of alcohol or other drugs, and never ride with a driver who is.
- Keep your car in good working order. Follow your vehicle manufacturer's maintenance recommendations. Make sure your brakes, tires, wipers, and window defrosters work well. Keep up with any safety recalls, such as the air bag recalls announced in 2013–2016; you can check for recalls using your vehicle's VIN at https://vinrcl.safercar.gov/vin/.
- Always allow enough following distance. Use the three-second rule: When the vehicle ahead passes a reference point, count out three seconds (say 1001, 1002, 1003). If you pass the reference point before you finish counting, drop back and allow more following distance. This rule works well at slower speeds when roads are dry and weather conditions are good. When traveling on highways or the interstate, use the four-second rule.
- Always increase your following distance and slow down if weather or road conditions are poor. In those kinds of situations, the minimum recommendation is to follow four seconds behind the car in front of you.
- Choose interstate highways rather than rural roads. Highways are much safer because of better visibility, wider lanes, and fewer surprises.

- Always signal when turning or changing lanes.
- Stop completely at stop signs. Follow all traffic laws.
- Take special care at intersections. Look left, right, and then left again. Make sure you have time to complete your maneuver in the intersection.
- Don't pass on two-lane roads unless you're in a designated passing area and have a clear view ahead.

Motorcycles and Motor Scooters   About one out of every seven traffic fatalities involves someone riding a motorcycle. In recent years, riders aged 50 years and over have represented one-third of these fatalities. The data also reveal that, per mile traveled, motorcycle riders are 26 times more likely to die in a crash than occupants of a car or other motor vehicle. Injuries from motorcycle collisions are generally more severe than those involving automobiles because motorcycles provide little, if any, protection.

People riding motor scooters face additional challenges. Such vehicles usually have a maximum speed of 35–40 mph and have less power for maneuverability, especially in an emergency.

Strategies for preventing motorcycle and motor scooter injuries include the following:

- Wear light-colored clothing, drive with your headlights on, and correctly position yourself in traffic.
- Develop the necessary skills. Lack of skill is a major factor in motorcycle and motor scooter injuries. Skidding from improper braking is the most common cause of loss of control.
- Wear a helmet. Helmets should be marked with the DOT symbol, certifying that they conform to federal safety standards established by the U.S. Department of Transportation. Helmet use is required by law in most states.
- Protect your eyes with goggles, a face shield, or a windshield.
- Drive defensively, particularly when changing lanes and at intersections, and never assume that other drivers can see you.

Bicycles   Bicycle injuries result primarily from riders not knowing or understanding the rules of the road, failing to follow traffic laws, not having sufficient skill or experience to handle traffic conditions, or being intoxicated. Bicycles are considered vehicles; bicyclists must obey all traffic laws that apply to automobile drivers, including stopping at traffic lights and stop signs.

Head injuries are involved in about three out of four bicycle-related deaths. Research shows that wearing a helmet reduces the risk of head injury by 66–88%. Safe cycling strategies include the following:

- Wear safety equipment, including a helmet, eye protection, gloves, and proper footwear. Secure the bottom of your pant legs with clips, and secure your shoelaces so that they don't get tangled in the chain.

- Wear light-colored, reflective clothing. Equip your bike with reflectors, and use lights, especially at night or when riding in wooded or other dark areas.
- Ride with the flow of traffic, not against it, and follow all traffic laws. Use bike paths when they are available.
- Ride defensively; never assume that drivers have seen you. Be especially careful when turning or crossing at corners and intersections. Watch for cars turning right.
- Stop at all traffic lights and stop signs. Know and use hand signals.

Pedestrians   About one in seven motor vehicle deaths involves pedestrians, and more than 66,000 pedestrians are injured each year. The highest rates of death and injury occur among the very young and the elderly. Pedestrians are hit more likely by the front of the vehicle than the rear or right or left side. Alcohol intoxication plays a significant role in up to half of all adult pedestrian fatalities. Walkers and runners should face traffic and cross only at marked cross-walks and intersections.

Leisure Injuries

Most people enjoy some form of leisure activities, so it is not surprising that **leisure injuries** are a significant health-related problem in the United States. Specific safety strategies for activities associated with leisure injuries include the following:

- Don't swim alone, in unsupervised places, under the influence of alcohol, or for an unusual length of time. Use caution when swimming in unfamiliar surroundings or in water colder than 70°F. Check the depth of water before diving. Make sure that residential pools are fenced, and never allow children to swim unsupervised.
- Always use a **personal flotation device** (also known as a life jacket) when on a boat.
- For all sports and recreational activities, make sure facilities are safe, follow the rules, and practice good sportsmanship. Develop adequate skill in the activity, and use proper safety equipment, including, where appropriate, a helmet, eye protection, correct footwear, and knee, elbow, and wrist pads (see the box "Head Injuries in Contact Sports").
- If using equipment such as skateboards, snowboards, mountain bikes, or all-terrain vehicles, wear a helmet

TERMS

leisure injuries   Unintentional injuries and deaths that occur in public places, or places used in a public way, not involving motor vehicles; include most sports and recreation deaths and injuries; examples are falls, drownings, burns, and heat and cold stress.

personal flotation device   A device designed to save a person from drowning by buoying up the body while in the water.

Reports of bizarre behavior, suicides, and middle-aged dementia among former professional football players, boxers, and soccer players have focused worldwide media attention on sports concussions. Death from chronic traumatic encephalopathy (CTE), a disease caused by repetitive brain trauma, was the diagnosis for the Super Bowl-winning quarterback from the Oakland Raiders, Kenny Stabler, and for former Minnesota Vikings linebacker Fred McNeill. They both died in 2015, in their 60s.

CTE has been found in younger athletes as well. An amateur football player in his early twenties suffered a variety of symptoms before dying at age 25. He had received repeated concussions since starting to play football at age six and continuing through college. He was an above-average student, but because of his symptoms—first, ongoing headaches, insomnia, anxiety, and difficulty with memory and concentration; and later, apathy, feelings of worthlessness, and suicidal thoughts—he had to stop both playing football and attending college. The diagnosis at his autopsy was CTE.

CTE can be diagnosed only on autopsy, whereas concussions, or mild traumatic brain injuries (MTBIs), can be diagnosed immediately or after some cognitive and neurological testing. An MTBI is a traumatic injury to the brain or spinal cord resulting from a direct blow to the head or indirect blows elsewhere that can cause violent brain movement in the skull. A concussion, for example, can result from a blow to the chest that makes the head snap forward. Symptoms include headache, nausea, vomiting, sleep disturbances, depression, and loss of concentration. Unconsciousness occurs in only 10% of concussions.

Forty million people worldwide suffer concussions every year. Concussions account for 5% of the nearly 225,000 sports injuries occurring in the United States each year. They are most common in football, hockey, skiing, wrestling, rugby, basketball, and soccer. The incidence is higher in men than in women, but women are at greater risk when playing the same sport—for example, soccer. Concussions and their neurodegenerative fallouts also occur in soldiers and, generally, in people of all ages and careers if they have a fall or sustain an injury in a motor vehicle crash.

Although the National Football League continues to downplay the risk of injury in football, researchers and journalists have documented that repeated concussions in childhood sports can cause progressive damage to the brain. Autopsies of deceased former high school, college, and professional football players show that 79% of all players and 97% of professional players showed evidence of CTE.

Can we predict brain injuries before they become fatal? Researchers are working to predict injury risk—both of MTBI in the moment it happens and of CTE as it develops. For example, bioengineers at Stanford University outfitted athletes with mouth guards that monitored symptoms of MTBI and recorded more than 500 moments of impact during regular sporting events. This is especially significant because athletes often fail to recognize—let alone report—that they have suffered an injury. Because sustaining a second injury shortly after the first can result in much greater damage, an instantaneous indication of concussion should require medical professionals to pull a player to the sidelines.

What can individuals do to reduce their risk of concussion? Always wear a helmet when cycling, skiing, snowboarding, rock climbing, or skateboarding. Wearing seat belts and ensuring that car airbags are functioning properly can also help. Older adults can reduce their risk of concussions by keeping living spaces free of clutter, wearing stable footwear, and maintaining strength and balance through regular exercise.

Preventing concussions in contact sports is more challenging. The pre-participation physical examination can identify athletes with a history of concussion and assess their readiness to compete. Helmets in sports like football and hockey protect the skull from impact injuries (fractures and lacerations) but have little effect on the incidence or severity of concussions. Coaching fundamentals can teach athletes to avoid dangerous techniques such as spear blocking and tackling but do little to change the nature of high-impact collision sports. Professional officiating can cut down on dangerous play. Rule changes such as eliminating zone coverage in football or heading in soccer might reduce the concussion rate. Recognizing concussion injuries is important for preventing long-term disability. Finally, education can teach athletes about the symptoms and seriousness of concussions.

SOURCES: Daneshvar, D. H., et al. 2013. *Clinics in Sports Medicine*. 30(1): 1–17; Gregory, S. 2016. The NFL still won't tackle brain trauma at the super bowl. *Time*, February 6 (http://time.com/4210564/nfl-super-bowl-brain-trauma-cte/); Harmon, K. G., et al. 2013. American Medical Society for Sports Medicine Position Statement: Concussion in sport. *British Journal of Sports Medicine* 47(1): 15–26; Hernandez, F., et al. 2015. Six degree-of-freedom measurements of human mild traumatic brain injury. *Annals of Biomedical Engineering* 43(8): 1918–1934; McCarthy, M. 2016. Chronic traumatic encephalopathy is reported in 25 year old former American football player. *British Medical Journal* 352: 7027; Misra, A. 2014. Common sports injuries: Incidence and average charges. *ASPE Issue Brief*, March 17 (https://aspe.hhs.gov/pdf-report/common-sports-injuries-incidence-and-average-charges).

and other safety equipment, and avoid excessive speeds and unsafe stunts. Use playground equipment only for those activities for which it is designed.

- If you are active in excessively hot and humid weather, drink plenty of fluids, rest frequently in the shade, and slow down or stop if you feel uncomfortable. Danger signals of heat stress include excessive perspiration, dizziness, headache, muscle cramps, nausea, weakness, rapid pulse, and disorientation.

- Do not use alcohol or other drugs during recreational activities—such activities require coordination and sound judgment.

Weather-Related Injuries

Even though conditions may seem harmless at times, they can become dangerous quickly, as noted here.

• *Heat.* Extreme heat is the leading weather-related killer in the United States, according to the National Weather Service. Heat-related illness such as heat stroke and heat exhaustion can be fatal, especially for children, older adults, and people who are dehydrated. The best way to deal with excessive heat is to stay indoors as much as possible, with a fan or air conditioner on. Wear lightweight, light-colored clothing; drink plenty of water to stay hydrated; and avoid heavy meals.

• *Cold.* Each year dozens of Americans die from exposure to cold temperatures. Conditions such as hypothermia (low body temperature) and frostbite (frozen skin or flesh) can be deadly. Most injuries and deaths in cold weather are due to a lack of preparedness or understanding of the dangers of low temperatures and wind chill. If you must go outdoors in very cold weather, dress in layers and cover your face, fingers, and ears to protect them from frostbite. Make sure your home and car are prepared with plenty of fuel, drinking water, warm clothes and blankets, batteries, and other emergency supplies.

• *Wind.* In extremely windy conditions, take cover in a sturdy shelter, preferably a permanent structure with a foundation. In a severe storm such as a tornado, move to the lowest portion of the building or to a small interior room away from windows. If you're outdoors when a severe storm or tornado strikes, lie flat in a low spot or ditch. Don't stay inside a car or hide under an open-sided structure such as a bridge; such structures can act as a funnel and make the wind more intense.

• *Lightning.* About 400 Americans are struck by lightning every year, and about 10% of them die. The National Weather Service recommends that you go indoors when conditions are right for lightning. You are safer in a house, as long as you avoid anything that conducts electricity, which includes corded telephones, electrical appliances, computers, plumbing, and metal doors and windows.

• *Flooding.* If you're near rapidly rising water, move to higher ground and call for help. Don't attempt to drive or walk through flooded streets, and don't traverse a bridge if it is being pounded by high, fast-moving water.

Work Injuries

The Bureau of Labor Statistics estimates that in 2014 over 1.5 million Americans suffered injuries on the job that resulted in days away from work, job transfer, or some kind of restriction. Certain types of **work injuries**, including skin disorders and repetitive strain injuries, are becoming more common. Although people who do extensive manual labor and lifting on the job make up less than half of the workforce, they account for more than 75% of all work-related injuries and illnesses. Most fatalities on the job involve crushing injuries, severe lacerations, burns, and electrocutions. In November 2013, OSHA proposed a new rule to improve

tracking of workplace injuries and illnesses through electronic submission of data on a quarterly basis.

Back problems accounted for over 200,000 work injuries in 2014. Many back injuries that occur on the job could be prevented through the use of proper lifting techniques:

• Avoid bending at the waist. Remain in an upright position and crouch down if you need to lower yourself to grasp the object. Bend at the knees and hips.

• Place feet securely about shoulder-width apart; grip the object firmly.

• Lift gradually, with straight arms. Avoid quick, jerky motions. Lift by standing up or pushing with your leg muscles. Keep the object close to your body.

• If you have to turn, change the position of your feet. Twisting is a common and dangerous cause of injury.

work injuries Unintentional injuries and deaths **TERMS** that arise out of and in the course of gainful work, such as falls, electrical shocks, exposure to radiation and toxic chemicals, burns, cuts, back sprains, and loss of fingers or other body parts in machines.

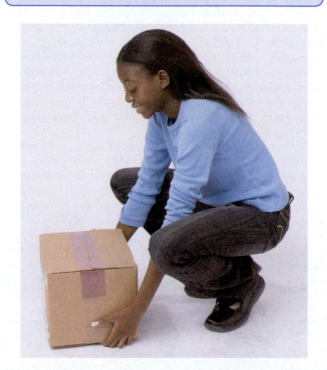

The correct lifting technique is to stay upright, bending at the knees and hips.

© McGraw-Hill Education/Ken Karp, photographer

Repetitive strain injuries (RSIs) impact the musculoskeletal and nervous systems of the body and affect many people around the world. Other terms to describe this condition include *repetitive motion disorder (RMD), cumulative trauma disorder (CTD),* and *occupational overuse syndrome (OOS).*

An RSI can be caused by a combination of physical and psychosocial stressors, but the injury typically involves some kind of repetitive action or forceful exertion on the body over time. Pain in the extremities as well as the back and shoulders is commonly cited and tends to worsen with extended activity.

The task associated with an RSI may be something relatively simple and non-exertive like typing, writing, or clicking a computer mouse. One of the most common work-related injuries is *carpal tunnel syndrome (CTS),* which is characterized by pressure on the median nerve in the wrist that also affects tendons and ligaments in the forearm. Symptoms of CTS include numbness, tingling, burning, and/or aching in the hand, particularly in the thumb and the first three fingers. The pain may worsen at night and may shoot up from the hand as far as the shoulder. If it does not clear up on its own, immobilization of the joint at night can be helpful; other options may involve anti-inflammatory drugs or even surgery in extreme cases.

In terms of physical activity by an athlete, examples include conditions commonly referred to as "golfer's elbow" or "tennis elbow," in which the joints are continually exposed to extreme stress in order to complete an action accurately with speed and force.

With new technologies being introduced every day, another type of RSI is now being recognized. Many people who use their thumbs to text are suffering from a condition referred to as "Blackberry thumb." Similarly, people who spend countless hours using handheld controls to play video games are experiencing "gamer's thumb."

In all cases, research indicates the primary risk factors are usually associated with poor posture, improper techniques for completing an activity, and overuse of a certain part of the body. The good news is that a person can make adjustments to reduce the risk of an RSI, either in what is being done or through modification of the environment. Warm up your wrists before you begin any repetitive motion activity, and take frequent breaks to stretch and flex your wrists and hands:

- Extend your arms out in front of you and stretch your wrists by pointing your fingers to the ceiling; hold for a count of five. Then straighten your wrists and relax your fingers for a count of five.

- With arms extended, make a tight fist with both hands and then bend your wrists so that your knuckles are pointed toward the floor; hold for a count of five. Then straighten your wrists and relax your fingers for a count of five.

Repeat these stretches several times, and finish by letting your arms hang loosely at your sides and shaking them gently for several seconds. It's also important to maintain a physically active lifestyle, take plenty of breaks to avoid hours of sedentary activity, stretch, apply proper ergonomic principles, and minimize other stress factors.

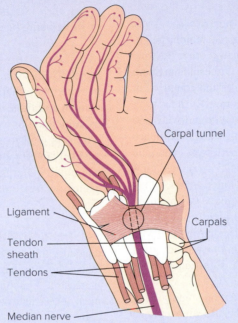

Carpal tunnel

Ligament

Tendon sheath

Tendons

Median nerve

Carpals

Plan ahead so that your pathway is clear and turning can be minimized.

- Put the object down gently, reversing the steps for lifting.

Musculoskeletal injuries and disorders in the workplace include **repetitive strain injuries (RSIs).** RSIs are caused by repeated strain on a particular part of the body. Twisting, vibrations, awkward postures, and other stressors may contribute to RSIs. **Carpal tunnel syndrome** is one type of RSI that has increased in recent years due to increased use of computers, both at work and in the home (see the box "Repetitive Strain Injury" for more information).

VIOLENCE AND INTENTIONAL INJURIES

Violence—the use of physical force with the intent to inflict harm, injury, or death upon yourself or another—is a major public health concern in the United States. According to the Federal Bureau of Investigation (FBI), 1.65 million violent

TERMS

repetitive strain injury (RSI) A musculoskeletal injury or disorder caused by repeated strain on the hand, arm, wrist, or other part of the body; also called *cumulative trauma disorder (CTD).*

carpal tunnel syndrome Compression of the median nerve in the wrist, often caused by repetitive use of the hands, such as in computer use; characterized by numbness, tingling, and pain in the hands and fingers; can cause nerve damage.

crimes occurred in the United States in 2014. Examples of violence are assault, homicide, sexual assault, domestic violence, suicide, and child abuse. In comparison to other industrialized countries, the United States has much higher rates of violence, with 4–10 times the homicide death rates found in similar countries.

Factors Contributing to Violence

Most intentional injuries and deaths are associated with an argument or a crime. However, there are many forms of violence, and no single factor can explain all of them.

Social Factors Rates of violence are not the same throughout society; they vary by geographic region, neighborhood, socioeconomic level, and many other factors. According to the FBI, violence rates were highest in the South in 2014, followed by the Midwest region of the country. For communities, increased rates of violence are associated with poverty and socioeconomic inequality and with prejudice and discrimination. In all racial/ethnic groups, rates of violence are highest for boys and young men in the lowest economic circumstances. In 2014, people under age 25 accounted for 4 out of 10 arrests for violent crime in the United States.

People who feel they are a part of society (with strong family and social ties), who are economically integrated (having a reasonable chance at getting a decent job), and who grow up in areas with a feeling of community (with good schools, parks, and neighborhoods) are significantly less likely to engage in violence.

Studies have shown that the environment on some college campuses also can contribute to violence. Because college campuses are transitory communities, some people may have less incentive to cooperate and coexist amicably.

Violence in the Media The mass media play a major role in exposing audiences of all ages to violence as an acceptable and effective means of solving problems. On average, children in the United States watch about four hours of television daily and may view as many as 10,000 violent acts on television and in movies each year. Computer and video games also include many violent acts, leading to concern that children's exposure to violence will make them more accepting or tolerant of it. The consequences of violence are depicted in the media much less frequently.

Researchers have found that exposure to media violence at least temporarily increases aggressive feelings in children, making them more likely to engage in violent or fearful behavior; the direct, short-term effects on teens and adults are less clear. Parents should monitor the TV shows, movies, video games, music, and other forms of media to which their children are exposed. Watching programs with children gives parents the opportunity to talk to them about violence and its consequences, to explain that violence is not the best way to resolve conflicts or solve problems, and to point out examples of positive behaviors such as kindness and cooperation.

Gender In most cases, violence is committed by men (Figure 16.1). Males are nine times more likely than females to commit murder, and three times more likely than females to be murdered. Male college students are twice as likely as female students to be the victims of violence.

Women do commit acts of violence, including a small but substantial proportion of murders of spouses. This fact has been used to argue that women have the same capacity to commit violence as men, but most researchers note substantial differences. Men often kill their wives as the culmination of years of violence or after stalking them; they may kill their entire families and themselves at the same time. Women virtually never kill in such circumstances; rather, they kill their husbands after repeated victimization or while being beaten.

Interpersonal Factors Although most people fear attack from strangers, the majority of victims are acquainted with their attackers. More than half of murders of women and three-fourths of sexual assaults are committed by someone the woman knows. Crime victims and violent criminals tend to share many characteristics—that is, they are likely to be young, male, and from a low-income minority community. Being a victim of teasing, bullying, or social exclusion (rejection) may lead to aggressive behavior or violence.

Alcohol and Other Drugs Substance misuse and dependence are consistently associated with interpersonal violence and suicide. Intoxication affects judgment and may increase aggression in some people, causing a small argument to escalate into a serious physical confrontation. On college campuses, alcohol is involved in about 95% of all violent crimes.

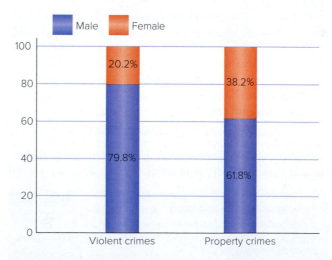

FIGURE 16.1 Arrests in the United States, 2014. Males were arrested significantly more often than females for both violent and property crimes.

SOURCE: Federal Bureau of Investigation. 2015. Crime in the United States 2014. Washington, DC: U.S. Department of Justice..

Firearms Many criminologists argue that the high rate of homicide in the United States is directly related to the fact that it is the only industrialized country in which handgun ownership is widespread and firearms are relatively easy to obtain. The use of a handgun can change a suicide attempt to a completed suicide and a violent assault to a murder.

Almost 120,000 deaths and injuries occur in the United States each year as a result of the use of firearms. Firearms are used in more than two-thirds of homicides, and studies reveal a strong correlation between the incidence of gun ownership and homicide rates for a given area of the country. Over half of all suicides involve a firearm, and people living in households in which guns are kept have a risk of suicide that is four or more times greater than that of people living in households without guns.

Assault

Assault is the use of physical force by a person or people to inflict injury or death on another. Homicide, aggravated assault, and robbery are examples of assault. Research indicates that the victims of assaultive injuries and their perpetrators tend to resemble one another in terms of ethnicity, educational background, psychological profile, and reliance on weapons.

Homicide

According to the CDC, nearly 16,000 Americans were murdered in 2014. Men, teenagers, young adults, and members of minority groups, particularly African Americans and Latinos, are most likely to be murder victims. Although homicide rates for African Americans have declined dramatically in the past 25 years, the death rate from homicide for black males is much higher than the rate for the U.S. population as a whole. Poverty and unemployment have been identified as key factors in homicide, and these factors may account for the high rates of homicide among blacks and other minority groups.

Most homicides are committed with a firearm, occur during an argument, and occur among people who know one another. Intrafamilial homicide, in which the perpetrator and the victim are related, accounts for about one out of every eight homicides. About 40% of family homicides are committed by spouses, usually following a history of physical and emotional abuse directed at the woman.

Although the data are incomplete, the CDC also separately tracks deaths due to "legal intervention"—killings by police or other peace officers—that are not technically classified as homicides. In 2014, 515 such deaths were reported to the CDC, 95% among men. By race and ethnicity among men, the greatest number of deaths due to legal intervention was among non-Hispanic whites (242 deaths); the highest rate was among non-Hispanic blacks (0.6 per 100,000 population, compared with 0.4 for Hispanics and 0.3 for non-Hispanic whites).

> **QUICK STATS**
>
> **300 million guns are owned by U.S. civilians, ranking the United States first out of 178 countries in the number of privately owned guns.**
> —Annals of Internal Medicine, 2015

Gang-Related Violence

Gangs are most frequently associated with large cities, but gang activity also extends to the suburbs and even to rural areas. It is estimated that about 1.4 million Americans belong to gangs. The average age for joining a gang is 14, so 40% of gang members are younger than 18 years of age.

Gangs are most common in areas where residents are poor and unemployment rates, population density, and crime rates are high. In these areas, young people may feel that legitimate success in life is out of reach and know that involvement in the drug market makes some gang members rich. Often gangs serve as a mechanism for companionship, self-esteem, support, and security. Indeed, gang membership may be viewed as the only possible means of survival in some areas.

Hate Crimes

When bias against another person's race or ethnicity, national origin, religion, sexual orientation, or disability motivates a criminal act, the offense is classified as a hate crime. Hate crimes may be committed against people or property. Those committed against people may include intimidation, assault, and even rape or murder. Crimes against property most frequently involve graffiti, the desecration of places of worship, cross burnings, and other acts of vandalism or property damage.

Over 6,400 hate crimes were reported in 2014; many more go unreported. Crimes against people made up about 60% of all incidents; intimidation and assault were the most common offenses. Racial or ethnic bias was cited as a motivation in nearly half of the hate crimes reported in 2014. Religion and sexual orientation were cited in 15% of cases.

Research indicates that a substantial number of hate crimes are committed by males under age 20. Hate crimes are frequently, but not always, associated with fringe groups that have extremist ideologies, such as the Ku Klux Klan and neo-Nazi groups. The Southern Poverty Law Center tracks hundreds of hate groups and group chapters currently active in the United States; the rapid growth of hate sites on the Internet is another area of concern.

School Violence

According to the National School Safety Center, over 300 school-associated violent deaths of students, faculty, and administrators occurred in the past decade. Most of these deaths occurred in urban areas or at high schools and involved use of a firearm. As with other types of violence, both victims and offenders were predominantly young men. Homicide and suicide are the most serious but least common types of violence in schools; an estimated 1,420,900 non-fatal victimizations occurred at schools in 2013, including theft, vandalism, and assault.

How risky is the school environment for students? Children have been safer at school than away from it, certainly in terms of serious and fatal victimization. Only 2% of all homicides among youths aged 5–19 occur at school, and between 1992 and 2008, crimes involving serious violence more often occurred away from school. Still, data from the National Crime Victimization Survey show that rates of serious violent victimizations against students aged 12–18 were the same at school or away from it, and the general rate of all violent incidents involving students aged 12–18 declined between 1992 and 2013, whether they occurred at or away from school.

Although schools are basically safe places overall, steps can be taken to identify at-risk youths and improve safety for all students. General characteristics of youths who have caused violent deaths in schools include uncontrollable angry outbursts, violent and abusive language and behavior, isolation from peers, depression and irritability, access to and preoccupation with weapons, and lack of support and supervision from adults.

Recommendations for reducing school violence include offering classroom training in anger management, social skills, and improved self-control; providing mental health and social services for students in need; developing after-school programs that help students build self-esteem and make friends; and keeping guns out of the hands of children and out of schools. Tragic incidents like the shooting that took place at Sandy Hook Elementary School in Newtown, Connecticut, in 2012 have also resulted in installation of security and surveillance systems in schools throughout the country, as well as new protocols for entry into school buildings.

Workplace Violence

Data show that workplace violence has decreased by 35% in the past decade, yet OSHA still reports that nearly 2 million American workers are victims of workplace violence each year, including about 500 homicides. In about 60% of cases, workplace violence is committed by strangers; acquaintances account for nearly 40% of cases; and intimates account for 1%. Most of the perpetrators of workplace violence are white males over age 21. Women's leading cause of death in the workplace is homicide. Firearms are used in nearly 80% of workplace homicides, and the majority of these homicides occur during the commission of a robbery or other crime.

Police and corrections officers have the most dangerous jobs, followed by taxi drivers, security guards, bartenders, mental health professionals, and workers at gas stations and convenience and liquor stores. According to the U.S. Department of Labor, workers in state government offices experience more workplace violence of all types than do workers in local government or private industry.

General crime prevention strategies, including use of surveillance cameras and silent alarms and limits on the amount of cash on hand, can help reduce workplace violence related to robberies. A highly stressed workplace is a risk factor in cases of violence between acquaintances or coworkers; clear guidelines about acceptable behavior and prompt action after any threats or incidents of violence can help control this type of workplace violence.

Terrorism

In 2001, more Americans died as a result of terrorism than in any year before or since; the attacks on September 11 killed more than 3000 people, including citizens of 78 countries. Acts of terrorism since 2001, including shootings at Fort Hood, in San Bernardino, and in Orlando, have killed more than 119 Americans on U.S. soil. The FBI defines *terrorism* as the unlawful use of force or violence against people or property to intimidate or coerce a government, the civilian population, or any segment thereof in furtherance of political or social objectives. Terrorism can be domestic, carried out by groups based in the United States, or international. It comes in many forms, including biological, chemical, nuclear, and cyber. Its intent is to promote helplessness by instilling fear of harm or destruction.

Terrorism-prevention activities occur at all levels of government. U.S. government efforts include close work with the diplomatic, law enforcement, intelligence, economic, and military communities. The mission of the U.S. Department of Homeland Security is to help prevent, protect against, and respond to acts of terrorism on U.S. territory. It coordinates efforts to protect electric and water supply systems, transportation, gas and oil supplies, emergency services, computer infrastructure, and other systems.

Individuals have a role in preventing terrorism by making sure they are prepared in case of a terrorist attack or a disaster. They can also be proactive by reporting anything they see or hear that is suspicious or threatening. The best approach is to take personal responsibility and not let the fear of terrorism immobilize or impede your ability to act.

Family and Intimate-Partner Violence

Family violence generally refers to any rough and illegitimate use of physical force, aggression, or verbal abuse by one family member toward another. Once referred to as domestic violence, the term **intimate-partner violence (IPV)** is now used to describe physical, social, or psychological harm imposed by a current partner or spouse. Based on reported cases, an estimated 6–8 million women and children in the United States are victimized each year as a result of IPV. Nearly five children die every day as a result of abuse and neglect.

intimate-partner violence (IPV) Physical, sexual, or psychological harm by a current or former partner or spouse.

TERMS

Battering Studies reveal that over 85% of intimate-partner violence victims are women; 20–35% of women who visit emergency departments are there for injuries related to ongoing abuse. Of all women murdered in the United States each year, about one-third are killed by an intimate partner. Violence against wives or intimate partners as a result of battering occurs at every level of society, although it is more common at lower socioeconomic levels. It occurs more frequently in relationships with a high degree of conflict—an apparent inability to resolve arguments through negotiation and compromise. Over 25% of women report having been physically assaulted or raped by an intimate partner, and more than 50% report having experienced some type of abuse—physical or psychological—in a relationship. In more than 10% of cases, the violence continues for 20 years or longer. The problem of intimate violence is apparent even among young people; 1 in 10 high school girls say they have been physically abused by a dating partner in the past year.

At the root of much of this abusive behavior is the need to control another person. Abusive partners (in most cases a man) are controlling partners. They not only want to have power over another person, but also believe they are entitled to it, no matter what the cost to the other person (see the box "Recognizing the Potential for Abusiveness in a Partner").

In abusive relationships, the abuser usually has a history of violent behavior, traditional beliefs about gender roles, and problems with alcohol abuse. He has low self-esteem and seeks to raise it by dominating and imposing his will on another person. Research has revealed a three-phase cycle of battering, consisting of a period of increasing tension, a violent explosion and loss of control, and a period of contriteness in which the man begs forgiveness and promises it will never happen again. The batterer is drawn back to this cycle over and over again, but he never succeeds in changing his feelings about himself.

Battered women often stay in violent relationships for years. They may be economically dependent on their partners, feel trapped or fear retaliation if they leave, believe their children need a father, or have low self-esteem themselves. They may love or pity their partner, or they may believe they'll eventually be able to stop the violence. They usually leave the relationship only when they become determined that the violence must end. Battered women's shelters offer physical protection, counseling, support, and other assistance.

Stalking and Cyberstalking

Stalking is a crime characterized by harassing behaviors such as following or spying on a person and making verbal, written, or implied threats. In the United States, it is estimated that 7 million women and men are stalked each year; about two-thirds of stalkers are men. About three out of four female victims are stalked by current or former intimate partners; of these, over two-thirds had been physically or sexually assaulted by that partner during the relationship. Weapons are used to threaten or harm victims in one out of five cases. Research indicates that stalking of female college students may be greater than that experienced by the general population. A stalker's goal may be to control or scare the victim or to keep her or him in a relationship. Most stalking episodes last a year or less.

The use of the Internet, e-mail, chat rooms, Facebook, Instagram, and other electronic means to stalk another person is known as **cyberstalking.** As with offline stalking, the majority of cyberstalkers are men, and the majority of victims are women, although there have been same-sex cyberstalking incidents.

Cyberstalkers may send harassing or threatening messages to the victim, or they may encourage others to harass the victim—for example, by impersonating the victim and posting inflammatory messages and personal information on bulletin boards or in chat rooms. Guidelines for staying safe online include the following:

- Avoid using your real name on the Internet. Select an age- and gender-neutral identity.
- Avoid filling out profiles for accounts with information that could be used to identify you.
- Do not share personal information in public spaces anywhere online or give it to strangers.
- Learn how to filter unwanted e-mail messages.
- Always use passwords that are unique and contain many characters—preferably an alphanumeric combination to make it more difficult for someone to hack into your account.
- If you use a social networking site, set your profile to "private" if that is an option.
- If you experience harassment online, do not respond to the harasser. Log off or go to a different site. If harassment continues, contact the harasser's Internet service provider (ISP) by identifying the domain of the stalker's account (after the "@" sign); most ISPs have an e-mail address for complaints. Often an ISP can try to stop the conduct by direct contact with the harasser or by closing his or her account. Save all communications for evidence, and contact your ISP and your local police department. Many states have laws against cyberstalking.

Violence against Children

Violence is also directed against children. In 2013, an estimated 679,000 children were abused or neglected in the United States. About 3.1 million children received preventive services from Child Protective Services.

TERMS

stalking Repeatedly harassing or threatening a person through behaviors such as following a person, appearing at a person's residence or workplace, leaving written messages or objects, making harassing phone calls, or vandalizing property; frequently directed at a former intimate partner.

cyberstalking The use of e-mail, chat rooms, bulletin boards, or other electronic communication devices to stalk another person.

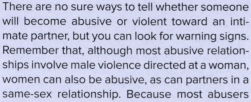

TAKE CHARGE
Recognizing the Potential for Abusiveness in a Partner

There are no sure ways to tell whether someone will become abusive or violent toward an intimate partner, but you can look for warning signs. Remember that, although most abusive relationships involve male violence directed at a woman, women can also be abusive, as can partners in a same-sex relationship. Because most abusers are male, the following material refers to the abuser as "he." If you are concerned that a person you are involved with has the potential for violence, observe his or her behavior, and ask yourself these questions:

• What is this person's attitude toward women? How does he treat his mother and his sister? How does he work with female students, female colleagues, or a female boss? How does he treat your women friends?

• What is his attitude toward your autonomy? Does he respect the work you do and the way you do it? Or does he mock it, tell you how to do it better, or encourage you to give it up? Does he tell you he'll take care of you?

• How self-centered is he? Does he want to spend leisure time on your interests or his? Does he listen to you? Does he remember what you say?

• Is he possessive or jealous? Does he want to spend every minute with you? Does he cross-examine you about things you do when you're not with him?

• What happens when things don't go the way he wants them to? Does he blow up? Does he always have to get his way?

• Is he moody, mocking, critical, or bossy? Do you feel as if you're walking on eggshells when you're with him?

• Do you feel you have to avoid arguing with him?

• Does he drink too much or use drugs?

• Does he refuse to use condoms or take other precautions for safer sex?

Listen to your own uneasiness, and stay away from any man who disrespects women, who wants or needs you intensely and exclusively, and who has a knack for getting his own way almost all the time.

If you are in a serious relationship with a controlling person, you may already have experienced abuse. Consider the following questions:

• Does your partner constantly criticize you, blame you for things that are not your fault, or verbally degrade you?

• Does he humiliate you in front of others?

• Is he suspicious or jealous? Does he accuse you of being unfaithful or monitor your mail or phone calls?

• Does he track all your time? Does he discourage you from seeing friends and family?

• Does he prevent you from getting or keeping a job or attending school? Does he control your shared resources or restrict your access to money?

• Has he ever pushed, pulled, slapped, hit, kicked, bitten, or restrained you? Thrown an object at you? Used a weapon on you or pointed one at you?

• Has he ever destroyed or damaged your personal property or sentimental items, or threatened to do so?

• Has he ever forced you to have sex or to do something sexually you didn't want to do?

• Does he anger easily when drinking or taking drugs?

• Has he ever threatened to harm you or your children, friends, pets, or property?

• Has he ever threatened to blackmail you if you leave?

If you answered yes to one or more of these questions, you may be experiencing intimate-partner violence. If you believe you or your children are in imminent danger, look in your local telephone directory for a women's shelter, or call 911. If you want information, referrals to a program in your area, or assistance, contact one of the organizations listed in the "For More Information" section at the end of the chapter.

Parents who abuse children tend to have low self-esteem, to believe in physical punishment, to have a poor marital relationship, and to have been abused themselves (although many people who were abused as children do not grow up to abuse their own children). Poverty, unemployment, and social isolation are characteristics of families in which children are abused. External stressors related to socioeconomic and environmental factors are most closely associated with neglect, whereas stressors related to interpersonal issues are more closely associated with physical abuse. Single parents, both men and women, are at especially high risk for abusing their children.

Elder Abuse   Each year over 4 million older adults are abused, exploited, or mistreated by someone who is supposed to be giving them care and protection; only one in 24 incidents is reported. Most abusers are family members who are serving as caregivers. Elder abuse can take different forms: physical, sexual, or emotional abuse; financial exploitation; neglect; or abandonment. Neglect accounts for about three out of five reported cases. Physical abuse accounts for about one out of six reported cases, and financial exploitation for about one out of eight reported cases.

Abuse often occurs when caring for a dependent adult becomes too stressful for the caregiver, especially if the

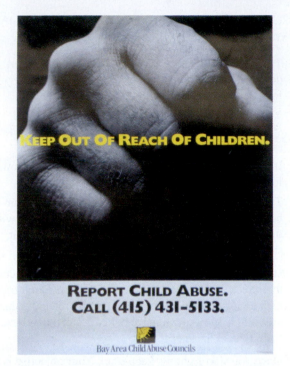

Education, counseling, and support can help the victims of family violence.

elder is incontinent, has suffered mental deterioration, or is violent. Abuse may become an outlet for frustration. Many observers believe that the solution to elder abuse is support in the form of greater social and financial assistance, such as adult day care centers and education and public care programs.

Sexual Violence

The use of force and coercion in sexual interactions is one of the most serious problems in human relationships. The most extreme manifestation of sexual coercion—forcing a person to submit to another's sexual desires—is rape, but sexual coercion occurs in many subtler forms, including sexual harassment.

Sexual Assault: Rape

Sexual assault is any unwanted sexual contact, including fondling and molestation. Rape is one type of sexual assault. Removing the term *forcible* from

> **QUICK STATS**
>
> **Out of every 1000 rapes, only an estimated 344 are reported to police and only 6 rapists will go to jail.**
>
> —Rape, Abuse, & Incest National Network (RAINN), 2016

> **TERMS**
>
> **sexual assault**   Any unwanted sexual contact.
>
> **rape**   Unwanted penetration—oral, anal, or vaginal.
>
> **statutory rape**   Sexual interaction with someone under the legal age of consent.
>
> **date rape**   Sexual assault by someone the victim knows or is dating; also called *acquaintance rape*.

the offense name, the FBI redefined **rape** in 2013 as "penetration, no matter how slight, of the vagina or anus with any body part or object, or oral penetration by a sex organ of another person, without consent of the victim." When the victim is younger than the legally defined age of consent, the act constitutes **statutory rape,** whether or not coercion is involved. Coerced sexual activity in which the victim knows or is dating the rapist is often referred to as **date rape,** or *acquaintance rape*. Most victims know their assailants, but fewer than 40% of all sexual crimes are reported.

Any woman—or man—can be a rape victim. Over 200,000 cases of rape are reported each year. An estimated 500,000 more women are raped each year, but those incidents are unreported. Estimates vary, but in surveys about 1 in 5 women and 1 in 71 men report having experienced an attempted or completed rape at some point in their lives. A study of college students also found that between one in four and one in five college women experience a completed or attempted rape during their college years. Most male-on-male rapes do not occur in prison.

WHO COMMITS RAPE?   Men who commit rape may be any age and come from any socioeconomic group. Some rapists are exploiters in the sense that they rape on the spur of the moment and mainly want immediate gratification. Some attempt to compensate for feelings of sexual inadequacy and an inability to obtain satisfaction otherwise. Others are more hostile and sadistic and are primarily interested in hurting and humiliating a particular woman or women in general. Often the rapist is more interested in dominance, control, and power than in sexual satisfaction.

Most women are in much less danger of being raped by a stranger than of being sexually assaulted by a man they know or date. Surveys suggest that as many as 25% of women have had experiences in which the men they were dating persisted in trying to force sex despite pleading, crying, screaming, or resisting. Surveys have also found that more than 60% of all rape victims were raped by a current or former spouse, boyfriend, or date.

Most cases of date rape are never reported to the police, partly because of the subtlety of the crime. Usually no weapons are involved, and direct verbal threats may not have been made. Rather than being terrorized, the victim usually is attracted to the man at first. Victims of date rape tend to shoulder much of the responsibility for the incident, questioning their own judgment and behavior rather than blaming the aggressor.

Strong evidence suggests that 15% of American women who have ever married have been raped by their husbands or ex-husbands; as many as 60% of battered women may have been raped by their husbands. A charge of spousal rape can now be taken to court in all states.

FACTORS CONTRIBUTING TO DATE RAPE   Although the general status of women in society has improved, the belief that nice women don't say yes to sex (even when they want to) and that real men don't take no for an answer is still prevalent among some groups.

Men and women also differ in their perception of romantic encounters and signals. In one study, researchers found that men interpreted women's actions on dates, such as smiling or talking in a low voice, as indicating an interest in having sex, whereas the women interpreted the same actions as being friendly. Men who rape their dates tend to have certain attributes, including hostility toward women, a belief that dominance alone is a valid motive for sex, and an acceptance of sexual violence.

DATE-RAPE DRUGS   About 5% of DFSA victims are given date-rape drugs. Also called predator drugs, the drugs include flunitrazepam (Rohypnol), gamma hydroxybutyrate (GHB), and ketamine ("Special K"). Rohypnol is not legal in the United States, but ketamine and GHB can be obtained legally because they are used for legitimate medical purposes.

These drugs have a variety of effects, including sedation; if slipped surreptitiously into a drink, they can incapacitate a person within about 20 minutes and make her or him more vulnerable to assault. Rohypnol, GHB, and other drugs also often cause anterograde amnesia, meaning victims have little memory of what happened while they were under the influence of the drug.

The Drug-Induced Rape Prevention and Punishment Act of 1996 adds up to 20 years to the prison sentence of any rapist who uses a drug to incapacitate a victim. Strategies such as the following can help ensure that your drink is not tampered with at a bar or party:

- Drink moderately and responsibly. Avoid group drinking and drinking games.
- Be wary of opened beverages—alcoholic or nonalcoholic—offered by strangers. When at an unfamiliar bar, watch the bartender pour your drink.
- Let your date be the first to drink from the punch bowl at a bar, club, or rave.
- If an opened beverage tastes, looks, or smells strange, do not drink it. If you leave your drink unattended, such as when you dance or use the restroom, get a fresh drink when you return to your table. Also, finish your food before leaving it unattended at the table.
- If you go to a party, club, or bar, go with friends. Arrange to arrive and leave together. Have a prearranged plan for checking on each other visually and verbally. If you feel giddy or lightheaded, get assistance.

Both males and females can take actions that will reduce the incidence of acquaintance rape; see the box "Preventing Date Rape" for specific suggestions.

DEALING WITH A SEXUAL ASSAULT   Each situation is unique, and a woman should respond in whatever way she thinks best. If you are threatened by a rapist and decide to fight back, here is what Women Organized Against Rape (WOAR) recommends:

- Trust your gut feeling. If you feel you are in danger, don't hesitate to run and scream. It is better to feel foolish than to be raped.
- Yell—and keep yelling. It will clear your head and start your adrenaline going; it may scare your attacker and also bring help.
- If an attacker grabs you from behind, use your elbows for striking his neck, his sides, or his stomach.
- Try kicking. Your legs are the strongest part of your body, and your kick is longer than his reach. Kick with the foot that is farther back and with the toe of your shoe. Aim low to avoid losing your balance.
- His most vulnerable spot is his knee; it's low, difficult to protect, and easily knocked out of place. Don't try to kick a rapist in the crotch; he has been protecting this area all his life and will have better protective reflexes there than at his knees.
- Once you start fighting, keep it up. Your objective is to get away as soon as you can.
- Remember that ordinary rules of behavior don't apply. It's OK to vomit, act crazy, or claim to have a sexually transmitted infection.

If you are raped, first get to a safe place. Call the police, tell them you were raped, and give your location. Try to remember as many facts as you can about your attacker; write down a description as soon as possible. Don't wash or change your clothes, or you may destroy important evidence. The police will take you to a hospital for a complete exam; show the physician any injuries. Tell the police simply, but exactly, what happened. If you decide that you don't want to report the rape to the police, be sure to see a physician as soon as possible. You need to be checked for pregnancy and STIs

THE EFFECTS OF RAPE   Rape victims suffer both physical and psychological injury. For most, physical wounds heal within a few weeks. Psychological pain may endure and be substantial. Even the most physically and mentally strong are likely to experience shock, anxiety, depression, shame, and a host of psychosomatic symptoms after being victimized. These psychological reactions following rape constitute rape trauma syndrome, which is characterized by fear, nightmares, fatigue, crying spells, and digestive upset. Self-blame is very likely; society has contributed to this tendency by perpetuating the myths that women can actually defend themselves and that no one can be raped if she doesn't want to be. Fortunately these false beliefs are dissolving in the face of evidence to the contrary.

Many organizations offer counseling and support to rape victims. Look in the telephone directory under Rape or Rape Crisis Center for a hotline number to call. Your campus may have counseling services or a support group.

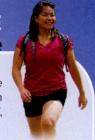

Guidelines for Women

• Believe in your right to control what you do. Set limits, and communicate these limits clearly, firmly, and early. Say no when you mean no.

• Be assertive with someone who is sexually pressuring you. Some men may interpret passivity as permission.

• If you are unsure of a new acquaintance, go on a group date or double date. If possible, provide your own transportation.

• Remember that some men assume sexy dress and a flirtatious manner mean a desire for sex.

• Remember that alcohol and drugs interfere with clear communication about sex. When drinking in a social situation, ask yourself, "Would I do this if I was sober?"

• Use the statement that has proven most effective in stopping date rape: "This is rape, and I'm calling the police."

Guidelines for Men

• Be aware of social pressure. It's OK not to "score."

• Understand that no means no. Don't continue making advances when your date resists or tells you she wants to stop. Remember that she has the right to refuse sex.

• Don't assume sexy dress and a flirtatious manner are invitations to sex, that previous permission for sex applies to the current situation, or that your date's relationships with other men constitute sexual permission for you.

• Remember that alcohol and drugs interfere with clear communication about sex. When drinking in a social situation, ask yourself, "Would I do this if I was sober?"

Guidelines for Bystanders

Everyone can help prevent sexual assaults. The Rape, Abuse, and Incest National Network (RAINN) recommends four strategies indicated by the acronym CARE for bystanders if they notice someone who looks at risk. Choose strategies that are appropriate for the situation, keep yourself and others safe, and act according to your comfort level:

• **Create a distraction.** Do what you can to interrupt a situation that doesn't seem right. A distraction can allow a person to leave a situation.

• **Ask directly.** Talk with a person who you think might be in trouble and make sure she or he gets to a safe place.

• **Refer to an authority.** Talk with a bartender, a security guard, or another employee about your concerns—for example, if someone is behaving aggressively.

• **Enlist others.** Ask another person for help or support. For example, ask someone who knows the person to check on her or him.

If appropriate, call 911. Visit the website for RAINN (https://www.rainn.org/safety-prevention) for additional suggestions on preventing sexual assault.

Child Sexual Abuse   Child sexual abuse is any sexual contact between an adult and a child who is below the legal age of consent. Adults and older adolescents are able to coerce children into sexual activity because of their authority and power over them. Threats, force, or the promise of friendship or material rewards may be used to manipulate a child. Sexual contacts are typically brief and consist of genital manipulation; genital intercourse is much less common.

Sexual abusers are usually male, heterosexual, and known to the victim. The abuser may be a relative, a friend, a neighbor, or another trusted adult acquaintance. Child abusers are often pedophiles, people who are sexually attracted to children. They may have poor interpersonal and sexual relationships with other adults and feel socially inadequate and inferior. One highly traumatic form of sexual abuse is **incest:** sexual activity between people too closely related to legally marry.

Child sexual abuse is often unreported. Surveys suggest that as many as 27% of women and 16% of men were sexually abused as children. An estimated 150,000–200,000 new cases of child sexual abuse occur each year. It can leave lasting scars; victims are more likely to suffer as adults from low self-esteem,

depression, anxiety, eating disorders, self-destructive tendencies, sexual problems, and difficulties in intimate relationships.

If you were a victim of sexual abuse as a child and feel it may be interfering with your functioning today, you may want to address the problem. A variety of approaches can help, such as joining a support group of people who have had similar experiences, confiding in a partner or friend, or seeking professional help.

Sexual Harassment   Unwelcome sexual advances, requests for sexual favors, and other verbal, visual, or physical conduct of a sexual nature constitute **sexual harassment** if

TERMS

incest   Sexual activity between close relatives, such as siblings or parents and their children.

sexual harassment   Unwelcome sexual advances, requests for sexual favors, and other conduct of a sexual nature that affects academic or employment decisions or evaluations; interferes with an individual's academic or work performance; or creates an intimidating, hostile, or offensive academic, work, or student living environment.

such conduct explicitly or implicitly affects academic or employment decisions or evaluations; interferes with an individual's academic or work performance; or creates an intimidating, hostile, or offensive academic, work, or student living environment.

Extreme cases of sexual harassment occur when a manager, a professor, or another person in authority uses his or her ability to control or influence jobs or grades to coerce people into having sex or to punish them if they refuse. A hostile environment can be created by conduct such as sexual gestures, display of sexually suggestive objects or pictures, derogatory comments and jokes, sexual remarks about clothing or appearance, obscene letters, and unnecessary touching or pinching.

If you have been the victim of sexual harassment, you can take action to stop it. Be assertive with anyone who uses language or actions you find inappropriate. If possible, confront your harasser and tell him or her that the situation is unacceptable to you and you want the harassment to stop. Be clear. "Do not *ever* make sexual remarks to me" is an unequivocal statement. If assertive communication doesn't work, assemble a file or log documenting the harassment, noting the details of each incident and information about any witnesses who may be able to support your claims. You may discover others who have been harassed by the same person, which will strengthen your case. Then file a grievance with the harasser's supervisor or employer.

If your attempts to deal with the harassment internally are not successful, you can file an official complaint with your city or state Human Rights Commission or Fair Employment Practices Agency, or with the federal Equal Employment Opportunity Commission. You may also wish to pursue legal action under the Civil Rights Act or under local laws prohibiting employment discrimination. Often the threat of a lawsuit or other legal action is enough to stop the harasser.

What You Can Do about Violence

Violence in our society is a serious threat to our collective health and well-being. This is especially true on college campuses, which in a sense are communities in themselves but sometimes lack the authority or guidance to tackle the issue of violence

directly (see the box "Staying Safe on Campus"). Schools are now providing training for conflict resolution and are educating people about the diverse nature of our society, thereby encouraging tolerance and understanding.

Reducing gun-related injuries may require changes in the availability, possession, and lethality of the 10–14 million firearms sold legally in the United States each year with the appropriate supporting documentation. As part of the Brady Handgun Violence Prevention Act, computerized instant background checks are performed for about 60% of gun sales (those by federally licensed dealers) to prevent purchases by convicted felons, people with a history of mental instability, and certain other groups. In some states, waiting periods are required in addition to the background checks. Some groups advocate bans on certain types of weapons, adoption of universal background checks (to cover private firearm sales), and background checks for ammunition sales.

Safety experts also advocate the adoption of consumer safety standards for guns, including features such as childproofing and indicators to show whether a gun is loaded. Technologies are now available to personalize handguns to help prevent unauthorized use. Owner identification through magnetic encoding, touch memory, radio frequency, or fingerprint reading can prevent others from using a personalized handgun. Education about proper storage is also important. Surveys indicate that more than 34% of homes with children contain guns. Data also show that in only 39% of those homes are firearms stored properly: locked, unloaded, and separate from ammunition. To be effective, any approach to firearm injury prevention must have the support of law enforcement and the community as a whole.

PROVIDING EMERGENCY CARE

A course in **first aid** can help you respond appropriately when someone is injured. One important benefit of first aid training is learning what *not* to do in certain situations. For example, a person with a suspected neck or back injury should not be moved unless there are other life-threatening conditions. A trained person can assess emergency situations accurately before acting.

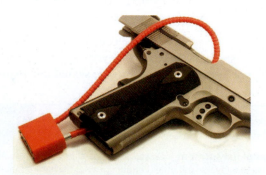

Safety strategies for gun owners include storing firearms and ammunition separately, storing unloaded guns in a locked box or gun safe, and using a cable or trigger lock.

© Keith Biros/123RF

first aid Emergency care given to an ill or injured person until medical care can be obtained. **TERMS**

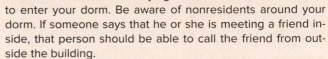

College campuses can be the site of criminal activity and violence, just as any other environment or living situation can be—and so they require the same level of caution and awareness that you would use in other situations. Two key points to remember: 80% of campus crimes are committed by one student against another, and alcohol or drug use is involved in 90% of campus felonies. Drinking or drug use can affect judgment and lower inhibitions, so be aware if you or another person is under the influence. Here are some suggestions for keeping yourself safe on campus:

• Don't travel alone after dark. Many campuses have shuttle buses that run from spots on campus such as the library and the dining hall to residence halls and other locations. Escorts are often available to walk with you at night.

• Be familiar with well-lit and frequently traveled routes around campus if you do need to walk alone.

• If you have a car, follow the usual precautions: Park in well-lit areas, keep the doors locked as you are driving, and never pick up hitchhikers.

• Always have your keys ready as you approach your residence hall, room, and car. Don't lend your keys to others.

• Let friends and family members know your schedule of classes and activities to create a sort of buddy system.

• Be sure the doors and windows of your dorm room have sturdy locks, and use them.

• Don't prop open doors or hold doors open for non-students or nonresidents trying to enter your dorm. Be aware of nonresidents around your dorm. If someone says that he or she is meeting a friend inside, that person should be able to call the friend from outside the building.

• Keep valuables and anything containing personal information—credit cards, wallets, jewelry, and so on—hidden. Secure expensive computer and stereo equipment with cables so that it can't be stolen easily. Use a quality U-shaped lock whenever you leave a bicycle unattended.

• Be alert when using an ATM, and don't display large amounts of cash.

• Stay alert and trust your instincts. Don't hesitate to call the police or campus security if something doesn't seem or feel right.

The Jeanne Clery Disclosure of Campus Security Policy and Campus Crime Statistics Act, named for a Lehigh University student who was murdered in her residence hall in 1986, requires colleges and universities to collect and report campus crime statistics. You can now review this information online at the Crime Statistics website of the U.S. Department of Education's Office of Postsecondary Education (ope.ed.gov/security/Search.asp).

Emergency rescue techniques can save the lives of people who are choking, who have stopped breathing, or whose hearts have stopped beating. As described earlier, the Heimlich maneuver is used when a victim is choking. Pulmonary resuscitation (also known as rescue breathing, artificial respiration, or mouth-to-mouth resuscitation) is used when a person is not breathing. Cardiopulmonary resuscitation (CPR) is used when a pulse cannot be found. In 2010, the American Heart Association made significant changes in its CPR guidelines for laypersons. Previous guidelines were to clear the airway, check for breathing, and begin chest compressions (ABC). The new guidelines are to begin chest compressions, clear the airway, and check for breathing (CAB). Starting with compressions gets the blood circulating, which is critical to keeping the person alive until help arrives. Compressions should be delivered fast, about 100 times a minute. The American Heart Association also authorizes use of a hands-only CPR technique on a teen or adult who suddenly collapses due to cardiac arrest; learn more and watch training videos at the association's website (heart.org/handsonlycpr). Courses in first aid and CPR are offered by the American Heart Association and the American Red Cross.

A new feature of some of these courses is training in the use of automated external defibrillators (AEDs), which monitor the heart's rhythm and, if appropriate, deliver an electrical shock to restart the heart. Because of the importance of early use of defibrillators in saving heart attack victims, these devices are being installed in public places, including casinos, airports, and many office buildings. As a person providing assistance, you are the first link in the **emergency medical services (EMS) system,** a system designed to network community resources for providing emergency care.

---

emergency medical services (EMS) system **TERMS**
A system designed to network community resources for providing emergency care.

Ask Yourself

QUESTIONS FOR CRITICAL THINKING AND REFLECTION

What kinds of emergency training have you had? What kinds of skills do you have that would enable you to help someone who was hurt, was trapped, or needed some other kind of assistance?

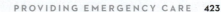

TIPS FOR TODAY AND THE FUTURE

Protecting yourself from injuries means taking sensible safety precautions every day, and preparing yourself to deal with an emergency.

RIGHT NOW YOU CAN:

- Check your home for any object or situation that could cause an injury, such as a tripping hazard, top-heavy shelves, and so on.
- Test the batteries in your home's smoke detectors, and change them if necessary. Test the detectors to make sure they work properly.
- If you ride a bike, check your helmet to ensure that it fits properly and will protect you in a crash. If you have any doubts, throw it away and buy a new one.

IN THE FUTURE YOU CAN:

- Get trained in CPR, rescue breathing, and the use of an automated external defibrillator. If you have already had such training, take a refresher course.
- Be watchful for hazardous situations at your school or workplace. If you notice anything suspicious, report it to an appropriate person right away.
- Prepare for a poisoning emergency by putting the number of your local poison control hotline in a conspicuous place.

SUMMARY

- Injuries are caused by a dynamic interaction of human and environmental factors. Risk-taking behavior is associated with a high rate of injury.

- The home can contain many poisonous substances, including medications, cleaning agents, plants, and fumes from cars and appliances.

- Most fall-related injuries occur on stairs. Alcohol, chairs, and ladders are also involved in a significant number of falls.

- Careless smoking and problems with cooking or heating equipment are common causes of home fires. Being prepared for fire emergencies means planning escape routes and installing smoke detectors.

- Performing the Heimlich maneuver can prevent someone from choking to death.

- The proper storage and handling of firearms can help prevent injuries; assume that any gun is loaded.

- Key factors in motor vehicle injuries include aggressive driving, speeding, a failure to wear seat belts, alcohol and drug intoxication, fatigue, and distraction.

- Motorcycle, motor scooter, and bicycle injuries can be prevented by developing appropriate skills, driving or riding defensively, and wearing proper safety equipment, especially a helmet.

- Many injuries during leisure activities result from the misuse of equipment, lack of experience, use of alcohol, and a failure to wear proper safety equipment.

- Most work-related injuries involve extensive manual labor; back problems and repetitive strain injuries are most common.

- Factors contributing to violence include poverty, the absence of strong social ties, the influence of the mass media, cultural attitudes about gender roles, problems in interpersonal relationships, alcohol and drug abuse, and the availability of firearms.

- Types of violence include assault, homicide, gang-related violence, hate crimes, school violence, workplace violence, terrorism, family and intimate-partner violence, and sexual violence.

- Battering occurs at every socioeconomic level. The core issue is the abuser's need to control other people.

- Most rape victims are women, and most know their attackers. Factors in date rape include different standards of appropriate sexual behavior for men and women and different perceptions of actions.

- Child sexual abuse often results in serious trauma; usually the abuser is a trusted adult.

- Sexual harassment is unwelcome sexual advances or other conduct of a sexual nature that affects academic or employment performance or evaluations or that creates an intimidating, hostile, or offensive academic, work, or student living environment.

- Strategies for reducing violence include conflict resolution training, social skills development, and education programs that foster tolerance and understanding among diverse groups.

- Steps in giving emergency care include making sure the scene is safe for you and the injured person, conducting a quick examination of the victim, calling for help, and providing emergency first aid.

FOR MORE INFORMATION

American Association of Poison Control Centers. Provides free, confidential, and expert advice related to poisoning.

800-222-1222

http://www.aapcc.org

American Automobile Association Foundation for Traffic Safety. Provides consumer information about all aspects of traffic safety; the website has online quizzes and extensive links.

http://www.aaafoundation.org/home

American Bar Association: Domestic Violence. Provides information about statistics, research, and laws relating to domestic violence.

http://www.americanbar.org/groups/domestic_violence
/resources/statistics.html

Consumer Product Safety Commission. Provides information and advice about safety issues relating to consumer products.

http://www.cpsc.gov

CyberAngels Internet Safety Program. Provides information about online safety and help and advice for victims of cyberstalking.

http://www.cyberangels.org

Governor's Highway Safety Association. Provides up-to-date information about cell phone and texting laws, as well as general information and publications related to traffic safety.

http://www.ghsa.org/html/stateinfo/laws/cellphone_laws.html

Insurance Institute for Highway Safety. Provides information about crashes on the nation's highways, as well as reports on topics such as speeding and crashworthiness of vehicles.

http://www.iihs.org

National Center for Injury Prevention and Control. Provides consumer-oriented information about unintentional injuries and violence.

http://www.cdc.gov/injury

National Center for Victims of Crime. An advocacy group for crime victims; provides statistics, news, safety strategies, tips on finding local assistance, and links to related sites.

http://www.victimsofcrime.org

National Children's Alliance. Helps local communities respond to allegations of child abuse.

http://nationalchildrensalliance.org

National Highway Traffic Safety Administration. Supplies materials about reducing deaths, injuries, and economic losses from motor vehicle crashes.

http://www.nhtsa.gov

National Safety Council. Provides information and statistics about preventing unintentional injuries.

http://www.nsc.org

National Violence Hotlines. Provide information, referral services, and crisis intervention.

800-799-SAFE (7233) (domestic violence), http://www.thehotline.org

800-422-4453 (child abuse), http://www.childhelp.org

800-656-HOPE (4673) (sexual assault), http://www.rainn.org

Occupational Safety and Health Administration. Provides information about topics related to health and safety issues in the workplace.

http://www.osha.gov

Prevent Child Abuse America. Provides statistics, information, and publications relating to child abuse, including parenting tips.

http://www.preventchildabuse.org

Rape, Abuse, and Incest National Network (RAINN). Provides guidelines for preventing and dealing with sexual assault and abuse.

http://www.rainn.org

Tolerance.Org. Offers suggestions for fighting hate and promoting tolerance; sponsored by the Southern Poverty Law Center.

http://www.tolerance.org

World Health Organization: Violence and Injury Prevention and Disability. Provides statistics and information about the consequences of intentional and unintentional injuries worldwide.

http://www.who.int/violence_injury_prevention

The following sites provide statistics and background information about violence and crime in the United States:

Bureau of Justice Statistics: http://www.bjs.gov

Federal Bureau of Investigation: http://www.fbi.gov

National Criminal Justice Reference Service: http://www.ncjrs.gov

SELECTED BIBLIOGRAPHY

Anderson, C. A., et al. 2010. Violent video game effects on aggression, empathy, and prosocial behavior in eastern and western countries: A meta-analytic review. *Psychological Bulletin* 136(2): 151–173.

Arnowitz, T. 2013. How safe are college campuses? *Journal of American College Health* 61(2): 57–59.

Bureau of Aircraft Accidents Archives. 2000–2016. *Death Rate Per Year* (http://www.baaa-acro.com/general-statistics/death-rate-per-year/)

Bureau of Labor Statistics. 2015. Nonfatal occupational injuries and illnesses requiring days away from work, 2014. *Economic News Release.* Washington, DC: U.S. Department of Labor.

Centers for Disease Control and Prevention. 2015. *Impaired Driving: Get the Facts. Injury Prevention and Control: Motor Vehicle Safety.* Atlanta, GA: Centers for Disease Control and Prevention.

Centers for Disease Control and Prevention. 2016. *Deaths: Final Data for 2013, Table 18.* Atlanta, GA: Centers for Disease Control and Prevention.

Centers for Disease Control and Prevention. 2016. *10 Leading Causes of Injury Deaths by Age Group Highlighting Unintentional Injury Deaths, United States—2014* (http://www.cdc.gov/injury/wisqars/leadingcauses.html).

Cramer, R., et al. 2013. An examination of sexual orientation and transgender-based hate crimes in the post-Matthew Shepard era. *Psychology, Public Policy, and Law* 19(3): 355–368.

Distraction.gov. 2016. *Facts and Statistics* (http://www.distraction.gov/stats-research-laws/facts-and-statistics.html).

Federal Bureau of Investigation. 2015. *Crime in the United States, 2014.* Washington, DC: U.S. Department of Justice

Federal Highway Administration, Office of Highway Policy Information. 2016. *Average Annual Miles per Driver by Age Group* (https://www.fhwa.dot.gov/ohim/onh00/bar8.htm).

Governors Highway Safety Association. 2016. *Child Passenger Safety Laws* (http://www.ghsa.org/html/stateinfo/laws/childsafety_laws.html).

Grinshteyn, E., and D. Hemenway. 2015. Violent death rates: The US compared with other high-income OECD countries, 2010. *American Journal of Medicine* [0002–9343].

Hemenway, D., and S. J. Solnick. 2015. Children and unintentional firearm death. *Injury Epidemiology* 2(1): 26

Insurance Institute for Highway Safety/Highway Loss Data Institute. 2015. *Motorcycles and ATVS: 2013.* Arlington, VA: Insurance Institute for Highway Safety/Highway Loss Data Institute.

Levinson, A. A., B. Lannert, and M. Yalch. 2012. The effects of intimate partner violence on women and children survivors: An attachment perspective. *Psychodynamic Psychiatry* 40(3): 397–433.

Miller, M., et al. 2015. Firearms and suicide in U.S. cities. *Injury Prevention* 21(e1): e116-e119.

Monuteaux, M. C., et al. 2015. Firearm ownership and violent crime in the U.S.: An ecological study. *American Journal of Preventive Medicine* 49(2): 207–214.

National Center for Health Statistics. 2015a. *Deaths from Unintentional Injury among Adults Aged 65 and Over: United States, 2000–2013* (NCHS Data Brief No. 199). Atlanta, GA: National Center for Health Statistics.

National Center for Health Statistics. 2015b. *Fact Sheet: NCHS Data on Drug Poisoning Deaths* (http://www.cdc.gov/nchs/data/factsheets/factsheet_drug_poisoning.pdf).

National Center for Health Statistics. 2015c. *National Estimates of the 10 Leading Causes of Nonfatal Injuries Treated in Hospital Emergency Departments, United States—2013* (http://www.cdc.gov/injury/images /lc-charts/leading_cause_of_nonfatal_injury_2013-a.gif).

National Center for Statistics and Analysis. 2015. *2014 Crash Data Key Findings* (Report No. DOT HS 812 219). Washington, DC: National Highway Traffic Safety Administration.

National Center for Statistics and Analysis. 2015. *Critical Reasons for Crashes Investigated in the National Motor Vehicle Crash Causation Survey* (Report No. DOT HS 812 115). Washington, DC: National Highway Traffic Safety Administration.

National Highway Traffic Safety Administration. 2015. *The Economic and Societal Impact of Motor Vehicle Crashes, 2010. (Revised)* (Report No. DOT HS 812 013). Washington, DC: National Highway Traffic Safety Administration.

National Safety Council. 2016. *Injury Facts.* Itasca, IL: National Safety Council.

Pew Research Center. 2014. The Demographics and Politics of Gun-Owning Households (http://www.pewresearch.org/fact-tank/2014/07/15/the -demographics-and-politics-of-gun-owning-households).

Pickrell, T. M., and E.-H. Choi. 2015. *Seat Belt Use in 2014—Overall Results* (Report No. DOT HS 812 113). Washington, DC: National Highway Traffic Safety Administration.

Robers, S., et al. 2015. *Indicators of School Crime and Safety: 2014* (NCES 2015–072/NCJ 248036). Washington, DC: National Center for Education Statistics, U.S. Department of Education, and Bureau of Justice Statistics, Office of Justice Programs, U.S. Department of Justice.

RAINN. 2016. *The Criminal Justice System: Statistics* (https://www.rainn .org/statistics/criminal-justice-system).

U.S. Equal Employment Opportunity Commission. 2016. *Charges Alleging Sexual Harassment FY 2010-FY 2015* (https://www.eeoc.gov/eeoc /statistics/enforcement/sexual_harassment_new.cfm).

U.S. Fire Administration. 2015. *Campus Fire Fatalities in Residential Buildings (2000–2015).* Washington, DC: U.S. Department of Homeland Security.

Webster, D., Crifasi, C. K., & J. S. Vernick. 2014. Effects of the repeal of Missouri's handgun purchaser licensing law on homicides. *Journal of Urban Health* 91(2): 293–302.

Weinberger, S. E., et al. 2015. Firearm-related injury and death in the United States: A call to action from 8 health professional organizations and the American Bar Association. *Annals of Internal Medicine* 162(7): 513–517.

World Health Organization. 2015. *Road Traffic Injuries* (Fact Sheet No. 358) (http://www.who.int/mediacentre/factsheets/fs358/en/).

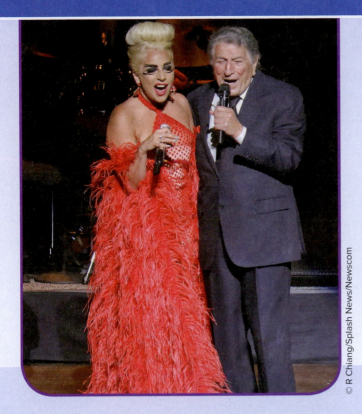

© R Chiang/Splash News/Newscom

CHAPTER OBJECTIVES

- List strategies for healthy aging
- Identify challenges that may accompany aging and explain how people can best confront them
- Explain the factors influencing life expectancy
- Understand the issues facing older adults in the United States
- Explain what death is
- List and describe personal considerations in planning for death
- Explain the challenges of coping with imminent death
- Explain the challenges of coping with loss
- Describe what it means to come to terms with death

CHAPTER **17**

The Challenge of Aging

Aging is the process of becoming older, a process that is genetically determined but also profoundly affected by your environment. Aging does not begin at some specific point in life, and there is no precise age at which a person becomes "old." Although youth is not entirely a state of mind, your attitude toward life and your attention to your health significantly affect the satisfaction you will get from life and even your ability to come to terms with death.

GENERATING VITALITY AS YOU AGE

Biological aging includes all the normal, progressive, irreversible changes to our bodies that begin at birth and continue until death. Psychological aging and social aging usually reflect more abrupt changes in circumstance and emotion: relocating, changing homes, losing a spouse and friends, retiring, having less income, and changing roles and social status. Although they may be challenging or difficult, these changes represent opportunities for growth throughout life.

Successful aging requires preparation. People need to establish good health habits in their teens and twenties. During their twenties and thirties, they usually develop important relationships and settle into a particular lifestyle. By their mid-forties, they generally know how much money they need to support the lifestyle they've chosen. At this point, they must assess their financial status and perhaps adjust their savings in order to continue enjoying that lifestyle after retirement. In their mid-sixties, they need to reevaluate their health insurance plans and may want to think about retirement housing. In their seventies and beyond, they need to consider ways of sharing their legacy with the next generation.

What Happens as You Age?

Many characteristics associated with aging are not due to aging at all. Rather, they result from the neglect and abuse of our bodies and minds. These assaults lay the foundation

aging A normal process of getting older, which includes physical, mental, and social changes, and a point past which there is a decline in function.

TERMS

for later psychological problems and chronic conditions such as arthritis, heart disease, diabetes, hearing loss, vision problems, and hypertension.

Even with the healthiest behavior and environment, aging inevitably occurs. It results from genetic and biochemical processes we don't yet fully understand. The physiological changes in organ systems are caused by a combination of gradual aging and impairment from disease. Because of redundancy in most organ systems, the body's ability to function is not affected until damage is fairly extensive. Studies of healthy people indicate that functioning remains essentially constant until after age 70. Further research may help pinpoint the causes of aging and develop therapies to repair damage to aging organs.

Life-Enhancing Measures: Age-Proofing

Through good habits you can prevent, delay, lessen, or even reverse some changes associated with aging. Simple, daily practices can make a great difference to your level of energy and vitality—your overall wellness.

Challenge Your Mind Numerous studies show that older adults who stay mentally active have lower levels of the brain protein linked to Alzheimer's and dementia. Reading, writing, doing puzzles, learning a language, and studying music are good ways to stimulate the brain. The more complex the activity, the more protective it may be.

Develop Physical Fitness Exercise significantly enhances both psychological and physical health. A review of more than 70 scientific studies cited in the 2008 *Physical Activity Guidelines Advisory Committee Report* found that

physically active people have about a 30% lower risk of dying prematurely compared with inactive people. Poor fitness and low physical activity levels were found to be better predictors of premature death than smoking, diabetes, or obesity. The committee found that about 150 minutes (2.5 hours) of physical activity per week is sufficient to decrease all causes of death and that it is the overall volume of energy expended, rather than the kinds of activities that require the energy expenditure, that makes a difference in risk of premature death.

The positive effects of exercise include lower blood pressure and healthier cholesterol levels; better protection against heart attacks and an increased chance of survival if one occurs; sustained or increased lung capacity; weight control through less accumulation of fat; maintenance of strength, flexibility, and balance; improved sleep; longer life expectancy; protection against osteoporosis and type 2 diabetes; increased effectiveness of the immune system; and maintenance of mental agility and flexibility, response time, memory, and hand–eye coordination.

The stimulus that exercise provides also seems to protect against the loss of **fluid intelligence,** which is the ability to find solutions to new problems. Fluid intelligence depends on rapidity of responsiveness, memory, and alertness. Individuals who exercise regularly are also less susceptible to depression and dementia.

Regular physical activity also fends off *sarcopenia,* which is age-related loss of muscle mass, strength, and function (see Chapter 10). The weaker a person becomes, the less he or she can do; this condition can rob you of self-sufficiency and lead to greater dependence on others. The muscle wasting that occurs in sarcopenia also leads to weight gain because muscle burns more calories than does fat, even at rest.

Regular physical activity is essential for healthy aging, as it is throughout life. The *2008 Physical Activity Guidelines for Americans* include recommendations for older adults that are the same as for all adults:

• All older adults should avoid inactivity. Some physical activity is better than none.

• For substantial health benefits, older adults should do at least 150 minutes a week of moderate-intensity activity, or 75 minutes a week of vigorous-intensity activity, or a combination of both. For additional and more extensive health benefits, older adults should increase their aerobic physical activity to 300 minutes a week of moderate-intensity, or 150 minutes a week of vigorous-intensity, aerobic physical activity.

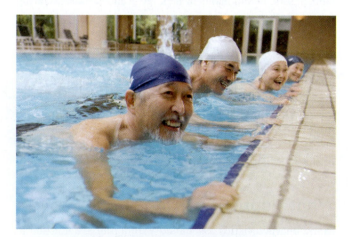

Regular exercise is a key to successful, healthy aging.
© Indeed/Getty Images

fluid intelligence   The capacity to analyze new problems, reason, and identify patterns and relationships, independent of past knowledge.   **TERMS**

Can Exercise Delay the Effects of Aging?

As people age, they often experience declines in functional health—the ability to perform the tasks of everyday life—and related declines in the quality of life. According to the Centers for Disease Control and Prevention (CDC), more than 24% of Americans over age 65 report their health as only "fair" or "poor." Similarly, according to a Medicare survey, 19% of men and 30% of women age 65 and over reported problems with basic physical tasks in 2010 (meaning they had difficulty with things such as walking two to three blocks, lifting 10 pounds, or stooping or kneeling).

Can physical activity and exercise combat the degenerative effects of aging in middle-aged and older adults? The evidence indicates that they can. In reviewing the research, the U.S. government's Physical Activity Guidelines Advisory Committee concluded that physical activity can prevent or delay the onset of limitations and declines in functional health in older adults, can maintain or improve functional health in those who already have limitations, and can reduce the incidence of falls and fall-related injuries.

One mechanism by which physical activity prevents declines in functional health is through maintenance or improvement of the physiological capacities of the body, such as aerobic power, muscular strength, and balance—in other words, through improvements in physical fitness. Declines in these physiological capacities occur with biological aging and are often compounded by disease-related disability. But evidence shows that older adults who participate in regular aerobic exercise are 30% less likely than inactive individuals to develop functional limitations (such as a limited ability to walk or climb stairs) or role limitations (such as a limited ability to be the family grocery shopper). Although studies found that both physical activity and aerobic fitness were associated with reduced risk of functional limitations, aerobic fitness was associated with a greater reduction of risk. Evidence also suggests that regular physical activity is safe and beneficial for older adults who already have functional limitations.

Numerous studies have shown that regular exercise—particularly strength training, balance training, and flexibility exercises—can improve muscular strength, muscular endurance, and stability and provide some protection against falls. Aerobic activity, especially walking, also helps reduce risk of falls, and some evidence indicates that tai chi exercise programs are beneficial as well. Regular exercise not only reduces the incidence of falls but also greatly enhances mobility, allowing older people to live more independently and with greater confidence. Research also shows that regular physical activity can reduce anxiety and depression in older adults. Exercise stimulates blood flow to the brain and can even increase brain mass, helping the brain to function more efficiently and improving memory. There is some evidence that exercise may stave off mental decline and the occurrence of age-related dementia.

Current physical activity recommendations for older adults from the American Heart Association and the American College of Sports Medicine include moderate- to vigorous-intensity aerobic activity, strength training, and flexibility exercises, as well as balance exercises for older adults at risk for falls. Unfortunately, more than 70% of Americans aged 65 and over do not get the recommended amounts of physical activity, and many get no exercise at all beyond the activities of daily living. Older adults are the least active group of Americans. Although it is important to exercise throughout life, the evidence indicates that older adults who become more active even late in life can experience improvements in physical fitness and functional health.

sources: Physical Activity Guidelines Advisory Committee. 2008. Physical Activity Guidelines Advisory Committee Report, 2008. Washington, DC: U.S. Department of Health and Human Services; Simonsick, E. M., et al. 2005. Just get out the door! Importance of walking outside the home for maintaining mobility: Findings from the Women's Health and Aging Study. *Journal of the American Geriatrics Society* 53(2): 198–203.

• Older adults should also do muscle-strengthening activities that are moderate or high intensity and involve all major muscle groups on two or more days a week because these activities provide additional health benefits.

There are also guidelines just for older adults:

• When older adults cannot do 150 minutes of moderate-intensity aerobic activity a week because of chronic conditions, they should be as physically active as their abilities and conditions allow.

• Older adults should do exercises that maintain or improve balance if they are at risk of falling.

• Older adults with chronic conditions should understand whether and how their conditions affect their ability to do regular physical activity safely.

• Older adults should perform flexibility exercises necessary for regular physical activity and activities of daily life.

For more about the beneficial effects of exercise for older adults, see the box "Can Exercise Delay the Effects of Aging?"

Eat Wisely   Good health at any age is enhanced by eating a varied diet full of nutrient-rich foods (see Chapter 9). For many adults, that means eating more fruits, vegetables, and whole grains while eating fewer foods high in saturated and trans fats and added sugars. Special guidelines for older adults include the following:

• Get enough vitamin B-12 and extra vitamin D from fortified foods or supplements.

• Limit sodium intake to 1500 mg per day (3/4 teaspoon salt), and get enough potassium (4700 mg per day).

Older adults tend to have higher blood pressure and to be salt-sensitive.

- Eat foods rich in dietary fiber and drink plenty of water to help prevent constipation.
- Pay special attention to food safety. Older adults are often more susceptible to foodborne illness.

Maintain a Healthy Weight Weight management is especially difficult if you have been overweight most of your life. A sensible program of expending more calories through exercise, cutting calorie intake, or a combination of both will work for most people who want to lose weight, but there is no magic formula. Obesity is not physically healthy, and it leads to premature aging (see Chapter 11).

Control Drinking and Overdependence on Medications Alcohol abuse ranks with depression as a common hidden mental health problem, affecting about 10% of older adults. (The ability to metabolize alcohol decreases with age.) The problem is often not identified because the effects of alcohol or drug dependence can mimic disease, such as Alzheimer's disease.

Signs of potential alcohol or drug dependence include unexplained falls or frequent injuries, forgetfulness, depression, and malnutrition. People who retire or lose a spouse and have few interests to replace their work lives are especially at risk. Problems can be avoided by not using alcohol to relieve anxiety or emotional pain and not taking medication when safer forms of treatment are available.

Don't Smoke The average pack-a-day smoker can expect to live about 13–14 fewer years than a nonsmoker. Furthermore, smokers suffer more illnesses that last longer, and they are subject to respiratory disabilities that limit their total vigor for many years before their death. Premature balding, skin wrinkling, and osteoporosis have been linked to cigarette smoking.

Schedule Physical Examinations to Detect Treatable Diseases When detected early, many diseases, including hypertension, diabetes, and many types of cancer, can be successfully controlled by medication and lifestyle changes. Regular testing for glaucoma after age 40 can prevent blindness from this eye disease. Recommended screenings and immunizations can protect against preventable chronic and infectious diseases.

Ask Yourself

QUESTIONS FOR CRITICAL THINKING AND REFLECTION
Where would you wish to spend your "golden years"? Do you look forward to this stage of your life, or are you anxious about it? What influences have shaped your feelings about aging?

Recognize and Reduce Stress Stress-induced physiological changes increase wear and tear on your body. Cut down on the stresses in your life. Don't wear yourself out through lack of sleep, substance abuse or misuse, or overwork. Practice relaxation using the techniques described in Chapter 2.

DEALING WITH THE CHANGES OF AGING

Just as you can act now to prevent or limit the physical changes of aging, you can also begin preparing yourself psychologically, socially, and financially for changes that may occur later in life.

Planning for Social Changes

Retirement marks a major change in the last quarter of life. As Americans' longevity has increased, people spend a larger proportion of their lives—17 years or more—in retirement. By 2030, 18% of the population will be over age 65, up from 13% in 2010. In 2056, for the first time, the older population (age 65 and over) is projected to outnumber the younger population (age 18 and under).

Changing Roles and Relationships Changes in social roles are a major feature of life as we age. Children become young adults and leave home, removing the duties of daily parenting. Parents experiencing this empty-nest syndrome must adapt to changes in their customary responsibilities and personal identities. And although retirement may be a desirable milestone for most people, it may also be viewed as a threat to prestige, purpose, and self-respect—the loss of a valued or customary role—and often requires some adjustment.

Retirement and the end of child rearing also bring about changes in the relationship between marriage partners. The amount of time a couple spends together will increase, and activities will change. Couples may need a period of adjustment in which they get to know each other as individuals again. Discussing what types of activities each partner enjoys can help couples set up a mutually satisfying routine of shared and independent activities.

Increased Leisure Time Although retirement confers the advantages of leisure time and freedom from deadlines, competition, and stress, many people do not know how to enjoy their free time. If you have developed diverse interests, retirement can be a joyful and fulfilling period of your life. It can provide opportunities for you to expand your horizons, try new activities, take classes, and meet new people. Volunteering in your community can enhance self-esteem through opportunities to contribute to society.

The Economics of Retirement Financial planning for retirement should begin early in life. People in their twenties and thirties should estimate how much money they need to support their standard of living, calculate their projected income, and begin a savings program. The earlier people begin such a program, the more money they will have at retirement.

Financial planning for retirement is especially critical for women. American women are much less likely than men to be covered by pension plans, 401(k) plans, and other retirement plans, reflecting the fact that many women have lower-paying jobs or work part time during their childbearing years. Although the gap is narrowing, women currently outlive men by about five to six years, and they are more likely to develop chronic conditions that impair their daily activities later in life. The net result of these factors is that older women are almost twice as likely as older men to live in poverty. Women should investigate their retirement plans and take charge of their finances to be sure they can provide for themselves as they age.

Adapting to Physical Changes

Some changes in physical functioning are inevitable, and successful aging involves anticipating and accommodating these changes. Decreased energy and changes in health mean that older people have to develop priorities for how to use their energy. Rather than curtailing activities to conserve energy, they need to learn how to generate energy. Generating energy usually involves saying yes to enjoyable activities and paying close attention to the need for rest and sleep. Adapting rather than giving up favorite activities may be the best strategy for dealing with physical limitations. For example, if arthritis interferes with playing an instrument, a person can continue to enjoy music by taking up a different instrument or attending concerts.

Hearing Loss   The loss of hearing is a common physical change that can have a particularly strong effect on the lives of older adults. Some people lose their hearing slowly as they age—a condition known as *presbycusis*. Hearing loss affects a person's ability to interact with others and can lead to a sense of isolation and depression. Hearing loss should be assessed and treated by a health care professional. In some cases, hearing can be restored completely by dealing with the underlying causes of the loss. In other cases, hearing aids may be prescribed.

Vision Changes   Vision usually declines with age. For some people, this can be traced to conditions such as **glaucoma** or **age-related macular degeneration (AMD)** that can be treated medically. Glaucoma is caused by increased pressure within the eye due to built-up fluid. The optic nerve can be damaged by this increased pressure, resulting in a loss of side vision and, if untreated, blindness. Medication can relieve the pressure by decreasing the amount of fluid produced or by helping it drain more efficiently. Laser and conventional surgery are other options. Of the more than 3 million Americans with glaucoma, only half know that they have it; others lose the opportunity to control it and preserve their sight. At risk are people over age 60, African Americans over age 40, and anyone with a family history of glaucoma.

AMD is a slow disintegration of the *macula*—the tissue at the center of the retina where fine, straight-ahead detail is distinguished. AMD usually occurs after age 60, but it affects more than 1.5 million Americans over age 40 and is the leading cause of blindness in people over age 75. Losing vision makes it difficult to read, drive, or perform other close-up activities. Risk factors for AMD are age, gender (women may be at higher risk than men), smoking, elevated cholesterol levels, and family history. Some cases of AMD can be treated with injections or laser surgery. Both glaucoma and AMD can be detected with regular screening.

By the time they reach their forties, many people have developed **presbyopia**—a gradual decline in the ability to focus on objects close to them. **Cataracts,** a clouding of the lens caused by lifelong oxidation damage (a by-product of normal body chemistry), may dim vision by the sixties.

Arthritis   More than 50 million American adults (about one in five) report having doctor-diagnosed **arthritis.** This degenerative disease causes joint inflammation leading to chronic pain, swelling, and loss of mobility.

There are more than 100 types of arthritis; osteoarthritis (OA) is by far the most common. It most often affects the hands and weight-bearing joints of the body—the knees, ankles, and hips.

Strategies for reducing the risk of arthritis and, for those who already have OA, for managing it include exercise, weight management, and avoidance of heavy or repetitive muscle use. Exercise lubricates joints and strengthens the muscles around them, protecting them from further damage. Swimming, walking, cross-country skiing, cycling, and tai chi are good low-impact exercises; knitting and crocheting are excellent for the hands.

Many people with OA take medication to relieve inflammation and reduce pain. Nonsteroidal anti-inflammatory drugs (NSAIDs) like ibuprofen can help but can irritate the digestive tract; prescription drugs that relieve pain without damaging the stomach may have other dangerous side effects. Acetaminophen can also reduce pain without upsetting the

TERMS

glaucoma   An increase in pressure in the eye due to fluid buildup that can result in loss of side vision and, if left untreated, blindness.

age-related macular degeneration (AMD)   A deterioration of the macula (the central area of the retina) leading to blurred vision and sensitivity to glare; some cases can lead to blindness.

presbyopia   The inability of the eyes to focus sharply on nearby objects, caused by a loss of elasticity of the lens that occurs with advancing age.

cataracts   Opacity of the lens of the eye that impairs vision and can cause blindness.

arthritis   Inflammation and swelling of a joint or joints, causing pain and swelling.

stomach, but exceeding the recommended dosage can cause liver damage.

Menopause   The natural process of menopause usually occurs during a woman's forties or fifties. The ovaries gradually stop functioning, estrogen levels drop, and eventually menstruation ceases. Several years before a woman stops menstruating, her periods usually become irregular, and she may experience hot flashes, vaginal dryness, sleep disturbances, and mood swings. This period, called *perimenopause,* can be troublesome for many women, some more than others.

Lifestyle strategies to reduce menopause-related problems include eating a healthy diet, exercising, losing weight, avoiding tobacco, and managing stress.

Sexual Functioning   The ability to enjoy sex can continue well into old age, particularly if people make the effort to understand and respond to the various changes that age brings to the natural pattern of sexual response. All too often, older people give up intercourse because they mistakenly interpret these changes as signs of impending impotence. Lovemaking may become a more leisurely affair as a couple gets older, but the benefits of maintaining the sexual aspect of the relationship into old age can be great.

Osteoporosis   As described in Chapter 9, **osteoporosis** is a condition in which bones become dangerously thin and fragile over time. Fractures are the most serious consequence of osteoporosis; up to 20% of all people who suffer a hip fracture die within a year. Other problems associated with osteoporosis are loss of height and a stooped posture due to vertebral fractures, severe back and hip pain, and breathing problems caused by changes in the shape of the skeleton.

More than 40 million people in the United States either already have osteoporosis or are at high risk due to low bone mass. Women are at greater risk for osteoporosis than are men because they have 10–25% less bone in their skeletons. As they lose bone mass with age, women's bones become dangerously thin sooner than men's bones (although more men will probably develop osteoporosis in the future as they live into their eighties and nineties). Bone loss accelerates in women during the first 5–10 years after the onset of menopause because of the drop in estrogen production. (Estrogen improves calcium absorption and reduces the amount of calcium the body excretes.) Black and Latino women have higher bone density and fewer fractures than white or Asian women but may be at increased risk of osteoporosis due to lack of vitamin D (a condition caused by high levels of melatonin). Other risk factors include a family history of osteoporosis, early menopause (before age 45), abnormal or irregular menstruation, a history of anorexia, and a thin, small frame. Regular con-

sumption of more than two alcoholic drinks a day increases the risk of osteoporosis, possibly because alcohol can interfere with the body's ability to absorb calcium. Thyroid medication, corticosteroid drugs for arthritis or asthma, and long-term use of certain contraceptives can also negatively affect bone mass.

Preventing osteoporosis requires building as much bone as possible during your young years and then maintaining it as you age. Girls aged 9–18 are in their critical bone-building years, and they should eat foods rich in calcium and vitamin D and get adequate exercise. Weight-bearing aerobic activities must be performed regularly throughout life to have lasting effects. Strength training improves bone density, muscle mass, strength, and balance, protecting against both bone loss and falls, a major cause of fractures. Even for people in their seventies, low-intensity strength training has been shown to improve bone density.

Two other lifelong strategies for reducing the effects of osteoporosis are avoiding tobacco use and managing depression and stress. Bone mineral density testing can be used to gauge an individual's risk of fracture and help determine if any treatment is needed.

Handling Psychological and Mental Changes

Many people associate old age with forgetfulness, and slowly losing memory. However, we now know that many older adults in good health remain mentally alert and retain their capacity to learn and remember new information. Occasional confusion or forgetfulness may indicate only temporary information overload, fatigue, or response to medications. Many people appear to become even smarter as they age and gain knowledge from life experience.

Dementia   **Dementia** is a loss of brain function that occurs with certain diseases. It affects memory, thinking, language, judgment, and behavior. Dementia affects about 1% of people aged 60–64 years and as many as 30–50% of people older than 85 years. Early symptoms of dementia include slight disturbances in a person's ability to grasp the situation he or she is in. As dementia progresses, memory failure becomes apparent, and the person may forget conversations,

> **QUICK STATS**
>
> Nearly **1 in 5** Medicare dollars is currently spent on people with Alzheimer's and other dementias. In 2050, it will be **1 in every 3** dollars.
> —Alzheimer's Association, 2016

the events of the day, or how to perform simple tasks. It is important to have any symptoms evaluated by a health care professional because some of the over 50 known causes of dementia are treatable.

The most common forms of dementia among older people—Alzheimer's disease, and multi-infarct dementia—are irreversible. The most common, **Alzheimer's disease (AD),** is a progressive brain disorder that damages and eventually destroys brain cells, leading to loss of memory, thinking, and other brain functions.

In 2013, an estimated 5.2 million Americans of all ages had Alzheimer's disease, which usually occurs in people over age 60 but can occur in people as young as age 40. By 2050, the number of people age 65 and over who currently have the disease may nearly triple from 5 million to a projected 13.8 million. Alzheimer's is ultimately fatal, and currently there is no cure.

Multi-infarct dementia results from a series of small strokes or changes in the brain's blood supply that deprive the brain of oxygen and destroy brain tissue. Symptoms may appear suddenly and worsen with additional strokes; they include disorientation in familiar locations; walking with rapid, shuffling steps; incontinence; laughing or crying inappropriately; difficulty following instructions; and problems handling money. High blood pressure, cigarette smoking, and high cholesterol are some of the risk factors for stroke that may be controlled to prevent vascular dementia.

Even for these incurable forms of dementia, treatment can improve an affected person's quality of life. Evidence indicates that some cases of dementia are hereditary, but experts say genetics are not always a sure sign that a person will develop the disease.

Grief   Another psychological and emotional challenge of aging is dealing with grief and mourning. Aging is associated with loss—the loss of friends, family and spouse, peers, physical appearance, possessions, and health. Grief is the process of getting through the pain of loss, and it can be one of the loneliest and most emotionally intense times in a person's life. It can take years to completely come to terms with the loss of a loved one. Unresolved grief can have serious physical and psychological or emotional health consequences and may require professional help.

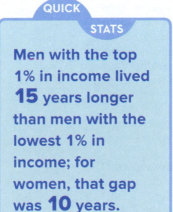

QUICK STATS

Men with the top 1% in income lived **15** years longer than men with the lowest 1% in income; for women, that gap was **10** years.

—Chetty et al, 2016

Depression and Suicide   Unresolved grief can lead to depression, a common problem in older adults (see Chapter 3). If you notice the signs of depression in yourself or someone you know, consult a mental health professional. A marked loss of interest in usually pleasurable activities, decreased appetite, insomnia, fatigue, and feelings of worthlessness are signs of depression. Listen carefully when an older friend or relative complains about being depressed; it may be a request for help.

Although the elderly (age 65 and over) comprise about 13% of the U.S. population, they account for over 18% of all suicides. People age 85 and over have the highest suicide rate of any age group. Older white men have a suicide rate almost six times that of the general population—more than women and minorities at any age. Depression is probably the single most significant factor associated with suicidal behavior in older adults.

LIFE IN AN AGING AMERICA

Life expectancy is the average length of time we can expect to live. It is calculated by averaging mortality statistics—the ages at death of a group of people over a certain period. In 2014, life expectancy for the total U.S. population was 78.8 years, but those who reach age 65 can expect to live even longer—about 20 more years. A man reaching age 65 today can expect to live, on average, until age 83. A woman turning age 65 today can expect to live, on average, until age 86. Women have a longer life expectancy than men do (see the box "Why Do Women Live Longer?").

As life expectancy increases, a larger proportion of Americans will be in their later years. This change will necessitate new government policies and changes in our general attitudes toward older adults.

America's Aging Minority

People over age 65 are a large minority in the American population—over 40.2 million people and about 14% of the total population in 2012. That number is expected to more than double by the year 2050.

The enormous increase in the over-65 population is markedly affecting our stereotypes of what it means to grow old. The misfortunes associated with aging—frailty, forgetfulness, poor health, isolation—occur in fewer people

Alzheimer's disease   A disease characterized by a progressive loss of mental functioning (dementia), caused by a degeneration of brain cells.

TERMS

life expectancy   The average length of time a person is expected to live.

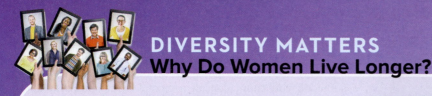

Women live longer than men in most countries around the world, even in places where maternal mortality rates are high. In the United States, women on average can expect to live about five years longer than men (see the table in this box). Worldwide, women comprise 85% of the population that is more than 100 years old.

The reason for the gender gap in life expectancy is not entirely understood but may be influenced by biological, social, and lifestyle factors. Medical consensus used to be that estrogen contributed to women's longevity. Not only has this theory been disproved, but research also indicates that estrogen supplements may be detrimental to postmenopausal women. However, estrogen production and other factors during a woman's younger years may protect her from early heart disease and from age-related declines in the heart's pumping power. Another theory suggests that menstruation has contributed to women's longer life expectancy. Because women excrete excess iron during menstruation, it is thought that women tend to experience a later onset of cardiovascular disease than do men. Men have higher iron levels in their bloodstreams throughout life, and iron can damage cells and cause free radicals to form, leading to cardiovascular conditions such as heart disease or stroke. Research findings made by a team of Japanese scientists suggest that women live longer than men partly because women's immune systems age more slowly. Additionally, women may have lower rates of stress-related illnesses because they cope more positively with stress.

The news for women is not all good, however, because not all their extra years are likely to be healthy years. They are more likely than men to suffer from chronic conditions like arthritis and osteoporosis. Women's longer life spans, combined with the facts that men tend to marry younger women and that widowed men remarry more often than widowed women do, mean there are many more single older women than men. Older men are more likely to live in family settings, whereas older women are more likely to live alone. Older women are also less likely to be covered by a pension or to have retirement savings, so they are more likely to be poor.

Social and behavioral factors may be more important than physiological causes in explaining the gender gap; for example, among the Amish, a religious sect that has strict rules against smoking and drinking, men usually live as long as women. This finding suggests that the longevity gap could be narrowed substantially through lifestyle

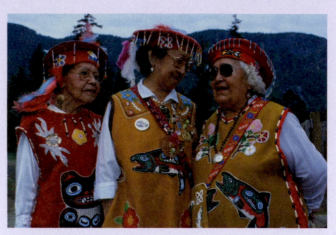

These Tlingit women participate in a traditional dance group, which helps them stay active and maintain social and community ties, enhancing wellness as they age.

changes. For example, men in general tend to take more risks than women—from driving more recklessly to using drugs and alcohol.

Life Expectancy

Year of Birth	Men	Women
Life expectancy at birth		
1900	46.3	48.3
1950	65.6	71.1
2000	74.1	79.3
2007	75.4	80.4
2010	76.2	81.1
Life expectancy at age 65		
1900	11.5	12.2
1950	12.8	15.0
2000	16.0	19.0
2010	17.7	20.3
2014	18.0	20.5

SOURCES: National Center for Health Statistics. 2016. *Health, United States, 2015.* Hyattsville, MD: National Center for Health Statistics; World Health Organization. 2012. *Gender, Health, and Aging.* Geneva: World Health Organization.

in their sixties and seventies and are shifting instead to burden the very old: those over age 85.

The homeownership rate exceeds 80% for those aged 65–84, declining slightly to about 76% for those older than 85. This rate is much higher than the homeownership rate for those under age 65 (about 65%). Older people's living expenses are lower after retirement because they no longer support children and have fewer work-related expenses; they consume and

buy less food. Some continue practicing their expertise for years after retirement and receive some income: Thousands of retired consultants, teachers, technicians, and craftspeople work until their middle and late seventies. They receive greater amounts of assistance, such as Medicare, pay proportionately lower taxes, and have greater net worth from lifetime savings.

As the aging population increases proportionately, however, the number of older people who are ill and dependent rises.

Health care remains the largest expense for older adults. On average, they visit a physician 10–12 times a year, are hospitalized more frequently, and require twice as many prescription drugs as the general population. Most older Americans have at least one chronic condition and many have multiple conditions.

Retirement finds many older people with incomes reduced to subsistence levels. The majority of older Americans live with fixed sources of income, such as pensions, that are eroded by inflation. Expenses tend to increase more rapidly, especially those resulting from circumstances over which people have little or no control, such as deteriorating health. **Social Security** is the major source of income for most of the elderly. Social Security was intended to serve as a supplement to personal savings and private pensions, not as a sole source of income. It is vital to plan for an adequate retirement income.

Family and Community Resources for Older Adults

With help from friends, family members, and community services, people in their later years can remain active and independent. Over half of noninstitutionalized older Americans live with a spouse; some live with a family member other than a spouse, and about 28% live alone. Only 3.4% live in institutional settings, but among those over age 85, about 10% live in a nursing home.

In about three out of four cases, a spouse, a grown daughter, or a daughter-in-law assumes a caregiving role for elderly relatives. Caregiving can be rewarding, but it is also hard work. If the experience is stressful and long term, family members may become emotionally exhausted. Corporations are increasingly responsive to the needs of their employees who are family caregivers by providing services such as referrals, flexible schedules and leaves, and on-site adult care.

Professional health care advice is another critical part of successful home care.

The best thing a family can do is talk honestly about the obligations, time, and commitment required for caregiving. Families should also explore community resources and professional assistance that may be available to reduce the stress associated with this difficult job.

Government Aid and Policies

The federal government helps older Americans through several programs, such as food assistance, housing subsidies, Social Security, Medicare, and Medicaid.

Medicare is a major health insurance program for older adults and disabled persons. It provides basic health care coverage for acute episodes of illness that require skilled professional care. It pays for some preventive services, including an initial physical exam, vaccinations, and screenings for cardiovascular disease, certain cancers, osteoporosis, diabetes, and glaucoma. It does not pay for many office visits, dental care, or dentures. Over 1.6 million older people currently live in nursing homes, but Medicare pays less than 2% of nursing home costs, and private insurers pay less than 1%, creating a tremendous financial burden for nursing home residents and their families. When their financial resources are exhausted, people may apply for Medicaid. Created by a 1965 amendment to the Social Security Act, Medicaid provides medical insurance to low-income people of any age.

Health care policy planners hope that rising medical costs for older adults will shrink dramatically through education and prevention. Health care professionals, including **gerontologists** and **geriatricians,** are beginning to practice preventive medicine, just as pediatricians do. They advise older people about how to avoid and, if necessary, how to manage disabilities.

Ask Yourself

QUESTIONS FOR CRITICAL THINKING AND REFLECTION

What do you want your life to be like when you are old? Do you hope to retire, or keep working indefinitely? Where would you like to live? How much time do you spend thinking about these questions? What have you planned for your later years?

WHAT IS DEATH?

Whether it is victims of a terrorist attack, an earthquake or a car crash, or a woman in her nineties dying peacefully with her family close by, images of death are all around us. Nevertheless, we rarely think about the inevitability of death in our own lives. Most of us live as if we are immortal, especially because in our 20s and 30s we haven't peaked yet on the arc toward death, and are not yet on the downhill. Accepting and dealing with death presents unique challenges to our sense of self, our relationships with others, and our understanding of the meaning of life itself.

Although pain and distress may accompany the dying process, facing death also presents an opportunity for growth as well as affirmation of the preciousness of our daily lives. Dealing with the death of a loved one can tear families apart, but it can also bring them together, healing old wounds in the process. The way we choose to confront death can greatly influence how we live.

Questions about the meaning of death and what happens when we die are central to the great religions and philosophies of the world. Some promise a better life after death. Others teach that everyone is evolving toward perfection or divinity, a goal reached after successive rounds of life, death and rebirth. Still others suggest that it is not possible to know what—if anything—happens after death and that any judgment about life's worth must be made on the basis of satisfactions or rewards we create for ourselves in our lifetimes.

Even for the most secular individuals, religious beliefs and traditions can shape attitudes and behaviors surrounding death. The mourning ceremonies associated with various religions ease the pangs of grief for many people. Dying and death are more than biological events; they have social and spiritual dimensions.

Senescence, the biological process of aging, is complex, rooted in genetics, and universal in all mammals, including humans. Organisms age on both a cellular and a whole-organism level, ultimately resulting in death. Although scientific understanding of senescence is progressing, and average life spans are increasing, death remains an inevitable event for humans.

Defining Death

Traditionally death has been defined as cessation of the flow of vital body fluids. This cessation occurs when the heart stops beating and breathing ceases, referred to as **clinical death.** These traditional signs are adequate for determining death in most cases. However, over the past several decades, the use of cardiopulmonary resuscitation (CPR) and other medical techniques have brought many "dead" people (by the traditional definition) back to life. The use of ventilators, artificial heart pumps, and other **life support systems** allow many body functions to be sustained artificially. In such cases, making a determination of death can be difficult and often controversial. The concept of **brain death** was

developed to determine whether a person is alive or dead when the traditional signs are inadequate because of supportive medical technology.

The Uniform Determination of Death Act, developed in 1981, provides criteria for determining brain death, which is defined as the complete and irreversible loss of function of the entire brain. The concept of brain death is particularly crucial for organ transplantation. Medical technologies such as ventilators are used so that organs will remain viable over the hours or days that are needed to arrange for transplantation. Some organs—hearts, most obviously—must be harvested from a human being who is legally determined to be dead. Timing is critical in removing a heart from someone who has been declared dead and transplanting it into a person whose life can thereby be saved.

Safeguards are necessary to ensure that the determination of death occurs without regard to any plans for subsequent transplantation of the deceased's organs. Several thorough examinations need to be performed over a period of time in order to determine that both higher brain and brain-stem functions (which regulate heartbeat and breathing) have ceased irreversibly. The American Academy of Neurology published guidelines in 2010 for determination of brain death, but a 2015 study showed that hospital policies and practices regarding brain death still vary considerably throughout the United States.

The way death is defined also has potential legal, ethical, and social consequences, including potential effects on criminal prosecution, inheritance, taxation, treatment of the corpse, and even mourning. Determining that someone is dead is simple and obvious in the vast majority of cases, but at times it can be difficult and controversial.

As medical and technological advances occur, it has become increasingly obvious that death consists of a series of biological events that occur over a period of time. In contrast to clinical death (irreversible cessation of heartbeat and breathing) or brain death, **cellular death** refers to a gradual process that occurs when heartbeat, respiration, and brain activity have stopped. Many cells throughout the body continue to survive for seconds, minutes, or hours after clinical and brain death, but gradually die as they utilize remaining

TERMS

senescence   The biological process of aging.

clinical death   The medical term applied to the point at which there is no longer blood flow in the body (the heart has stopped beating) and breathing has ceased.

life support systems   Medical technologies, such as a ventilator, that allow vital body functions to be sustained artificially.

brain death   A complete and irreversible cessation of brain activity indicated by various diagnostic criteria; this medical determination may be necessary when intensive hospital-based life support systems have been used to artificially sustain organ systems in the body.

cellular death   The breakdown of metabolic processes at the level of the body's cells.

oxygen and glucose. Cellular death encompasses the breakdown of metabolic processes and results in complete non-functionality at the cellular level. In a biological sense, therefore, death can be defined as the cessation of life due to irreversible changes in cell metabolism.

Learning about Death

Our understanding of death changes as we grow and mature, as do our attitudes toward it. Very young children view death as an interruption and an absence, but their lack of a mature time perspective means that they do not understand death as final and irreversible. A child's understanding of death evolves greatly from about age 6 to age 9. During this period, most children begin to understand that death is final, universal, and inevitable. A person who consciously recognizes these facts is said to possess a **mature understanding of death.**

However, even individuals who possess a mature understanding of death commonly also hold nonempirical ideas about it. Such nonempirical ideas—that is, ideas not subject to scientific proof—deal mainly with the notion that human beings survive in some form beyond the death of the physical body. What happens to an individual's personality after he or she dies? Does the self or soul continue to exist after the death of the physical body? If so, what is the nature of this afterlife? Developing personally satisfying answers to such questions, which involve what Mark Speece and Sandor Brent term **noncorporeal continuity,** is also part of the process of acquiring a mature understanding of death.

In the United States, with its relative affluence and orderliness, death is not a part of the day-to-day existence of most young people. There are exceptions, however, especially among those who have grown up in relatively dangerous environments, such as neighborhoods in the inner city, where violent deaths among young people may be agonizingly frequent. Rural kids may also experience close encounters with death at a young age, as they lose loved ones to fatal automotive crashes on dangerous country roads. However, even when death strikes those around us, many of us continue to feel a sense of invulnerability—that is, "It won't happen to me." By the time we reach old age, reminders of aging and death are frequent, especially as older adults experience the loss of many of their contemporaries. The very old have often lost nearly everyone of significance in their lives. Coping with the death of loved ones and contemplating their own impending deaths are central developmental tasks for the very elderly.

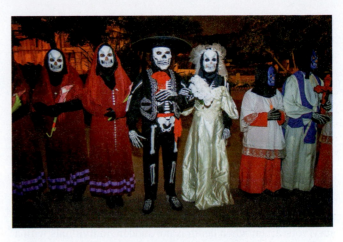

In Mexico, individuals publicly celebrate departed loved ones on the annual holiday *Día de los Muertos* (Day of the Dead).
© fitopardo.com/Getty Images

Denying versus Acknowledging Death

The ability to find meaning and comfort in the face of mortality depends not only on having an understanding of the facts of death but also on our attitudes toward it. Many people avoid any thought or mention of death. The sick and old are often isolated in hospitals and nursing homes. Relatively few Americans have been present at the death of a loved one. Where the reality of death is concerned, "out of sight, out of mind" is often the rule of the day.

Although some commentators characterize the predominant attitude toward death in the United States as "death denying," others are reluctant to generalize so broadly. People often maintain conflicting or ambivalent attitudes toward death. Those who view death as a relief or release from insufferable pain may have at least a sense that death is sometimes welcomed, but few people wholly avoid or wholly welcome death. In the past several decades, attitudes toward death in our culture have begun to change slowly. The hospice movement (discussed in this chapter) has provided support and guidance for many families who choose to be present during the dying process of their loved ones, often in their own homes.

Not all cultures are reluctant to publicly acknowledge death. For example, traditional Mexican culture honors the dead by remembering them often and even including them in

mature understanding of death The recognition that death is universal and irreversible, that it involves the cessation of all physiological functioning, and that there are biological reasons for its occurrence.

noncorporeal continuity The notion that human beings survive in some form after the death of the physical body.

TERMS

Ask Yourself

QUESTIONS FOR CRITICAL THINKING AND REFLECTION

What situations or events make you think seriously about your own mortality? Is this something you consider now and then, or do you avoid thinking about death? What has influenced your willingness or reluctance to think about death?

family activities. *Día de los Muertos* (Day of the Dead) is an annual holiday in Mexico, in which families celebrate their departed loved ones. This holiday is festive, tinged with some sadness, but mostly full of love, fun, and good humor. Similar celebrations that honor the dead in a festive manner are common in many cultures throughout the world.

PLANNING FOR DEATH

Acknowledging the inevitability of death allows us to plan for it. Adequate planning can help ensure that a sudden, unexpected death is not made even more difficult for survivors. Even when death is not sudden, individuals with a debilitating illness may become unable to make decisions. Many decisions can be anticipated, considered, and discussed with close relatives and friends.

Making a Will

Surveys indicate that about 55% of adult Americans do not have a will. A **will** is a legal instrument expressing a person's intentions and wishes for the disposition of his or her property after death. It is a declaration of how your **estate**—that is, money, property, and other possessions—will be distributed after death. During the life of the **testator** (the person making the will), a will can be changed, replaced, or revoked. When the testator dies, it becomes a legal instrument governing the distribution of the estate.

When a person dies **intestate**—that is, without having left a valid will—property is distributed according to rules set up by the state. If you haven't yet made a will, start thinking about how you'd like your property distributed in the case of your death. If you have a will, consider whether it needs to be updated in response to a key life event such as marriage, the birth of a child, or the purchase of a home.

A person making a will can also help family members by completing a *testamentary letter*. This document includes information about personal affairs, such as bank accounts, credit cards, insurance policies, the location of documents and keys, the names of professional advisers, passwords for online accounts, the names of people who should be notified of the death, and so on.

Considering Options for End-of-Life Care

As life draws to a close, care may involve any combination of home care, hospital stays, nursing home care, and hospice care. By becoming aware of the options, we and our families are empowered to make informed, meaningful choices.

Home Care   The majority of people express a preference for at-home care during the end of life. An obvious advantage of home care is the fact that the person is in a familiar setting, ideally in the company of family and friends. Family

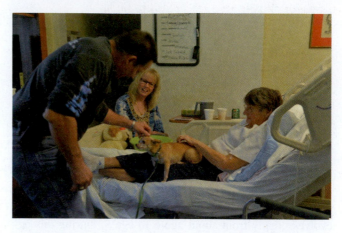

Hospice care focuses on relieving pain and other distressing symptoms in dying people and on providing support for family members.
© Jahi Chikwendiu/The Washington Post/Getty Images

members may or may not be capable of providing the level of care that is needed. Currently about 25% of Americans die at home, about 25% die in nursing facilities, and about 50% die in hospitals, including more than 20% in intensive care units.

Hospice Programs.   Terminally ill people who wish to die at home, in their assisted-living residence, or in a more peaceful hospital environment are often aided by **hospice** programs, which are widely available throughout the United States and are providing a growing number of terminally ill patients with much-needed assistance.

Hospice is a system of **palliative care,** a collaborative, team-based approach to treatment that aims to prevent and relieve suffering in patients with serious or life-threatening illness. The overarching goal of palliative care is to improve the quality of life for the patient and his or her family during this period in their lives.

About two-thirds of hospice patients receive care in the place they call "home," which is most frequently their private residence, but also can be a nursing home or a residential facility. Hospice care is also offered in hospitals and freestanding hospice facilities. Hospice care is available to

---

TERMS

will   A legal instrument expressing a person's intentions and wishes for the disposition of his or her property after death.

estate   The money, property, and other possessions belonging to a person.

testator   The person who makes a will.

intestate   Not having made a legal will.

hospice   A system of palliative care specifically for patients who are likely to die within six months, often at home, to optimize the quality of life for dying patients and their families.

palliative care   A collaborative, team-based approach to treatment that aims to prevent and relieve suffering in patients with serious or life-threatening illness.

people of all ages who are judged to be in their last six months of life.

More than 45% of people who died in the United States in 2014 were under the care of a hospice program. About 67% of hospice patients are over 75 years old, although hospice programs take care of patients of all ages, including children. In addition to helping patients achieve a good and peaceful death, an important gift of hospice care is the potential to help patients and families discover how much can be shared at the end of life through personal and spiritual connections.

Difficult Decisions at the End of Life

Modern medicine can sometimes keep the human organism alive despite the cessation of normal heart, brain, respiratory, or kidney function. But should a patient without any hope of recovery be kept alive by means of artificial machine support? At what point does such treatment become futile? What if a patient has fallen into a **persistent vegetative state,** a state of profound unconsciousness, lacking any sign of normal reflexes and unresponsive to external stimuli, with no reasonable hope of improvement?

Ethical questions about a person's right to die have become prominent since the landmark case of Karen Ann Quinlan in 1975. At age 22 she was admitted in a comatose state to an intensive care unit, where her breathing was sustained by a mechanical ventilator. When she remained unresponsive, in a persistent vegetative state, her parents asked that the respirator be disconnected, but the medical staff responsible for Karen's care denied their request. The request to withdraw treatment eventually reached the New Jersey Supreme Court, which ruled that artificial respiration could be discontinued.

Since then, courts have ruled on removing other types of life-sustaining treatment, including artificial feeding mechanisms that provide nutrition and hydration to permanently comatose patients who are able to breathe on their own. Notable was the case of Terri Schiavo in 2003. Terri had been diagnosed as being in a persistent vegetative state. Contending that she would not want to continue living on life support, Terri's husband requested that her feeding tube be removed. Terri's parents contested the request, and a series of legal actions ensued. Finally, in 2005, after intervention by the U.S. Supreme Court, physicians were allowed to remove the tube. Cases like this highlight the importance of expressing your wishes about life-sustaining treatment, in writing, before the need arises.

Withholding or Withdrawing Treatment   The right of a competent patient to refuse unwanted treatment is now generally established in both law and medical practice. The consensus is that there is no medical or ethical distinction between withholding (not starting) a treatment and withdrawing (stopping) a treatment once it has been started. The right to refuse treatment remains constitutionally protected even when a patient is unable to communicate. Although specific requirements vary, all states authorize some type of written legal document, referred to as an advance directive, in which individuals can record their wishes, and those wishes will be honored if and when those individuals cannot speak for themselves.

Physician-Assisted Death and Voluntary Active Euthanasia   In contrast to withdrawing or withholding treatment, *physician-assisted death* and *voluntary active euthanasia* refer to practices that intentionally hasten the death of a person; both assume the full informed consent of the patient. Physician-assisted death is legal in five states in the United States (Oregon, Washington, Vermont, Montana, and California). Some form of voluntary active euthanasia is legal in the Netherlands, Luxemburg, Belgium, Columbia, and Canada (as of February 2016).

Physician-assisted death (PAD) occurs when a physician provides a prescription for a lethal dose of medication (usually a sedative medication)—at the patient's request—with the understanding that the patient plans to use the medication to end his or her life. The patient chooses if and when he or she wishes to take the fatal dose, usually in a home setting without the physician present.

Oregon was the first state to legalize PAD following a citizens' initiative called the Death with Dignity Act, which Oregon voters approved in 1994 and again in 1997. Even though PAD has been legally available in Oregon since 1994, the practice remains rare; in 2015, only 125 deaths occurred in Oregon in this way.

An important Supreme Court ruling on PAD, in 1997, involved the concept of **double effect** in the medical

persistent vegetative state   A condition of profound unconsciousness in which a person lacks normal reflexes and is unresponsive to external stimuli, lasting for an extended period with no reasonable hope of improvement.

physician-assisted death (PAD)   The practice of a physician intentionally providing, at the patient's request, a lethal overdose of drugs or other means for a patient to hasten death with the understanding that the patient plans to use them to end his or her life. The patient administers the drugs to himself or herself.

double effect   A situation in which a harmful effect occurs as an unintended side effect of a beneficial action, such as when medication intended to control a patient's pain has the unintended result of causing the patient's death.

TERMS

management of pain. The doctrine of double effect states that a harmful effect of treatment, even if it results in death, is permissible if the harm is not intended and occurs as a side effect of a beneficial action. Sometimes the dosages of medication needed to relieve a patient's pain (especially those in the end stage of some diseases) must be increased to levels that can cause respiratory depression, which could hasten the patient's death. Thus, the relief of suffering, the intended good effect, may have a potential bad effect, which is foreseen but is not the primary intention. The Court said that giving medication as needed to control pain, even if it hastens death, is not considered PAD if the intent is to relieve pain. The doctrine of double effect allows physicians throughout the United States to do what is necessary to relieve a patient's pain, even if there is a chance that the medication may hasten death.

Unlike PAD, **active euthanasia** is the intentional act of killing someone who would otherwise suffer from an incurable and painful disease. *Voluntary euthanasia* (also known as voluntary active euthanasia, or VAE) is the intentional termination of life at the patient's request by someone other than the patient. In practice, this generally means that a competent patient requests direct assistance to die, and he or she receives assistance from a qualified medical practitioner. Voluntary active euthanasia is legal under very strict guidelines in Belgium, Luxembourg, the Netherlands, and Canada (as of February 2016) but is currently unlawful in the United States and the rest of the world. In the United States, taking active steps to end someone's life is a crime—even if the motive is mercy.

When a patient is near death and still suffering despite optimal treatment with pain medications, sometimes **palliative sedation** will be used. Palliative sedation involves giving a sedative that keeps the patient in an unconscious or semiconscious state until pain is brought under control or the patient dies as a result of his or her underlying disease. Palliative sedation is not meant to hasten death; rather it is used as a last resort when physician, patient, and family agree that this is the best way to relieve otherwise intractable suffering.

Completing an Advance Directive

To make your preferences known about medical treatment, you need to document them through a written **advance directive,** which becomes a legal document. Two forms of advance directives are legally important. First is the **living will,** which enables individuals to provide instructions about the kind of medical care they wish to receive or prohibit if they become incapacitated or otherwise unable to participate in treatment decisions.

The second important form of advance directive is the **health care proxy,** which is also known as a *durable power of attorney for health care.* This document makes it possible to appoint another person to make decisions about medical treatment if you become unable to do so. This decision maker may be a family member, a close friend, or an attorney with whom you have discussed your treatment preferences. The proxy is expected to act in accordance with your wishes as stated in an advance directive or as otherwise made known.

For advance directives to be of value, you must do more than merely complete the paperwork. Discuss your wishes ahead of time with caregivers and family members as well as with your physician.

Giving the Gift of Life

Each day about 79 people receive an organ transplant, but another 22 people on the waiting lists die because not enough organs are available. As of January 2016, more than 123,000 Americans were waiting for organ transplants.

If you decide to become an organ donor, the first step is to indicate your wish by completing a **Uniform Donor Card** (Figure 17.1); alternatively, in many states you can indicate your wish on your driver's license. Because

---

QUICK STATS

One deceased donor can save up to 8 lives through organ donation and can save or improve the quality of **100 more** people's lives through tissue donation.

—American Transplant Foundation, 2016

TERMS

active euthanasia   A deliberate act intended to end another person's life; voluntary active euthanasia involves the practice of a physician's administering—at the request of a patient—medication or some other intervention that causes death.

palliative sedation   The practice of using a sedative medication to keep a patient in an unconscious or semiconscious state until pain is brought under control or the patient dies as a result of the underlying disease.

advance directive   Any legally recognized statement made by a competent person about his or her choices for medical treatment should he or she become unable to make such decisions or communicate them in the future.

living will   A type of advance directive that allows individuals to provide instructions about the kind of medical care they wish to receive, or not receive, if they become unable to participate in treatment decisions.

health care proxy   A type of advance directive that allows an individual to appoint another person as an agent in making health care decisions in the event he or she becomes unable to participate in treatment decisions; also known as a *durable power of attorney for health care.*

Uniform Donor Card   A consent form authorizing the use of the signer's body parts for transplantation or medical research upon his or her death.

Organ/Tissue Donor Card

I wish to donate my organs and tissues. I wish to give:

☐ any needed organs and tissues
☐ only the following organs and tissues:

_____

Donor
Signature _____ Date _____

Witness _____

Witness _____

FIGURE 17.1   A sample organ/tissue donor card.

SOURCE: U.S. Department of Health and Human Services (http://www.organdonor.gov/index.html).

relatives are called on to make decisions about organ and tissue donation at the time of a loved one's death, your second step is to discuss your decision with your family.

Planning a Funeral or Memorial Service

Funerals and memorial services are rites of passage that commemorate a person's life and acknowledge his or her passing from the community. Funerals and memorials allow survivors to support one another as they cope with their loss and express their grief. The presence of death rites in every human culture suggests that these ceremonies serve innate human needs.

Disposition of the Body   People generally have a preference about the final disposition of their own body. For most Americans, the choice is either burial or cremation. *Burial* involves a grave dug into the earth or entombment in a mausoleum. If the body is to be buried and the family wishes that the body be viewed during a wake or in an open-casket funeral, **embalming** is generally done.

Cremation involves subjecting a body to intense heat, thereby reducing its organic components to a mineralized skeleton. The remaining bone fragments are then usually put through a cremulator, which reduces them to a granular state, often referred to as ashes (which actually resemble coarse sand). In some parts of the United States, especially in the West, cremation is now more common than burial. Cremation is acceptable to many, but not all, religions (for more on cremation, see the box, "A Consumer Guide to Funerals").

Arranging a Service   A funeral or memorial service can be a healing experience that allows loved ones to share memories and support one another. The more the service fits the personality of the deceased person and meets the practical needs of the family, the better.

People who have a terminal illness sometimes find comfort and satisfaction in helping to plan for their own memorial services. A memorial service can be the joint creation of the dying person and family members who wish

to be part of the project. Making at least some plans ahead of time can help ease the burden on survivors, who will undoubtedly face a great number of tasks and decisions when the death occurs.

COPING WITH IMMINENT DEATH

There is no one right way to live with or die of a life-threatening illness. Every disease has its own set of problems and challenges, and each person copes with these problems and challenges in his or her own way. Much suffering experienced by people with a life-threatening illness comes from overwhelming feelings of loss on all levels.

Living with an illness that is life-threatening and incurable can be described as a living–dying experience. Honesty and hope are often delicately balanced—honesty to face reality as it is, and hope for a positive outcome—a state that psychiatrist Avery Weisman described as **middle knowledge.** The early hope that the symptoms are not really serious gives way to hope that a cure is possible. When the illness is deemed incurable, there is hope for more time. As time begins to run out, one hopes for a pain-free death—a "good death."

The Tasks of Coping

In her groundbreaking 1969 book *On Death and Dying,* Elisabeth Kübler-Ross, a Swiss American psychiatrist and one of the first medical experts to focus on the topic of end of life, suggested that the response to an awareness of imminent death involves five psychological stages: denial, anger, bargaining, depression, and acceptance. Individuals go back and forth among the stages during the course of an illness, and stages can occur simultaneously. Today the notion of stages has been deemphasized in favor of highlighting the tasks that

> **embalming**   The process of removing blood and other fluids and replacing them with chemicals to disinfect and temporarily retard deterioration of a corpse; some of the chemicals used, such as formaldehyde, are toxic.
>
> **TERMS**
>
> **middle knowledge**   A state of knowing in which a person both acknowledges the reality of a threatening situation and maintains hope for a positive outcome.

CRITICAL CONSUMER
A Consumer Guide to Funerals

A traditional funeral with a casket costs about $7000, and many funerals cost $10,000 or more. When no preplanning has been done, as often occurs, family members have to make decisions under time pressure and in the grip of strong feelings. As a result, they may make poor decisions and spend more than they need to. To avoid these problems, millions of consumers are now making funeral arrangements in advance, comparing prices and services so that they can make well-informed purchasing decisions. Many people see funeral planning as an extension of will and estate planning.

Alternatives to traditional funerals exist. Cremation is now used in nearly 50% of deaths in the United States, with the rate of cremation increasing rapidly in recent years. Cremation is also a much less expensive alternative to a traditional burial. A direct cremation (no service or visitation at the funeral home) can cost as little as $600 in some cities and has a lower environmental impact than traditional burial. Cremated remains can be buried, placed in a columbarium niche, put into an urn kept by the family, interred in an urn garden, or scattered at sea or on land.

Whole-body donation (usually to a medical school) is another option chosen by many people for altruistic reasons, as well as for the fact that there is usually no cost. Another alternative to an expensive traditional funeral is a more personalized, "do-it-yourself" family-centered funeral, with minimal costs because most or all of the tasks needed to care for the deceased person are provided by family and friends.

To ensure that you make the best possible decisions when planning a funeral, follow these guidelines:

- Plan ahead. Think about what type of funeral you want, and ask your loved ones about their preferences.

- Shop around. If you are going to use a funeral home, look for one that belongs to the National Funeral Directors Association (NFDA), and compare prices from at least two funeral homes.

- Ask for a price list. The Funeral Rule requires funeral directors to give you an itemized price list when you ask either in person or over the telephone. Many funeral homes offer package funerals that cost less than individual items, but you may not need or want everything included in the package.

- Decide on the goods and services you want. Basic services include planning the funeral and coordinating arrangements with the cemetery or crematory. Embalming is not necessary or legally required if the body is buried or cremated shortly after death. The casket is usually the single most expensive item; an average casket costs slightly more than $2000, but some caskets sell for as much as $10,000. You do not have to buy the casket from the funeral home you use. Many "big box" stores now sell caskets at much lower cost than funeral homes. Special body bags are also used and can cost under $1000.

- Resist pressure to buy goods and services you don't really want or need. Funeral directors are required to inform you that you need buy only those goods and services you want. If you feel you are being pressured, go elsewhere.

- In choosing a cemetery, consider its location, religious affiliation, if any, the types of monuments allowed, and cost. Visit the cemetery ahead of time to make sure it's suitable. If cremation is chosen, use of a cemetery is optional.

- Once decisions have been made, put them in writing, give copies to family members, and keep a copy accessible. Review these decisions every few years and revise them if necessary.

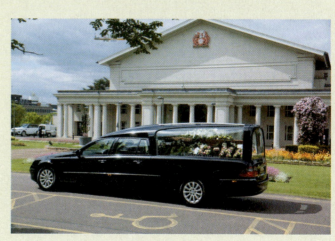

© David Warren/Alamy

require attention in order to cope well with a life-threatening illness. Psychologist and author Charles Corr, for example, distinguishes four primary dimensions in coping with dying:

1. *Physical.* Satisfying bodily needs and minimizing physical distress

2. *Psychological.* Maximizing a sense of security, self-worth, autonomy, and richness in living

3. *Social.* Sustaining significant relationships and addressing the social implications of dying

4. *Spiritual.* Identifying, developing, or reaffirming sources of meaning and fostering hope

Some people with life-threatening illness respond with a fighting spirit that views the illness not only as a threat but also as a challenge. These people strive to inform themselves about their illness and take an active part in treatment decisions, as much as they are able. They are optimistic and have a capacity to discover positive meaning in ordinary events. Holding to a positive outlook despite distressing circumstances, these people attempt to continue to accomplish

Ask Yourself

QUESTIONS FOR CRITICAL THINKING AND REFLECTION

What is your notion of a "good death?" In what setting does it take place, and who is there? In the last days of your life, what do you think you'll need to say, and to whom will you want to say it? If you were terminally ill, what would be the most supportive things others could do for you?

goals, maintain relationships, and sustain a sense of personal vitality, competence, and power despite life-threatening illness. Other people with terminal disease, particularly in the later stages, tend to withdraw, and sometimes find their peace in quietly letting go of striving. Many people who are nearing the end of life develop dementia or delirium, which can greatly limit their ability to cope cognitively and emotionally with the challenges of dying.

Supporting a Person in the Last Phase of Life

People often feel uncomfortable in the presence of a person who is in the final stage of life. How should we act? What can we say? Perhaps the most important and comforting thing we can do for a dying person is to simply be present. Sitting quietly and listening carefully, we can take our cues from the person who is dying. If the person is capable of speaking, and wishes to talk, attentive listening is an act of great kindness. If the person doesn't wish to talk, or is not able to, physical touch such as holding hands or putting a hand on the person's shoulder can be the most effective way to express your love and concern.

As death is drawing near, simple steps—such as repositioning the patient, covering him or her with a light blanket, dimming the room's lighting, playing soft favorite music, or holding hands—can provide great relief and reassurance in the last moments.

COPING WITH LOSS

Even if you have not experienced the death of someone close, you have experienced loss because of changes and endings. The loss of a job, the ending of a relationship, transitions from one school or neighborhood to another—these are the kinds of losses that occur in all our lives. Such losses are sometimes called little deaths, and in varying degrees they all involve grief.

Experiencing Grief

Grief is the reaction to loss. It encompasses thoughts and feelings as well as physical and behavioral responses. Mental distress may involve disbelief, confusion, anxiety, disorganization, and depression. The emotions that can be present in normal grief include not only sorrow and sadness, but also relief, anger, guilt, and self-pity, among others. Bereaved people experience a range of feelings, even conflicting ones. Observing the faces of families at the funeral of a beloved relative often reveals smiles and moments of laughter in addition to solemn expressions and tears. Recognizing that grief can involve many feelings—not just sadness—makes us more able to cope with it. Common behaviors associated with grief include crying and talking repetitively about the deceased and the circumstances of the death. Bereaved people may be restless, as if not knowing what to do with themselves. Outward signs of grief may involve frequent sighing, crying, inappropriate laughter, insomnia, loss of appetite, and marked fatigue. Grief may also evoke a reexamination of religious or spiritual beliefs as a person struggles to make meaning of the loss. Guilt is a common emotion after the death of a loved one. People may blame themselves in some way for the death, or for not doing enough for the deceased, or for feeling a sense of relief that their loved one is gone. All such manifestations of grief can be present as part of our total response to **bereavement**—that is, the event of loss.

Mourning is closely related to grief and is often used as a synonym for it. However, mourning refers not so much to the *reaction* to loss but to the *process* by which a bereaved person adjusts to loss and incorporates it into his or her life. How this process is managed is determined, at least partly, by cultural and gender norms for the expression of grief.

The Course of Grief Grieving, like dying, is highly individual. In the first hours or days following a death, a bereaved person is likely to experience shock and numbness, as well as a sense of disbelief, especially if the death was unexpected. The cause or mode of death—natural, accidental, homicide, or suicide—influences how grief is experienced. Even when a death is anticipated, grief is not necessarily diminished when the loss becomes real.

The death of a loved one is frequently a severe physical as well as emotional stressor. Grieving people often have difficulty sleeping, may neglect to eat nourishing food, and may forget to take their usual medications. These factors add to the health risks associated with recent loss. Recent loss also has a cognitive impact on many grievers. People often report that they feel confused and have difficulty concentrating following a significant loss.

After the initial shock begins to fade, the course of grief is characterized by anxiety, apathy, and pining for the deceased.

TERMS

grief A person's reaction to loss as manifested physically, emotionally, mentally, and behaviorally.

bereavement The objective event of loss.

mourning The process whereby a person actively copes with grief in adjusting to a loss and integrating it into his or her life.

The pangs of grief are felt as the bereaved person deeply experiences the pain of separation. Mourners often experience despair as they repeatedly go over the events surrounding the loss, perhaps fantasizing that somehow everything could be undone and be as it was before.

As time goes on, the acute pain and emotional turmoil of grief begin to subside. Physical and mental balance are reestablished. The bereaved person becomes increasingly reintegrated into his or her social world. Sadness doesn't go away completely, but it recedes into the background much of the time. Although reminders of the loss stimulate waves of active grieving from time to time, the main focus is the present, not the past. Adjusting to loss may sometimes feel like a betrayal of the deceased loved one, but it is healthy to engage again in ongoing life and the future.

Social support for the bereaved is as critical during the later course of grief as it is during the first days after a loss. In offering support, we can reassure the grieving person that grief is normal, permissible, and appropriate. The anniversary of the loved one's death, birthdays, and major holidays following a significant loss can renew grieving, and the support of others is important and appreciated. Knowing that others remember the loss and that they take time to connect is usually perceived as comforting.

Bereaved people may find it helpful to share their stories and concerns through organized support groups. Hospices provide bereavement support groups and counseling, usually for 13 months after the death. Many online and in-person support groups are organized around specific types of bereavement, such as the loss of a child, the loss or a parent, or the loss of a loved one to suicide.

There is no hard and fast "normal" amount of time that grief should last, but when the duration and intensity far exceed what is usually expected, it is often referred to as **complicated grief.** If the griever remains seriously impacted by disabling grief many months or years after a death, she or he may be experiencing complicated grief. Rates of complicated grief in Western countries tend to be highest when a child is lost, or when the death was violent and unexpected (see box "Surviving the Violent Death of a Loved One"). A history of depression or other mood disorder increases the risk for complicated grief. People who experience complicated grief are at increased risk for suicide and serious functional impairment. Psychotherapy is recommended for the treatment of complicated grief.

Supporting a Grieving Person

When a person finds out that a loved one has died, the initial reaction may be profound shock and overwhelming distress. Such a person may initially respond best to the physical comfort of hugging and holding. Later, simply listening may be the most effective way to help. Talking about a loss is an important way that many survivors cope with the changed reality, and they may need to tell their story over and over. The key to being a good listener is to avoid speaking too much, and to refrain from making judgments about whether the thoughts and feelings expressed by a survivor are right or wrong, good or bad.

If a grieving friend or relative talks about suicide, or seems in danger of causing harm to himself or herself or others, seek professional help right away. The recent loss of a loved one is a major risk factor for suicide and self-harm. Be alert to signs that a grieving person is in serious danger.

When a Young Adult Loses a Friend

Among young people aged 18-24 in the United States, the three leading causes of death tend to be sudden and unexpected: unintentional injuries, homicide, and suicide. Losing a close friend to an unexpected death can be particularly traumatic. As a friend, you may feel unsupported and left out of the family's grieving. Also, you may blame yourself in some way for your friend's death or feel you should have somehow prevented the tragedy. If you lose a friend, be sure to look for support from friends, family, clergy, or health professionals, especially if the intense sadness or guilt feelings last for more than a few days or weeks. Friends can often help each other by working together to create their own way of celebrating the life of their lost friend.

Helping Children Cope with Loss

Children tend to cope with loss in a healthier fashion when they are included as part of their family's experience of grief and mourning. Although adults may be uncomfortable about sharing potentially disturbing or painful news with children, a child's natural curiosity usually negates the option of withholding information. Mounting evidence shows that it is best to include children from the beginning—as soon as a terminal prognosis is made, for example—to help them understand what is happening. Children should spend time with the dying person, if possible, to learn, share, offer, and receive comfort.

In talking about death with children, the most important guideline is to be honest. Offer an explanation at the child's level of understanding. Find out what the child wants to know. Keep the explanation simple, stick to basics, and verify what the child has understood from your explanation.

complicated grief Grief that is unusually intense, prolonged, and debilitating. **TERMS**

Ask Yourself

QUESTIONS FOR CRITICAL THINKING AND REFLECTION
Have you ever been in a close relationship with a bereaved person? What kind of support did he or she seem to appreciate most? Why do you think that was the case? How did the experience affect you?

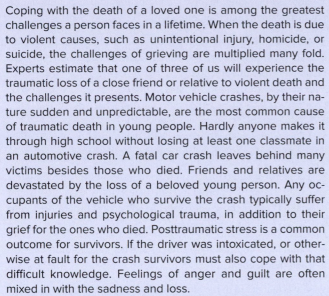

Coping with the death of a loved one is among the greatest challenges a person faces in a lifetime. When the death is due to violent causes, such as unintentional injury, homicide, or suicide, the challenges of grieving are multiplied many fold. Experts estimate that one of three of us will experience the traumatic loss of a close friend or relative to violent death and the challenges it presents. Motor vehicle crashes, by their nature sudden and unpredictable, are the most common cause of traumatic death in young people. Hardly anyone makes it through high school without losing at least one classmate in an automotive crash. A fatal car crash leaves behind many victims besides those who died. Friends and relatives are devastated by the loss of a beloved young person. Any occupants of the vehicle who survive the crash typically suffer from injuries and psychological trauma, in addition to their grief for the ones who died. Posttraumatic stress is a common outcome for survivors. If the driver was intoxicated, or otherwise at fault for the crash survivors must also cope with that difficult knowledge. Feelings of anger and guilt are often mixed in with the sadness and loss.

Although homicide is far less common in the United States than motor vehicle crashes, young people who grow up in high-crime neighborhoods all too often experience the loss of relatives, friends, or acquaintances due to killings. When a loved one is murdered, grievers may agonize over the circumstances of the crime and imagine the horrible suffering their loved one might have endured. Survivors may be haunted by memories of the person's mangled body or may obsess over missing details of the crime. Survivors may also fear for their own safety. The police and legal system may add to the trauma through insensitivity at best, and offensive behavior toward survivors at worst.

People who survive a loved one's suicide also experience great suffering as a result of the stigma attached to suicide. They often feel terrible guilt, wondering if they were in part responsible for their loved one's distress, or whether they could have done something to prevent the suicide. Perhaps the most difficult aspect of coping with violent death, and suicide in particular, is the societal stigma frequently directed at the survivors. The spouse or parent of someone who has committed suicide is often suspected of having been a source of the victim's unhappiness, or at least guilty for not sensing the trouble and doing something about it.

Thus, beyond the challenges of coping with a "natural" death, those who lose a loved one to a violent death face many additional sources of anguish. The sense of the world as a benevolent, safe, and predictable place is often lost when loved ones die in traumatic circumstances. Survivors often face questions of blame, legal issues, financial distress, and lack of social support. A grieving survivor may be called upon to relive the trauma and its horrifying memories over and over again during encounters with police and in legal proceedings. Moreover, friends and community members often avoid survivors, or respond with morbid curiosity or judgmental comments, rather than providing the loving support that is so desperately needed. Or they may back away from someone whose loss is too frightening to contemplate. The instinct to blame the deceased and the survivors for some aspect of a violent death is also common and often represents our attempt to reassure ourselves that if only we are vigilant, and do the right thing, this kind of tragedy won't happen to us or our loved ones.

Some experts refer to the grief experience related to violent loss as "traumatic grief," a term used by Marilyn Armour, a prominent researcher in the field. Traumatic grief involves symptoms of separation-related distress, resulting from the loss of a loved one, as well as symptoms of traumatic distress related to the horrible ordeal the mourner has experienced. Posttraumatic stress often complicates a survivor's ability to recover, and severe, prolonged grief may result. Finding meaning in a sudden and violent death is much more challenging than in a death from old age or a lengthy illness. When someone dies of natural causes, the survivors are often comforted by the belief that at least their loved one is no longer suffering or that the person "died peacefully." In the case of violent death, there are no similar thoughts to soften the blow.

Despite the great challenges, most of those who lose someone to a violent death do eventually recapture a sense of normalcy. Helping survivors starts with all of us reaching out with nonjudgmental love and kindness. For all survivors, the support of friends and community is crucial for regaining a sense of peace. A number of excellent organizations support survivors of loved ones' deaths through accidents, suicide, homicide, and other types of violent death (see "For More Information" at the end of this chapter). Most of these organizations provide information about joining online and in-person support groups, as well as finding professional help for those who are having difficulty coping with traumatic loss.

COMING TO TERMS WITH DEATH

We may wish we could keep death out of view and protect others from the pain associated with it. But this wish cannot be fulfilled. With the death of a beloved friend or relative, we are confronted with emotions and thoughts that relate not only to the immediate loss but also to our own mortality.

Our encounters with dying and death teach us that relationships are more important than material possessions and that life offers no guarantees. In discovering the meaning of death in our own lives, we find that life is both precious and precarious.

Allowing ourselves to make room for death, we discover that it touches not only the dying or bereaved person and his or her family and friends but also the wider community of which we are all part. We recognize that dying and death offer opportunities for extraordinary growth in the midst of loss. Denying death, it turns out, results in denying life.

TIPS FOR TODAY AND THE FUTURE

The best way to ensure a high-quality life in later years is by cultivating healthy habits, including a clear-sighted view of death, in your younger years.

RIGHT NOW YOU CAN:

- Review your financial situation, and start thinking about a plan for the future.
- Think about any unhealthy habits you have and resolve to change them. Review the information in this text to devise strategies for change.
- Don't miss out on opportunities to let your friends and loved ones know that you care for them. Let your awareness of death guide you into leading a loving and purposeful life.
- Consider organ donation as a lasting gift of life to others. If you want to be an organ donor, make the appropriate arrangements now, as described in this chapter.

IN THE FUTURE YOU CAN:

- Learn a new skill, such as speaking a new language or playing a new instrument or game of strategy.
- Volunteer with a nonprofit group in your community; consider a literacy campaign, a soup kitchen, a youth mentoring program, or a group that helps the elderly in some manner.
- Talk to your parents or grandparents about their wishes for the end of life. Let them know you care for them and want to be involved. Suggest that you look together at an advanced directive form; see For More Information for resources.

SUMMARY

- People who take charge of their health during their youth have greater control over the physical and mental aspects of aging.

- Biological aging takes place over a lifetime, but some other changes associated with aging are more abrupt.

- A lifetime of interests and hobbies helps maintain creativity and intelligence.

- Exercise and a healthful diet throughout life enhance physical and psychological health.

- Alcohol abuse is a common but often hidden problem among older adults, as is overdependence on medications. Tobacco use shortens life and also may cause severe health impairment for many years.

- Regular physical examinations help detect conditions that can shorten life and make old age less healthy.

- Stress increases wear and tear on the body; getting enough sleep, avoiding drugs, and practicing relaxation help reduce stress.

- Retirement can be a fulfilling and enjoyable time of life for those who adjust to their new roles, enjoy participating in a variety of activities, and have planned ahead for financial stability.

- Successful aging involves anticipating and accommodating physical changes and limitations.

- Slight confusion and forgetfulness are not signs of a serious illness; however, severe symptoms may indicate Alzheimer's disease or another form of dementia.

- Resolving grief and mourning and dealing with depression are important tasks for older adults.

- Older adults can be role models for the successful integration of life's experiences and the ability to adapt to challenges.

- People over age 65 form a large minority in the United States, and their status is improving. But older adults who are ill and dependent—often those who were already poor—experience major social and economic problems.

- Family and community resources can help older adults stay active and independent.

- Government aid to the elderly includes food assistance, housing subsidies, Social Security, Medicare, and Medicaid.

- Although death makes rational sense in terms of species survival and evolution, there may be no completely satisfying answer to the question of why death exists from a personal point of view.

- Dying and death are more than biological events; they have social and spiritual dimensions.

- The traditional criteria for determining death focus on vital signs such as breathing and heartbeat. Brain death is an irreversible cessation of brain activity indicated by various diagnostic criteria.

- A mature understanding of death can include ideas about the survival of the human personality or soul after death. Problems arise when avoidance or denial of death fosters the notion that it happens only to others.

- A will is a legal instrument that governs the distribution of a person's estate after death.

- End-of-life care may involve a combination of home care, hospital stays, and hospice or palliative care.

- Palliative care is a team-based approach to making dying patients comfortable by controlling pain and relieving suffering.

- Hospice programs are a type of palliative care specifically for patients who are likely to die within six months, often at home, to optimize the quality of life of dying patients and their families.

- Exercising choices about end-of-life care can involve making decisions about attempting to prolong life or choosing to allow natural death with comfort care.

- The right of a competent patient to refuse unwanted treatment is now generally established in both law and medical practice.

- Physician-assisted death occurs when a physician provides lethal drugs or other interventions, at a patient's request, with the understanding that the patient plans to use them to end his or her life. Voluntary active euthanasia refers to the intentional ending of a patient's life, at his or her request, by someone other than the patient.

• Advance directives, such as living wills, are used to express people's wishes about the use of life-sustaining treatment and how they wish to be treated if they cannot speak for themselves.

• People can donate their bodies or specific organs for transplantation and other medical uses after death. People of all ages can make their wishes to donate their organs known on their driver's license or other state forms. They also need to let their families know that they wish to be organ donors.

• Bereaved people usually benefit from participating in a funeral or other type of memorial service to commemorate a loved one's life and death.

• For Americans, the decision about what to do with the body after death usually involves choosing between burial or cremation.

• Coping with dying involves physical, psychological, social, and spiritual dimensions.

• In offering support to a dying person, the gift of listening and loving touch can be especially important.

• Grief encompasses thoughts and feelings as well as physical and behavioral responses.

• Mourning, the process by which a person integrates a loss into his or her life, is determined partly by social and cultural norms for expressing grief.

• Children tend to cope with death in a healthier fashion when they are included in their family's experience of grief and mourning.

• Dying and death offer opportunities for growth in the midst of loss.

FOR MORE INFORMATION

AARP. Provides information about all aspects of aging, including health promotion, health care, and retirement planning.

http://www.aarp.org

Administration on Aging. Provides fact sheets, statistical information, and Internet links to other resources on aging.

http://www.aoa.gov

Aging Well. A practical resource for seniors that includes information about diet, exercise, safety, and medical care.

http://www.aging.ny.gov

Aging with Dignity: Five Wishes. Source for an advanced directive that includes designation of a health care proxy (durable power of attorney), the kind of medical treatment you want or want to avoid, your wishes about pain control, how you want people to treat you, and what you want your loved ones to know when you are dying.

http://www.agingwithdignity.org/five-wishes.php

Alliance for Aging Research. A nonprofit organization that supports medical and psychological research on aging.

http://www.agingresearch.org

Alzheimer's Association. Offers tips for caregivers and patients and information on the causes and treatment of Alzheimer's disease.

http://www.alz.org

American Association of Suicidology. Provides information and help for people who have lost loved ones to suicide. Contains a variety of resources, including a directory of support groups.

http://www.suicidology.org/suicide-survivors/suicide-loss
-survivors

Arthritis Foundation. Provides information about arthritis, including free brochures, referrals to local services, and research updates.

http://www.arthritis.org

Association for Death Education and Counseling (ADEC). Provides resources for education, bereavement counseling, and care of the dying.

http://www.adec.org

Caring Connections (a program of the National Hospice and Palliative Care Organization). Provides resources for end-of-life decision making with the goal of planning before a crisis occurs, including information about state-specific advance directives. A hotline and multilingual line are available.

http://www.caringinfo.org

The Compassionate Friends. Provides grief support after the death of a child, including local chapters and online support groups.

http://www.compassionatefriends.org

The Dougy Center. Offers education about childhood bereavement and support groups for bereaved children, teens, young adults, and parents.

http://www.dougy.org

Funeral Consumers Alliance. A site with extensive information about how to plan a dignified family-centered funeral, details of cremation and burial, and dealing with death and grief.

http://www.funerals.org

GRASP: Grief Recovery After a Substance Passing. Website for friends and family of people who have died as a result of substance use. Local and online support groups are available.

http://grasphelp.org

GriefNet. A site where you can communicate with others via e-mail support groups in the areas of death, grief, and major loss. You can create a memorial on this website.

http://www.griefnet.org

Healthy Aging: U.S. Department of Health and Human Services. Lists numerous significant resources for all aspects of aging healthfully: brain and mental health, nutrition, exercise training, networking, how to locate benefits and find care, retirement planning, and many other aspects.

http://www.hhs.gov/aging/healthy-aging/index.html#

Hospice Foundation of America. Promotes the hospice concept of care through education and leadership.

http://www.hospicefoundation.org

LeadingAge. Provides information about living and care arrangements available for older adults.

http://www.leadingage.org

Medicare. Provides signup information; listings to compare doctors, providers, hospitals, plans, and suppliers available through the program; and details on costs and coverage.

http://www.medicare.gov

National Cancer Institute: Grief, Bereavement and Coping with Loss. Provides extensive information about types of grief reactions, complicated grief, treatment for complicated grief, children and loss, and cultural aspects of grief.

http://www.cancer.gov/about-cancer/advanced-cancer/caregivers/planning/bereavement-pdq

National Council on Aging. Provides helpful information about retirement planning, health promotion, and lifelong learning.

http://www.ncoa.org

National Funeral Directors Association (NFDA). Provides resources related to funerals and funeral costs, body disposition, and bereavement support.

http://www.nfda.org

National Hospice and Palliative Care Organization (NHPCO). Provides information about hospice care and advance directives, including an online national directory of hospices listed by state and city.

http://www.nhpco.org

National Institute on Aging. Provides fact sheets and brochures about aging-related topics.

http://www.nia.nih.gov

http://nihseniorhealth.gov

https://go4life.nia.nih.gov (plans for balanced workouts and snack activities)

National Osteoporosis Foundation. Provides information about the causes, prevention, detection, and treatment of osteoporosis.

http://www.nof.org

Nolo Press: Wills and Estate Planning. Provides answers to questions about planning for death, from writing a basic will to organ donation.

http://www.nolo.com

The following organizations provide information about organ donation and donor cards:

Coalition on Donation (http://www.donatelife.net)

Organ Procurement and Transplantation Network (http://www.organdonor.gov/index.html)

SELECTED BIBLIOGRAPHY

AARP Public Policy Institute and National Alliance for Caregiving. 2015. *Caregiving in the United States 2015* (http://www.aarp.org/ppi/info-2015/caregiving-in-the-united-states-2015.html).

Administration on Aging. 2014. *A Profile of Older Americans: 2014* (http://www.aoa.acl.gov/Aging_Statistics/Profile/2014/docs/2014-Profile.pdf).

Agency for Healthcare Research and Quality. 2016. *Statistical Brief #491: National Health Care Expenses in the U.S. Civilian Noninstitutionalized Population, Distributions by Type of Service and Source of Payment, 2013* (https://meps.ahrq.gov/data_files/publications/st491/stat491.shtml).

Alzheimer's Association. 2016. *2063 Alzheimer's Disease Facts and Figures* (http://www.alz.org/facts/overview.asp).

American Academy of Hospice and Palliative Medicine. 2014. *Palliative Sedation Position Statement* (http://aahpm.org/positions/palliative-sedation).

American Transplant Foundation. 2016. *Facts and Myths* (http://www.americantransplantfoundation.org/about-transplant/facts-and-myths/).

Armour, M. 2016. *Aftermath of Violent Death* (http://www.survivorresources.org/grief-knowledge/articles-survivors/aftermath-of-violent-death/).

Bratton, C., et al. 2011. Racial disparities in organ donation and why. *Current Opinion in Organ Transplantation* 16(2): 243-249.

Burkle, C. M., et al. 2014. Why brain death is considered death and why there should be no confusion. *Neurology,* September 12 (epub).

Callanan, M., and P. Kelley. 1992. *Final Gifts: Understanding the Special Awareness, Needs, and Communications of the Dying.* New York: Bantam Books.

Chetty, R., et al. 2016. The association between income and life expectancy in the United States, 2001–2014. *Journal of the American Medical Association* 315(16): 1750–1766.

Death with Dignity National Center. 2016. *Death with Dignity around the U.S.* (http://www.deathwithdignity.org/advocates/national/).

Gawande, A. 2014. *Being Mortal: Medicine and What Matters in the End.* New York: Metropolitan Books/Henry Holt & Company.

Greer, D. M., et al. 2016. Variability of brain death policies in the United States. *JAMA Neurology* 73(2): 213-218.

Gurian, M. 2013. *The Wonder of Aging: A New Approach to Embracing Life after Fifty.* New York: Atria Books.

National Cancer Institute. 2013. *Grief, Bereavement, and Coping with Loss* (http://www.cancer.gov/cancertopics/pdq/supportivecare/bereavement/HealthProfessional).

National Council on Aging. 2015. *Falls Free: 2015 National Falls Prevention Action Plan* (www.ncoa.org/wp-content/uploads/FallsActionPlan_2015-FINAL.pdf).

National Funeral Directors Association. 2016. *Statistics* (http://nfda.org/media-center/statistics.html#cremationburial).

National Hospice and Palliative Care Organization. 2015. *History of Hospice Care* (http://www.nhpco.org/history-hospice-care).

National Hospice and Palliative Care Organization. 2015. *NHPCO's Facts and Figures: Hospice Care in America* (http://www.nhpco.org/sites/default/files/public/Statistics_Research/2015_Facts_Figures.pdf).

National Institute on Aging. 2016. *World's Older Population Grows Dramatically* (https://www.nia.nih.gov/newsroom/2016/03/worlds-older-population-grows-dramatically)

National Kidney Foundation. 2015. *Organ Donation and Transplantation Statistics* (https://www.kidney.org/news/newsroom/factsheets/Organ-Donation-and-Transplantation-Stats).

Nuland, S. 1993. *How We Die: Reflections on Life's Final Chapter.* New York: Random House.

Oregon Death with Dignity Act: 2015 Data. Summary (https://public.health.oregon.gov/ProviderPartnerResources/EvaluationResearch/DeathwithDignityAct/Documents/year18.pdf).

Oregon Health Authority. 2016. *Frequently Asked Questions about the Death with Dignity Act* (http://public.health.oregon.gov/ProviderPartnerResources/EvaluationResearch/DeathwithDignityAct/Pages/faqs.aspx).

Ortman, J. M., V. A. Velkoff, and H. Hogan. 2014. *Aging Nation: The Older Population in the U.S.* (http://www.census.gov/prod/2014pubs/p25-1140.pdf).

Parkes, C., P. Laungani, and W. Young (Eds.). 2015. *Death and Bereavement across Cultures,* 2nd ed. New York: Routledge.

Sacks, O. 2015. *Gratitude.* Canada: Knopf.

Simon, S. 2015. *Unforgettable: A Son, a Mother, and the Lessons of a Lifetime.* New York: Flatiron Books, Macmillan.

Social Security Administration. 2015. *Fast Facts & Figures About Social Security, 2015* (SSA Publication No. 13-11785). Washington, DC: Social Security Administration.

Smith, T. J., and B. E. Hillner. 2011. Bending the cost curve in cancer care. *New England Journal of Medicine* 364: 2060–2065.

Steinhauser, K. E., et al. 2000. In search of a good death: Patients, families and providers. *Annals of Internal Medicine* 132(10): 825–832.

U.S. Department of Health and Human Services. 2015. *The Need Is Real: Data* (http://www.organdonor.gov/about/data.html).

U.S. Department of Health and Human Services. 2016. *Why Minority Donors Are Needed* (http://www.organdonor.gov/whydonate/minorities.html).

White House. 2015. *2015 White House Conference on Aging* (http://www.whitehouseconferenceonaging.gov/2015-WHCOA-Final-Report.pdf).

INDEX

Rapid eye movement sleep, **40**–41, 41f
Rapid HIV tests, 348b
Rationalization, 55t
Raw foods, 242b, 243
Reaction formation, 55t
Readiness to change, 16–17
Realistic goals, 18–19
Rebound relationships, 78–79
Reciprocity, 75
Recognition, in immune response, 331
Recommended Dietary Allowance, 227, 230f
Rectal cancer, 318–319. *See also* Colorectal cancer
Rectum, 216f
Recycling, **372**–373
Red Bull, 188b
"Reduced harm" cigarettes, 201
Refined grains, 220
Refractory periods, 103
Reframing, 56
Refrigeration, 242b
Registered nurses, 387
Regulatory T cells, 332
Reiki, **395**
Reinforcement, **66**, 162
Relapses, 17–18, 177
Relationships. *See* Intimate relationships
Relative risk, 386b
Relaxation, 37, 45, 100
Religion, 67, 150, 436
Remission, **312**
Renewable energy sources, 366
Repetitions in strength training, 261
Repetitive strain injuries, 413b, **413**
Repression, 55t
Reproduction. *See also* Pregnancy
    fertility and infertility, 112–114
    hormones and life cycle, 97–101
    impact of alcohol misuse, 190f
    sexual anatomy, 93–96
    tobacco use and, 204
Rescue breathing, 423
Research, 15b, 386b
Reservoirs, **335**
Resilience, **28**
Resistance exercise, **260**–261
Resistance stage, 29
Resolution phase, 103
Respect, 75
Respiratory diseases, 6t
Respiratory system, 249, 250f, 330
Response, defined, **66**
Responsible drinking, 197b
Responsiveness of parents, 88
Rest, 258
Restatement, 81b
Resting metabolic rate, **278**, 284b
Restless leg syndrome, **44**
Rest pain, 310
Retinoic acid, 121
Retirement, 430–431, 434, 435
Reversibility, **258**
Rewards for behavior change, 17, 19
Rheumatic fever, **311**
Rheumatic heart disease, 311
Rheumatoid arthritis, 343
Rh factor, **120**
Rh-immune globulin, 120
Riboflavin, 224t
R-I-C-E principle, 266
Rickettsia, 339
Right atrium, **295**
Right to die, 439
Right ventricle, **295**
Ring (contraceptive), 137f, 139–140
Risk factors defined, **1**
Ritalin, 168t, 172
Rituals, 90
Robberies, 416
Roberts, Dorothy, 149b
Rocky Mountain spotted fever, 339
Roe v. Wade decision, 150, 154
Rohypnol, **170**, 420
Role models, 16

Romantic partners, choosing, 82–85
Rotavirus vaccines, 333
Roundup, 375
Routines, 90
Rubella virus, 121, 333, 340
Rural areas, health disparities in, 11

Safe injection facilities, 178
Safer sex, 109b, 362b
Safe sex, 111
Safety. *See also* Injuries
    emergency care and, 422–423
    firearms, 407
    of foods, 4f, 120–121, 240–243, 242b, 343
    of herbal products, 393
    home injuries, 404–407
    motor vehicle accidents, 7t, 42, 407–410
    prescription drug, 390
    in sports and leisure activities, 410–411, 411b
    of vaccines, 333
    workplace, 412–413
Salivary glands, 216f
Salmonella, 240
Salovey, Peter, 77
Salt, reducing in diet, 298–299
Same-sex relationships
    basic features, 84–85
    changing attitudes, 75
    HIV/AIDS risk and, 346b, 347–348
    marriage, 86b
    sexuality in, 107–108
San Bernardino shootings (2015), 35b
Sanitary landfills, **372**
Sarcomas, **318**
Sarcopenia, 428
Satiety, 284b
Saturated fatty acids, 217, 218b, 219t, 231b
Savings, 5b
Saw palmetto, 394t
Saxenda, 286
Scabies, **358**
Scanning technologies, 272, 309
Schiavo, Terri, 439
Schizophrenia, 58t, **62**–63, 67
School violence, 415–416
Schwartz, Gary, 29–30
Scientific journals, 386b
Scientific method, 384–385
Scooters, 410
Scotomata, 123
Scrotum, 95f, **95**, 147
Scurvy, 223
Seasonal affective disorder, **62**
Seat belts, 409
Secondary hypertension, 297
Secondary reinforcers, **199**
Secondary syphilis, 357
Secondary tumors, 313
Secondhand smoke, 206, 297
Second-trimester abortions, 153
Second-trimester development, 118
Secure attachment, 74, 128–129
Sedation, **169**, 440
Sedative effects of nicotine, 198
Sedative-hypnotics, **169**–171
Sedentary lifestyle, 251, 254–255, 300, 315
Seizures, 193
Selective estrogen receptor modulators, 320
Selective serotonin reuptake inhibitors, 100
Selenium, 223, 225t, 226
Self-acceptance, 3, 73–74
Self-actualization, **50**
Self-assessment, 48b, 265, 380
Self-blame for rape, 420
Self-care, 380–382
Self-concept, **50**, 51–57, 73–74
Self-confidence, 3, 252

Self-disclosure, 80
Self-efficacy, **15**–16, 252
Self-esteem
    in abusive relationships, 417
    defined, 3, **50**
    developing, 52–54
    exercise effects, 252
    intimacy and, 73–74
    jealousy and, 78
    obesity's impact, 282
Self-examination for cancer, 316, 323, 324b, 324f
Self-harm, 6t, 65b. *See also* Suicide
Self-help, 67
Self-medication, 381–382
Self-talk, 16, 17, 54b, **54**, 72b, 282
Self-treatment, 381–382
Seligman, Martin, 50
Selye, Hans, 29
Semen, **95**, 147
Seminal vesicles, 95f, **96**
Senescence, **436**
Senses, alcohol's effects, 190f
Separation, 88
September 11 attacks, 416
Septicemia, 6t
Serotonin, 62, 286
Set-point theory, 277
Sets in strength training, 261
Sewage, 371
Sex. *See also* Gender
    bone loss and, 432
    cancer incidence and, 313
    cardiovascular disease risk and, 303, 304b
    defined, 9
    effects on BAC, 185
    exercise effects and, 261
    HIV/AIDS risk and, 346b
    life expectancy and, 434b
    psychological disorders and, 58t
    relation to wellness, 9
    as risk factor for trying drugs, 164
    role in stress responses, 28–29
    tobacco use and, 197, 198f, 204
    toxin exposure and, 374b
    violence and, 414, 419–420
Sex addiction, 163
Sex chromosomes, **97**
Sexting, 111
Sexual anatomy, 93–96
Sexual assault, 112, **419**–421
Sexual behaviors
    alcohol use and, 83b, 189
    among college students, 13b, 134b
    deaths linked to, 5, 7t
    gender differences, 76
    hooking up, 82, 83b
    in loving relationships, 75–76
    variations, 108–112
Sexual coercion, **110**
Sexual dysfunctions, **104**–106
Sexual harassment, **421**–422
Sexual identity, 74
Sexual intercourse
    alcohol use and, 189
    among college students, 134b
    casual encounters, 82, 83b
    defined, **95**
    in later adulthood, 100, 432
    preparation for, 110
Sexuality
    aging and, 432
    behavioral expressions, 108–112
    defined, **93**
    gender roles and, 106–107
    hormones and reproductive life cycle, 97–101
    impact of alcohol misuse, 190f
    in loving relationships, 75–76
    physical and psychological problems, 103–106
    self-assessment, 109b
    sexual orientation and, 107–108
    stimulation and response, 102–103

Sexually transmitted infections
    alcohol use and, 189
    from anal intercourse, 110
    chlamydia, 351–353
    circumcision benefits, 96b
    condoms' effectiveness against, 140–141, 142, 148, 352b
    contraceptive methods and, 136, 138, 139, 140, 146t
    defined, **133**, **344**
    general prevention, 352b, 358
    genital herpes, 355–356
    gonorrhea, 353
    hepatitis B, 316, 341, 356
    HIV/AIDS, 345–351. *See also* HIV/AIDS
    human papillomavirus, 316, 321, 333, 341, 353–355
    pelvic inflammatory disease, 353
    pregnancy and, 121–122
    syphilis, 356–357
    understanding risks, 109b, 111
Sexual orientation
    defined, **84**
    health disparities and, 11–12
    in intimate relationships, 75, 84–85
    marriage and, 86b
    origins, 108
    sexuality and, 107–108
Sexual response cycle, 102–103
Sexual violence, 419–422
Sex work, **111**
Shapiro, Shauna, 30
Shingles, 340
Shin splints, 265t
Shoes for exercise, 264b
Shopping, compulsive, 163
Short-acting reversible contraception, 137–146
Short-term benefits of behavior change, 14, 15
Shyness, 72b
Sickle-cell disease, 10
Side effects, 165, 333, 351
Side stitch, 265t
Sidestream smoke, **201**, 206
Sigmoidoscopies, 317t
Silent infections, hepatitis, 356
Silent Spring (Carson), 373
Silent strokes, 309
Simple carbohydrates, 220
Singlehood, 85–87
Single parents, 89–90
Sinoatrial node, 295
Sinsemilla, 173
Sipuleucel-T, 321
Skill-related fitness, **253**, 262
Skin, 190f, 250f, 329
Skin cancer, 313, 322–324
Skinfold measurement, 272
Skin patches. *See* Patch (contraceptive)
Skyla, 135, 136
Sleep
    deficits and driving, 42, 409
    disorders, 43–45
    effect on body fat levels, 279
    exercise effects, 251
    health and, 34, 42
    immune system benefits, 344
    improving, 45–46, 48b
    physiology of, 40–42
Sleep apnea, 44f, **44**–45
Sleep cycles, 41
Sleep deprivation, **42**
Sleep logs, 48b
Sleep restriction, 48b
Slowdown, in immune response, 332
Small-for-dates babies, 124
Small intestine, 216f
SMART goals, 18–19
Smartphones, 43b, 111
Smog, **367**
Smoke detectors, 406
Smoke-free places, 207, 208
Smoke inhalation, 406